eturned

WITHDRAWN

Essentials of Nursing Research

Appraising Evidence for Nursing Practice

DENISE F. POLIT, PhD

President, Humanalysis, Inc., Saratoga Springs, New York
and Adjunct Professor, Griffith University School of Nursing,
Gold Coast, Australia
(www.denisepolit.com)

CHERYL TATANO BECK, DNSc, CNM, FAAN

Distinguished Professor, School of Nursing,
University of Connecticut
Storrs, Connecticut

 Wolters Kluwer | Lippincott Williams & Wilkins
Health

Philadelphia · Baltimore · New York · London
Buenos Aires · Hong Kong · Sydney · Tokyo

CD-ROM available

Acquisitions Editor: Hilarie Surrena
Managing Editor: Helen Kogut
Director of Nursing Production: Helen Ewan
Senior Managing Editor / Production: Erika Kors
Production Editor: Mary Kinsella
Art Director, Design: Joan Wendt
Art Director, Illustration: Brett McNaughton
Manufacturing Coordinator: Karin Duffield
Production Services / Compositor: Aptara

Seventh Edition

9 8 7 6 5 4 3 2 1

Printed in China

Library of Congress Cataloging-in-Publication Data

Polit, Denise F.
   Essentials of nursing research : appraising evidence for nursing practice / Denise F. Polit, Cheryl Tatano Beck. — 7th ed.
      p. ; cm.
   Includes bibliographical references and index.
   ISBN-13: 978-1-6091-3004-6
   1. Nursing—Research.   I. Beck, Cheryl Tatano.   II. Title.
   [DNLM: 1. Nursing Research.   WY 20.5 P769eg 2008]
   RT81.5.P63 2008
   610.73072—dc22   2008047112

Care has been taken to confirm the accuracy of the information presented and to describe generally accepted practices. However, the authors, editors, and publisher are not responsible for errors or omissions or for any consequences from application of the information in this book and make no warranty, expressed or implied, with respect to the currency, completeness, or accuracy of the contents of the publication. Application of this information in a particular situation remains the professional responsibility of the practitioner; the clinical treatments described and recommended may not be considered absolute and universal recommendations.

The authors, editors, and publisher have exerted every effort to ensure that drug selection and dosage set forth in this text are in accordance with the current recommendations and practice at the time of publication. However, in view of ongoing research, changes in government regulations, and the constant flow of information relating to drug therapy and drug reactions, the reader is urged to check the package insert for each drug for any change in indications and dosage and for added warnings and precautions. This is particularly important when the recommended agent is a new or infrequently employed drug.

Some drugs and medical devices presented in this publication have Food and Drug Administration (FDA) clearance for limited use in restricted research settings. It is the responsibility of the health care provider to ascertain the FDA status of each drug or device planned for use in his or her clinical practice.

To Our Students From Around the World
Whose interests, passions, and curiosity have fueled our dedication to good teaching and to high-quality research

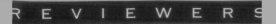

Kathleen Barta, EdD, RN
Associate Professor
University of Arkansas
Fayetteville, Arkansas

Mary Bennett, RN, MS, DNSc, FNP
Assistant Dean; Associate Professor
Indiana State University
Terre Haute, Indiana

Carolyn Blue, RN, PhD, CHES
Professor
University of North Carolina
Greensboro, North Carolina

Diane Breckenridge, PhD, RN
Associate Professor
La Salle University
Philadelphia, Pennsylvania

Becky Christian, PhD, RN
Associate Professor; Division Chair
University of Utah
Salt Lake City, Utah

Linda Cook, RN, BC
Associate Professor
Bloomsburg University of Pennsylvania
Bloomsburg, Pennsylvania

Bernadette Curry, PhD
Molloy College
Rockville Centre, New York

Barbara Davis, PhD, RN
Professor
University of Southern Indiana
Evansville, Indiana

Velma Edmonds, DNS, MSN, BSN, RN
Assistant Professor
University of Texas
El Paso, Texas

Kay Foland, PhD, APRN, BC, CNP
Associate Professor
South Dakota State University
Rapid City, South Dakota

Sharon George, PhD
University of Alabama
Huntsville, Alabama

Marilyn Handley, RN, PhD
Associate Professor
University of Alabama
Tuscaloosa, Alabama

Grace E. Hardie, RN, PhD
Assistant Professor; Assistant Clinical Professor;
Collaborative Researcher
San Francisco State University;
University of San Francisco
San Francisco, California

Susan Hendricks, PhD
Indiana University
Kokomo, Indiana

Elizabeth Hill
Duke University
Durham, North Carolina

Ann Hilton, RN, PhD
Professor and Coordinator of MSN Program
University of British Columbia
Vancouver, British Columbia

Barbara J. Hoerst, RN, PhD
Assistant Professor
La Salle University
Philadelphia, Pennsylvania

Karyn Holm, PhD, RN, FAAN
Professor
DePaul University
Chicago, Illinois

Debra Horoho, MSN
Indiana University
Kokomo, Indiana

Ann Jacobson, PhD, RN
Associate Professor
Kent State University
Kent, Ohio

Peggy Leapley, PhD, RN, FNP, CNS, APRN, BC
Professor and Chair of Nursing
California State University
Bakersfield, California

Gayle Lee, PhD, FNP-C, CCRN
Nursing Faculty
Brigham Young University, Idaho
Rexburg, Idaho

Margaret Louis, PhD
University of Nevada
Las Vegas, Nevada

Nelda Martinez, PhD, RN
Associate Professor; Senior Fellow
University of Texas, El Paso; Hispanic Health Disparities
Research Center
El Paso, Texas

Carrie McCoy, PhD, MSPH, RN, CEN
Professor; Director of ABSN Program
Northern Kentucky University
Highland Heights, Kentucky

Marylou K. McHugh, RN, EdD
Adjunct Faculty
Drexel University; Temple University
Philadelphia, Pennsylvania

Nancy Menzel, PhD, APRN-BC, COHN-S, CNE
Associate Professor
University of Nevada, Las Vegas
Las Vegas, Nevada

Ruby Morrison
University of Alabama
Tuscaloosa, Alabama

Donna Musser, PhD, RN
Assistant Professor
University of Central Arkansas
Conway, Arkansas

Sarah Newton, PhD, RN
Associate Professor
Oakland University
Rochester, Michigan

Priscilla C. O'Connor, PhD, APRN, BC
Lecturer
Temple University
Philadelphia, Pennsylvania

Nicole Ouellet, PhD, RN
Professor
Université du Québec à Rimouski
Rimouski, Quebec

Elizabeth Petit De Mange, RN, PhD
Assistant Professor
Drexel University
Philadelphia, Pennsylvania

Pammla Petrucka, RN, BSc, BScN, MN, PhD
Associate Professor
University of Saskatchewan
Regina, Saskatchewan

Janice Polizzi, MSN, RN
Associate Professor
Florida Hospital College
Orlando, Florida

Patsy Riley
Troy University
Troy, Alabama

Denise Robinson, PhD, RN, FNP
Interim Chair and Regents Professor
Northern Kentucky University
Highland Heights, Kentucky

Nancy Schlapman
Indiana University
Kokomo, Indiana

Joanne Serembus, EdD, RN, CCRN, CNE
Clinical Associate Professor
Drexel University
Philadelphia, Pennsylvania

Sandra L. Siedlecki, RN, CNS, PhD
Senior Nurse Researcher
Cleveland Clinic Foundation
Cleveland, Ohio

Matthew Sorenson, PhD, RN
Assistant Professor
DePaul University
Chicago, Illinois

Valmi Sousa, PhD
University of North Carolina
Charlotte, North Carolina

Amy Spurlock, PhD, RN
Associate Professor
Troy State University
Troy, Alabama

Thomas Stenvig, RN, PhD, MPH, CNAA
Associate Professor
South Dakota State University
Brookings, South Dakota

Marliyn Stoner, RN, PhD
Associate Professor
California State University
San Bernardino, California

Helene Sylvain, PhD
Université du Québec à Rimouski
Rimouski, Quebec

Jane Tarnow
DePaul University
Chicago, Illinois

Becky Thiel
Shawnee State University
Portsmouth, Ohio

Molly Walker, PhD, RN, CNS
Associate Professor
Angelo State University
San Angelo, Texas

Karen Ward, PhD
Middle Tennessee State University
Murfreesboro, Tennessee

Gail Washington, DNS, RN
Assistant Professor
California State University
Los Angeles, California

Joan Wasserman, PhD, MBA, RN
Assistant Professor
University of Texas, Houston
Houston, Texas

Latricia Weed, PhD
Troy State University
Troy, Alabama

Katherine Willock, PhD, APRN, BC
Associate Professor and Director of Graduate Programs
Indiana University-Purdue University
Fort Wayne, Indiana

Evelyn Wills, BSN, MSN, PhD
Professor
University of Louisiana
Lafayette, Louisiana

Mary Woo, DNSc, RN
Professor
University of California
Los Angeles, California

Geri L. Wood, PhD, RN, FAAN
Associate Professor
University of Texas Health Science Center
Houston, Texas

Patti Rager Zuzelo, EdD, APRN, BC, CNS
Associate Professor & CNS Track Coordinator;
Associate Director of Nursing for Research
La Salle University; Albert Einstein Healthcare Network
Philadelphia, Pennsylvania

This book marks the seventh time we have worked on this textbook, which is designed to teach students how to read research reports and critique the methods used in nursing studies. It is perhaps difficult to imagine that writing a seventh edition of a textbook on research methods could be *fun*—but that is exactly the right word to describe our experience in working on this new edition. We have made many changes to the content and organization of this textbook, and the revisions kept our enthusiasm and energy for this project at a very high level. We are confident that we have introduced numerous improvements—but at the same time, we have retained many features that have made this book a classic throughout the world. We think that this edition will make it easier and more satisfying for nurses to pursue a professional pathway that incorporates thoughtful appraisals of evidence.

NEW TO THIS EDITION

Up-front, Consistent Emphasis on Evidence-Based Practice

To an even greater extent than in the past, we emphasize in this edition that research is a crucial enterprise for building an evidence base for nursing practice. We have given the topic of evidence-based practice (EBP) greater prominence by making the chapter on EBP the second chapter of the book (previously the last chapter), and by expanding its content. We emphasize throughout that high quality evidence is a product of researchers' decisions in designing and executing a study. Every chapter offers guidance on how to appraise research evidence for its utility in informing nurses' clinical decisions. We have also added a new chapter on how to read, interpret, and critique systematic reviews, which are considered by many to be a cornerstone of EBP The *Study Guide* that supplements this textbook includes a full report of an EBP project. The increased focus on EBP prompted us to modify the book's title to emphasize the important link between *research* and *evidence*.

New Material Relating to Medical Research Methodology

Nurse researchers have tended to use methods and jargon that originated in the social sciences, but the push for EBP in medicine has led to methodologic innovations that are relevant to all healthcare research. Moreover, nurses can profit from familiarity with medical research terms and approaches so they can comfortably read articles in a broad range of health care journals. This edition offers a more balanced presentation of medical and social science methods and nomenclature.

Improved Content on Qualitative Methods

In every new edition we have expanded content on qualitative research methods, and this edition is no exception. We are especially pleased to include a new chapter on the issue of quality and trustworthiness in qualitative inquiry, Chapter 18. We believe that the content and breadth of this important chapter is unparalleled in other general textbooks on research methods for nurses.

Greater Assistance With Interpretation

Many books on research methods describe the techniques used to generate evidence, but they typically offer little or no guidance on interpreting research results. We have made efforts to address this deficiency by offering an interpretive framework for both quantitative (Chapter 16) and qualitative (Chapter 18) research.

Additional Support for Research Appraisals—The Toolkit

Each chapter of the book includes questions to aid students in reading and appraising research journal articles. In this edition, these critiquing guidelines are also available on the accompanying Student CD-ROM and thePoint. With electronic files of these resources, students can download the guidelines, adapt them as needed, and then enter their answers to the questions directly, without having to photocopy pages from the book. Many faculty have told us that the general critiquing guidelines (which we have put in an earlier chapter than in previous editions) are useful as handouts, and now they are more readily accessible.

ORGANIZATION OF THE TEXT

The content of this edition is organized into five main parts.

➢ **Part I—Overview of Nursing Research and Its Role in Evidence-Based Practice** introduces fundamental concepts in nursing research. Chapter 1 summarizes the history and future of nursing research, discusses the philosophical underpinnings of qualitative research versus quantitative research, and describes major purposes of nursing research. Chapter 2 offers guidance on using research to build an EBP. Chapter 3 introduces readers to key research terms, and presents an overview of steps in the research process for both qualitative and quantitative studies. Chapter 4 focuses on research reports, explaining what they are and how to read them. Chapter 5 discusses ethics in nursing studies.

➢ **Part II—Preliminary Steps in the Appraisal of Evidence** further sets the stage for learning about the research process by considering aspects of a study's conceptualization. Chapter 6 focuses on the development of research questions and the formulation of research hypotheses. Chapter 7 discusses how to prepare and critique literature reviews. Chapter 8 presents information about theoretical and conceptual frameworks.

➢ **Part III—Designs for Nursing Research** presents material on the design of qualitative and quantitative nursing studies. Chapter 9 describes some fundamental design principles and discusses many specific aspects of quantitative research design. Chapter 10 addresses the various research traditions that have contributed to the growth of naturalistic inquiry and qualitative research. Chapter 11 provides an introduction to some specific types of research (e.g., evaluations, surveys, secondary analyses), and also describes mixed method studies that integrate qualitative and quantitative components. Chapter 12 introduces designs for sampling study participants.

➤ **Part IV—Data Collection** concerns the gathering of data to address research questions. Chapter 13 discusses a range of data collection options for nurse researchers, including both qualitative and quantitative approaches. Chapter 14 describes the concept of *measurement* and criteria for assessing data quality in quantitative studies.

➤ **Part V—Data Analysis and Interpretation** discusses analytic methods for qualitative and quantitative research. Chapter 15 reviews methods of quantitative analysis. The chapter assumes no prior instruction in statistics and focuses primarily on helping readers to understand why statistics are needed, what tests might be appropriate in a given situation, and what statistical information in a research report means. Chapter 16 discusses ways of appraising rigor in quantitative studies, and approaches to interpreting statistical results. Chapter 17 presents a discussion of qualitative analysis, with an emphasis on ethnographies, phenomenologic studies, and grounded theory studies. Chapter 18 elaborates on criteria for appraising integrity and quality in qualitative studies. Finally, Chapter 19 describes systematic reviews, including how to understand and appraise both meta-analyses and metasyntheses.

KEY FEATURES

This edition, like its predecessors, is focused on the art—and science—of research critiques. It offers guidance to students who are learning to appraise research reports and use research findings in practice. Among the basic principles that helped to shape this and earlier editions of this book are (1) an assumption that competence in doing and appraising research are critical to the nursing profession; (2) a conviction that research inquiry is intellectually and professionally rewarding to nurses; and (3) an unswerving belief that learning about research methods need be neither intimidating nor dull. Consistent with these principles, we have tried to present research fundamentals in a way that both facilitates understanding and arouses curiosity and interest.

General Features

We have retained many of the key features that were successfully used in previous editions to assist consumers of nursing research:

➤ **Clear, "User-Friendly" Style.** Our writing style is designed to be easily digestible and nonintimidating. Concepts are introduced carefully and systematically, difficult ideas are presented clearly, and readers are assumed to have no prior knowledge of technical terms.

➤ **Critiquing Guidelines.** Each chapter includes guidelines for conducting a critique of various aspects of a research report. The guidelines sections provide a list of questions that walk students through a study, drawing attention to aspects of the study that are amenable to appraisal by research consumers. Electronic versions of the guidelines are available on the accompanying student CD-ROM and thePoint.

➤ **Research Examples.** Each chapter concludes with one or two actual research examples designed to highlight critical points made in the chapter and to sharpen the reader's critical thinking skills. In addition, many research examples are used to illustrate key points in the text and to stimulate students' thinking about areas of research inquiry. We have chosen many international examples to communicate to students that nursing research is growing in importance worldwide.

➤ **Tips for Consumers.** The textbook is filled with practical guidance and "tips" on how to translate the abstract notions of research methods into more concrete applications. In these tips, we have paid special attention to helping students *read* research reports, which are often daunting to those without specialized research training.

➤ **Graphics.** Colorful graphics, in the form of supportive tables, figures, and examples, reinforce the text and offer visual stimulation.

Features for Student Learning

We have used many features to enhance and reinforce learning—and, especially, to facilitate the development of critiquing skills. These include the following:

➤ **Student Objectives.** Learning objectives are identified in the chapter opener to focus students' attention on critical content.

➤ **Key Terms.** New terms are defined in context (and bolded) when used for the first time in the text. Each chapter concludes with a list of new terms, and we have made the list less daunting by including only *key* new terms. A *glossary* at the end of the book provides additional support for those needing to look up the meaning of a methodologic term.

➤ **Bulleted Summary Points.** A succinct list of summary points that focus on salient chapter content is included at the end of each chapter.

➤ **Full-Length Research Articles.** In this edition, the textbook includes four recent full-length studies—two quantitative and two qualitative—that students can read, analyze, and critique. Two appear in the appendices of the textbook, and two are on the CD-ROM packaged with the book and thePoint.

➤ **Critiquing Supports.** Each chapter of the textbook concludes with "Critical Thinking Activities"—exercises that provide opportunities to practice critiquing. Some exercises are based on the studies that are included in their entirety in the appendices of the book, while others are based on studies that are summarized at the end of the chapters. Importantly, students can then consult the accompanying CD-ROM and thePoint to find our "answers" (our expert thoughts about each question), so that *students can get immediate feedback about their grasp of material in the chapter.* (In some cases, there are also thoughtful comments by the actual researchers who conducted the studies). This edition also includes full critiques of the two studies on the CD-ROM and thePoint, which students can use as models for a comprehensive research critique. Many more critiquing opportunities are available in the *Study Guide*, which includes seven studies in their entirety in the appendices and exercises in each chapter that guide students in reading, understanding, and critiquing these studies.

TEACHING-LEARNING PACKAGE

Essentials of Nursing Research: Appraising Evidence for Nursing Practice, seventh edition, has an ancillary package designed with both students and instructors in mind.

➤ **The** *Study Guide* augments the text and provides students with application exercises for each text chapter. Critiquing skills are emphasized, but there are also activities to support the learning of fundamental research terms and principles. Seven recent studies—including one report of an EBP project—are included in the appendices, and many chapter exercises are based on these studies. The studies represent a range of research types, including a clinical trial, a survey, an evaluation of an EBP project, a grounded theory study, a feminist study, a meta-analysis, and a metasynthesis.

➤ **Free CD-ROM.** The textbook includes a CD-ROM that has many important resources. First, as noted, we provide our answers to the Critical Thinking Activities from the textbook. Critiquing guidelines for each chapter, as well as some other resources, are included as a toolkit in electronic files for downloading, adapting, and printing. Next, the CD-ROM provides hundreds of review questions to assist students in self-testing. This review program provides a rationale for both correct and incorrect answers, helping students to identify areas of strength and areas needing further study. Finally, the CD-ROM has lists of relevant and useful websites for each chapter, which can be "clicked" on directly without having to retype the URL and risk a typographical error. All of these resources are also available on thePoint.

➤ **The Instructor's Resource CD-ROM (IRCD)** includes a chapter corresponding to every chapter in the textbook. Each IRCD chapter contains the following: Statement of Intent, Special Class Projects, Answers to Selected *Study Guide* Exercises, and Test Questions and Answers. In the special class projects, we offer opportunities for students to develop a quantitative and (or) a qualitative data set. With regard to test questions to evaluate student learning, we offer multiple choice and true/false questions and, importantly, we have added questions specifically designed to test students' ability to comprehend research reports. In addition, PowerPoint slides summarizing key points in each chapter are available in a format that permits easy adaptation. All of this content is also available on thePoint.

It is our hope and expectation that the content, style, and organization of this seventh edition of *Essentials of Nursing Research* will be helpful to those students desiring to become skillful and thoughtful readers of nursing studies and to those wishing to enhance their clinical performance based on research findings. We also hope that this textbook will help to develop an enthusiasm for the kinds of discoveries and knowledge that research can produce.

DENISE F. POLIT, PhD

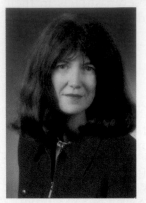

CHERYL TATANO BECK, DNSc, CNM, FAAN

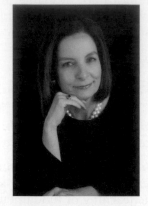

ACKNOWLEDGMENTS

This seventh edition, like the previous six editions, depended on the contribution of many generous people. Many faculty and students who used the text have made invaluable suggestions for its improvement, and to all of you we are very grateful. Suggestions were made to us both directly in personal interactions (mostly at the University of Connecticut and Griffith University in Australia), and via the wonderful communication tool of email correspondence. In addition to all those who assisted us during the past three decades with the earlier editions, there are some who deserve special mention for this new work.

We would like to acknowledge the comments of the reviewers of the previous edition of *Essentials*, whose anonymous feedback influenced our revisions. Several of the comments triggered several important changes, and for this we are indebted.

Other individuals made specific contributions. Although it would be impossible to mention all, we note with thanks the nurse researchers who shared their work with us as we developed examples, including work that in some cases was not yet published. Through the Internet, we worked with authors of the reports that appear in the appendices. We shared with them our critiques and "answers" to the critiquing exercises to make sure that we had not misread or misinterpreted their reports, and they gave generously of their time in reviewing our material. Special thanks to Carol Howell, Marti Rice, Linda Walsh, and Michael McGillion for their help. We also got extraordinary cooperation from the authors of studies that were summarized at the end of the chapters, and we are grateful to them all.

We extend our warm thanks as well to those who helped to turn the manuscript into a finished product. The staff at Lippincott Williams & Wilkins has been of tremendous assistance in the support they have given us over the years. We are indebted to Hilarie Surrena, Helen Kogut, Mary Kinsella, Annette Ferran, Joan Wendt, and all the others behind the scenes for their fine contributions.

Finally, we thank our family, our loved ones, and our friends, who provided ongoing support and encouragement throughout this endeavor and who were tolerant when we worked long into the night, over weekends, and during holidays to get this seventh edition finished.

C O N T E N T S

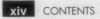

APPENDICES: RESEARCH REPORTS

Overview of Nursing Research and Its Role in Evidence-Based Practice

CHAPTER

1 Introduction to Nursing Research in an Evidence-Based Practice Environment

STUDENT OBJECTIVES

On completing this chapter, you will be able to:

➤ Describe why research is important in the nursing profession and discuss the need for evidence-based practice

➤ Describe historic trends and future directions in nursing research

➤ Describe alternative sources of evidence for nursing practice

➤ Describe major characteristics of the positivist and naturalistic paradigm, and discuss similarities and differences between the traditional scientific method (quantitative research) and naturalistic methods (qualitative research)

➤ Identify several purposes of qualitative and quantitative research

➤ Define new terms in the chapter

...G RESEARCH IN PERSPECTIVE

It is an exciting—and challenging—time to be a nurse. Nurses are performing their clinical responsibilities at a time when the nursing profession and larger health care systems require an extraordinary range of skills and talents of them. Nurses are expected to deliver competent, high-quality care in a compassionate but also cost-effective manner. To accomplish these diverse goals, nurses continually need to access and evaluate new information, and incorporate it into their clinical decision-making. In today's world, *nurses must become lifelong learners*, capable of reflecting on, evaluating, and modifying their clinical practice based on emerging knowledge from systematic nursing and health care research.

What Is Nursing Research?

Research is systematic inquiry that uses disciplined methods to answer questions and solve problems. The ultimate goal of research is to develop, refine, and expand a body of knowledge.

Nurses are increasingly engaged in disciplined studies that benefit the profession and its clients. **Nursing research** is systematic inquiry designed to develop trustworthy evidence about issues of importance to the nursing profession, including nursing practice, education, administration, and informatics.

In this book, we emphasize **clinical nursing research,** that is, research designed to guide nursing practice and to improve the health and quality of life of nurses' clients. Clinical nursing research typically begins with questions stemming from practice-related problems—problems such as ones you may have already encountered.

Examples of nursing research questions:
➤ Among current smokers, are more sources of secondhand smoke exposure associated with higher nicotine dependence and lower intention to quit smoking? (Okoli, Browning, Rayens, & Hahn, 2008)
➤ What are the late effects of cancer treatment among long-term cancer survivors, and what are ways in which survivors find support and information that are not provided via follow-up care? (Klemm, 2008)

The Importance of Research to Evidence-Based Nursing Practice

In all parts of the world, nursing has experienced a profound culture change over the past few decades. Nurses are increasingly expected to understand and conduct research, and to base their professional practice on emerging evidence from research—that is, to adopt an **evidence-based practice (EBP).** EBP is broadly defined as the use of the best clinical evidence in making patient care decisions, and such evidence typically comes from research conducted by nurses and other health care professionals.

Evidence for EBP can come from various sources, but there is widespread agreement that research findings from rigorous studies provide especially strong evidence for informing nurses' decisions and actions. Nurses are accepting the need to base specific nursing actions and decisions on evidence indicating that the actions are clinically appropriate, cost-effective, and result in positive outcomes for clients.

In the United States, research has come to play an important role in nursing in terms of credentialing and status. The American Nurses Credentialing Center—an arm of the American Nurses Association—has developed a Magnet Recognition Program® to recognize health care organizations that provide very high-quality nursing care, and to elevate the standards and reputation of the nursing profession. As noted by Turkel and colleagues (2005), to achieve Magnet status, it is essential for nurse leaders to create, advance, and sustain a practice environment grounded in EBP and nursing research.

Changes to nursing practice are occurring regularly because of EBP efforts. Often these practice changes are local initiatives, many of which are not publicized, but broader clinical changes are also occurring based on accumulating research evidence about beneficial practice innovations.

Example of evidence-based practice:

"Kangaroo care," the holding of diaper-clad preterm infants skin-to-skin, chest-to-chest by parents, is now widely practiced in neonatal intensive care units (NICUs) in the United States and elsewhere, but this is a new trend. As recently as the early 1990s, only a minority of NICUs offered kangaroo care options. The adoption of this practice reflects the mounting evidence that early skin-to-skin contact has clinical benefits without any apparent negative side effects (Dodd, 2005; Galligan, 2006). Some of the accumulated evidence was developed in rigorous studies by nurse researchers in the United States, Australia, Canada, Taiwan, Korea, and other countries (e.g., Chwo et al., 2002; Ludington-Hoe et al., 2004, 2006; Moore & Anderson, 2007).

Roles of Nurses in Research

With the current emphasis on EBP, it has become every nurse's responsibility to engage in one or more roles along a continuum of research participation. At one end of the continuum are users (*consumers*) *of nursing research*—nurses who read research reports to develop new skills and to keep up to date on relevant findings that may affect their practice. Nurses are now expected to maintain this level of involvement with research, at a minimum. EBP depends on well-informed nursing research consumers.

At the other end of the continuum are the *producers of nursing research*—nurses who actively participate in designing and implementing studies. At one time, most nurse researchers were academics who taught in schools of nursing, but research is increasingly being conducted by practicing nurses who want to find what works best for their clients.

Between these two endpoints on the consumer–producer continuum lie a rich variety of research activities in which nurses may engage. Even if you never conduct a study, you may well do one or more of the following:

rticipate in a journal club in a practice setting, which involves meetings to discuss and critique research articles

- ↗ Attend research presentations at professional conferences
- ➤ Solve clinical problems and make clinical decisions based on rigorous research
- ➤ Help to develop an idea for a clinical study
- ➤ Review a proposed research plan and offer clinical expertise to improve the plan
- ➤ Assist researchers by recruiting potential study participants or collecting research information (e.g., distributing questionnaires to clients)
- ➤ Provide information and advice to clients about participation in studies
- ➤ Discuss the implications and relevance of research findings with clients

Example of research publicized in the mass media:
Here is a headline about a health study that was publicized in newspapers and major television networks in the United States and Canada in April, 2007: "Study doesn't back abortion-cancer link." According to the study, which involved more than 100,000 nurses who were followed for over a decade, having an abortion does not raise a woman's risk of breast cancer.

What would you say if clients asked you about this study? Would you be able to comment on the believability of the findings, based on your assessment of how rigorously the study was conducted? This book should enable you to do this.

In all the possible research-related activities, nurses who have some research skills are better able than those without them to make a contribution to nursing and to EBP. An understanding of nursing research can improve the depth and breadth of every nurse's professional practice.

NURSING RESEARCH: PAST, PRESENT, AND FUTURE

Although nursing research has not always had the prominence and importance it enjoys today, its long and interesting history portends a distinguished future. Table 1.1 summarizes some of the key events in the historic evolution of nursing research.

The Early Years: From Nightingale to the 1970s

Most people would agree that research in nursing began with Florence Nightingale. Her landmark publication, *Notes on Nursing* (1859), describes her early interest in environmental factors that promote physical and emotional well-being—an interest that continues among nurses 150 years later. Based on her skillful analysis of factors affecting soldier mortality and morbidity during the Crimean War, she was successful in effecting some changes in nursing care—and, more generally, in public health.

For many years after Nightingale's work, the nursing literature contained little research. Studies began to be published in the early 1900s, mostly concerning

TABLE 1.1	HISTORIC LANDMARKS IN NURSING RESEARCH
YEAR	**EVENT**
1859	Nightingale's *Notes on Nursing* is published
1900	*American Nursing Journal* begins publication
1923	Columbia University establishes first doctoral program for nurses
	Goldmark Report with recommendations for nursing education published
1930s	*American Journal of Nursing* publishes clinical cases studies
1936	Sigma Theta Tau awards first nursing research grant in the United States
1948	Brown publishes report on inadequacies of nursing education
1952	The journal *Nursing Research* begins publication
1955	Inception of the American Nurses' Foundation to sponsor nursing research
1957	Establishment of nursing research center at Walter Reed Army Institute of Research
1963	*International Journal of Nursing Studies* begins publication
1965	American Nurses' Association (ANA) begins sponsoring nursing research conferences
1969	*Canadian Journal of Nursing Research* begins publication
1971	ANA establishes a Commission on Research
1972	ANA establishes its Council of Nurse Researchers
1976	Stetler and Marram publish guidelines on assessing research for use in practice
1978	The journals *Research in Nursing & Health* and *Advances in Nursing Science* begin publication
1979	*Western Journal of Nursing Research* begins publication
1982	The Conduct and Utilization of Research in Nursing (CURN) project publishes report
1983	*Annual Review of Nursing Research* begins publication
1985	ANA Cabinet on Nursing Research establishes research priorities
1986	National Center for Nursing Research (NCNR) established within U.S. National Institutes of Health
1988	The journal *Applied Nursing Research* begins publication
1989	U.S. Agency for Health Care Policy and Research (AHCPR) is established (renamed Agency for Healthcare Research and Quality or AHRQ in 1999)
1993	NCNR becomes a full institute, the National Institute of Nursing Research (NINR)
	The Cochrane Collaboration is established
1994	The journal *Qualitative Health Research* begins publication
1995	The Joanna Briggs Institute, an international EBP collaborative, is established in Australia
1997	Canadian Health Services Research Foundation is established with federal funding
2000	NINR's annual funding exceeds $100 million
	The Canadian Institute of Health Research is launched
2004	The journal *Worldviews on Evidence-Based Nursing* begins publication
2005	Sigma Theta Tau International publishes research priorities

nurses' education. As more nurses received university-based education, studies concerning nursing students—their characteristics, problems, and satisfactions—became a major focus. During the 1940s, government-initiated studies of nursing education continued, spurred on by the unprecedented demand for nursing personnel during World War II. When hospital staffing patterns changed, fewer students were available over a 24-hour period. As a consequence, researchers focused their investigations not only on the supply and demand of nurses but also on the amount of time required to perform certain nursing activities.

A number of forces combined during the 1950s to put nursing research on a rapidly accelerating upswing in the United States. An increase in the number of nurses with advanced degrees and better research training, an increase in the availability of funds from the government and private foundations, and the establishment of the journal *Nursing Research* are a few of the forces propelling nursing research at mid-century.

During the 1960s, practice-oriented research on various clinical topics began to emerge in the literature and nursing research advanced worldwide: the *International Journal of Nursing Studies* began publication in 1963, and both the *Journal of Nursing Scholarship* and the *Canadian Journal of Nursing Research* were first published in the late 1960s.

Example of nursing research breakthroughs in the 1960s:
Jeanne Quint Benoliel began a program of research that had a major impact on medicine, medical sociology, and nursing. Quint explored the subjective experiences of patients after diagnosis with a life-threatening illness (1967). Of particular note, physicians in the early 1960s usually did not advise women that they had breast cancer, even after a mastectomy. Quint's (1963) seminal study of the personal experiences of women after radical mastectomy contributed to changes in communication and information control by physicians and nurses.

During the 1970s, there was a decided change in emphasis in nursing research from areas such as teaching and nurses themselves to improvements in client care. Nurses also began to pay attention to the utilization of research findings in nursing practice. A seminal article by Stetler and Marram (1976) offered guidance on assessing research for application in practice settings. By the 1970s, the growing number of nurses conducting studies and the discussions of theoretic and contextual issues surrounding nursing research created the need for additional communication outlets. Several journals that focus on nursing research were established in the 1970s, including *Research in Nursing & Health*, the *Journal of Advanced Nursing*, and the *Western Journal of Nursing Research*.

Example of nursing research breakthroughs in the 1970s:
Kathryn Barnard's research led to breakthroughs in the area of neonatal and child development. Her research program focused on the identification and assessment of children at risk of developmental and health problems, such as abused and neglected children and failure-to-thrive children (Barnard, 1973; Barnard, Wenner, Weber, Gray, & Peterson, 1977). Her research contributed to early interventions for children with disabilities, and also to the field of developmental psychology.

Nursing Research Since 1980

The 1980s brought nursing research to a new level of development. Several events contributed to the momentum. For example, the first volume of the *Annual Review of Nursing Research* was published in 1983. These annual reviews include summaries of current research evidence on selected areas of research practice and encourage utilization of research findings. Of particular importance in the United States was the establishment in 1986 of the National Center for Nursing Research (NCNR) at the National Institutes of Health (NIH). The purpose of NCNR was to promote—and financially support—research projects and training relating to patient care. Funding for nursing research also became available in Canada in the 1980s through the National Health Research Development Program (NHRDP) and the Medical Research Council of Canada.

Also in the 1980s, nurses began to conduct formal projects specifically designed to increase research utilization, such as the Conduct and Utilization of Research in Nursing (CURN) project. Additional research-related journals were established in the 1980s, including *Applied Nursing Research* and, in Australia, the *Australian Journal of Nursing Research*.

Several forces outside of nursing in the late 1980s helped to shape today's nursing research landscape. A group from the McMaster Medical School in Canada designed a clinical learning strategy that was called evidence-based medicine (EBM). EBM, which promulgated the view that research findings were far superior to the opinions of authorities as a basis for clinical decisions, constituted a profound shift for medical education and practice, and has had a major effect on all health care professions.

In 1989, the U.S. government established the Agency for Health Care Policy and Research (AHCPR). AHCPR (renamed the Agency for Healthcare Research and Quality, or AHRQ, in 1999) is the federal agency that has been charged with supporting research specifically designed to improve the quality of health care, reduce health costs, and enhance patient safety, and thus plays a pivotal role in supporting EBP.

Example of nursing research breakthroughs in the 1980s:
A team of researchers headed by Dorothy Brooten engaged in studies that led to the development and testing of a model of site transitional care. For example, Brooten and her colleagues (1986, 1988) conducted studies of nurse specialist-managed home follow-up services for very-low-birth-weight infants who were discharged early from the hospital, and demonstrated a significant cost savings—with comparable health outcomes. The site transitional care model, which was developed in anticipation of government cost-cutting measures, has been used as a framework for patients who are at health risk as a result of early discharge from hospitals, and has been recognized by numerous health care disciplines.

Nursing research was strengthened and given more national visibility when NCNR was promoted to full institute status within the NIH: in 1993, the **National Institute of Nursing Research (NINR)** was established. The birth of NINR helped put nursing research more into the mainstream of research activities enjoyed by other health disciplines. Funding for nursing research has also grown. In 1986, the NCNR had a budget of $16 million, whereas by fiscal year 1999, the budget for NINR had grown to about $70 million. Funding opportunities expanded in other countries as well. For example, the Canadian Health Services Research Foundation (CHSRF) was established in 1997 with an endowment from federal funds, and plans for the Canadian Institute for Health Research got underway. Beginning in 1999, the CHSRF allocated $25 million for nursing research.

In addition to growth in funding opportunities, the 1990s witnessed the birth of several more journals for nurse researchers, including *Qualitative Health Research*, *Clinical Nursing Research*, and *Clinical Effectiveness*. These journals emerged in response to the growth in clinically oriented and in-depth research among nurses, and interest in EBP. Another major contribution to EBP was inaugurated in 1993: the Cochrane Collaboration, an international network of institutions and individuals that maintains and updates **systematic reviews** of hundreds of clinical interventions to facilitate EBP. International cooperation around the issue of EBP in nursing also began to develop in the 1990s. For example, Sigma Theta Tau International began to focus attention on research utilization, and sponsored the first international research utilization conference, in cooperation with the faculty of the University of Toronto, in 1998.

Example of nursing research breakthroughs in the 1990s:
Many studies that Donaldson (2000) identified as *breakthroughs* in nursing research were conducted in the 1990s. This reflects, in part, the growth of **research programs** in which teams of researchers engage in a series of related research on important topics, rather than discrete and unconnected studies. As but one example, several nurse researchers had breakthroughs during the 1990s in the area of psychoneuroimmunology, which has been adopted as the model of mind–body interactions. Swanson and Zeller, for example, conducted several studies relating to human immunodeficiency virus (HIV) infection and neuropsychologic function (Swanson, Cronin-Stubbs, Zeller, Kessler, & Bielauskas, 1993; Swanson, Zeller & Spear, 1998) that have led to discoveries in environmental management as a means of improving immune system status.

Directions for Nursing Research in the New Millennium

Nursing research continues to develop at a rapid pace and will undoubtedly flourish in the 21st century. Funding continues to grow; for example, NINR funding in fiscal year 2008 was nearly $140 million, more than twice what funding levels were in 1999. Broadly speaking, the priority for nursing research in the future will be the promotion of excellence in nursing science. Toward this end, nurse researchers and practicing nurses will be sharpening their research skills, and using those skills to address emerging issues of importance to the profession and its clientele.

Certain trends for the 21st century are evident from developments taking shape in the early years of the millennium:

➤ *Heightened focus on EBP.* Concerted efforts to use research findings in practice are sure to continue, and nurses at all levels will be encouraged to engage in evidence-based patient care. In turn, improvements will be needed both in the quality of nursing studies and in nurses' skills in locating, understanding, critiquing, and using relevant study results. Relatedly, there is an emerging interest in *translational research*—research on how findings from studies can best be translated into nursing practice.

➤ *Stronger evidence base through more rigorous methods and multiple, confirmatory strategies.* Practicing nurses rarely adopt an innovation on the basis of weakly designed or isolated studies. Strong research designs are essential, and confirmation is usually needed through deliberate replication (i.e., repeating) of studies with different clients, in different clinical settings, and at different times to ensure that the findings are robust. Another confirmatory strategy is the conduct of multisite studies by researchers in several locations.

➤ *Greater emphasis on systematic reviews.* Systematic reviews are a cornerstone of EBP, and undoubtedly will increase in importance in all health disciplines. Systematic reviews amass and integrate comprehensive research information on a topic to draw conclusions about the state of evidence.

➤ *Expanded local research in health care settings.* There will almost certainly be an increase of small, localized research designed to solve immediate problems. In the United States, this trend will be reinforced as more hospitals apply for (and are recertified for) Magnet status. Mechanisms need to be developed to ensure that evidence from these small projects becomes available to others facing similar problems.

➤ *Strengthening of multidisciplinary collaboration.* Interdisciplinary collaboration of nurses with researchers in related fields (as well as intradisciplinary collaboration among nurse researchers) is likely to continue to expand in the 21st century as researchers address fundamental problems at the biobehavioral and psychobiologic interface.

➤ *Expanded dissemination of research findings.* The Internet and other electronic communications have a big impact on the dissemination of research information, which in turn helps to promote EBP. Through such technologic advances as electronic location and retrieval of research articles; on-line publishing (e.g., the *Online Journal of Knowledge Synthesis for Nursing*); on-line resources such as Lippincott's NursingCenter.com; e-mail; and electronic mailing lists, information about innovations can be communicated more widely and more quickly than ever before.

➤ *Increasing the visibility of nursing research.* Efforts to increase the visibility of nursing research will likely expand. Most people are unaware that nurses are scholars and researchers. Nurse researchers internationally must market themselves and their research to professional organizations, consumer organizations, governments, and the corporate world to increase support for their research.

➤ *Increased focus on cultural issues and health disparities.* The issue of health disparities has emerged as a central concern in nursing and other health disciplines, and this in turn has raised consciousness about the ecologic validity and cultural sensitivity of health interventions. *Ecologic validity* refers to the extent to which study designs and findings have relevance and meaning in a variety of real-world contexts. There is growing awareness that research must be sensitive to the health beliefs, behaviors, epidemiology, and values of culturally and linguistically diverse populations.

Research priorities for the future are under discussion, both by nursing specialty organizations and by broader groups and institutions. In 2005, Sigma Theta Tau International issued a position paper on nursing research priorities that incorporated priorities from nursing organizations internationally, including NINR. This synthesis of global nursing priorities identified the following: (1) health promotion and disease prevention; (2) promotion of health of vulnerable and marginalized communities; (3) patient safety; (4) development of evidence-based practice and translational research; (5) promotion of the health and well-being of older people; (6) patient-centered care and care coordination; (7) palliative and end-of-life care; (8) care implications of genetic testing and therapeutics; (8) capacity development of nurse researchers; and (9) nurses' working environments (Sigma Theta Tau International, 2005).

Examples of landmark nursing studies of the 21st century:
Celebrating its 20th anniversary, NINR published a report in 2006 on 10 landmark studies that had been supported with NINR funds. The 10 selected studies encompassed a wide range of research, including a study on the relationship between nurse staffing and patient well-being by Aiken and colleagues (2002); a test of a clinical intervention to improve metabolic outcomes for adolescents with type I diabetes by Grey and colleagues (2001); and an evaluation of a multidisciplinary project to reduce high blood pressure in inner-city hypertensive men by Hill and colleagues (2003).

TIP

All websites cited in this chapter, plus additional websites with useful content relating to the foundations of nursing research, are in the "Useful Websites for Chapter 1" file on the accompanying CD-ROM. This will allow you to simply use the "Control/Click" feature to go directly to the website, without having to type in the URL and risk a typographic error. Websites corresponding to the content of most chapters of the book are also in files on the CD-ROM.

SOURCES OF EVIDENCE FOR NURSING PRACTICE

As a nursing student, you are gaining skills on how to practice nursing, but it is important to recognize that learning about best-practice nursing will continue throughout your career. Some of what you have learned thus far is based on systematic research, but much of it is not. Only a little over a decade ago, Millenson (1997) estimated that a full 85% of health care practice was not scientifically validated. Although the percentage of validated practices may have increased since 1997, there is widespread support for the idea that nursing practice should rely more heavily on evidence from research. Information sources for clinical practice vary in dependability and validity. Increasingly there are discussions of **evidence hierarchies** that acknowledge that certain types of evidence are superior to others. A brief discussion of some alternative sources of evidence shows how research-based information is different.

Tradition and Authority

Within Western culture and within the nursing profession, certain beliefs are accepted as truths—and certain practices are accepted as effective—simply based on custom. Tradition may, however, undermine effective problem solving. Traditions may be so entrenched that their validity or usefulness is not questioned or evaluated. There is growing concern that many nursing interventions are based on tradition, customs, and "unit culture" rather than on sound evidence.

Another common source of knowledge is an authority, a person with specialized expertise and recognition for that expertise. Reliance on nursing authorities (e.g., nursing faculty) is to some degree unavoidable; however, like tradition, authorities as a source of information have limitations. Authorities are not infallible (particularly if their expertise is based primarily on personal experience), yet their knowledge often goes unchallenged.

Clinical Experience, Trial and Error, and Intuition

Clinical experience is a familiar and functional source of knowledge. The ability to recognize regularities, and to make predictions based on observations is a hallmark of the human mind. Nevertheless, personal experience has limitations as a source of evidence for practice because each nurse's experience is typically too narrow to be generally useful, and personal experiences are often colored by biases.

Related to clinical experience is the method of trial and error. In this approach, alternatives are tried successively until a solution to a problem is found. Trial and error may be practical in some cases, but it is often fallible and inefficient. The method tends to be haphazard and the solutions may be idiosyncratic.

Finally, intuition is a type of knowledge that cannot be explained on the basis of reasoning or prior instruction. Although intuition and hunches undoubtedly play a role in nursing practice—as they do in the conduct of research—it is difficult to develop policies and practices for nurses on the basis of intuition.

Logical Reasoning

Solutions to many problems are developed by logical reasoning, which combines experience, intellectual faculties, and formal systems of thought. **Inductive reasoning** is the process of developing generalizations from specific observations. For example, a nurse may observe the anxious behavior of (specific) hospitalized children and conclude that (in general) children's separation from their parents is stressful. **Deductive reasoning** is the process of developing specific predictions from general principles. For example, if we assume that separation anxiety occurs in hospitalized children (in general), then we might predict that (specific) children in a local hospital whose parents do not room-in will manifest symptoms of stress.

Both types of reasoning are useful as a means of understanding phenomena, and both play a role in nursing research. However, reasoning in and of itself is limited because the validity of reasoning depends on the accuracy of the information (or premises) with which one starts.

Assembled Information

In making clinical decisions, health care professionals also rely on information that has been assembled for a variety of purposes. For example, local, national, and international **bench-marking data** provide information on such issues as the rates of using various procedures (e.g., rates of cesarean deliveries) or rates of infection (e.g., nosocomial pneumonia rates), and can serve as a guide in evaluating clinical practices. **Quality improvement and risk data**, such as medication error reports, can be used to assess practices and determine the need for practice changes. Such sources, although offering some information that can be used in practice, provide no mechanism for determining whether improvements in patient outcomes result from their use.

Disciplined Research

Research conducted within a disciplined format is the most sophisticated method of acquiring knowledge that humans have developed. Nursing research combines aspects of logical reasoning with other features to create evidence that, although fallible, tends to be more reliable than other methods of knowledge acquisition. Cumulative findings from rigorous, systematically appraised research are at the pinnacle of most evidence hierarchies. The current emphasis on evidence-based health care requires nurses to base their clinical practice—to the extent possible—on research-based findings rather than on tradition, authority, intuition, or personal experience, although nursing will always remain a rich blend of art and science.

PARADIGMS FOR NURSING RESEARCH

A **paradigm** is a world view, a general perspective on the complexities of the real world. Disciplined inquiry in the field of nursing is being conducted mainly (although not exclusively, as described in Chapter 10) within two broad paradigms, both of which have legitimacy for nursing research. This section describes the two paradigms and broadly outlines the research methods associated with them.

The Positivist Paradigm

The paradigm that has dominated nursing research for decades is known as **positivism** (sometimes referred to as *logical positivism*). Positivism is rooted in 19th century thought, guided by such philosophers as Comte, Newton, and Locke. Positivism is a reflection of a broader cultural phenomenon (*modernism*) that emphasizes the rational and the scientific.

As shown in Table 1.2, a fundamental assumption of positivists is that there is a reality *out there* that can be studied and known. (An **assumption** is a principle that is believed to be true without proof or verification.) Adherents of positivism assume that nature is basically ordered and regular and that an objective reality exists independent of human observation. In other words, the world is assumed not to be merely a creation of the human mind. The related assumption of **determinism** refers to the positivists' belief that *phenomena* (observable facts and events) are

TABLE 1.2 ▶	MAJOR ASSUMPTIONS OF THE POSITIVIST AND NATURALISTIC PARADIGMS	
TYPE OF ASSUMPTION	**POSITIVIST PARADIGM**	**NATURALISTIC PARADIGM**
The nature of reality	Reality exists; there is a real world driven by real natural causes	Reality is multiple and subjective, mentally constructed by individuals
Relationship between researcher and those being researched	The inquirer is independent from those being researched	The inquirer interacts with those being researched; findings are the creation of the interactive process
The role of values in the inquiry	Values and biases are to be held in check; objectivity is sought	Subjectivity and values are inevitable and desirable
Best methods for obtaining evidence	➤ Deductive processes ➤ Emphasis on discrete, specific concepts ➤ Focus on the objective and quantifiable ➤ Verification of researchers' predictions ➤ Fixed, prespecified design ➤ Outsider knowledge—researcher as external ➤ Control over context ➤ Measured, quantitative information; statistical analysis ➤ Seeks generalizations ➤ Focus on the product	➤ Inductive processes ➤ Emphasis on the whole ➤ Focus on the subjective and nonquantifiable ➤ Emerging insight grounded in participants' experiences ➤ Flexible, emergent design ➤ Insider knowledge—researcher as internal ➤ Context bound, contextualized ➤ Narrative information; qualitative analysis ➤ Seeks in-depth understanding ➤ Focus on the product and the process

not haphazard or random, but rather have antecedent causes. If a person has a cerebrovascular accident, the scientist in a positivist tradition assumes that there must be one or more reasons that can be potentially identified. Within the **positivist paradigm**, much research activity is directed at understanding the underlying causes of natural phenomena.

Because of their belief in an objective reality, positivists seek to be objective. Their approach involves the use of orderly, disciplined procedures with tight controls over the research situation to test hunches about the nature of phenomena being studied and relationships among them.

Strict positivist thinking has been challenged and undermined, and few researchers adhere to the tenets of pure positivism. In the *postpositivist paradigm*, there is still a belief in reality and a desire to understand it, but postpositivists recognize the impossibility of total objectivity. They do, however, see objectivity as a goal and strive to be as neutral as possible. Postpositivists also appreciate the impediments to knowing reality with certainty and therefore seek probabilistic evidence (i.e., learning what the true state of a phenomenon *probably* is, with a high and ascertainable degree of likelihood). This modified positivist position remains a dominant force in nursing research. For the sake of simplicity, we refer to it as positivism.

The Naturalistic Paradigm

The **naturalistic paradigm** (sometimes called the *constructivist paradigm*) began as a countermovement to positivism with writers such as Weber and Kant. The naturalistic paradigm represents a major alternative system for conducting disciplined research in nursing. Table 1.2 compares four major assumptions of the positivist and naturalistic paradigms.

For the naturalistic inquirer, reality is not a fixed entity but rather a construction of the individuals participating in the research; reality exists within a context, and many constructions are possible. Naturalists take the position of relativism: If there are always multiple interpretations of reality, then there is no process by which the ultimate truth or falsity of the constructions can be determined.

The naturalistic paradigm assumes that knowledge is maximized when the distance between the inquirer and the participants in the study is minimized. The voices and interpretations of those under study are crucial to understanding the phenomenon of interest, and subjective interactions are the primary way to access them. The findings from a naturalistic inquiry are the product of the interaction between the inquirer and the participants.

Paradigms and Methods: Quantitative and Qualitative Research

Research methods are the techniques researchers use to structure a study and to gather and analyze information relevant to the research question. The alternative paradigms have strong implications for the research methods to be used to develop evidence. The methodologic distinction typically focuses on differences between **quantitative research**, which is most closely allied with the positivist tradition, and **qualitative research**, which is associated with naturalistic inquiry—although positivists sometimes undertake qualitative studies, and naturalistic researchers sometimes collect quantitative information. This section provides an overview of the methods linked to the two alternative paradigms.

The Scientific Method and Quantitative Research

The traditional, positivist **scientific method** entails a set of orderly, disciplined procedures used to acquire information. Quantitative researchers use deductive reasoning to generate predictions that are tested in the real world. They typically move in a systematic fashion from the definition of a problem and the selection of concepts on which to focus, to the solution of the problem. By *systematic*, we mean that investigators progress logically through a series of steps, according to a prespecified plan. Quantitative researchers use mechanisms designed to control the research situation so that biases are minimized and precision and validity are maximized.

Quantitative researchers gather **empirical evidence**—evidence that is rooted in objective reality and gathered directly or indirectly through the senses rather than through personal beliefs or hunches. Evidence for a study in the positivist paradigm is gathered systematically, using formal instruments to collect needed information. Usually (but not always) the information gathered is **quantitative**—that is, numeric information that results from some type of formal measurement and that is analyzed with statistical procedures. Scientists strive to go beyond the specifics of a research situation; the ability to generalize research findings to individuals other than those who participated in the study (referred to as **generalizability**) is an important goal.

The traditional scientific method has enjoyed considerable stature as a method of inquiry, and it has been used productively by nurse researchers studying a wide range of nursing problems. This is not to say, however, that this approach can solve all nursing problems. One important limitation—common to both quantitative and qualitative research—is that research methods cannot be used to answer moral or ethical questions. Many persistent and intriguing questions about the human experience fall into this area (e.g., should euthanasia be practiced?). Given the many moral issues linked to health care, it is inevitable that the nursing process will never rely exclusively on scientific information.

The traditional research approach also must contend with problems of *measurement*. To study a phenomenon, scientists attempt to measure it, that is, to attach numeric values that express quantity. For example, if the phenomenon of interest were patient morale, researchers might want to assess if morale is high or low, or higher under certain conditions. Although physiologic phenomena such as blood pressure and cardiac activity can be measured with considerable accuracy and precision, the same cannot be said of psychological phenomena, such as morale or self-esteem.

Another issue is that nursing research tends to focus on human beings, who are inherently complex and diverse. The traditional scientific method typically focuses on a relatively small portion of the human experience (e.g., weight gain, depression, chemical dependency) in a single study. Complexities tend to be controlled and, if possible, eliminated rather than studied directly. This narrow focus can sometimes obscure insights. Finally and relatedly, quantitative research conducted in the positivist paradigm has sometimes been accused of a narrowness and inflexibility of vision, a problem that has been called a *sedimented view* of the world that does not fully capture the reality of experiences.

Naturalistic Methods and Qualitative Research

Naturalistic methods of inquiry deal with the issue of human complexity by exploring it directly. Researchers in naturalistic traditions emphasize the inherent depth of humans, their ability to shape and create their own experiences, and the idea that truth is a composite of realities. Consequently, naturalistic investigations emphasize understanding the human experience as it is lived, usually through the careful collection and analysis of **qualitative** materials that are narrative and subjective.

Researchers who reject the traditional scientific method believe that a major limitation of the classical model is that it is *reductionist*—that is, it reduces human experience to only the few concepts under investigation, and those concepts are defined in advance by the researcher rather than emerging from the experiences of those under study. Naturalistic researchers tend to emphasize the dynamic, holistic, and individual aspects of phenomena and attempt to capture those aspects in their entirety, within the context of those who are experiencing them.

Flexible, evolving procedures are used to capitalize on findings that emerge in the course of the study. Naturalistic inquiry usually takes place in the **field** (i.e., in naturalistic settings), often over an extended period. The collection of information and its analysis typically progress concurrently; as researchers sift through information, insights are gained, new questions emerge, and further evidence is sought to amplify or confirm the insights. Through an inductive process, researchers integrate information to develop a theory or description that helps explicate the phenomena under observation.

Naturalistic studies yield rich, in-depth information that can potentially clarify the varied dimensions of a complicated phenomenon (e.g., the process by which mid-life women adapt to menopause). The findings from in-depth qualitative research are typically grounded in the real-life experiences of people with first-hand knowledge of a phenomenon. Nevertheless, the approach has several limitations. Human beings are used directly as the instrument through which information is gathered, and humans are extremely intelligent and sensitive—but fallible—tools. The subjectivity that enriches the analytic insights of skillful researchers can yield trivial "findings" among less competent ones.

Another potential limitation involves the subjective nature of the inquiry, which can raise questions about the idiosyncratic nature of the conclusions. Would two naturalistic researchers studying the same phenomenon in similar settings arrive at similar conclusions? The situation is further complicated by the fact that most naturalistic studies involve a relatively small study group. Thus, the generalizability of findings from naturalistic inquiries can sometimes be challenged.

TIP

Researchers often do not discuss the underlying paradigm of their studies in their reports. Qualitative researchers are more likely to explicitly mention the naturalistic paradigm (or to say they have undertaken a naturalistic inquiry) than are quantitative researchers to mention positivism.

Multiple Paradigms and Nursing Research

Paradigms are lenses that help to sharpen our focus on phenomena of interest, not blinders that limit intellectual curiosity. The emergence of alternative paradigms for the study of nursing problems is, in our view, a healthy and desirable trend in the pursuit of new evidence for practice. Nursing knowledge would be meager without a rich array of methods available within the two paradigms—methods that are often complementary in their strengths and limitations.

We have emphasized differences between the two paradigms and their associated methods to make their distinctions more understandable. It is equally important, however, to note that these two paradigms have many features in common, some of which are mentioned here:

➤ *Ultimate goals*. The ultimate aim of disciplined research, regardless of the paradigm, is to gain understanding. Both quantitative and qualitative researchers seek to capture the truth with regard to an aspect of the world in which they are interested, and both can make noteworthy—and mutually beneficial—contributions to nursing practice.

➤ *External evidence*. Although the word *empiricism* has come to be allied with the classic scientific method, researchers in both traditions gather and analyze evidence empirically, that is, through their senses. Neither qualitative nor quantitative researchers are armchair analysts, relying on their own beliefs to generate their evidence.

➤ *Reliance on human cooperation*. Because evidence for nursing research comes primarily from humans, human cooperation is essential. To understand people's characteristics and experiences, researchers must persuade them to participate in the investigation *and* to speak and act candidly.

➤ *Ethical constraints*. Research with human beings is guided by ethical principles that sometimes interfere with research goals. For example, if researchers want to test a potentially beneficial intervention, is it ethical to withhold the treatment from some people to see what happens? As discussed in Chapter 5, ethical dilemmas often confront researchers, regardless of paradigms or methods.

➤ *Fallibility of disciplined research*. Virtually all studies—in either paradigm—have limitations. Every research question can be addressed in many different ways, and inevitably there are trade-offs. Financial constraints are often an issue, but limitations often exist even in well-funded research. This does not mean that small, simple studies have no value. *It means that no single study can ever definitively answer a research question*. Each completed study adds to a body of accumulated evidence. The fallibility of any single study makes it important to understand and critique researchers' methodologic decisions when evaluating the quality of their evidence.

Thus, despite philosophic and methodologic differences, researchers using the traditional scientific method or naturalistic methods often share overall goals and face many similar constraints and challenges. The selection of an appropriate method depends on researchers' philosophy and world view, but also on the research question. If a researcher asks, "What are the effects of cryotherapy on nausea and oral mucositis in patients undergoing chemotherapy?" the researcher really needs to express the effects through the careful quantitative assessment of patients. On the other hand, if a researcher asks, "What is the process by which parents learn to cope with the death of a child?" the researcher would be hard pressed to quantify such a process. Personal world views of researchers help to shape their questions.

In reading about the alternative paradigms for nursing research, you likely were more attracted to one of the two paradigms—the one that corresponds most closely to your view of the world and of reality. It is important, however, to learn about and respect both approaches to disciplined inquiry, and to recognize their respective strengths and limitations. In this textbook, we describe methods associated with both qualitative and quantitative research.

HOW-TO-TELL TIP

How can you tell if a study is qualitative or quantitative? As you progress through this book, you should be able to identify most studies as qualitative versus quantitative based simply on the title, or based on terms in the abstract at the beginning of the report. At this point, though, it may be easiest to distinguish the two types of studies based on how many *numbers* appear in the report, especially in tables. Qualitative studies may have no tables with quantitative information, or only one numeric table describing participants' characteristics (e.g., the percentage who were male or female). Quantitative studies typically have several tables with numbers and statistical information. Qualitative studies often have "word tables" or diagrams and figures illustrating processes inferred from the narrative information gathered.

PURPOSES OF NURSING RESEARCH

The general purpose of nursing research is to answer questions or solve problems of relevance to the nursing profession. Sometimes a distinction is made between basic and applied research. As traditionally defined, **basic research** is undertaken to extend the base of knowledge in a discipline. For example, a researcher may perform an in-depth study to better understand normal grieving processes, without having explicit applications in mind. **Applied research** focuses on finding solutions to existing problems. For example, an applied study might assess the effectiveness of a nursing intervention to ease grieving. Basic research is appropriate for discovering general principles of human behavior and biophysiologic processes; applied research is designed to indicate how these principles can be used to solve problems in nursing practice.

Specific purposes can be classified in a number of different ways. We present two systems, primarily so that we can illustrate the range of questions that nurse researchers have addressed.

Research to Achieve Varying Levels of Explanation

One way to classify research purposes concerns the extent to which studies are designed to provide explanatory information. Although specific study goals can range along an explanatory continuum, a fundamental distinction that is especially relevant in quantitative research is between studies whose primary intent is to *describe* phenomena and how they are interrelated, and those that are **cause-probing**—that is, designed to illuminate the underlying causes of phenomena. Evidence hierarchies such as those we will discuss in Chapter 2 are fundamentally concerned with evidence on *causes* of health-related outcomes.

Using a descriptive or explanatory framework, the specific purposes of nursing research include identification, description, exploration, prediction or control and explanation. For each purpose, various types of question are addressed by nurse researchers—some more amenable to qualitative than to quantitative inquiry, and vice versa.

Identification and Description

Qualitative researchers sometimes study phenomena about which little is known. In some cases, so little is known that the phenomenon has yet to be clearly identified or named or has been inadequately defined or conceptualized. The in-depth, probing nature of qualitative research is well suited to the task of answering such questions as, "What is this phenomenon?" and "What is its name?" (Table 1.3). In quantitative research, by contrast, researchers begin with a phenomenon that has been previously studied or defined—sometimes in a qualitative study. Thus, in quantitative research, identification typically precedes the inquiry.

TABLE 1.3 ▶ RESEARCH PURPOSES AND TYPES OF RESEARCH QUESTIONS		
PURPOSE	TYPES OF QUESTIONS: QUANTITATIVE RESEARCH	TYPES OF QUESTIONS: QUALITATIVE RESEARCH
Identification		What is this phenomenon? What is its name?
Description	How prevalent is the phenomenon? How often does the phenomenon occur? What are the characteristics of the phenomenon?	What are the dimensions of the phenomenon? What is important about the phenomenon?
Exploration	What factors are related to the phenomenon? What are the antecedents of the phenomenon?	What is the full nature of the phenomenon? What is really going on here? What is the process by which the phenomenon evolves or is experienced?
Prediction and Control	If phenomenon X occurs, will phenomenon Y follow? How can we make the phenomenon occur or alter its prevalence? Can the phenomenon be prevented or controlled?	
Explanation	What is the underlying cause of the phenomenon or the causal pathway through which the phenomenon unfolds? Does the theory explain the phenomenon?	How does the phenomenon work? Why does the phenomenon exist? What does the phenomenon mean? How did the phenomenon occur?

Qualitative example of identification:
Giske and Gjengedal (2007) conducted an in-depth study of how patients coped while going through a gastric diagnosis, pending the results of diagnostic workups. They identified a process that they called *preparative waiting* that described how patients braced themselves.

Description of phenomena is an important purpose of research. In descriptive studies, researchers observe, count, delineate, elucidate, and classify. Nurse researchers have described a wide variety of phenomena. Examples include patients' stress, pain responses, and health beliefs. Quantitative description focuses on the prevalence, incidence, size, and measurable attributes of phenomena. Qualitative researchers, on the other hand, describe the dimensions, variations, and importance of phenomena. Table 1.3 compares descriptive questions posed by quantitative and qualitative researchers.

Quantitative example of description:
Carls (2007) described the prevalence of stress urinary incontinence in young female athletes participating in high impact sports, and the rate at which they had told someone of their problem.

Exploration
Like descriptive research, exploratory research begins with a phenomenon of interest; but rather than simply observing and describing it, exploratory researchers investigate the full nature of the phenomenon, the manner in which it is manifested, and the other factors to which it is related—including potential factors that might be *causing* it. For example, a *descriptive* quantitative study of patients' preoperative stress might seek to document the degree of stress patients experience before surgery and the percentage of patients who experience it. An *exploratory* study might ask: What factors diminish or increase a patient's stress? Is a patient's stress related to behaviors of the nursing staff? Is stress related to the patient's cultural backgrounds? Qualitative methods are useful for exploring the full nature of little-understood phenomena. Exploratory qualitative research is designed to shed light on the various ways in which a phenomenon is manifested and on underlying processes.

Qualitative example of exploration:
Im and colleagues (2008) explored the experience of cancer pain in African American patients with cancer through a 6-month online forum.

Prediction and Control
Many phenomena defy explanation and resist efforts to understand their causes. Yet it is frequently possible to make predictions and to control phenomena based on research findings, even in the absence of complete understanding. For example, research has shown that the incidence of Down syndrome in infants increases with the age of the mother. We can thus predict that a woman aged 40 years is at higher risk of bearing a child with Down syndrome than is a woman aged 25 years. We can partially control the outcome by educating women about the risks and offering

amniocentesis to women older than 35 years of age. Note, however, that the ability to predict and control in this example does not depend on an explanation of what *causes* older women to be at a higher risk of having an abnormal child. In many nursing and health-related studies—typically, quantitative ones—prediction and control are key objectives. Although explanatory studies are powerful in an EBP environment, studies whose purpose is prediction and control are also critical in helping clinicians make decisions.

Quantitative example of prediction:
Harton and colleagues (2007) conducted a study to identify factors that predicted return to preoperative incentive spirometry volume following cardiac surgery.

Explanation
The goals of explanatory research are to understand the underpinnings of specific natural phenomena—often, to explain what *caused* them. Explanatory research is often linked to **theories**, which represent a method of organizing and integrating ideas about phenomena and their interrelationships. Whereas descriptive research provides new information, and exploratory research provides promising insights, explanatory research attempts to offer understanding of the underlying causes or full nature of a phenomenon. In quantitative research, theories or prior findings are used deductively to generate hypothesized explanations that are then tested empirically. In qualitative studies, researchers may search for explanations about how or why a phenomenon exists or what a phenomenon means as a basis for *developing* a theory that is grounded in rich, in-depth, experiential evidence.

Quantitative example of explanation:
Blue (2007) tested a theoretic model to explain physical activity and dietary patterns among adults at risk for diabetes. The model purported to explain positive health behaviors on the basis of theoretically relevant concepts, such as subjective norms and perceived behavioral control.

Qualitative example of explanation:
Coughlan and Ward (2007) conducted a study that sought to explain the meaning of "quality of care" for recently relocated residents from two older hospital-style facilities to a new long-term care facility in Canada.

Research Purposes Linked to EBP

Most nursing studies can be described in terms of a purpose on the descriptive-explanatory dimension just described, but some studies do not fall into such a system. For example, a study to develop and rigorously test a new instrument to screen women for domestic violence could not easily be classified using this categorization.

In both nursing and medicine, several books have been written to facilitate evidence-based practice, and these books categorize studies in terms of the types of information needed by clinicians (e.g., DiCenso et al., 2005; Guyatt & Rennie, 2002;

Melnyk & Fineout-Overholt, 2005). These writers focus on several types of clinical concerns: Treatment, therapy, or intervention; diagnosis and assessment; prognosis; harm and etiology; and meaning. Not all nursing studies have these purposes, but many of them do, and such studies have great potential for EBP.

Treatment, Therapy, or Intervention

Nurse researchers are increasingly undertaking studies designed to help nurses make evidence-based treatment decisions. Such studies range from evaluations of highly specific treatments (e.g., comparing two types of cooling blankets for febrile patients) to complex multi-component interventions designed to effect behavioral changes (e.g., nurse-led smoking cessation interventions). Such **intervention research,** which can involve interventions for both treating and preventing health problems and adverse outcomes, plays a critical role in EBP. Before intervening with patients, nurses have a responsibility to determine the benefits and risks of the intervention, and also whether the expenditure of resources for the intervention is justifiable.

Example of a study aimed at treatment/therapy:
Yeh and colleagues (2008) tested the effectiveness of an intervention that included acupressure and interactive multimedia on visual acuity in school-aged children with visual impairment.

Diagnosis and Assessment

A burgeoning number of nursing studies concern the rigorous development and evaluation of formal instruments to screen, diagnose, and assess patients and to measure important clinical outcomes. High-quality instruments with documented accuracy are essential both for clinical practice and for research.

Example of a study aimed at diagnosis/assessment:
Vanderwee and colleagues (2007) evaluated two methods of assessing the need for pressure ulcer prevention in a sample of more than 1,600 hospitalized patients. They compared the efficacy of beginning preventive measures when nonblanchable erythema appeared, compared with when scores on a standard assessment tool achieved the recommended cutoff score.

Prognosis

Studies of prognosis examine the outcomes of a disease or health problem, estimate the probability the outcomes will occur, explore factors that can modify the prognosis, and indicate when (and for which types of people) the outcomes are most likely. Such studies facilitate the development of long-term care plans for patients. They also provide valuable information that can guide patients to make important lifestyle choices or to be vigilant for key symptoms. Prognostic studies can also play a role in resource allocation decisions.

Example of a study aimed at prognosis:
Wakefield and Holman (2007) studied factors associated with different functional trajectories and with functional decline in hospitalized older adults.

Harm and Etiology

It is difficult, and sometimes impossible, to prevent harm or treat health problems if we do not know what causes them. For example, there would be no smoking cessation programs if research had not provided firm evidence that smoking cigarettes causes or contributes to a wide range of health problems. Thus, determining the factors and exposures that affect or cause illness, mortality, or morbidity is an important purpose of many studies.

Example of a study aimed at studying harm:
Albers and co-researchers (2007) studied whether epidural use was associated with spontaneous genital tract lacerations in normal vaginal births.

Meaning and Processes

Designing effective interventions, motivating people to comply with treatments and to engage in health promotion activities, and providing sensitive advice to patients are among the many health care activities that can greatly benefit from understanding the clients' perspectives. Research that provides evidence about what health and illness mean to clients, what barriers they face to positive health practices, and what processes they experience in a transition through a health care crisis is important to evidence-based nursing practice.

Example of a study aimed at studying meaning:
Vellone and colleagues (2008) studied the meaning of *quality of life* for caregivers of patients with Alzheimer's disease.

TIP

Most of these EBP-related purposes (except *diagnosis* and *meaning*) fundamentally call for *cause-probing* research. For example, research on interventions focuses on whether an intervention *causes* improvements in key outcomes. Prognosis research asks if a disease or health condition *causes* subsequent adverse outcomes. And etiology research seeks explanations about the underlying *causes* of health problems.

ASSISTANCE FOR CONSUMERS OF NURSING RESEARCH

This book is designed to help you develop skills that will allow you to read, evaluate, and use nursing studies (i.e., to become skillful consumers and users of nursing research). In each chapter of this book, we present information relating to the methods used by nurse researchers and provide specific guidance in several ways. First, interspersed throughout the chapters, we offer tips on what you can expect to

---

**BOX 1.1   QUESTIONS FOR A PRELIMINARY OVERVIEW
              OF A RESEARCH REPORT**

1. How relevant is the research problem to the actual practice of nursing? Does the study focus on a topic that is considered a priority area for nursing research?
2. Is the research quantitative or qualitative?
3. What is the underlying purpose (or purposes) of the study—identification, description, exploration, prediction/control, or explanation? Does the purpose correspond to an EBP focus such as treatment, diagnosis, prognosis, harm and etiology, or meaning?
4. What might be some clinical implications of this research? To what type of people and settings is the research most relevant? If the findings are accurate, how might the results of this study be used by *me*?

---

find in actual research articles with regard to the content in the chapter, identified by the icon 🔖 . These include special "how-to-tell" tips that help you find concepts discussed in this book in research reports. These tips are identified with this icon: 💡 . Second, we include guidelines for critiquing those aspects of a study covered in each chapter. Each set of critiquing guidelines is included in the Toolkit section ⚙ on the accompanying CD-ROM ⏵ so that you can "fill in" answers on a computer, or adapt questions to suit your needs. The questions in Box 1.1 are designed to assist you in using the information in this chapter in an overall preliminary assessment of a research report. And third, we offer opportunities to apply your newly acquired skills. The critical thinking activities at the end of each chapter guide you through appraisals of real research examples (some of which are presented in their entirety in the appendix) of both qualitative and quantitative studies. These activities also challenge you to think about how the findings from these studies could be used in nursing practice.

RESEARCH EXAMPLES AND CRITICAL THINKING ACTIVITIES

Each chapter of this book presents brief descriptions of actual studies conducted by nurse researchers, focusing on key terms and concepts discussed in the chapters. The descriptions are followed by some questions to guide critical thinking. A review of the full journal articles would prove useful for learning more about study methods and findings.

EXAMPLE 1 ■ Quantitative Research

Study

Depression and anxiety in women with breast cancer and their partners (Badger et al., 2007).

Study Purpose

The purpose of the study was to evaluate the effectiveness of telephone-delivered psychosocial interventions in decreasing depression and anxiety in women with breast cancer and their partners.

Study Methods

A total of 96 women with breast cancer and their partners were recruited to participate in the study. Two different, but complementary, interventions were implemented using a telephone delivery method. The 6-week telephone interpersonal counseling intervention (TIP-C) combined cancer education with interpersonal counseling that targeted the social support behavior of both cancer survivors and their partners. The other 6-week telephone intervention focused on self-managed exercise (EX). Study participants were allocated, based on a lottery-type system, to either one of the two interventions or to a control group that received neither treatment but that got printed information and brief weekly calls (CON). All study participants, including partners, were interviewed before the study began, and then 6 weeks and 10 weeks later. The interviews included scales that measured levels of depression and anxiety.

Key Findings

The analysis suggested that anxiety was reduced, for both the women and their partners, in both the TIP-C and EX intervention groups but not in the control group. Depression decreased over time in all three groups.

Conclusions

Badger and colleagues concluded that both telephone-delivered interventions were effective in improving psychological quality of life when compared with nonreceipt of either intervention.

CRITICAL THINKING SUGGESTIONS*:

*See the Student Resource CD-ROM for a discussion of these questions. 💿

1. Answers the questions from Box 1.1 regarding this study.
2. Also consider the following targeted questions, which may assist you in assessing aspects of the study's merit:
    a. Why do you think the researchers decided to have a third group that did not get either intervention?
    b. Why do you think the control group participants received brief weekly phone calls?
    c. Could this study have been undertaken as a qualitative study? Why or why not?

👤 EXAMPLE 2 ■ Qualitative Research

Study

Living with risk: Mothering a child with food-induced anaphylaxis (Gillespie et al., 2007).

Study Purpose

The purpose of this study was to develop a narrative description of the underlying meaning of mothers' lived experience of parenting a child with food-induced anaphylaxis (FIA).

Study Methods

Six mothers of children 6 to 12 years of age who were considered at risk for FIA were recruited to participate in the study. The number and type of food allergies varied, but peanut was the most common. Two in-depth interviews, each lasting 1½ to 2 hours, were conducted with each mother in her own home. The interviews, which were audiotaped and then transcribed, focused on what it was like for the mothers to have a child with a life-threatening food allergy.

Key Findings

"Living with risk" was identified as the essence of the mothers' experience, and was supported by five themes: (1) living with fear; (2) worrying about well-being; (3) looking for control; (4) relying on resources; and (5) it is hard, but it is not. Each theme was supported with rich narrative descriptions from the in-depth interviews.

Conclusions

The researchers concluded that the themes describing mothers' fears and concerns would be useful in assisting nurses to meet families' education and support needs related to FIA.

CRITICAL THINKING SUGGESTIONS:

1. Answer the questions in Box 1.1 regarding this study.
2. Also consider the following targeted questions, which may assist you in assessing aspects of the study's merit:
   a. Why do you think that the researchers audiotaped and transcribed their in-depth interviews with study participants?
   b. Do you think it would have been appropriate for the researchers to conduct this study using quantitative research methods? Why or why not?

EXAMPLE 3 ■ Quantitative Research in Appendix A

1. Read the abstract and the introduction from Howell and colleagues' (2007) study ("Anxiety, anger, and blood pressure in children") in Appendix A of this book, and then answer the relevant questions in Box 1.1.
2. Also consider the following targeted questions, which may further sharpen your critical thinking skills and assist you in assessing aspects of the study's merit:
   a. What gap in the existing research was the study designed to fill?
   b. Would you describe this study as applied or basic, based on information provided in the abstract?
   c. Could this study have been undertaken as a qualitative study? Why or why not?
   d. Who helped to pay for this research? (This information appears at the end of the report).

EXAMPLE 4 ■ Qualitative Research in Appendix B

1. Read the abstract and the introduction from Beck's (2006) study ("Anniversary of Birth Trauma") in Appendix B of this book and then answer the questions in Box 1.1.
2. Also consider the following targeted questions, which may further sharpen your critical thinking skills and assist you in assessing aspects of the study's merit:
   a. What gap in the existing research was the study designed to fill?
   b. Was Beck's study conducted within the positivisit paradigm or the naturalistic paradigm? Provide a rationale for your choice.

CHAPTER REVIEW

••

Key new terms introduced in the chapter, together with a summary of major points, are presented in this section. Chapter 1 of the accompanying *Study Guide for Essentials of Nursing Research,* 7th edition also offers exercises and study suggestions for reinforcing the concepts presented in this chapter. For additional review, see self study questions on the CD-ROM provided with this book. ●

Key New Terms

••

Assumption	Evidence hierarchy	Positivist paradigm
Cause-probing research	Generalizability	Qualitative research
Clinical nursing research	Inductive reasoning	Quantitative research
Deductive reasoning	Intervention research	Research methods
Determinism	Naturalistic paradigm	Research program
Empirical evidence	Nursing research	Scientific method
Evidence-based practice	Paradigm	Systematic review

Summary Points

••

⇴ **Nursing research** is systematic inquiry to develop evidence on problems of importance to nurses.

⇴ Nurses in various settings are adopting an **evidence-based practice** (**EBP**) that incorporates research findings into their decisions and their interactions with clients.

⇴ Knowledge of nursing research enhances the professional practice of all nurses—including both *consumers of research* (who read and evaluate studies) and *producers of research* (who design and undertake studies).

⇴ Nursing research began with Florence Nightingale, but developed slowly until its rapid acceleration in the 1950s. Since the 1980s, the focus has been on **clinical nursing research**—that is, on problems relating to clinical practice.

⇴ The **National Institute of Nursing Research** (NINR), established at the U.S. National Institutes of Health (NIH) in 1993, affirms the stature of nursing research in the United States.

⇴ Future emphases of nursing research are likely to include EBP projects, **replications** of research, research integration through **systematic reviews**, multisite and interdisciplinary studies, expanded dissemination efforts, and increased focus on health disparities.

⇴ Disciplined research stands in contrast to other sources of evidence for nursing practice, such as tradition, authority, personal experience, trial and error, intuition, and logical reasoning; rigorous research is at the pinnacle of an **evidence hierarchy** as a basis for making clinical decisions.

➢ Although logical reasoning is, in itself, insufficient as an evidence base, both **deductive reasoning** (the process of developing specific predictions from general principles) and **inductive reasoning** (the process of developing generalizations from specific observations) are used in research.

➢ Disciplined inquiry in nursing is conducted mainly within two broad **paradigms**—world views with underlying **assumptions** about the complexities of reality: the positivist paradigm and the naturalistic paradigm.

➢ In the **positivist paradigm,** it is assumed that there is an objective reality and that natural phenomena are regular and orderly. The related assumption of **determinism** refers to the belief that phenomena are the result of prior causes and are not haphazard.

➢ In the **naturalistic paradigm,** it is assumed that reality is not a fixed entity but is rather a construction of human minds, and thus "truth" is a composite of multiple constructions of reality.

➢ The positivist paradigm is associated with **quantitative research**—the collection and analysis of numeric information. Quantitative research is typically conducted within the traditional **scientific method,** which is a systematic and controlled process. Quantitative researchers base their findings on **empirical evidence** (evidence collected by way of the human senses) and strive for **generalizability** of their findings beyond a single setting or situation.

➢ Researchers within the naturalistic paradigm emphasize understanding the human experience as it is lived through the collection and analysis of subjective, narrative materials using flexible procedures that evolve in the **field;** this paradigm is associated with **qualitative research.**

➢ **Basic research** is designed to extend the base of information for the sake of knowledge. **Applied research** focuses on discovering solutions to immediate problems.

➢ A fundamental distinction that is especially relevant in quantitative research is between studies whose primary intent is to *describe* phenomena and those that are **cause-probing** (i.e., designed to illuminate underlying causes of phenomena). Specific purposes on the description/explanation continuum include identification, description, exploration, prediction/control and explanation.

➢ Many nursing studies can also be classified in terms of a key EBP aim: treatment or therapy or intervention; diagnosis and assessment; prognosis; harm and etiology; and meaning and process.

STUDIES CITED IN CHAPTER 1[1]

Aiken, L., Clarke, S., Sloane, D., Sochalski, J., & Silber, J. (2002). Hospital nurse staffing and patient mortality, nurse burnout, and job dissatisfaction. *Journal of the American Medical Association, 288,* 1987–1993.

---

[1] This citation list contains only *studies* that were cited in this chapter. Citations for all methodologic, theoretic, or other nonempirical work cited in this and subsequent chapters are in a separate section at the end of the book. See Methodologic and Theoretic References, beginning on page 541.

Albers, L., Migliaccio, L., Bedrick, E., Teaf, D., & Peralta, P. (2007). Does epidural analgesia affect the rate of spontaneous obstetric lacerations in normal births? *Journal of Midwifery and Women's Health*, *52*, 31–36.

Badger, T., Segrin, C., Dorros, S., Meek, P., & Lopez, A.M. (2007). Depression and anxiety in women with breast cancer and their partners. *Nursing Research, 56*, 44–53.

Barnard, K. E. (1973). The effects of stimulation on the sleep behavior of the premature infant. In M. Batey (Ed.), *Communicating nursing research* (Vol. 6, pp. 12–33). Boulder, CO: WICHE.

Barnard, K. E., Wenner, W., Weber, B., Gray, C., & Peterson, A. (1977). Premature infant refocus. In P. Miller (Ed.), *Research to practice in mental retardation: Vol. 3, Biomedical aspects*. Baltimore, MD: University Park Press.

Blue, C. L. (2007). Does the theory of planned behavior identify diabetes-related cognitions for intention to be physically active and eat a healthy diet? *Public Health Nursing, 24*, 141–150.

Brooten, D., Kumar, S., Brown, L. P., Butts, P., Finkler, S., Bakewell-Sachs, S. et al. (1986). A randomized clinical trial of early hospital discharge and home follow-up of very low birthweight infants. *New England Journal of Medicine, 315*, 934–939.

Brooten, D., Brown, L. P., Munro, B. H., York, R., Cohen, S., Roncoli, M. et al. (1988). Early discharge and specialist transitional care. *Image: Journal of Nursing Scholarship, 20*, 64–68.

Carls, C. (2007). The prevalence of stress urinary incontinence in high school and college-age female athletes in the Midwest. *Urologic Nursing, 27*, 21–24.

Chwo, M. J., Anderson, G. C., Good, M., Dowling, D. A., Shiau, S. H., & Chu, D. M. (2002). A randomized controlled trial of early kangaroo care for preterm infants: Effects on temperature, weight, behavior, and acuity. *Journal of Nursing Research, 10*, 129–142.

Coughlan, R., & Ward, L. (2007). Experiences of recently relocated residents of a long-term care facility in Ontario. *International Journal of Nursing Studies, 44*, 47–57.

Dodd, V. L. (2005). Implications of kangaroo care for growth and development in preterm infants. *Journal of Obstetric, Gynecologic, & Neonatal Nursing, 34*, 218–232.

Galligan, M. (2006). Proposed guidelines for skin-to-skin treatment of neonatal hypothermia. *MCN: The American Journal of Maternal-Child Nursing, 31*, 298–304.

Gillespie, C., Woodgate, R., Chalmers, K., & Watson, W. (2007). "Living with risk": Mothering a child with food-induced anaphylaxis. *Journal of Pediatric Nursing, 22*, 30–42.

Giske, T., & Gjengedal, E. (2007). "Preparative waiting" and coping theory with patients going through gastric diagnosis. *Journal of Advanced Nursing, 57*, 87–94.

Grey, M., Davidson, M., Boland, E., & Tamborlane, W. (2001). Clinical and psychosocial factors associated with achievement of treatment goals in adolescents with diabetes mellitus. *Journal of Adolescent Health, 28*, 377–385.

Harton, S., Grap, M., Savage, L., & Elswick, R. (2007). Frequency and predictors of return to incentive spirometry volume baseline after cardiac surgery. *Progress in Cardiovascular Nursing, 22*, 7–12.

Hill, M., Han, H., Dennison, C., Kim, M., Roary, M., Blumenthal, R. et al. (2003). Hypertension care and control in underserved urban African American men. *American Journal of Hypertension, 16*, 906–913.

Im, E. O., Lim, H., Clark, M., & Chee, W. (2008). African American cancer patients' pain experience. *Cancer Nursing, 31*, 38–46.

Klemm, P. (2008). Late effects of treatment for long-term cancer survivors: Qualitative analysis of an online support group. *Computers, Informatics, Nursing, 26*, 49–58.

Ludington-Hoe, S. M., Anderson, G. C., Swinth, J. Y., Thompson, C., & Hadeed, A. J. (2004). Randomized controlled trial of kangaroo care: Cardiorespiratory and thermal effects on healthy preterm infants. *Neonatal Network, 23*, 39–48.

Ludington-Hoe, S., Johnson, M., Morgan, K., Lewis, T., Gutman, J., Wilson, P. et al. (2006). Neurophysiologic assessment of neonatal sleep organization: Preliminary results of a randomized, controlled trial of skin contact with preterm infants. *Pediatrics, 117*, 909–923.

Moore, E., & Anderson, G. (2007). Randomized controlled trial of very early mother-infant skin-to-skin contact and breastfeeding status. *Journal of Midwifery & Women's Health, 52*, 116–125.

Nightingale, F. (1859). *Notes on nursing: What it is, and what it is not*. Philadelphia: J. B. Lippincott.

Okoli, C., Browning, S., Rayens, M., & Hahn, E. (2008). Secondhand tobacco smoke exposure, nicotine dependence, and smoking cessation, *Public Health Nursing, 25*, 46–56.

Quint, J. C. (1963). The impact of mastectomy. *American Journal of Nursing, 63*, 88–91.

Quint, J. C. (1967). *The nurse and the dying patient*. New York: Macmillan.

Swanson, B., Cronin-Stubbs, D., Zeller, J. M., Kessler, H. A., & Bielauskas, L. A. (1993). Characterizing the neuropsychological functioning of persons with human immunodeficiency virus infection. *Archives of Psychiatric Nursing, 7*, 82–90.

Swanson, B., Zeller, J. M., & Spear, G. (1998). Cortisol upregulates HIV p24 antigen in cultured human monocyte-derived macrophages. *Journal of the Association of Nurses in AIDS Care, 9*, 78–83.

Vanderwee, K., Grypdonck, M., & DeFloor, M. (2007). Non-blanchable erythema as an indicator for the need for pressure ulcer prevention. *Journal of Clinical Nursing, 16*, 325–335.

Vellone, E., Piras, G., Talucci, C., & Cohen, M. (2008). Quality of life for caregivers of people with Alzheimer's disease. *Journal of Advanced Nursing, 61*, 222–231.

Wakefield, B., & Holman, J. (2007). Functional trajectories associated with hospitalization in older adults. *Western Journal of Nursing Research, 29*, 161–177.

Yeh, M., Chen, C., Chen, H., & Lin, K. (2008). An intervention of acupressure and interactive multimedia to improve visual health among Taiwanese schoolchildren. *Public Health Nursing, 25*, 10–17.

2 Evidence-Based Nursing Practice: Fundamentals

STUDENT OBJECTIVES

On completing this chapter, you will be able to:

➤ Distinguish research utilization (RU) and evidence-based practice (EBP), and discuss their current status within nursing

➤ Identify several resources available to facilitate EBP in nursing practice

➤ Identify several models that have relevance for RU and EBP

➤ Discuss the five major steps in undertaking an EBP effort for individual nurses

➤ Identify the components of a well-worded clinical question and be able to frame such a question

➤ Discuss strategies for undertaking an EBP project at the organizational level

➤ Define new terms in the chapter

Evidence-based practice (EBP) is the conscientious use of current best evidence in making clinical decisions about patient care (Sackett et al., 2000). A basic feature of EBP as a clinical problem-solving strategy is that it de-emphasizes decisions based on custom, authority, or ritual; the emphasis is on identifying the best available research evidence and *integrating* it with other factors. Advocates of EBP do not minimize the importance of clinical expertise. Rather, they argue that evidence-based decision making should integrate best research evidence with clinical expertise, patient preferences and circumstances, and awareness of the clinical setting and resource constraints. EBP involves efforts to personalize evidence to fit a specific patient's needs and a particular clinical situation.

This book will help you to develop the methodologic skills you need for evaluating research evidence for nursing practice. Before we elaborate on methodologic techniques, we discuss key aspects of EBP to further clarify the key role that research now plays in nursing.

BACKGROUND OF EVIDENCE-BASED NURSING PRACTICE

This section provides a context for understanding evidence-based nursing practice. Part of this context involves a discussion of a closely related concept, research utilization.

Research Utilization

The terms *research utilization* and *evidence-based practice* are sometimes used synonymously. Although there is overlap between the two concepts, they are distinct. **Research utilization** (RU) is the use of findings from disciplined research in a practical application that is unrelated to the original research. In RU, the emphasis is on translating empirically derived knowledge into real-world applications; the genesis of the process is a research-based innovation or new evidence.

Evidence-based practice is broader than RU because it integrates research findings with other factors, as just noted. Also, whereas RU begins with the research itself (How can I put this innovation to good use in my clinical setting?), the start-point in EBP is a clinical question (What does the evidence say is the best approach to solving this problem?).

Research utilization was an important concept in nursing before the EBP movement took hold. This section provides a brief overview of RU in nursing.

The Research Utilization Continuum

The start-point of research utilization is the emergence of new knowledge and new ideas. Research is conducted and, over time, evidence on a topic accumulates. In turn, the evidence works its way into use—to varying degrees and at differing rates.

Theorists who have studied the phenomenon of knowledge development and the diffusion of ideas typically recognize a continuum in terms of the specificity of the use to which research findings are put. At one end of the continuum are discrete, clearly identifiable attempts to base specific actions on research findings (e.g., placing infants in supine instead of prone sleeping position to minimize the risk of sudden infant death syndrome). Research findings can, however, be used in a more diffuse manner—in a way that reflects cumulative awareness, understanding, or enlightenment. Thus, a practicing nurse may read a qualitative research report describing *courage* among individuals with long-term health problems as a dynamic process that includes efforts fully to accept reality and to develop problem-solving skills. The study may make the nurse more observant and sensitive in working with patients with long-term illnesses, but it may not necessarily lead to formal changes in clinical actions.

Estabrooks (1999) studied research utilization by collecting information from 600 nurses in Canada. She found evidence to support three distinct types of RU: (1) *indirect research utilization* (sometimes call *conceptual utilization*), involving changes in nurses' thinking; (2) *direct research utilization* (sometimes called *instrumental utilization*), involving the direct use of findings in giving patient care; and (3) *persuasive utilization*, involving the use of findings to persuade others (typically those in decision-making positions) to make changes in policies or practices relevant to nursing care. These varying ways of thinking about RU clearly suggest a role for both qualitative and quantitative research.

The History of Research Utilization in Nursing Practice

During the 1980s, research utilization emerged as an important buzz word, and several changes in nursing education and nursing research were prompted by the desire to develop a knowledge base for nursing practice. In education, nursing schools increasingly began to include courses on research methods so that students would become skillful research consumers. In the research arena, there was a shift in focus toward clinical nursing problems.

These changes helped to sensitize the nursing community to the desirability of using research as a basis for practice, but there were mounting concerns about the limited use of research findings in the delivery of nursing care. Some of these concerns were based on studies that suggested that practicing nurses were unaware of (or ignored) important research findings (e.g., Ketefian, 1975). The need to reduce the gap between research and practice led to formal attempts to bridge the gap. The best-known of several early nursing RU projects is the **Conduct and Utilization of Research in Nursing (CURN) Project**, a 5-year project awarded to the Michigan Nurses' Association by the Division of Nursing in the 1970s. The major objective of CURN was to increase the use of research findings in nurses' daily practice by disseminating current research findings, facilitating organizational changes needed to implement innovations, and encouraging collaborative clinical research. The CURN project staff saw RU as primarily an organizational process, with the commitment of organizations that employ nurses as essential to RU (Horsley, Crane, & Bingle, 1978). The CURN project team concluded that RU by practicing nurses was feasible, but only if the research was relevant to practice and if the results were broadly disseminated.

During the 1980s and 1990s, RU projects were undertaken by a growing number of organizations, and project descriptions appeared regularly in nursing journals. These projects were generally institutional attempts to implement changes in nursing practice on the basis of research findings, and to evaluate the effects of the innovations. Although there were studies that continued to document a gap between research and practice, the findings suggested some improvements in nurses' utilization of research (e.g., Coyle & Sokop, 1990; Rutledge, Greene, Mooney, Nail, & Ropka, 1996). During the 1990s, however, the call for research utilization began to be superseded by the push for EBP.

Evidence-Based Practice in Nursing

The EBP movement has given rise to considerable debate, with both advocates and critics. Supporters argue that EBP offers a solution to improving health care quality in our current cost-constrained environment. They argue that a rational approach is needed to provide the best possible care to the most people, with the most cost-effective use of resources. Advocates also note that EBP provides an important framework for self-directed lifelong learning that is essential in an era of rapid clinical advances and the information explosion. Critics worry that the advantages of EBP are exaggerated and that individual clinical judgments and patient inputs are being devalued. They are also concerned that insufficient attention is being paid to the role of qualitative research. Although there is a need for close scrutiny of how the EBP journey unfolds, it seems likely that the EBP path is one that health care professions will follow in the years ahead.

Overview of the Evidence-Based Practice Movement

A keystone of the EBP movement is the Cochrane Collaboration, which was founded in the United Kingdom based on the work of British epidemiologist Archie Cochrane. Cochrane published an influential book in the early 1970s that drew attention to the dearth of solid evidence about the effects of health care. He called for efforts to make research summaries about interventions available to physicians and other health care providers. This eventually led to the development of the Cochrane Center in Oxford in 1993, and the international **Cochrane Collaboration**, with centers now established in over a dozen locations throughout the world. Its aim is to help providers make good decisions about health care by preparing, maintaining, and disseminating systematic reviews of the effects of health care interventions.

At about the same time that the Cochrane Collaboration got under way, a group from McMaster Medical School in Canada developed a clinical learning strategy they called *evidence-based medicine*. The evidence-based medicine movement, pioneered by Dr. David Sackett, has broadened to the use of best evidence by *all* health care practitioners in a multidisciplinary team.

EBP has been considered a major paradigm shift for health care education and practice. In the EBP environment, a skillful clinician can no longer rely on a repository of memorized information, but rather must be adept in accessing, evaluating, synthesizing, and using new research evidence.

Types of Evidence and Evidence Hierarchies

No consensus exists about what constitutes usable evidence for EBP, but there is general agreement that findings from rigorous research are paramount. There is, however, some debate about what constitutes *"rigorous"* research and what qualifies as *"best"* evidence.

In the initial phases of the EBP movement, there was a definite bias toward reliance on information from a type of study called a *randomized controlled trial* (or, sometimes, a *randomized clinical trial*, RCT). This bias stemmed, in part, from the fact that the Cochrane Collaboration initially focused on evidence about the effectiveness of interventions, rather than about health care issues more generally. As we explain in Chapter 9, the strategies used in RCTs are especially well-suited for drawing conclusions about the effects of health care interventions. The bias in ranking sources of evidence primarily in terms of questions about effective treatments led to some resistance to EBP by nurses who felt that evidence from qualitative and non-RCT studies would be ignored.

Positions about the contribution of various types of evidence are less rigid than previously. Nevertheless, most published **evidence hierarchies**, which rank evidence sources according to the strength of the evidence they provide, look something like the one shown in Figure 2.1. This figure, adapted from schemes presented in several references on EBP (DiCenso et al., 2005; Melnyk & Fineout-Overholt, 2005) shows a seven-level hierarchy that has systematic reviews of RCTs at its pinnacle. Systematic reviews of nonrandomized clinical trials (Level Ib) offer less powerful evidence. The second rung of the hierarchy is individual RCT

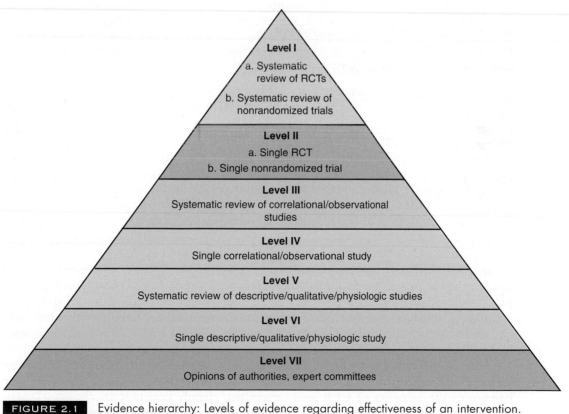

Level I
a. Systematic review of RCTs
b. Systematic review of nonrandomized trials

Level II
a. Single RCT
b. Single nonrandomized trial

Level III
Systematic review of correlational/observational studies

Level IV
Single correlational/observational study

Level V
Systematic review of descriptive/qualitative/physiologic studies

Level VI
Single descriptive/qualitative/physiologic study

Level VII
Opinions of authorities, expert committees

FIGURE 2.1   Evidence hierarchy: Levels of evidence regarding effectiveness of an intervention.

studies, and so on (the terms in this figure are explained in subsequent chapters of this book). At the bottom of this evidence hierarchy is found opinions from experts.

Of course, *within* any level in an evidence hierarchy, evidence quality can vary considerably. For example, an individual RCT (Level IIa) could be well designed, yielding persuasive evidence, or it could be so flawed that the evidence would be useless. We must also emphasize that the hierarchy in Figure 2.1 is not universally appropriate—a point that is not always made sufficiently clear. This hierarchy has merit for ranking evidence for certain clinical questions, but not others. In particular, this hierarchy is appropriate with regard to *cause-probing* questions, especially questions about the effects of clinical interventions. For example, evidence about the efficacy of massage therapy on pain in cancer patients would be classified according to this hierarchy, but the hierarchy would not be relevant for ranking evidence relating to such questions as the following: What is the experience of pain like for patients with cancer? What percentage of cancer patients experience intense pain, and for how long does the pain persist?

Thus, in nursing, *best evidence* refers generally to findings from research that are methodologically appropriate, rigorous, and clinically relevant for answering pressing questions—questions not only about the efficacy, safety, and cost-effectiveness of nursing interventions, but also about the reliability of nursing assessment measures, the determinants of health and well-being, the meaning of health or illness, and the nature of patients' experiences. Confidence in the evidence is enhanced when the research methods are compelling, when there have been multiple confirmatory replication studies, and when the evidence has been systematically evaluated and synthesized.

Barriers to Research Utilization and Evidence-Based Practice

Nurses have completed many studies about EBP and the translation of research into practice, including research on factors that hinder or facilitate EBP. This is an important area of research, because the findings indicate ways in which EBP efforts can be promoted or undermined, and thus suggest issues that need to be addressed in advancing evidence-based nursing. Studies that have explored barriers to research use have yielded remarkably similar results in numerous countries about constraints clinical nurses face. Most barriers fall into one of three categories: (1) quality and nature of the research, (2) nurses' characteristics, and (3) organizational factors.

With regard to the research itself, the main problem is that for some practice areas, availability of high-quality research evidence is limited. There remains an ongoing need for research that directly addresses pressing clinical problems, for methodologically strong and generalizable studies, and for replication of studies in a range of settings. Another issue is that nurse researchers need to improve their ability to communicate their findings (and the clinical implications of their findings) to practicing nurses.

Nurses' attitudes and education consistently have emerged as potential barriers to RU and EBP. Studies have found that some nurses do not value research or believe in the benefits of EBP, and others are simply resistant to change. Fortunately, there is growing evidence from international surveys that many nurses *do* value research and want to be involved in research-related activities. Additional barriers, however, are that many nurses do not know how to access research information and do not possess the skills to critically evaluate research findings—and even those who do may not know how to effectively incorporate research evidence into clinical decision making.

Finally, many of the impediments to using research in practice are organizational. "Unit culture" has been found to be a major factor in research use (Pepler, Edgar, Frisch, Rennick, Swidzinsky, White, et al., 2005), and administrative and other organizational barriers have repeatedly been found to play a role. Although many organizations support the idea of EBP in theory, they do not always provide the necessary supports in terms of staff release time and resources. EBP will become part of organizational norms only if there is a commitment on the part of managers and administrators. Strong leadership in health care organizations is essential to making EBP happen.

RESOURCES FOR EVIDENCE-BASED PRACTICE

The translation of research evidence into nursing practice is an ongoing challenge, but it is a challenge to which the nursing profession has risen. In this section, we describe some of the resources that are available to support evidence-based nursing practice.

Systematic Reviews

Evidence-based practice relies on meticulous integration of research evidence on a topic. The emphasis on *best evidence* implies that all key evidence about a clinical problem has been gathered, evaluated, and synthesized so that conclusions can be drawn about effective practices. A systematic review is not just a literature review, such as ones we describe in Chapter 7. A systematic review is in itself a methodic, scholarly inquiry that follows many of the same steps as those for other studies. Chapter 19 offers some basic guidance on reading and critiquing systematic reviews.

Systematic reviews can take various forms. Until fairly recently, the most common type of systematic review was a traditional narrative (qualitative) integration that merged and synthesized findings, much like a thorough literature review. Narrative reviews of quantitative studies increasingly are being replaced by a type of systematic review known as a meta-analysis.

Meta-analysis is a technique for integrating quantitative research findings statistically. In essence, meta-analysis treats the findings from a study as one piece of information. The findings from multiple studies on the same topic are combined and then all of the information is analyzed statistically in a manner similar to that in a usual study. Thus, instead of study participants being the *unit of analysis* (the most basic entity on which the analysis focuses), individual studies are the unit of analysis in a meta-analysis. Meta-analysis provides a convenient, objective method of integrating a body of findings and of observing patterns that might not have been detected.

Example of a meta-analysis:
Rawson and Newburn-Cook (2007) conducted a meta-analysis to analyze evidence on the effectiveness of low-dose warfarin for reducing the incidence of thrombosis in patients with cancer who have a central venous catheter. Integrating results from four intervention studies, the researchers concluded that prophylactic use of low-dose warfarin may not prevent thrombus formation.

Efforts are also underway to develop techniques for qualitative metasynthesis. A **metasynthesis** involves integrating qualitative findings on a specific topic that are themselves interpretive syntheses of narrative information. A metasynthesis is distinct from a quantitative meta-analysis; a metasynthesis is less about reducing information and more about amplifying and interpreting it. A new group within the Cochrane Collaboration, the Qualitative Research Methods Group, now undertakes and disseminates metasyntheses.

Example of a metasynthesis:
Downe and colleagues (2007) undertook a metasynthesis exploring the skills and practices related to expert intrapartum nonphysician maternity care. Their metasynthesis, which examined qualitative studies published between 1970 and 2006, identified three intersecting themes in seven relevant studies: wisdom, skilled practice, and enacted vocation.

Fortunately, systematic reviews on various clinical topics are increasingly available. Such reviews are published in professional journals that can be accessed using standard literature search procedures (see Chapter 7), and are also available in databases that are dedicated to such reviews. In particular, the Cochrane Database of Systematic Reviews (CDSR) contains thousands of systematic reviews relating to health care interventions. Another resource for those wishing to access systematic reviews is the Agency for Healthcare Research and Quality (AHRQ). This agency awarded contracts to establish EBP centers at institutions in the United States and Canada. Each center issues *evidence reports* that are based on rigorous systematic reviews of relevant literature.

TIP

Websites with useful content relating to EBP, including ones for locating systematic reviews, are in the "Useful Websites for Chapter 2" file on the accompanying CD-ROM for you to access simply by using the "Control/Click" feature.

Other Preappraised Evidence

Preappraised evidence is evidence that has been selected from primary studies and evaluated for use in clinical situations. Systematic reviews are one such resource, and *clinical practice guidelines* (discussed later in this chapter) are another. We mention a few additional resources that might be useful.

DiCenso and colleagues (2005) described a hierarchy of preprocessed evidence that puts clinical practice guidelines at the top as being especially useful. On the next rung are synopses of systematic reviews, followed by systematic reviews themselves, and then synopses of single studies. Synopses of systematic reviews and of single studies are available in evidence-based abstract journals. For example, the *Evidence-Based Nursing* journal, published quarterly, presents critical summaries of studies and systematic reviews published in more than 150 journals. The summaries include commentaries on the clinical implications of each reviewed study. *Evidence-Based Nursing* has been linked to other health care abstraction journals (e.g., *Evidence-Based Mental Health)* into one electronic resource, *Evidence-Based Medicine Reviews*. Another journal-based resource is the "evidence digest" feature in each issue of *Worldviews on Evidence-Based Nursing.*

In some journals and also in some practice settings, tools called **critically appraised topics (CATs)** are becoming available. A CAT is a quick summary of a clinical question and an appraisal of the best evidence, and it typically begins with a "clinical bottom line"—that is, what the best-practice recommendation is. Sackett and colleagues (2000) advocate the creation and use of CATs as a teaching/learning tool for EBP.

Models of the Evidence-Based Practice Process

A number of different models and theories of EBP and RU have been developed and are important resources. These models offer frameworks for understanding the EBP process and for implementing an EBP project in a practice setting. Some models focus on the use of research from the perspective of individual clinicians (e.g., the Stetler Model), while some focus on institutional EBP efforts (e.g., the Iowa Model). Models that offer a framework for guiding an EBP or RU effort include the following:

❧ Advancing Research and Clinical Practice Through Close Collaboration (ARCC) Model (Melnyk & Fineout-Overholt, 2005)

❧ Diffusion of Innovations Theory (Rogers, 1995)

❧ Framework for Adopting an Evidence-Based Innovation (DiCenso et al., 2005)

❧ Iowa Model of Research in Practice (Titler et al., 2001)

❧ Johns Hopkins Nursing EBP Model (Newhouse et al., 2005)

❧ Ottawa Model of Research Use (Logan & Graham, 1998)

❧ Promoting Action on Research Implementation in Health Services (PARIHS) Model, (Rycroft -Malone et al., 2002, 2007)

❧ Stetler Model of Research Utilization (Stetler, 2001)

Although each model offers different perspectives on how to translate research findings into practice, several of the steps and procedures are similar across the models. The most prominent of these models have been the **Diffusion of Innovations Theory**, the **PARIHS Model**, the **Stetler Model**, and the **Iowa Model**. The latter two, developed by nurses, were originally crafted in an environment that emphasized RU, but they have been updated to incorporate EBP processes. For those wishing to follow a formal EBP model, the cited references should be consulted. Several of the models are also nicely synthesized by Melnyk and Fineout-Overholt (2005). We provide an overview of key activities and processes in EBP efforts, based on a distillation of common elements from the various models, in a subsequent section of this chapter. We rely especially heavily on the Iowa Model, a diagram for which is shown in Figure 2.2.

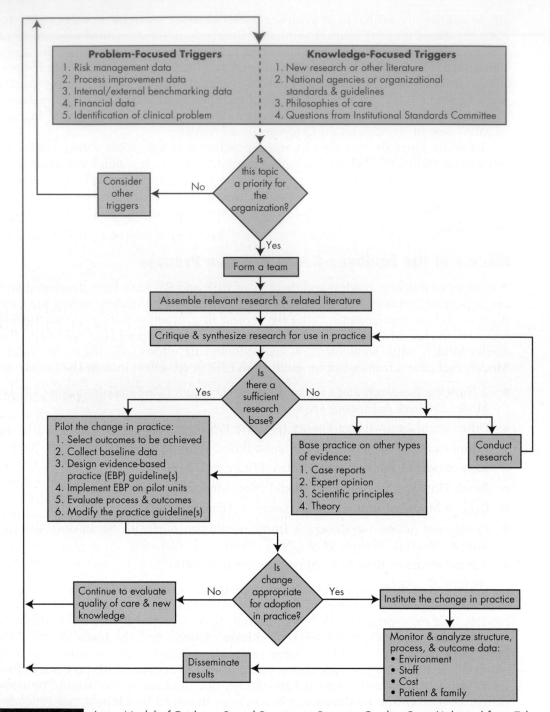

Problem-Focused Triggers
1. Risk management data
2. Process improvement data
3. Internal/external benchmarking data
4. Financial data
5. Identification of clinical problem

Knowledge-Focused Triggers
1. New research or other literature
2. National agencies or organizational standards & guidelines
3. Philosophies of care
4. Questions from Institutional Standards Committee

Is this topic a priority for the organization?

Consider other triggers — No

Yes

Form a team

Assemble relevant research & related literature

Critique & synthesize research for use in practice

Is there a sufficient research base?

Yes — No

Pilot the change in practice:
1. Select outcomes to be achieved
2. Collect baseline data
3. Design evidence-based practice (EBP) guideline(s)
4. Implement EBP on pilot units
5. Evaluate process & outcomes
6. Modify the practice guideline(s)

Base practice on other types of evidence:
1. Case reports
2. Expert opinion
3. Scientific principles
4. Theory

Conduct research

Is change appropriate for adoption in practice?

Continue to evaluate quality of care & new knowledge — No

Yes — Institute the change in practice

Monitor & analyze structure, process, & outcome data:
• Environment
• Staff
• Cost
• Patient & family

Disseminate results

FIGURE 2.2 Iowa Model of Evidence-Based Practice to Promote Quality Care (Adapted from Titler, et al. [2001]. The Iowa Model of Evidence-Based Practice to Promote Quality Care. *Critical Care Nursing Clinics of North America, 13,* 497–509.

EVIDENCE-BASED PRACTICE IN INDIVIDUAL NURSING PRACTICE

In the years ahead, you are likely to engage in individual and institutional efforts to use research as a basis for clinical decisions. This will almost assuredly be the case if you work in a hospital that is aspiring to or has attained Magnet status. In any EBP activity, you will be well served by having skills in finding, understanding, and critiquing research.

This and the following sections, which are based on various models of EBP, provide an overview of how research can be put to use in clinical settings. More extensive guidance is available in textbooks devoted to evidence-based nursing (e.g., DiCenso et al., 2005; Melnyk & Fineout-Overholt, 2005). We first discuss strategies and steps for individual clinicians and then describe activities used by organizations or teams of nurses.

Clinical Scenarios and the Need for Evidence

Individual nurses make many decisions and are called on to provide health care advice, and so they have ample opportunity to put research into practice. Here are four clinical scenarios that provide examples of such opportunities:

➤ *Clinical Scenario 1.* You are working on a hemodialysis unit and one of your patients with type 2 diabetes develops severe foot ulceration that ultimately leads to amputation of several toes. You want to know if there is a reliable assessment tool for the earlier detection of foot complications so that the risk of amputation for patients with end-stage renal disease would be reduced.

➤ *Clinical Scenario 2.* You are an Advance Practice Registered Nurse (APRN) working in a rehabilitation hospital and one of your elderly patients, who had total hip replacement, tells you that she is planning a long airplane trip to visit her daughter after her rehabilitation treatments are completed. You know that a long plane ride will increase the patient's risk of deep vein thrombosis and wonder if compression stockings are really an effective in-flight treatment and should be recommended. You decide to look for the best possible evidence to answer this question.

➤ *Clinical Scenario 3.* You are working in an allergy clinic and notice how difficult it is for many children to undergo allergy scratch tests. You wonder if there is an effective intervention to help allay children's fears about the skin tests.

➤ *Clinical Scenario 4.* You are caring for a hospitalized patient who, a week before hospitalization, was given a prescription for a selective serotonin reuptake inhibitor (SSRI) antidepressant. He confides in you that he is ashamed to fill the prescription because he feels it is "unmanly." You wonder if there is any evidence about what it feels like to begin an SSRI regimen so that you can better understand how to address your patient's concerns.

In these and thousands of other clinical situations, research evidence can be put to good use to improve the quality of nursing care. Some situations might lead to unit-wide or institution-wide scrutiny of current practices, but in other situations individual nurses can personally investigate the evidence to help address specific problems.

For individual EBP efforts, the major steps in EBP include the following:

1. Asking clinical questions that are answerable with research evidence
2. Searching for and collecting relevant evidence
3. Appraising and synthesizing the evidence
4. Integrating the evidence with your own clinical expertise, patient preferences, and local context
5. Assessing the effectiveness of the decision, intervention, or advice.

Asking Well-Worded Clinical Questions

Books on evidence-based practice typically devote considerable attention to the first EBP step of asking an answerable clinical question. Authors of books on EBP often distinguish between background and foreground questions. **Background questions** are foundational questions about a clinical issue, for example: What is cancer cachexia (progressive body wasting) and what is its pathophysiology? Answers to background questions are typically found in textbooks. **Foreground questions**, by contrast, are those that can be answered based on current best research evidence on diagnosing, assessing, or treating patients, or on understanding the meaning, cause, or prognosis of their health problems. For example, we may wonder, is a fish-oil enhanced nutritional supplement effective in stabilizing weight in patients with advanced cancer? The answer to such a question may provide guidance on how best to treat patients with cachexia—that is, the answer provides an opportunity for EBP.

DiCenso and colleagues (2005) advise that, for questions that call for quantitative information (e.g., about the effectiveness of a treatment), three components should be identified:

1. The *population* (What are the characteristics of the patients or clients?)
2. The *intervention* or *exposure* (What are the treatments or interventions of interest? or, What are the potentially harmful exposures that concern us?)
3. The *outcomes* (What are the outcomes or consequences in which we are interested?)

If we applied this scheme to our question about cachexia, we would say that our *population* is cancer patients with advanced cancer or cachexia; the *intervention* is fish-oil enhanced nutritional supplements; and the *outcome* is weight stabilization. As another example, in the first clinical scenario about foot complications cited earlier, the population is diabetic patients undergoing hemodialysis; the intervention is a foot assessment tool; and the outcome is detection of foot problems.

For questions that can best be answered with qualitative information (e.g., about the meaning of an experience or health problem), DiCenso et al. (2005) suggest two components:

1. The *population* (What are the characteristics of the patients or clients?)
2. The *situation* (What conditions, experiences, or circumstances are we interested in understanding?)

For example, suppose our question was, What is it like to suffer from cachexia? In this case, the question calls for rich qualitative information; the *population* is patients with advanced cancer and the *situation* is the experience of cachexia.

Fineout-Overholt and Johnston (2005) suggested a five-component scheme for formulating EBP questions and used an acronym (PICOT) as a guide. The five components are population (P), intervention or issue (I), comparison of interest (C), outcome (O), and time (T). Their scheme contrasts an intervention with a specific comparison, such as an alternative treatment. For example, we might specifically be interested in learning whether fish-oil enhanced supplements are better than melatonin in stabilizing weight in cancer patients. In some cases, it is important to designate a specific comparison, whereas in others we might be interested in uncovering evidence about *all* alternatives to the intervention of primary interest. That is, in searching for evidence about the effectiveness of fish-oil supplements, we might want to search for studies that have compared such supplements with melatonin, placebos, other treatments, or no treatments. The final component in the Fineout-Overholt and Johnston scheme is a timeframe, that is, the timeframe in which the question occurs. As with the "C" component, the "T" is not always essential.

Table 2.1 offers some question templates for asking well-framed clinical questions in selected circumstances. The right-hand panel includes questions with an explicit comparison, and the left-hand panel does not.

TIP

The Toolkit section of Chapter 2 on the accompanying CD-ROM includes Table 2.1 in a Word file that can be adapted for your use, so that the template questions can be readily "filled in."

Finding Research Evidence

By asking clinical questions in the forms suggested, you should be able to more effectively search the research literature for the information you need. For example, by using the templates in Table 2.1, the information you insert into the blanks constitute *keywords* that can be used in an electronic search.

For an individual EBP endeavor, the best place to begin is by searching for evidence in a systematic review, clinical practice guideline, or other preprocessed source because this approach leads to a quicker answer—and, if your methodologic skills are limited, potentially a superior answer as well. Researchers who prepare reviews and clinical guidelines typically are well trained in research methods and usually use exemplary standards in evaluating the evidence. Moreover,

TABLE 2.1   QUESTION TEMPLATES FOR SELECTED CLINICAL FOREGROUND QUESTIONS

TYPE OF QUESTION	QUESTION TEMPLATE FOR QUESTIONS *WITHOUT* AN EXPLICIT COMPARISON	QUESTION TEMPLATE FOR QUESTIONS *WITH* AN EXPLICIT COMPARISON
Treatment/Intervention	In _____ (population), what is the effect of _____ (intervention) on _____ (outcome)?	In _____ (population), what is the effect of _____ (intervention), in comparison to _____ (comparative/alternative intervention), on _____ (outcome)?
Diagnosis/Assessment	For _____ (population), does _____ (tool/procedure) yield accurate and appropriate diagnostic/assessment information about _____ (outcome)?	For _____ (population), does _____ (tool/procedure) yield more accurate or more appropriate diagnostic/assessment information than _____ (comparative tool/procedure) about _____ (outcome)?
Prognosis	For _____ (population), does _____ (disease or condition) increase the risk of or influence _____ (outcome)?	For _____ (population), does _____ (disease or condition), relative to _____ (comparative disease or condition) increase the risk of or influence _____ (outcome)?
Etiology/Harm	Does _____ (exposure or characteristic) increase the risk of _____ (outcome) in _____ (population)?	Does _____ (exposure or characteristic) increase the risk of _____ (outcome) compared with _____ (comparative exposure or condition) in _____ (population)?
Meaning/Process	What is it like for _____ (population) to experience _____ (condition, illness, circumstance)? **OR** What is the process by which _____ (population) cope with, adapt to, or live with _____ (condition, illness, circumstance)?	(Explicit comparisons are not typical in these types of question)

BOX 2.1   QUESTIONS FOR APPRAISING THE EVIDENCE   ⊗

What is the quality of the evidence (i.e., how rigorous and reliable is it)?
What is the evidence—what is the magnitude of effects?
How precise is the estimate of effects?
What evidence is there of any side effects or side benefits?
What is the financial cost of applying (and not applying) the evidence?
Is the evidence relevant to my particular clinical situation?

---

preprocessed evidence is often prepared by a team, which means that the conclusions are cross-checked and fairly objective. Thus, when preprocessed evidence is available to answer a clinical question, you may not need to look any further—unless the review is outdated. When preprocessed evidence cannot be located or is old, you will need to look for best evidence in primary studies, using strategies we describe in Chapter 7.

Appraising the Evidence

After locating appropriate evidence, it should be appraised before taking clinical action. The critical appraisal of evidence for the purposes of EBP may involve several types of assessments (Box 2.1). The thoroughness of your appraisal usually depends on several factors, the most important of which is the nature of the clinical action for which evidence is being sought. Some clinical actions have implications for patient safety, whereas others affect patients' satisfaction. While using best evidence to guide nursing practice is important for a wide range of outcomes, the appraisal standards would clearly be especially strict for evidence that could affect patient safety and morbidity.

Evidence Quality

The first appraisal issue is the extent to which the findings are valid. That is, were the study methods sufficiently rigorous that the evidence can be believed? We offer guidance on critiquing studies and evaluating the strength of research evidence throughout this book. If there are several primary studies and no existing systematic review, you would need to draw conclusions about the body of evidence taken as a whole. Clearly, you would want to put the most weight on the most rigorous studies.

Magnitude of Effects

You would also need to assess what the results actually *are,* and whether they are clinically important. This criterion considers not whether the results are likely to be "real," but what they are and how powerful the effects are. For example, consider clinical scenario number 2 cited earlier, which suggests the following clinical question: Does the use of compression stockings lower the risk of flight-related deep vein thrombosis for high-risk patients? In our search for evidence, we find a relevant meta-analysis of nine RCTs (Hsieh & Lee, 2005). The conclusion of the meta-analysis is that compression stockings are fairly effective and the evidence is strong, suggesting that advice about the use of compression stockings may be appropriate, pending an appraisal of other factors.

Determining the magnitude of the effect for quantitative findings is especially important when an intervention is costly or when there are potentially negative side effects. If, for example, there is strong evidence that an intervention is only modestly effective in improving a health problem, it would be important to consider other factors (e.g., evidence on the effects on quality of life). There are various ways to quantify the magnitude of effects, several of which are described later in this book.

Precision of Estimates

Another consideration, relevant when the evidence is quantitative, is how precise the estimate of effect is. This level of appraisal requires some statistical sophistication and so we postpone our discussion of *confidence intervals* to Chapter 15. Research results provide only an *estimate* of effects and it may be useful to understand not only the exact estimate, but the range within which the actual effect probably lies.

Peripheral Effects

If the evidence is judged to be valid and the magnitude of effects suggests that further consideration is warranted, there are situations in which supplementary information is important in guiding decisions. One issue concerns peripheral benefits and costs, evidence for which would typically have emerged during your search. In framing your clinical question, you would have identified the key outcomes in which you were interested—for example, weight stabilization or weight gain for an intervention to address cancer cachexia. Research on this topic, however, would likely have considered other outcomes that would need to be taken into account—for example, quality of life, comfort, side effects, satisfaction, and so on.

Financial Issues

Another issue concerns the financial cost of applying the evidence. In some cases, the costs may be small or nonexistent. For example, in clinical scenario 4, where the question concerned the experience of initiating an SSRI treatment, nursing action would presumably be cost neutral because the evidence would be used primarily to provide information and reassurance to the patient. Some interventions and assessment protocols, however, are costly and so the amount of time and resources needed to put best evidence into practice would need to be estimated and factored into any decision. Of course, while the cost of a clinical decision needs to be considered, the cost of *not* taking action is equally important.

Clinical Relevance

Finally, it is important to appraise the evidence in terms of its relevance for the clinical situation at hand—that is, for *your* patient in a specific clinical setting. Best practice evidence can most readily be applied to an individual patient in your care if he or she is sufficiently similar to people in the study or studies under review. Would your patient have qualified for participation in the study—or is there some factor such as age, illness severity, mental status, or comorbidity that would have excluded him or her? DiCenso and colleagues (2005), who advised clinicians to ask whether there is a compelling reason to conclude that results may *not* be applicable in their clinical situation, have written some useful tips on applying evidence to individual patients.

Actions Based on Evidence Appraisals

Appraisals of the evidence may lead you to different courses of action. You may reach this point on your EBP path and conclude that the evidence base is not sufficiently sound, or that the likely effect is too small or nonexistent, or that the cost of applying the evidence is too high to merit consideration. The appraisal information may suggest that "usual care" is the best strategy—or it may suggest the need for a new EBP inquiry. For instance, in the example about cachexia, you likely would have learned that recent evidence suggests that fish-oil enhanced nutritional supplements may be an ineffective treatment (Jatoi, 2005). However, during your search you may have come across a Cochrane review that concluded that megestrol acetate improves appetite and weight gain in patients with cancer (Berenstein & Ortiz, 2005). This may lead to a new evidence inquiry and to discussions with other members of your health care team about developing a nutrition-focused protocol for your clinical setting. If, however, the initial appraisal of evidence suggests a promising clinical action, then you can proceed to the next step.

Integrating Evidence

As the definition for EBP implies, research evidence needs to be integrated with other types of information, including your own clinical expertise and knowledge of your clinical setting. You may be aware of factors that would make implementation of the evidence, no matter how sound and how promising, inadvisable.

Patient preferences and values are also important. A discussion with the patient may reveal strong negative attitudes toward a potentially beneficial course of action, or contraindications (e.g., previously unsuspected comorbidities), or possible impediments (e.g., lack of health insurance). Also, if the resources needed to apply the evidence are not routinely available, you would need to determine the feasibility of obtaining needed resources.

One final issue is the desirability of integrating evidence from qualitative research. Qualitative research can provide rich insights about how patients experience a problem, or about barriers to complying with a treatment. A potentially beneficial intervention may fail to achieve desired outcomes if it is not implemented with sensitivity to a patient's perspective. As Morse (2005) has noted, evidence from an RCT may tell whether a pill is effective, but qualitative research can help you understand why patients may not swallow the pill.

Implementing the Evidence and Evaluating Outcomes

After the first four steps of the EBP process have been completed, you can use the integrated information to make an evidence-based decision or to provide evidence-based advice. Although the steps in the process, as just described, may seem complicated, in reality the process can be quite efficient—*if* there is adequate evidence, and especially if it has been skillfully preprocessed. EBP is most challenging when findings from research are contradictory, inconclusive, or "thin"—that is, when better quality evidence is needed.

One last step in an individual EBP effort concerns evaluation. Part of the evaluation process involves following up to determine if your actions or decisions achieved the desired outcome. Another part, however, concerns an evaluation of how well you are performing EBP. Sackett and colleagues (2000) offer self-evaluation questions to appraise your efforts. The questions relate to the previous EBP steps, such as asking answerable questions (Am I asking any clinical questions at all? Am I asking well-formulated questions?) and finding external evidence (Do I know the best sources of current evidence? Am I becoming more efficient in my searching?). A self-appraisal may lead to the conclusion that at least some of the clinical questions of interest to you are best addressed as a group effort.

EVIDENCE-BASED PRACTICE IN AN ORGANIZATIONAL CONTEXT

For some clinical scenarios, individual nurses may be able to implement evidence-based strategies on their own (e.g., providing advice about using compression stockings on an upcoming flight). However, there are many situations in which decisions must be made at the organizational level, or are best made among a team of nurses working together to solve a recurrent clinical problem. This section describes some additional considerations that are relevant to institutional efforts at EBP—efforts designed to result in a formal policy or protocol affecting the practice of many nurses.

Many of the steps in organizational EBP projects are similar to the ones described in the previous section. For example, gathering and appraising evidence are key activities in both. However, additional issues are relevant at the organizational level.

Selecting a Problem for an Institutional Evidence-Based Practice Project

Some EBP projects are "bottoms-up" efforts that originate in deliberations among clinicians who have encountered a problem and propose problem-solving activities to their supervisors. Others, however, are "top-down" efforts in which administrators take steps to stimulate creative thought and the use of research evidence among clinicians. This latter approach is increasingly likely to occur in U.S. hospitals as part of the Magnet recognition process.

Example of EBP within the Magnet recognition process:
Turkel and colleagues (2005) described a model used by Northwest Community Hospital in Illinois to advance EBP as part of the hospital's pursuit of Magnet status. The five steps that were part of this process included establishing a foundation for EBP, identifying areas of concern, creating internal expertise, implementing EBP, and contributing to a study.

Several models of EBP, such as the Iowa Model, have distinguished two types of stimulus ("triggers") for an EBP endeavor—(1) *problem-focused triggers*—the identification of a clinical practice problem in need of solution, or (2) *knowledge-focused triggers*—readings in the research literature. Problem-focused triggers may arise in the normal course of clinical practice (as in the case of the clinical scenarios described earlier) or in the context of quality-assessment or quality-improvement efforts. This problem identification approach is likely to have staff support if the selected problem is one that numerous nurses have encountered, and is likely to be clinically relevant because a specific clinical situation generated interest in the problem in the first place.

Gennaro and colleagues (2001) advised nurses to begin by clarifying the practice problem that needs to be solved and framing it as a broad question. The goal can be finding the best way to anticipate a problem (how to *diagnose* it) or how best to solve it (how to *intervene*). Initial questions may well take the form of "What is the best way to . . . ?"—for example, "What is the best way to stabilize weight in patients with advanced cancer?" These initial questions would have to be transformed to more focused clinical questions capable of being answered through a search for (and appraisal of) evidence, as previously described.

A second catalyst for an EBP project is the research literature (i.e., knowledge-focused triggers). Sometimes this catalyst takes the form of a new clinical guideline, or the impetus could emerge from discussions in a journal club. With knowledge-focused triggers, an assessment might need to be made of the clinical relevance and applicability of the research. The central issue is whether a problem of significance to nurses in that particular setting will be solved by making a change or introducing an innovation. Titler and Everett (2001) offer suggestions for selecting interventions to test, using concepts from Rogers' Diffusion of Innovations Model.

With both types of triggers, there should be a general consensus about the importance of the problem and the need for improving practice. The first decision point in the Iowa Model (Figure 2.2) is determining whether the topic is a priority for the organization considering practice changes. Titler and colleagues (2001) advise considering the following issues before finalizing a topic for EBP: the topic's fit with the organization's strategic plan; the magnitude of the problem; the number of people invested in the problem; support of nurse leaders and of those in other disciplines; costs; and possible barriers to change.

TIP

In the early stages of an EBP effort, some practical matters should be resolved. A major issue concerns team organization. A motivated and motivational team leader is essential, and the recruitment of EBP team members often requires an interdisciplinary perspective. Identifying tasks to be undertaken, developing a realistic timetable and budget, assigning members to specific tasks, and scheduling meetings are necessary to ensure that the effort will progress.

Finding and Appraising Evidence: Clinical Practice Guidelines

Evidence-based **clinical practice guidelines** represent an effort to distill a body of evidence into a usable form. Unlike systematic reviews, clinical practice guidelines (which are often *based* on systematic reviews) give specific recommendations for evidence-based decision making. Guideline development typically involves the consensus of a group of researchers, experts and clinicians. We focus in this section on clinical practice guidelines because, for an organizational EBP effort, the best possible scenario involves identifying appropriate clinical practice guidelines that have been prepared based on rigorous research evidence. Of course, for many problem areas, clinical guidelines will need to be *developed* based on the evidence, and not just implemented or adapted for use.

Example of a nursing clinical practice guideline:

In 2007, the Registered Nurses Association of Ontario issued a best practice guideline (a revised version of one issued in 2004) on adult asthma care. Developed by an interdisciplinary panel under the leadership of Lisa Cicutto, the guideline's purpose is to provide nurses working in diverse settings with an evidence-based summary of strategies to promote asthma control in adults.

Finding Clinical Practice Guidelines

It can be challenging to find clinical practice guidelines because there is no single guideline repository. A standard search for such guidelines in bibliographic databases such as MEDLINE (see Chapter 7) will yield many references—but could produce a frustrating mixture of citations to not only the actual guidelines, but also to commentaries, implementation studies, and so on.

> **TIP**
>
> When using bibliographic databases, search terms such as the following can be used: practice guideline, clinical practice guideline, best practice guideline, evidence-based guideline, standards, and consensus statement.

Another recommended approach is to search for guidelines in guideline databases, or through specialty organizations that have sponsored guideline development. It would be impossible to list all possible sources, but a few deserve special mention. In the United States, nursing and other health care guidelines are maintained by the National Guideline Clearinghouse (www.guideline.gov). In Canada, the Registered Nurses Association of Ontario (RNAO) (www.rnao.org/bestpractices) maintains information about clinical practice guidelines. In the United Kingdom, two sources for clinical guidelines are the Translating Research Into Practice (TRIP) database and the National Institute for Clinical Excellence. Professional societies and organizations also maintain collections of guidelines of relevance to their area of specialization. For example, the Association of Women's Health, Obstetric and Neonatal Nursing (AWHONN) has developed a host of clinical practice guidelines.

Many topics exist for which practice guidelines have not yet been developed, but the opposite problem is also true; the dramatic increase in the number of guidelines means that there are sometimes multiple guidelines on the same topic from which clinicians must chose. Worse yet, because of variation in the rigor of guideline development and in the interpretation of evidence, different guidelines sometimes offer different or even conflicting recommendations (Lewis, 2001). Thus, those who wish to adopt clinical practice guidelines are urged to appraise them critically to identify ones that are based on the strongest evidence, have been meticulously developed, are user friendly, and are appropriate for local use or adaptation.

Appraising Clinical Practice Guidelines

Several appraisal instruments are available to facilitate the evaluation of clinical practice guidelines. The one that seems to have the broadest support is the Appraisal of Guidelines Research and Evaluation (AGREE) instrument (AGREE Collaboration, 2001). This tool has been translated into over a dozen languages and has been endorsed by the World Health Organization.

The AGREE instrument (www.agreecollaboration.org) consists of ratings of quality on a four-point scale (strongly agree, agree, disagree, and strongly disagree) for 23 quality dimensions organized in six domains: Scope and purpose; stakeholder involvement; rigor of development; clarity and presentation; application; and editorial independence. As examples, one dimension in the Scope and Purpose domain is "The patients to whom the guideline is meant to apply are specifically described"; and one in the Rigor of Development domain is "The guideline has been externally reviewed by experts prior to its publication." The AGREE instrument should be applied to the guideline under review by a team of two to four appraisers.

One final issue is that the guidelines change more slowly than the evidence. If a guideline is not recent, it is advisable to determine whether more up-to-date evidence would alter (or strengthen) the guideline's recommendations.

Actions Based on Evidence Appraisals

In the Iowa Model, the synthesis and appraisal of research evidence provides the basis for a second major decision. The crux of the decision concerns whether the research base is sufficient to justify an EBP change—for example, whether an existing clinical practice guideline is of sufficient high quality that it can be used or adapted locally, or whether the research evidence is sufficiently rigorous to recommend a practice innovation.

Coming to conclusions about the adequacy of the evidence can lead to different pathways for further action. If the research evidence is weak or inconclusive, the team could abandon the EBP project, or they could assemble nonresearch evidence (e.g., through consultation with experts, client surveys) to ascertain the desirability of a practice change. Another possibility is to pursue an original study to address the practice question, thereby gathering new evidence and contributing to practice knowledge. This last course of action may be impractical for many, and would clearly result in years of delay before any further conclusions could be drawn. If, on the other hand, there is a solid research base or a high-quality clinical practice guideline, then the team would develop plans for moving forward with implementing a practice innovation.

Assessing Implementation Potential

In some EBP models, the next step is the development and testing of the innovation, followed by an assessment of organizational "fit." Other models recommend steps to assess the appropriateness of innovation within the specific organizational context before implementing it. In some cases, such an assessment (or aspects of it) may be warranted even before embarking on efforts to assemble best evidence. A preliminary assessment of the **implementation potential** (or, *environmental readiness*) of a clinical innovation is often sensible, although there may be situations with little need for a formal assessment.

In determining the implementation potential of an innovation in a particular setting, several issues should be considered, particularly the transferability of the innovation, the feasibility of implementing it, and its cost-to-benefit ratio.

➤ *Transferability*. The transferability issue concerns whether it makes sense to implement the innovation in your practice setting. If some aspect of the setting is fundamentally incongruent with the innovation—in terms of its philosophy, types of client served, or administrative structure—then it might not be prudent to try to adopt the innovation, even if it is clinically effective in other contexts.

➤ *Feasibility*. Feasibility concerns such practicalities as the availability of staff and resources and the organizational climate. An important issue is whether nurses will have (or will share) control over the innovation. If nurses will not have full control, the interdependent nature of the project should be identified early so that the EBP team has interdisciplinary representatives.

➤ *Cost-to-benefit ratio*. A critical part of any decision to proceed with an EBP project is a careful assessment of the costs and benefits of the change. The assessment should encompass likely costs and benefits to clients, staff, and the overall organization. Clearly, if the degree of risk to clients is high, then the potential benefits must be great and the evidence must be very sound. The assessment should consider the costs and benefits of *not* instituting an innovation as well. It is sometimes easy to forget that the status quo bears its own risks and that failure to change—especially when such change is based on a firm evidence base—is costly to clients and to others.

If the implementation assessment suggests that there might be problems in testing the innovation in that particular practice setting, then the team can either identify a new problem and begin the process anew or consider adopting a plan to improve the implementation potential (e.g., seeking external resources if costs are prohibitive).

TIP

The Toolkit for this chapter, on the accompanying CD-ROM, has a list of some relevant assessment questions for assessing implementation potential.

Developing Evidence-Based Guidelines or Protocols

If the implementation criteria are met and the evidence base is adequate, the team can prepare an action plan for designing and piloting the new clinical practice. In most cases, a key activity will involve developing a local evidence-based clinical practice protocol or guideline, or adapting an existing one.

If an existing clinical practice guideline is of sufficient quality and relevance, the EBP team needs to decide whether to (1) adopt it in its entirety, (2) adopt only certain recommendations, while disregarding others (e.g., recommendations for which the evidence base is less sound), or (3) adapt the guidelines by making changes deemed necessary based on local circumstances.

If no clinical practice guideline exists (or if an existing guideline is weak), the team will need to develop its own protocol or guideline reflecting accumulated research evidence. Strategies for developing clinical practice guidelines are suggested in DiCenso et al. (2005) and Melnyk and Fineout-Overholt (2005). Whether a guideline is developed "from scratch" or adapted from an existing one, independent peer review is advisable, to ensure that the guidelines are clear, comprehensive, and congruent with best existing evidence.

Implementing and Evaluating the Innovation

Once the EBP product has been developed, the next step is to **pilot test** it (give it a trial run) in a clinical setting and to evaluate the outcome. Building on the Iowa Model, this phase of the project likely would involve the following activities:

1. Developing an evaluation plan (e.g., identifying outcomes to be achieved, determining how many clients to include, deciding when and how often to measure outcomes)

2. Measuring client outcomes before implementing the innovation, to establish a comparison against which the outcomes of the innovation can be assessed

3. Training relevant staff in the use of the new guideline and, if necessary, "marketing" the innovation to users so that it is given a fair test

4. Trying the guideline out on one or more units or with a group of clients

5. Evaluating the pilot project, in terms of both process (e.g., How was the innovation received? To what extent were the guidelines followed? What problems were encountered?) and outcomes (e.g., How were client outcomes affected? What were the costs?)

A variety of research strategies and designs can be used to evaluate the innovation, as described in our discussion of evaluation research in Chapter 11. A fairly informal evaluation usually will be adequate, for example, comparing outcome information before and after the innovation, and gathering information about patient and staff satisfaction. Qualitative information can also contribute considerably because a qualitative perspective can uncover subtleties about the implementation process and help to explain research findings.

> **TIP**
>
> Every nurse can play a role in using research evidence. Here are some strategies:
>
> ➤ *Read widely and critically.* Professionally accountable nurses keep up to date on important developments and read journals relating to their specialty, including research reports in them.
>
> ➤ *Attend professional conferences.* Many nursing conferences include presentations of studies that have clinical relevance. Conference attendees get opportunities to meet researchers and to explore practice implications.
>
> ➤ *Insist on evidence that a procedure is effective.* Every time nurses or nursing students are told about a standard nursing procedure, they have a right to ask the question: Why? Nurses need to develop expectations that the decisions they make in their clinical practice are based on sound evidence-based rationales.
>
> ➤ *Become involved in a journal club.* Many organizations that employ nurses sponsor journal clubs that discuss research articles that have potential relevance to practice. The traditional approach for a journal club (nurses coming together as a group to discuss and critique an article), in some settings, has been replaced with electronic online journal clubs that acknowledge time constraints and the inability of nurses from all shifts to come together at one time.
>
> ➤ *Pursue and participate in RU/EBP projects.* Several studies have found that nurses who are involved in research-related activities (e.g., a utilization project or data collection activities) develop more positive attitudes toward research and better research skills.

⊙ RESEARCH EXAMPLES AND CRITICAL THINKING ACTIVITIES

EXAMPLE 1 ■ Research Translation Project

Hundreds of projects to translate research evidence into nursing practice are underway worldwide, and many that have been described in the nursing literature offer good information about planning and implementing such an endeavor. In this section, we summarize such a project. The article appears in its entirely in the accompanying *Study Guide*.

Study

Translating best practices in nondrug postoperative pain management (Tracy et al., 2006).

Background

A team of researchers and clinicians observed that nondrug methods of relieving pain, many of which have been empirically validated as being beneficial, are underused as standard postoperative pain management practices in most hospitals. They cited evidence that nursing knowledge about pain and pain relief is typically inadequate.

Purpose

The purpose of the project was to use an RU model—the Collaborative Research Utilization (CRU) Model—to translate research into practice in a hospital in Rhode Island, using nondrug pain management protocols for postoperative pain of older adults as the example.

Model

The CRU Model is a six-step model adapted from the CURN project, underpinned by Rogers' (1995) Diffusion of Innovation Theory. The model involves student and staff nurses in each step. The use of nursing students to evaluate the strength of research evidence and assist in generating best-practice protocols is unique to this model.

Method

The first step in the model was to identify a clinical problem and assess the evidence base. Using both qualitative and quantitative approaches, the team ascertained the desirability of addressing the underuse of nondrug treatments for pain management in the study hospital. Interventions (massage, music, and self-guided imagery) were selected based on an AHRQ evidence summary, and undergraduate nursing students performed a literature search on these therapies. Step 2 involved evaluating the relevance of the research vis-à-vis the problem, agency values, and potential costs and benefits. Roundtable discussions, held on surgical and rehabilitative care units, resulted in the generation of 22 specific recommendations. In Step 3, the recommendations were transformed into three best-practice protocols for a tailored teaching intervention by a team of clinicians and researchers. A 12-member nursing Comfort Therapy Service was formed and trained in the use of the protocols. Step 4 involved the implementation and evaluation of the protocols for feasibility, usefulness, and effectiveness. This step included both a pilot study, which was the focus of the 2006 report, and a larger study that was still in progress when the paper was published. The pilot study examined, for 46 surgical patients, changes in knowledge of, attitudes toward, and use of the three interventions, from preadmission to the third postoperative day. In Step 5 of the model, the team presented pilot results to nursing staff and administration for decisional consideration. The final step is dissemination of the project results.

Findings

The team found that, in the pilot study, there were gains in patients' knowledge, attitudes, and use of the three nondrug interventions for pain management. At the time the paper was written, more than 300 patients had used the comfort therapy services. Nurses reported that implementing the protocols did not interfere with their other responsibilities, and that the time required to implement them was about 15 minutes.

Conclusions

Although administrators had not yet made a decision about the ongoing use of the protocols, hospital volunteers at the study site agreed to help in ensuring that nurses and patients have the supplies needed to carry out the comfort protocols. The team concluded that preliminary results were encouraging, but noted the desirability of conducting further studies with the intervention in sites with a more heterogeneous group of patients.

CRITICAL THINKING SUGGESTIONS*:

*See the Student Resource CD-ROM for a discussion of these questions. 💿

1. Of the EBP-focused purposes described in Chapter 1, which purpose did this project address?

2. How does the CRU Model used in this project compare with the Iowa Model (Figure 2.1)?

3. Would you say that this project had a knowledge-focused or problem-focused trigger?

EXAMPLE 2 ■ Quantitative Research in Appendix A

1. Read the abstract and the introduction from Howell and colleagues' (2007) study ("Anxiety, anger, and blood pressure in children") in Appendix A of this book. Identify one or more clinical foreground question that, if posed, would be addressed by this study. Which PICOT components does your question capture?
2. How, if at all, might evidence from this study be used in an EBP project (individual or organizational)?

EXAMPLE 3 ■ Qualitative Research in Appendix B

1. Read the abstract and the introduction from Beck's (2006) study ("Anniversary of birth trauma") in Appendix B of this book. Identify one or more clinical foreground questions that, if posed, would be addressed by this study. Which PICOT components does your question capture?
2. How, if at all, might evidence from this study be used in an EBP project (individual or organizational)?

CHAPTER REVIEW

Key new terms introduced in the chapter, together with a summary of major points, are presented in this section. Chapter 2 of the accompanying *Study Guide for Essentials of Nursing Research,* 7th edition also offers exercises and study suggestions for reinforcing the concepts presented in this chapter. For additional review, see self-study questions on the CD-ROM provided with this book.

Key New Terms

Background question
Clinical practice
  guideline
Cochrane Collaboration
Critically appraised topic
  (CAT)

Diffusion of Innovations
  Theory
Evidence hierarchy
Evidence-based practice
Foreground question
Implementation potential

Iowa Model
Meta-analysis
Metasynthesis
Pilot test
Stetler Model
Systematic review

Summary Points

➤ **Evidence-based practice (EBP)** is the conscientious use of current best evidence in making clinical decisions about patient care; it is a clinical problem-solving strategy that de-emphasizes decision making based on custom and emphasizes the integration of research evidence with clinical expertise and patient preferences.

❧ **Research utilization (RU)** and EBP are overlapping concepts that concern efforts to use research as a basis for clinical decisions, but RU *starts* with a research-based innovation that gets evaluated for possible use in practice.

❧ Research utilization exists on a continuum, with direct utilization of some specific innovation at one end and, at the other end, more diffuse use in which people are influenced in their thinking about an issue based on research findings.

❧ Nurse researchers have undertaken several major utilization projects (e.g., the **Conduct and Utilization of Research in Nursing** or **CURN project**), which demonstrated that RU can be increased but also shed light on barriers to utilization.

❧ Two underpinnings of the EBP movement are the **Cochrane Collaboration** (which is based on the work of British epidemiologist Archie Cochrane), and the clinical learning strategy called *evidence-based medicine* developed at the McMaster Medical School.

❧ EBP typically involves weighing various types of evidence in an effort to determine *best evidence*; often an **evidence hierarchy** is used to rank study findings and other information according to the strength of evidence provided. Hierarchies for evaluating evidence about health care interventions typically put systematic reviews of *randomized clinical trials* (RCTs) at the pinnacle and expert opinion at the base.

❧ Researchers have found that EBP/RU efforts often face a variety of barriers, including the quality of the evidence, nurses' characteristics (limited training in research and EBP) and organizational factors (e.g., lack of organizational support).

❧ Resources to support EBP are growing at a phenomenal pace. Among the resources are systematic reviews (and electronic databases that make them easy to locate); evidence-based clinical practice guidelines and other decision support tools; a wealth of other *preappraised evidence* that makes it possible to practice EBP efficiently; and models of RU and EBP that provide a framework for undertaking EBP efforts.

❧ **Systematic reviews**, a cornerstone of EBP, are rigorous integrations of research evidence from multiple studies on a topic. Systematic reviews can involve either qualitative, narrative approaches to integration (including **metasynthesis** of qualitative studies), or quantitative methods **(meta-analysis)** that integrate findings statistically.

❧ Many models of RU and EBP have been developed, including models that provide a framework for individual clinicians (e.g., the **Stetler Model**) and others for organizations or teams of clinicians (e.g., the **Iowa Model** of Evidence-Based Practice to Promote Quality Care). Another widely used model in RU/EBP efforts is Rogers' **Diffusion of Innovations Theory**.

❧ Individual nurses have regular opportunity to put research into practice. The five basic steps for individual EBP are (1) framing an answerable clinical question; (2) searching for relevant research-based evidence; (3) appraising and synthesizing the evidence; (4) integrating evidence with other factors; and (5) assessing effectiveness.

❧ One scheme for asking well-worded clinical questions involves five components, an acronym for which is PICOT: population (P), intervention or issue (I), comparison of interest (C), outcome (O), and time (T).

➤ An appraisal of the evidence involves such considerations as the validity of study findings; their clinical importance; the precision of estimates of effects; associated costs and risks; and utility in a particular clinical situation.

➤ EBP in an organizational context involves many of the same steps as an individual EBP effort, but tends to be more formalized and must take organizational and interpersonal factors into account. *Triggers* for an organizational project include both pressing clinical problems and existing knowledge.

➤ Team-based or organizational EBP projects typically involve the implementation, development, or adaptation of clinical practice guidelines or clinical protocols. Evidence-based **clinical practice guidelines** combine a synthesis and appraisal of research evidence with specific recommendations for clinical decision making. Clinical practice guidelines should be carefully and systematically appraised, for example using the Appraisal of Guidelines Research and Evaluation (AGREE) instrument.

➤ Before an EBP-based guideline or protocol can be tested, there should be an assessment of the **implementation potential** of the innovation, which includes the dimensions of transferability of findings, feasibility of using the findings in the new setting, and the cost-to-benefit ratio of a new practice.

➤ Once an evidence-based protocol or guideline has been developed and deemed worthy of implementation, the team can move forward with a **pilot test** of the innovation and an assessment of the outcomes before widespread adoption.

STUDIES CITED IN CHAPTER 2

Berenstein, E. G., & Ortiz, Z. (2005). Megestrol acetate for the treatment of anorexia-cachexia syndrome. *Cochrane Database of Systematic Reviews*, No. CD004310.

Coyle, L. A., & Sokop, A. G. (1990). Innovation adoption behavior among nurses. *Nursing Research, 39*, 176–180.

Downe, S., Simpson, L., & Trafford, K. (2007). Expert intrapartum maternity care: A meta-synthesis. *Journal of Advanced Nursing, 57*, 127–140.

Estabrooks, C. A. (1999). The conceptual structure of research utilization. *Research in Nursing & Health, 22*, 203–216.

Hsieh, H. F., & Lee, F. P. (2005). Graduated compression stockings as prophylaxis for flight-related venous thrombosis: Systematic literature review. *Journal of Advanced Nursing, 51*, 83–98.

Jatoi, A. (2005). Fish oil, lean tissue, and cancer: Is there a role for eicosapentaenoic acid in treating the cancer/anorexia/weight loss syndrome? *Critical Review of Oncology & Hematology, 55*, 37–43.

Ketefian, S. (1975). Application of selected nursing research findings into nursing practice. *Nursing Research, 24*, 89–92.

Pepler, C. J., Edgar, L., Frisch, S., Rennick, J., Swidzinski, M., White, C. et al. (2005). Unit culture and research-based nursing practice in acute care. *Canadian Journal of Nursing Research, 37*, 66–85.

Rawson, K., & Newburn-Cook, C. (2007). The use of low-dose warfarin as prophylaxis for central venous catheter thrombosis in patients with cancer: A meta-analysis. *Oncology Nursing Forum, 34*, 1037–1043.

Rutledge, D. N., Greene, P., Mooney, K., Nail, L. M., & Ropka, M. (1996). Use of research-based practices by oncology staff nurses. *Oncology Nursing Forum, 23*, 1235–1244.

Tracy, S., Dufault, M., Kogut, S., Martin, V., Rossi, S., & Willey-Temkin, C. (2006). Translating best practices in nondrug postoperative pain management. *Nursing Research, 55*, S57–S67.

3 Key Concepts and Steps in Qualitative and Quantitative Research

STUDENT OBJECTIVES

On completing this chapter, you will be able to:

➤ Distinguish terms associated with quantitative and qualitative research

➤ Distinguish experimental and nonexperimental research

➤ Identify the three main disciplinary traditions for qualitative nursing research

➤ Describe the flow and sequence of activities in quantitative and qualitative research, and discuss why they differ

➤ Define new terms presented in the chapter

THE BUILDING BLOCKS OF RESEARCH

Research, as with any discipline, has its own language—its own *jargon*. Some terms are used by both qualitative and quantitative researchers, but others are used mainly by one or the other group. To make matters even more complex, most research jargon used in nursing research has its roots in the social sciences, but sometimes different terms for the same concepts are used in medical research; we cover both but acknowledge that social scientific jargon predominates.

The Faces and Places of Research

When researchers address a problem or answer a question through disciplined research—regardless of the underlying paradigm—they are doing a **study** (or an *investigation* or *research project*).

HOW-TO-TELL TIP

How can you tell if an article appearing in a nursing journal is a *study*? In journals that specialize in research (e.g., the journal *Nursing Research*), most articles are original research reports, but in specialty journals there is usually a mix of research and nonresearch articles. Sometimes you can tell by the title, but sometimes you cannot. For example, Fontenot (2007) wrote an article entitled "Transition and adaptation to adoptive motherhood" in *Journal of Obstetric, Gynecologic, & Neonatal Nursing*. This article discusses research findings, but it is not a study. Look at the major headings of an article, and if there is no heading called "Method" or "Research Design" (the section that describes what a researcher *did*) and no heading called "Findings" or "Results" (the section that describes what a researcher *learned*), then it is probably not a study.

Studies with humans involve two sets of people: those who do the research and those who provide the information. In a quantitative study, the people being studied are called **subjects** or **study participants**, as shown in Table 3.1. (People who provide information by answering questions—e.g., by filling out a questionnaire—may be called **respondents**.) In a qualitative study, the individuals cooperating in the study play an active rather than a passive role, and are therefore referred to as **informants** or study participants. The person who conducts the research is the *researcher* or *investigator*. Studies are often undertaken by a research team rather than by a single researcher.

Research can be undertaken in a variety of *settings* (the specific places where information is gathered) and in one or more sites. Some studies take place in **naturalistic settings**—in the field; at the other extreme, some studies are done in highly controlled laboratory settings. Qualitative researchers are especially likely to engage in **fieldwork** in natural settings because they are interested in the contexts of people's lives and experiences. A *site* is the overall location for the research—it could be an entire community (e.g., a Haitian neighborhood in Miami) or an institution within a community (e.g., a clinic in Seattle). Researchers sometimes engage

TABLE 3.1 ⓘ KEY TERMS USED IN QUANTITATIVE AND QUALITATIVE RESEARCH		
CONCEPT	QUANTITATIVE TERM	QUALITATIVE TERM
Person Contributing Information	Subject Study participant Respondent	— Study participant Informant, key informant
Person Undertaking the Study	Researcher Investigator Scientist	Researcher Investigator —
That Which Is Being Investigated	— Concepts Constructs Variables	Phenomena Concepts — —
System of Organizing Concepts	Theory, theoretical framework Conceptual framework, conceptual model	Theory Conceptual framework, sensitizing framework
Information Gathered	Data (numeric values)	Data (narrative descriptions)
Connections Between Concepts	Relationships (cause-and-effect, functional)	Patterns of association
Logical Reasoning Processes	Deductive reasoning	Inductive reasoning

in **multisite studies** because the use of multiple sites usually offers a larger or more diverse sample of study participants.

Example of a multisite collaborative study:

Champion and an interdisciplinary team of nurses and physicians (2007) tested an intervention to increase mammography adherence. Study participants included 1,244 women from two sites: a general medicine clinic and a Health Maintenance Organization (HMO).

Phenomena, Concepts, and Constructs

Research involves abstractions. For example, the terms *pain*, *spirituality*, and *resilience* are all abstractions of particular aspects of human behavior and characteristics. These abstractions are called **concepts** or, in qualitative studies, **phenomena**.

Researchers may also use the term **construct**. As with a concept, a construct refers to an abstraction or mental representation inferred from situations or behaviors. Kerlinger and Lee (2000) distinguish concepts from constructs by noting that constructs are abstractions that are deliberately and systematically invented (or constructed) by researchers for a specific purpose. For example, *self-care* in Orem's model of health maintenance is a construct. The terms *construct* and *concept* are sometimes used interchangeably, although by convention, a construct often refers to a slightly more complex abstraction than a concept.

Theories and Conceptual Models

A **theory** is a systematic, abstract explanation of some aspect of reality. In a theory, concepts are knitted together into a coherent system to describe or explain some aspect of the world. Theories play a role in both qualitative and quantitative research.

In a quantitative study, researchers often start with a theory or a **conceptual model** (the distinction is discussed in Chapter 8) and, using deductive reasoning, make predictions about how phenomena would behave in the real world *if the theory were true*. The specific predictions are then tested through research, and the results are used to support, reject, or modify the theory.

In qualitative research, theories may be used in various ways. Sometimes conceptual or *sensitizing frameworks*—derived from various qualitative research traditions that we describe later in this chapter—offer an orienting world view with clear conceptual underpinnings. In other qualitative studies, theory is the *product* of the research: The investigators use information from study participants inductively to develop a theory firmly rooted in the participants' experiences. The goal is to develop a theory that explains phenomena *as they exist*, not as they are preconceived. Theories generated in qualitative studies are sometimes subjected to controlled testing in quantitative studies.

Variables

In quantitative studies, concepts are usually called **variables**. A variable, as the name implies, is something that varies. Weight, anxiety, and body temperature are all variables—each varies from one person to another. In fact, nearly all aspects of human beings are variables. If everyone weighed 150 pounds, weight would not be a variable; it would be a **constant**. But it is precisely because people and conditions *do* vary that most research is conducted. Most quantitative researchers seek to understand how or why things vary, and to learn how differences in one variable are related to differences in another. For example, lung cancer research is concerned with the variable of lung cancer, which is a variable because not everybody has this disease. Researchers have studied factors that might be linked to lung cancer, such as cigarette smoking. Smoking is also a variable because not everyone smokes. A variable, then, is any quality of a person, group, or situation that varies or takes on different values—typically, numeric values. Variables are the central building blocks of quantitative studies.

Variables are often inherent characteristics of people, such as their age, blood type, or weight. Sometimes, however, researchers *create* a variable. For example, if a researcher tests the effectiveness of patient-controlled analgesia compared with intramuscular analgesia in relieving pain after surgery, some patients would be given one type of analgesia and others would receive the other. In the context of this study, method of pain management is a variable because different patients are given different analgesic methods.

Some variables take on a wide range of values that can be represented on a continuum (e.g., a person's age or weight). Other variables take on only a few values; sometimes such variables convey quantitative information (e.g., number of children) but others simply involve placing people into categories (e.g., male, female, or blood type A, B, AB, or O).

TIP

Every study focuses on one or more phenomena, concepts, or variables, but these terms per se are not necessarily used in research reports. For example, a report might say: "The purpose of this study is to examine the effect of primary nursing on patient satisfaction." Although the researcher has not explicitly labeled anything a concept, the concepts (variables) under study are type of nursing and patient satisfaction. Key concepts or variables are often indicated right in the study title.

Dependent and Independent Variables

As noted in Chapter 1, many studies are aimed at understanding causes of phenomena. Does a nursing intervention *cause* improvements in patient outcomes? Does smoking *cause* lung cancer? The presumed cause is the **independent variable**, and the presumed effect is the **dependent variable**.

Variation in the dependent variable (sometimes called the **outcome variable**) is presumed to *depend on* variation in the independent variable. For example, researchers investigate the extent to which lung cancer (the dependent variable) depends on smoking (the independent variable). Or, investigators might examine the extent to which patients' pain (the dependent variable) depends on different nursing actions (the independent variable). The dependent variable is the variable researchers want to understand, explain, or predict, and corresponds to the *outcome* from the PICOT scheme described in Chapter 2. The independent variable corresponds to the *intervention* or *exposure* within evidence-based practice (EBP)-focused questions.

Frequently, the terms *independent variable* and *dependent variable* are used to indicate *direction of influence* rather than cause and effect. For example, suppose a researcher studied the mental health of caregivers caring for spouses with Alzheimer's disease and found better mental health outcomes for wives than for husbands. The researcher might be unwilling to conclude that caregivers' mental health was *caused* by gender. Yet, the direction of influence clearly runs from gender to mental health: it makes *no* sense to suggest that caregivers' mental health influenced their gender! Although in this example the researcher does not infer a cause-and-effect connection, it is appropriate to conceptualize mental health as the dependent variable and gender as the independent variable.

TIP

Few research reports explicitly label variables as dependent and independent, despite the importance of this distinction. Moreover, variables (especially independent variables) are sometimes not fully spelled out. Take the following research question: What is the effect of exercise on heart rate? In this example, heart rate is the dependent variable. Exercise, however, is not in itself a variable. Rather, exercise versus something else (e.g., no exercise) is a variable; "something else" is implied rather than stated in the research question. Note that, if exercise were not compared with something else, such as no exercise or different amounts of exercise, then exercise would not be a variable.

Many dependent variables studied by nurse researchers have multiple causes or antecedents. If we were studying factors that influence people's weight, for example, we might consider height, physical activity, and diet as independent variables. Two or more *dependent* variables (outcomes) also may be of interest to researchers. For example, a researcher may compare the effectiveness of two methods of nursing care for children with cystic fibrosis. Several dependent variables could be used to assess treatment effectiveness, such as length of hospital stay, recurrence of respiratory infections, presence of cough, and so forth. It is common to design studies with multiple independent and dependent variables.

Variables are not *inherently* dependent or independent. A dependent variable in one study could be an independent variable in another. For example, a study might examine the effect of a nurse-initiated exercise intervention (the independent variable) on osteoporosis (the dependent variable). Another study might investigate the effect of osteoporosis (the independent variable) on bone fracture incidence (the dependent variable). In short, whether a variable is independent or dependent is a function of the role that it plays in a particular study.

Example of independent and dependent variables:
Research question: What is the effect of elk velvet antler on joint pain and swelling in persons with rheumatoid arthritis following standard treatment? (Allen, Oberle, Grace, Russell, & Aderwale, 2008)
Independent variable: Receipt or nonreceipt of elk velvet antler
Dependent variables: Joint pain and swelling

Conceptual and Operational Definitions

Concepts in a study need to be defined and explicated, and dictionary definitions are almost never adequate. Two types of definition are relevant in a study— conceptual and operational.

The concepts in which researchers are interested are abstractions of observable phenomena, and researchers' world view shapes how those concepts are defined. A **conceptual definition** presents the abstract or theoretic meaning of the concepts being studied. Even seemingly straightforward terms need to be conceptually defined by researchers. The classic example of this is the concept of *caring*. Morse and colleagues (1990) scrutinized the works of numerous nurse researchers and theorists to determine how *caring* was defined, and identified five different categories of conceptual definitions: as a human trait, a moral imperative, an affect, an interpersonal relationship, and a therapeutic intervention. Researchers undertaking studies of caring need to clarify which conceptual definition they have adopted. In qualitative studies, conceptual definitions of key phenomena may be the major end product, reflecting an intent to have the meaning of concepts defined by those being studied.

In quantitative studies, however, researchers must define concepts at the outset, because they must decide how the variables will be observed and measured. An **operational definition** of a concept specifies the operations that researchers must perform to collect the required information. Operational definitions should be congruent with conceptual definitions.

Variables differ in the ease with which they can be operationalized. The variable weight, for example, is easy to define and measure. We might operationally define weight as follows: the amount that an object weighs in pounds, to the nearest full pound. Note that this definition designates that weight will be measured using one measuring system (pounds) rather than another (grams). We could also specify that subjects' weight will be measured to the nearest pound using a spring scale with subjects fully undressed after 10 hours of fasting. This operational definition clearly indicates what we mean by the variable *weight*.

Unfortunately, few variables are operationalized as easily as weight. There are multiple methods of measuring most variables, and researchers must choose the one that best captures the variables as they conceptualize them. For example, *anxiety* is a concept that can be defined in terms of both physiologic and psychological functioning. For researchers choosing to emphasize physiologic aspects of anxiety, the operational definition might involve a measure such as the Palmar Sweat Index. If, on the other hand, researchers conceptualize anxiety as primarily a psychological state, the operational definition might involve a paper-and-pencil measure such as the State Anxiety Scale. Readers of research reports may not agree with how investigators conceptualized and operationalized variables, but definitional precision has the advantage of communicating exactly what terms mean within the context of the study.

Example of conceptual and operational definitions:

Schim, Doorenbos, and Borse (2006) tested an intervention designed to expand cultural competence among hospice workers. Cultural competence was composed of several aspects, such as *cultural awareness,* which was conceptually defined as a care provider's knowledge about areas of cultural expression in which cultural groups may differ. The researchers measured their constructs with an instrument they developed, called Cultural Competence Assessment (CCA). Operationally, the CCA captures cultural awareness by having health care staff indicate their level of agreement with such statements as, "I understand that people from different cultural groups may define the concept of 'health care' in different ways."

Data

Research **data** (singular, datum) are the pieces of information obtained in a study. All the pieces of data that researchers gather in a study comprise their **data set.**

BOX 3.1   EXAMPLE OF QUANTITATIVE DATA

Question: Thinking about the past week, how depressed would you say you have been on a scale from 0 to 10, where 0 means "not at all" and 10 means "the most possible?"

Data: 9   (Subject 1)

0   (Subject 2)

4   (Subject 3)

In quantitative studies, researchers identify the variables of interest, develop conceptual and operational definitions of those variables, and then collect relevant data from subjects. The actual *values* of the study variables constitute the data. Quantitative researchers collect primarily **quantitative data**—information in numeric form. For example, suppose we conducted a quantitative study in which a key variable was *depression*. In such a study, we would need to measure how depressed participants were. We might ask, "Thinking about the past week, how depressed would you say you have been on a scale from 0 to 10, where 0 means 'not at all' and 10 means 'the most possible'?" Box 3.1 presents quantitative data for three fictitious respondents. The subjects provided a number along the 0 to 10 continuum corresponding to their degree of depression—*9* for subject 1 (a high level of depression), *0* for subject 2 (no depression), and *4* for subject 3 (little depression). The numeric values for all subjects, collectively, would comprise the data on depression.

In qualitative studies, researchers collect primarily **qualitative data**, that is, narrative descriptions. Narrative data can be obtained by having conversations with participants, by making notes about how participants behave in naturalistic settings, or by obtaining narrative records, such as diaries. Suppose we were studying depression qualitatively. Box 3.2 presents qualitative data for three participants responding

---

BOX 3.2   EXAMPLE OF QUALITATIVE DATA

Question: Tell me about how you've been feeling lately—have you felt sad or depressed at all, or have you generally been in good spirits?

Data: ➤ "Well, actually, I've been pretty depressed lately, to tell you the truth. I wake up each morning and I can't seem to think of anything to look forward to. I mope around the house all day, kind of in despair. I just can't seem to shake the blues, and I've begun to think I need to go see a shrink." (Participant 1)

➤ "I can't remember ever feeling better in my life. I just got promoted to a new job that makes me feel like I can really get ahead in my company. And I've just gotten engaged to a really great guy who is very special." (Participant 2)

➤ "I've had a few ups and downs the past week, but basically things are on a pretty even keel. I don't have too many complaints." (Participant 3)

conversationally to the question, "Tell me about how you've been feeling lately—have you felt sad or depressed at all, or have you generally been in good spirits?" Here, the data consist of rich narrative descriptions of participants' emotional state.

Relationships

Researchers usually study phenomena in relation to other phenomena—they examine relationships. A **relationship** is a bond or connection between two or more phenomena; for example, researchers repeatedly have found that there is a *relationship* between cigarette smoking and lung cancer. Both qualitative and quantitative studies examine relationships, but in different ways.

In quantitative studies, researchers are primarily interested in the relationship between independent variables and dependent variables. Variation in the dependent variable is presumed to be systematically related to variation in the independent variable. Relationships are often explicitly expressed in quantitative terms, such as *more than*, *less than*, and so on. For example, let us consider as our dependent variable a person's weight. What variables are related to (associated with) a person's weight? Some possibilities include height, caloric intake, and exercise. For each of these independent variables, we can make a prediction about its relationship to the dependent variable:

Height: Taller people will weigh more than shorter people.

Caloric intake: People with higher caloric intake will be heavier than those with lower caloric intake.

Exercise: The lower the amount of exercise, the greater will be the person's weight.

Each statement expresses a predicted relationship between weight (the dependent variable) and a measurable independent variable. Most quantitative research is conducted to determine whether relationships do or do not exist among variables, and often to quantify how strong the relationship is.

TIP

Relationships are expressed in two basic forms. First, relationships can be expressed as "if more of Variable X, then more of (or less of) Variable Y." For example, there is a relationship between height and weight: With more height, there tends to be more weight (i.e., taller people tend to weigh more than shorter people). The second form is sometimes confusing to students because there is no explicit relational statement. The second form involves relationships expressed as group differences. For example, there is a relationship between gender and height: Men tend to be taller than women.

Variables can be related to one another in different ways. One type of relationship is a **cause-and-effect (causal) relationship.** Within the positivist paradigm, natural phenomena are assumed not to be haphazard; they have antecedent causes that are presumably discoverable. In our example about a person's weight, we might speculate that there is a causal relationship between caloric intake and weight: all else being equal, eating more calories causes weight gain. As noted in Chapter 1, many quantitative studies are *cause-probing*—they seek to illuminate the causes of phenomena.

Example of a study of causal relationships:
Lengacher and colleagues (2008) studied whether the use of relaxation and guided imagery caused lower stress and better immune function in patients undergoing treatment for breast cancer.

Not all relationships between variables can be interpreted as cause-and-effect relationships. There is a relationship, for example, between a person's pulmonary artery and tympanic temperatures: People with high readings on one tend to have high readings on the other. We cannot say, however, that pulmonary artery temperature *caused* tympanic temperature, nor that tympanic temperature *caused* pulmonary artery temperature, despite the relationship that exists between the two variables. This type of relationship is sometimes referred to as a *functional* (or *associative*) *relationship* rather than a causal one.

Example of a study of functional relationships:
Liu and colleagues (2008) examined the relationship between health-related quality of life on one hand, and gender and age on the other, among adult kidney transplant recipients.

Qualitative researchers are not concerned with quantifying relationships, nor in testing and confirming causal relationships. Rather, qualitative researchers may seek patterns of association as a way of illuminating the underlying meaning and dimensionality of phenomena of interest. Patterns of interconnected themes and processes are identified as a means of understanding the whole.

Example of a qualitative study of patterns:
Clark and Redman (2007) studied the expectations for children's health services among mothers of Mexican descent living in the United States. Differences and similarities in expectations and health care access among mothers of varying acculturation levels and lengths of time in the country were observed.

MAJOR CLASSES OF QUANTITATIVE AND QUALITATIVE RESEARCH

Researchers usually work within a paradigm that is consistent with their world view, and that gives rise to the types of question that excite their curiosity. In this section, we briefly describe broad categories of quantitative and qualitative research.

Quantitative Research: Experimental and Nonexperimental Studies

A basic distinction in quantitative studies is the difference between experimental and nonexperimental research. In **experimental research**, researchers actively introduce an intervention or treatment. In **nonexperimental research**, on the other hand, researchers are bystanders—they collect data without introducing treatments or making changes. For example, if a researcher gave bran flakes to one group of subjects and prune juice to another to evaluate which method facilitated elimination more effectively, the study would be experimental because the researcher intervened in the normal course of things. If, on the other hand, a researcher compared elimination patterns of two groups whose regular eating patterns differed—for example, some normally took foods that stimulated bowel elimination and others did not—there is no intervention. Such a study is nonexperimental. In medical and epidemiologic research, an experimental study usually is called a **controlled trial** or **clinical trial**, and a nonexperimental inquiry is called an **observational study.** (As we discuss in Chapter 11, a randomized controlled trial [RCT] is a particular type of clinical trial.)

Experimental studies are explicitly designed to test causal relationships—to test whether the intervention *caused* changes in the dependent variable. Sometimes nonexperimental studies also seek to elucidate causal relationships, but doing so is tricky and usually is less conclusive because experimental studies offer the possibility of greater control over confounding influences.

Example of experimental research:
Tseng and colleagues (2007) tested the effectiveness of a range-of-motion exercise intervention aimed at improving joint flexibility, activity function, and pain in stroke survivors. Some study participants received the intervention—a 4-week exercise program—whereas others did not.

In this example, the researchers intervened by designating that some patients would receive the special exercise intervention, and that others would not be given this opportunity. In other words, the researcher *controlled* the independent variable, which in this case was the exercise intervention.

Example of nonexperimental research:
Sweeney, Glaser, and Tedeschi (2007) studied the relationship between inner-city adolescents' physical activity and eating habits on the one hand and demographic characteristics of the adolescents (e.g., gender, ethnicity, household type) on the other.

In this nonexperimental study, the researchers did not intervene in any way. They were interested in exercise, as in the previous example, but their intent was to describe the status quo and explore existing relationships rather than to test a potential solution to a problem.

Qualitative Research: Disciplinary Traditions

Many qualitative studies are rooted in research traditions that originated in the disciplines of anthropology, sociology, and psychology. Three such traditions have had especially strong influences on qualitative nursing research and are briefly described here so that we can explain similarities and differences throughout the book. Chapter 10 provides a fuller discussion of qualitative research traditions and the methods associated with them.

The **grounded theory** tradition seeks to describe and understand the key social, psychological, and structural processes that occur in a social setting. Grounded theory was developed in the 1960s by two sociologists, Glaser and Strauss (1967). Most grounded theory studies focus on a developing social experience—the social and psychological stages and phases that characterize a particular event or episode. A major component of grounded theory is the discovery of a *core variable* that is central in explaining what is going on. Grounded theory researchers strive to generate comprehensive explanations of phenomena that are grounded in reality.

Example of a grounded theory study:
Lewis and colleagues (2007) studied the process of practicing spirituality in relation to health promotion and disease management among African Americans.

Phenomenology, rooted in a philosophic tradition developed by Husserl and Heidegger, is concerned with the lived experiences of humans. Phenomenology is an approach to thinking about what life experiences of people are like and what they mean. The phenomenological researcher asks the questions: What is the *essence* of this phenomenon as experienced by these people?, or, What is the meaning of the phenomenon to those who experience it?

Example of a phenomenological study:
Hinck (2007) studied the lived experience and meaning of *time* in the oldest old. The study involved in-depth interviews with 19 elders older than 85 years.

Ethnography, the primary research tradition within anthropology, provides a framework for studying the patterns, lifeways, and experiences of a defined cultural group in a holistic fashion. Ethnographers typically engage in extensive fieldwork, often participating to the extent possible in the life of the culture under study. The aim of ethnographers is to *learn from* (rather than to *study*) members of a cultural group to understand their world view as they perceive and live it.

Example of an ethnographic study:
Holmes, O'Byrne, and Gastaldo (2007) conducted ethnographic fieldwork in three gay bathhouses in two Canadian metropolitan areas to explore how sexual desire intersects with the bathhouse environment and with health imperatives.

MAJOR STEPS IN A QUANTITATIVE STUDY

In quantitative studies, researchers move from the beginning point of a study (the posing of a question) to the end point (the obtaining of an answer) in a reasonably linear sequence of steps that is broadly similar across studies (Figure 3.1). This section describes that flow, and the next section describes how qualitative studies differ.

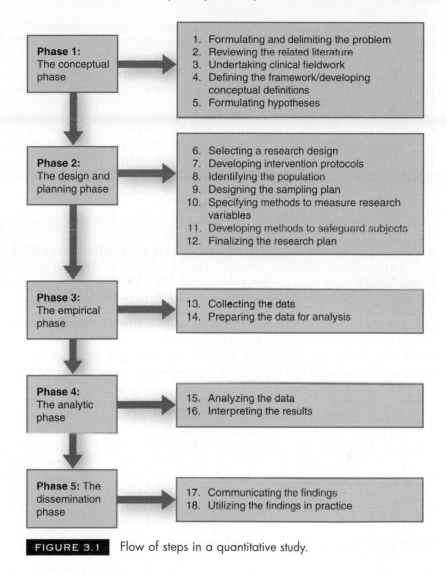

Phase 1:
The conceptual phase

1. Formulating and delimiting the problem
2. Reviewing the related literature
3. Undertaking clinical fieldwork
4. Defining the framework/developing conceptual definitions
5. Formulating hypotheses

Phase 2:
The design and planning phase

6. Selecting a research design
7. Developing intervention protocols
8. Identifying the population
9. Designing the sampling plan
10. Specifying methods to measure research variables
11. Developing methods to safeguard subjects
12. Finalizing the research plan

Phase 3:
The empirical phase

13. Collecting the data
14. Preparing the data for analysis

Phase 4:
The analytic phase

15. Analyzing the data
16. Interpreting the results

Phase 5: The dissemination phase

17. Communicating the findings
18. Utilizing the findings in practice

FIGURE 3.1   Flow of steps in a quantitative study.

Phase 1: The Conceptual Phase

The early steps in a quantitative research project typically involve activities with a strong conceptual or intellectual element. During this phase, researchers call on such skills as creativity, deductive reasoning, and a grounding in existing research evidence on the topic of interest.

Step 1: Formulating and Delimiting the Problem

Quantitative researchers begin by identifying an interesting, significant research problem and formulating good **research questions**. In developing research questions, nurse researchers must pay close attention to substantive issues (Is this research question important, given the evidence base?); theoretic issues (Is there a conceptual context for enhancing understanding of this problem?); clinical issues (Could study findings be useful in clinical practice?); methodologic issues (How can this question best be answered to yield high-quality evidence?); and ethical issues (Can this question be rigorously addressed in an ethical manner?).

Step 2: Reviewing the Related Literature

Quantitative research is typically conducted within the context of previous knowledge. Quantitative researchers typically strive to understand what is already known about a topic by undertaking a thorough **literature review** before any data are collected.

Step 3: Undertaking Clinical Fieldwork

Researchers embarking on a clinical study often benefit from spending time in appropriate clinical settings, discussing the topic with clinicians and health care administrators, and observing current practices. Such clinical fieldwork can provide perspectives on recent clinical trends, current diagnostic procedures, and relevant health care delivery models; it can also help researchers better understand clients' perspectives and the settings in which care is provided.

Step 4: Defining the Framework and Developing Conceptual Definitions

When quantitative research is performed within the context of a conceptual framework, the findings may have broader significance and utility. Even when the research question is not embedded in a theory, researchers must have a conceptual rationale and a clear vision of the concepts under study.

Step 5: Formulating Hypotheses

Hypotheses state researchers' expectations about relationships among study variables. Hypotheses are predictions of expected outcomes; they state the relationships researchers expect to observe in the study data. The research question identifies the concepts under investigation and asks how the concepts might be related; a hypothesis is the predicted answer. Most quantitative studies are designed to test hypotheses through statistical analysis.

Phase 2: The Design and Planning Phase

In the second major phase of a quantitative study, researchers make decisions about the study site and about the methods and procedures to be used to address the research question. Researchers typically have considerable flexibility in designing a study and make many methodologic decisions. These decisions have crucial implications for the integrity and generalizability of the study findings.

Step 6: Selecting a Research Design

The **research design** is the overall plan for obtaining answers to the questions being studied and for handling various challenges to the worth of the study evidence. In designing the study, researchers decide which specific design will be adopted and what they will do to minimize bias and enhance the interpretability of results. In quantitative studies, research designs tend to be highly structured and controlled. Research designs also indicate other aspects of the research—for example, how often data will be collected, what types of comparisons will be made, and where the study will take place. The research design is the architectural backbone of the study.

Step 7: Developing Protocols for the Intervention

In experimental research, researchers create the independent variable, which means that participants are exposed to different treatments or conditions. An **intervention protocol** for the study would need to be developed, specifying exactly what the intervention will entail (e.g., who would administer it, how frequently and over how long a period the treatment would last, and so on) *and* what the alternative condition would be. The goal of well-articulated protocols is to have all subjects in each group treated in the same way. In nonexperimental research, of course, this step is not necessary.

Step 8: Identifying the Population

Quantitative researchers need to know what characteristics the study participants should possess, and clarify the group to whom study results can be generalized— that is, they must identify the population to be studied. A **population** is *all* the individuals or objects with common, defining characteristics. For example, the population of interest might be all adult male patients undergoing chemotherapy in Dallas.

Step 9: Designing the Sampling Plan

Researchers typically collect data from a **sample**, which is a subset of the population. Using samples is clearly more practical and less costly than collecting data from an entire population, but the risk is that the sample might not adequately reflect the population's traits. In a quantitative study, a sample's adequacy is assessed by the criterion of *representativeness* (i.e., how typical or representative the sample is of the population). The **sampling plan** specifies in advance how the sample will be selected and how many subjects there will be.

Step 10: Specifying Methods to Measure Variables

Quantitative researchers must develop or borrow methods to measure the research variables as accurately as possible. Based on the conceptual definitions, researchers select or design methods to operationalize the variables and collect their data. A variety of quantitative data collection approaches exist; the primary methods are *self-reports* (e.g., interviews), *observations* (e.g., observing children's behavior), and *biophysiologic measurements*. The task of measuring research variables and developing a **data collection plan** is a complex and challenging process.

Step 11: Developing Methods to Safeguard Human/Animal Rights

Most nursing research involves human subjects, although some involve animals. In either case, procedures need to be developed to ensure that the study adheres to ethical principles. Each aspect of the study plan needs to be scrutinized to determine whether the rights of subjects have been adequately protected.

Step 12: Reviewing and Finalizing the Research Plan

Before actually collecting data, researchers often perform a number of "tests" to ensure that procedures will work smoothly. For example, they may evaluate the *readability* of written materials to determine if participants with low reading skills can comprehend them, or they may *pretest* their measuring instruments to assess their adequacy. Researchers usually have their research plan critiqued by reviewers to obtain substantive, clinical, or methodologic feedback before implementing the plan. Researchers seeking financial support submit a **proposal** to a funding source, and reviewers usually suggest improvements.

Phase 3: The Empirical Phase

The empirical portion of quantitative studies involves collecting research data and preparing the data for analysis. The empirical phase is often the most time-consuming part of the study. Data collection may require months of work.

Step 13: Collecting the Data

The actual collection of data in a quantitative study often proceeds according to a pre-established plan. The researcher's plan typically articulates procedures for training data collection staff, describing the study to participants, the actual collection of data (e.g., where and when the data will be gathered), and recording information.

Step 14: Preparing the Data for Analysis

Data collected in a quantitative study are rarely amenable to direct analysis. Preliminary steps are needed. One such step is **coding**, which is the process of translating verbal data into numeric form (e.g., coding gender information as "1" for females and "2" for males). Another preliminary step involves transferring the data from written documents onto computer files for analysis.

Phase 4: The Analytic Phase

Quantitative data gathered in the empirical phase are not reported as a mass of numbers. They are subjected to analysis and interpretation, which occurs in the fourth major phase of a project.

Step 15: Analyzing the Data

To answer research questions and test hypotheses, researchers need to analyze their data in an orderly, coherent fashion. Quantitative information is analyzed through **statistical analyses,** which include some simple procedures (e.g., computing an average) as well as complex and sophisticated methods.

Step 16: Interpreting the Results

Interpretation is the process of making sense of study results and of examining their implications. Researchers attempt to explain the findings in light of prior evidence, theory, and their own clinical experience—and in light of the adequacy of the methods they used in the study. Interpretation also involves determining how the findings can best be used in clinical practice, or what further research is needed before utilization can be recommended.

Phase 5: The Dissemination Phase

In the analytic phase, researchers come full circle: the questions posed at the outset are answered. The researchers' job is not completed, however, until the study results are disseminated.

Step 17: Communicating the Findings

A study cannot contribute evidence to nursing practice if the results are not communicated. Another—and often final—task of a research project, therefore, is the preparation of a **research report** that can be shared with others. We discuss research reports in the next chapter.

Step 18: Putting the Evidence into Practice

Ideally, the concluding step of a high-quality study is to plan for its use in practice settings. Although nurse researchers may not themselves be in a position to implement a plan for utilizing research findings, they can contribute to the process by developing recommendations regarding how the evidence could be incorporated into nursing practice, by ensuring that adequate information has been provided for a meta-analysis, and by vigorously pursuing opportunities to disseminate the findings to practicing nurses.

ACTIVITIES IN A QUALITATIVE STUDY

Quantitative research involves a fairly linear progression of tasks—researchers plan in advance the steps to be taken to maximize study integrity and then follow those steps as faithfully as possible. In qualitative studies, by contrast, the progression is closer to a circle than to a straight line. Qualitative researchers are continually examining and interpreting data and making decisions about how to proceed based on what has already been discovered (Figure 3.2).

Because qualitative researchers have a flexible approach to the collection and analysis of data, it is impossible to define the flow of activities precisely—the flow varies from one study to another, and researchers themselves do not know ahead of time exactly how the study will unfold. We try to provide a sense of how qualitative studies are conducted by describing some major activities and indicating how and when they might be performed.

Conceptualizing and Planning a Qualitative Study

Identifying the Research Problem

Qualitative researchers usually begin with a broad topic area, often focusing on an aspect of a topic that is poorly understood and about which little is known. They therefore may not pose refined research questions at the outset. Qualitative researchers often proceed with a fairly broad initial question that allows the focus to be sharpened and delineated more clearly once the study is underway.

Doing a Literature Review

Qualitative researchers do not all agree about the value of doing an upfront literature review. Some believe that researchers should not consult the literature before collecting data. Their concern is that prior studies might influence the conceptualization of the phenomena under study. According to this view, the phenomena should be elucidated based on participants' viewpoints rather than on prior information. Others believe that researchers should conduct at least a brief

Planning the study
- Identifying the research problem
- Doing a literature review
- Developing an overall approach
- Selecting and gaining entrée into research sites
- Developing methods to safeguard participants

Disseminating findings
- Communicating findings
- Utilizing (or making recommendations for utilizing) findings in practice and future research

Developing data collection strategies
- Deciding what type of data to gather and how to gather them
- Deciding from whom to collect the data
- Deciding how to enhance trustworthiness

Gathering and analyzing data
- Collecting data
- Organizing and analyzing data
- Evaluating data: making modifications to data collection strategies, if necessary
- Evaluating data: determining if saturation has been achieved

FIGURE 3.2   Flow of activities in a qualitative study.

literature review at the outset. In any case, qualitative researchers typically find a relatively small body of relevant previous work because of the type of questions they ask.

Selecting and Gaining Entrée into Research Sites

Before going into the field, qualitative researchers must identify a site that is consistent with the research topic. For example, if the topic is the health beliefs of the urban poor, an inner-city neighborhood with a concentration of low-income residents must be identified. In some cases, researchers may have access to the selected site, but in others they need to **gain entrée** into the site. Gaining entrée typically involves negotiations with **gatekeepers** who have the authority to permit entry into their world.

TIP

The process of gaining entrée is usually associated with doing fieldwork in qualitative studies, but quantitative researchers often need to gain entrée into sites for collecting data as well.

Developing an Overall Approach

Quantitative researchers do not collect data before finalizing the research design. Qualitative researchers, by contrast, use an **emergent design**—a design that emerges during the course of data collection. Certain design features are guided by the study's qualitative tradition, but qualitative studies rarely have rigidly structured designs that prohibit changes while in the field.

Addressing Ethical Issues

Qualitative researchers, like quantitative researchers, must also develop plans for addressing ethical issues—and, indeed, there are special concerns in qualitative studies because of the more intimate nature of the relationship that typically develops between researchers and study participants.

Conducting a Qualitative Study

In qualitative studies, the tasks of sampling, data collection, data analysis, and interpretation typically take place iteratively. Qualitative researchers begin by talking with or observing people who have first-hand experience with the phenomenon under study. The discussions and observations are loosely structured, allowing participants to express a full range of beliefs, feelings, and behaviors. Analysis and interpretation are ongoing, concurrent activities that guide choices about the kinds of people to question next and the types of question to ask or observations to make.

The actual process of data analysis involves clustering together related types of narrative information into a coherent scheme. As analysis and interpretation progress, researchers begin to identify **themes** and categories, which are used to build a rich description or theory of the phenomenon. The kinds of data obtained become increasingly focused and purposeful as the theory emerges. Concept development and verification shape the sampling process—as a conceptualization or theory develops, the researcher seeks participants who can confirm and enrich the theoretic understandings, as well as participants who can potentially challenge them and lead to further theoretic insight.

Quantitative researchers decide in advance how many subjects to include in the study, but qualitative researchers' sampling decisions are guided by the data themselves. Many qualitative researchers use the principle of **saturation**, which occurs when themes and categories in the data become repetitive and redundant, such that no new information can be gleaned by further data collection.

Quantitative researchers seek to collect high-quality data by using measuring instruments that have been demonstrated to be accurate and valid. Qualitative researchers, by contrast, *are* the main data collection instrument and must take steps to demonstrate the *trustworthiness* of the data while in the field. The central feature of these efforts is to confirm that the findings accurately reflect the experiences and viewpoints of participants, rather than researchers' perceptions. One confirmatory activity, for example, involves going back to participants and sharing preliminary interpretations with them so that they can evaluate whether the researcher's thematic analysis is consistent with their experiences.

Qualitative nursing researchers also strive to share their findings at conferences and in journal articles. Qualitative findings often are the basis for formulating

---

BOX 3.3   ADDITIONAL QUESTIONS FOR A PRELIMINARY REVIEW OF A STUDY

1. What is the study all about? What are the main phenomena, concepts, or constructs under investigation?
2. If the study is quantitative, what are the independent and dependent variables (if applicable)?
3. Did the researchers examine relationships or patterns of association among variables or concepts? Does the report imply the possibility of a causal relationship?
4. Are key concepts clearly defined, both conceptually and operationally?
5. What type of study does it appear to be, in terms of types described in this chapter—experimental or nonexperimental/observational? grounded theory? phenomenology? ethnography?
6. Does the report provide any information to suggest how long the study took to complete?

---

hypotheses that are tested by quantitative researchers, for developing measuring instruments for both research and clinical purposes, and for designing effective nursing interventions. Qualitative studies help to shape nurses' perceptions of a problem or situation, their conceptualizations of potential solutions, and their understanding of patients' concerns and experiences.

GENERAL QUESTIONS IN REVIEWING A STUDY

Most of the remaining chapters of this book contain guidelines to help you evaluate different aspects of a research report critically, focusing primarily on the methodologic decisions that the researcher made in conducting the study. Box 3.3 presents some further questions related to performing a preliminary overview of a research report, drawing on concepts explained in this chapter. These guidelines supplement those presented in Box 1.1, Chapter 1.

RESEARCH EXAMPLES AND CRITICAL THINKING ACTIVITIES

In this section, we illustrate the progression of activities and discuss the time schedule of two studies (one quantitative and the other qualitative) conducted by the second author of this book.

EXAMPLE 1 ■ Project Schedule for a Quantitative Study

Study

Further validation of the Postpartum Depression Screening Scale (Beck & Gable, 2001).

Study Purpose

Beck and Gable undertook a study to assess the Postpartum Depression Screening Scale (PDSS), an instrument designed for use by clinicians and researchers to screen mothers for postpartum depression.

Study Methods

This study required nearly 3 years to complete. Key activities and methodologic decisions included the following:

Phase 1. Conceptual Phase: 1 Month. This phase was the shortest, in large part because much of the conceptual work had been done in Beck and Gable's (2000) first study, in which they actually developed the screening scale. The literature had already been reviewed, so they only needed to update it. The same framework and conceptual definitions that had been used in the first study were used in the new study.

Phase 2. Design and Planning Phase: 6 Months. The second phase was time-consuming. It included not only fine-tuning the research design, but gaining entrée into the hospital from which subjects were recruited and obtaining approval from the hospital's human subjects review committee. During this period, Beck met with statistical consultants and with Gable, an instrument development specialist, numerous times to finalize the study design.

Phase 3. Empirical Phase: 11 Months. Data collection took almost a year to complete. The design called for administering the PDSS to 150 mothers who were 6 weeks postpartum, and then scheduling them for a psychiatric diagnostic interview to determine if they were suffering from postpartum depression. Women were recruited into the study during prepared childbirth classes. Recruitment began 4 months before data collection, and then the researchers had to wait until 6 weeks after delivery to gather data. The nurse psychotherapist, who had her own clinical practice, was able to come to the hospital only 1 day a week to conduct the diagnostic interviews; this contributed to the time required to achieve the desired sample size.

Phase 4. Analytic Phase: 3 Months. Statistical tests were performed to determine a cut off score on the PDSS above which mothers would be identified as having screened positive for postpartum depression. Data analysis also was undertaken to determine the accuracy of the PDSS in predicting diagnosed postpartum depression. During this phase, Beck met with Gable and with statisticians to interpret results.

Phase 5. Dissemination Phase: 18 Months. The researchers prepared and submitted their report to the journal *Nursing Research* for possible publication. It was accepted within 4 months, but it was "in press" (awaiting publication) for 14 months before being published. During this period, the authors presented their findings at regional and international conferences. The researchers also had to prepare a summary report for submission to the agency that funded the research.

CRITICAL THINKING SUGGESTIONS*:

*See the Student Resource CD-ROM for a discussion of these questions. 🔘

1. Answer the questions from Box 3-3 regarding this study.
2. Also consider the following targeted questions, which may further sharpen your critical thinking skills and assist you in understanding this study:
   a. What do you think is the *population* for this study?
   b. Would you describe the method of data collection as *self-report* or *observation*?
   c. How would you evaluate Beck and Gable's dissemintation plan?

  d. Do you think an appropriate amount of time was allocated to the various phases and steps in this study?

  e. Would it have been appropriate for the researchers to address the research question using qualitative research methods? Why or why not?

3. If the results of this study are valid and generalizable, what might be some of the uses to which the findings could be put in clinical practice?

EXAMPLE 2 ■ Project Schedule for a Qualitative Study

Study

Birth trauma: In the eye of the beholder (Beck, 2004).

Study Purpose

The purpose of this study was to understand the experience of birth trauma from the mothers' own perspectives.

Study Methods

The total time required to complete this study was nearly 3 years. Beck's key activities included the following:

Phase 1. Conceptual Phase: 3 Months. Beck, who is renowned for her program of research on postpartum depression, became interested in birth trauma when she was invited to deliver the keynote address at the September 2001 Australasian Marce Society Biennial Scientific Meeting in New Zealand. She was asked to speak on perinatal anxiety disorders. In reviewing the literature to prepare the address, Beck located only a few published studies describing birth trauma and its resulting post-traumatic stress disorder (PTSD). Following her keynote speech, a mother made a riveting presentation about her experience of PTSD due to a traumatic birth. The mother, Sue Watson, was one of the founders of Trauma and Birth Stress (TABS), a charitable trust in New Zealand. Before Watson had finished her presentation, Beck realized that she wanted to do research on birth trauma. Later that day, Watson and Beck discussed the possibility of Beck conducting a qualitative study with the mothers who were members of TABS. Gaining entrée into TABS was facilitated by Watson who, with other founders of TABS, approved the study.

Phase 2. Design and Planning Phase: 3 Months. Beck selected a phenomenological design for this research. She corresponded by email with Watson to design an approach for recruiting mothers. Plans were made for Beck to write an introductory letter explaining the study, and for Watson to write a letter endorsing the study. Both letters would be sent to the mothers who were members of TABS, asking for their cooperation. Once the basic design was finalized, Beck obtained approval by the human subjects committee at her university.

Phase 3. Empirical/Analytic Phases 24 months. Data for the study were collected over an 18-month period. During that period, 40 mothers sent their stories of birth trauma to Beck via e-mail attachments. For an additional 6 months Beck analyzed the mothers' stories. Four themes emerged from data analysis: (1) To care for me: Was that too much to ask? (2) To communicate with me: Why was this neglected? (3) To provide safe care: You betrayed my trust and I felt powerless. and (4) The end justifies the means: At whose expense? At what price?

Phase 4 Dissemination Phase: 5+ Months. A manuscript describing this study was submitted to the journal *Nursing Research* in April 2003. In June, Beck received a letter from the journal's editor indicating that the reviewers' of her manuscript recommended she revise and resubmit it. Six weeks later Beck resubmitted a revised manuscript that incorporated the reviewers' recommendations. In September 2003 Beck received notification that her revised manuscript had been accepted for publication. The article was published in the January/February 2004 issue. Additionally, Beck has presented the findings at numerous national and international research conferences.

CRITICAL THINKING SUGGESTIONS:

1. Answer the questions from Box 3.3 regarding this study.
2. Also consider the following targeted questions, which may further sharpen your critical thinking skills and assist you in understanding this study:
   a. Given the study purpose, was a phenomenological approach appropriate for this study?
   b. Do you think an appropriate amount of time was allocated to the various phases and steps in this study?
   c. How would you evaluate Beck dissemination plan?
   d. Would it have been appropriate for Beck to address the research question using quantitative research methods? Why or why not?

EXAMPLE 3 ■ Quantitative Research in Appendix A

1. Read the abstract and the introduction from Howell and colleagues' (2007) study ("Anxiety, anger, and blood pressure in children") in Appendix A of this book, and then answer the relevant questions in Box 3.3.
2. Also consider the following targeted questions, which may further sharpen your critical thinking skills and assist you in assessing aspects of the study's merit:
   a. Could any of the variables in this study be considered *constructs?*
   b. Did this report present any actual *data* from the study participants?
   c. Would it have been possible for the researchers to use an experimental design for this study?

EXAMPLE 4 ■ Qualitative Research in Appendix B

1. Read the abstract and introduction from Beck's (2006) study ("Anniversary of birth trauma") in Appendix B of this book and then answer the relevant questions in Box 3.3.
2. Also consider the following targeted questions, which may further sharpen your critical thinking skills and assist you in assessing aspects of the study's merit:
   a. Find an example of actual *data* in this study (You will need to look at the "Results" section of this study).
   b. How long did it take Beck to collect the data for this study? (You will find this information in the "Procedure" section.)
   c. How much time elapsed between when the paper was accepted for publication and when it was actually published? (You will find relevant information at the end of the paper).

CHAPTER REVIEW

Key new terms introduced in the chapter, together with a summary of major points, are presented in this section. Chapter 3 of the accompanying *Study Guide for Essentials of Nursing Research*, 7th edition also offers exercises and study suggestions for reinforcing the concepts presented in this chapter. For additional review, see self-study questions on the CD-ROM provided with this book.

Key New Terms

Cause-and-effect (causal) relationship	Gaining entrée	Population
Clinical trial	Grounded theory	Qualitative data
Concept	Hypothesis	Quantitative data
Conceptual definition	Independent variable	Relationship
Construct	Intervention protocol	Research design
Data	Literature review	Sample
Dependent variable	Nonexperimental research	Sampling plan
Emergent design	Observational research	Saturation
Ethnography	Operational definition	Statistical analysis
Experimental research	Outcome variable	Study participant
Fieldwork	Phenomenology	Subject
		Variable

Summary Points

➤ The people who provide information to the **researchers** (investigators) in a *study* are referred to as **subjects, study participants,** or **respondents** in quantitative research, or study participants or **informants** in qualitative research; collectively they comprise the **sample.**

➤ The *site* is the overall location for the research; researchers sometimes engage in **multisite studies**. *Settings* are the more specific places where data collection will occur. Settings for nursing research can range from totally naturalistic environments to formal laboratories.

➤ Researchers investigate **concepts** and **phenomena** (or **constructs**), which are abstractions or mental representations inferred from behavior or characteristics.

➤ Concepts are the building blocks of **theories,** which are systematic explanations of some aspect of the real world.

➤ In quantitative studies, concepts are called variables. A **variable** is a characteristic or quality that takes on different values (i.e., varies from one person or object to another).

➤ The **dependent** (or **outcome**) **variable** is the behavior, characteristic, or outcome the researcher is interested in understanding, explaining, predicting, or affecting. The **independent variable** is the presumed cause of, antecedent to, or influence on the dependent variable.

➤ A **conceptual definition** describes the abstract or theoretical meaning of the concepts being studied. An **operational definition** specifies the procedures required to measure a variable.

➤ **Data**—the information collected during the course of a study—may take the form of narrative information (**qualitative data**) or numeric values (**quantitative data**).

➤ A **relationship** is a bond or connection (or pattern of association) between two variables. Quantitative researchers examine the relationship between the independent variables and dependent variables.

➤ When the independent variable causes or affects the dependent variable, the relationship is a **cause-and-effect (causal) relationship**. In a *functional* or *associative relationship*, variables are related in a noncausal way.

➤ A basic distinction in quantitative studies is between **experimental research**, in which researchers actively intervene, and **nonexperimental** (or **observational**) **research,** in which researchers make observations of existing phenomena without intervening.

➤ Qualitative research often is rooted in research traditions that originate in other disciplines. Three such traditions are grounded theory, phenomenology, and ethnography.

➤ **Grounded theory** seeks to describe and understand key social psychological and structural processes that occur in a social setting.

➤ **Phenomenology** focuses on the lived experiences of humans and is an approach to gaining insight into what the life experiences of people are like and what they mean.

➤ **Ethnography** provides a framework for studying the meanings, patterns, and lifeways of a culture in a holistic fashion.

➤ In a quantitative study, researchers usually progress in a linear fashion from asking research questions to answering them. The main phases in a quantitative study are the conceptual, planning, empirical, analytic, and dissemination phases.

➤ The *conceptual phase* involves (1) defining the problem to be studied; (2) doing a **literature review;** (3) engaging in **clinical fieldwork** for clinical studies; (4) developing a framework and conceptual definitions; and (5) formulating **hypotheses** to be tested.

➤ The *planning phase* entails (6) selecting a **research design;** (7) developing **intervention protocols** if the study is experimental; (8) specifying the **population;** (9) developing a **sampling plan;** (10) specifying methods to measure the research variables; (11) developing strategies to safeguard the rights of subjects; and (12) finalizing the research plan (e.g., conferring with colleagues, *pretesting* instruments).

➤ The *empirical phase* involves (13) collecting data; and (14) preparing data for analysis (e.g., *coding* data).

➤ The *analytic phase* involves (15) analyzing data through **statistical analysis;** and (16) interpreting the results.

➤ The *dissemination phase* entails (17) communicating the findings; and (18) efforts to promote the use of the study evidence in nursing practice.

➤ The flow of activities in a qualitative study is more flexible and less linear. Qualitative studies typically involve an **emergent design** that evolves during **fieldwork**.

➤ Qualitative researchers begin with a broad question regarding a phenomenon of interest, often focusing on a little-studied aspect. In the early phase of a qualitative study, researchers select a site and seek to **gain entrée** into it, which typically involves enlisting the cooperation of **gatekeepers** within the site.

➤ Once in the field, researchers select informants, collect data, and then analyze and interpret them in an iterative fashion; field experiences help in an ongoing fashion to shape the design of the study.

➤ Early analysis in qualitative research leads to refinements in sampling and data collection, until **saturation** (redundancy of information) is achieved. Analysis typically involves a search for critical **themes.**

➤ Both qualitative and quantitative researchers disseminate their findings, most often by publishing their research reports in professional journals.

STUDIES CITED IN CHAPTER 3

Allen, M., Oberle, K., Grace, M., Russell, A., & Aderwale, A. (2008). A randomized clinical trial of elk velvet antler in rheumatoid arthritis. *Biological Research for Nursing, 9,* 254–261.

Beck, C. T. (2004). Birth trauma: In the eye of the beholder. *Nursing Research, 53*(1), 28–35.

Beck, C. T., & Gable, R. K. (2000). Postpartum Depression Screening Scale: Development and psychometric testing, *Nursing Research, 49,* 272–282.

Beck, C. T., & Gable, R. K. (2001). Further validation of the Postpartum Depression Screening Scale. *Nursing Research, 50,* 155–164.

Champion, V., Skinner, C., Hui, S., Monahan, P., Juliar, B., Daggy, J., et al. (2007). The effect of telephone versus print tailoring for mammography adherence. *Patient Education and Counseling, 65,* 416–423.

Clark, L., & Redman, R. (2007). Mexican immigrant mothers' expectations for children's health services. *Western Journal of Nursing Research, 29,* 670–690.

Fontenot, H. B. (2007). Transition and adaptation to adaptive motherhood. *Journal of Obstetric, Gynecologic, and Neonatal Nursing, 36,* 175–182.

Hinck, S. M. (2007). The meaning of time in oldest-old age. *Holistic Nursing Practice, 21,* 35–41.

Holmes, D., O'Byrne, P., & Gastaldo, D. (2007). Setting the space for sex: Architecture, desire and health issues in gay bathhouses. *International Journal of Nursing Studies, 44,* 273–284.

Lengacher, C., Bennett, M., Gonzales, L., Gilvary, D., Cox, C., Cantor, A., et al. (2008). Immune responses to guided imagery during breast cancer treatment. *Biological Research for Nursing, 9,* 205–214.

Lewis, L., Hankin, S., Reynolds, D., & Ogedegbe, G. (2007). African American spirituality: A process of honoring God, others, and self. *Journal of Holistic Nursing, 25,* 16–23.

Liu, H., Feurer, I., Dwyer, K., Speroff, T., Shaffer, D., & Wright-Pinson, C. (2008). The effects of gender and age on health-related quality of life following kidney transplantation. *Journal of Clinical Nursing, 17,* 82–89.

Schim, S., Doorenbos, A., & Borse, N. (2006) Enhancing cultural competence among hospice staff. *The American Journal of Hospice & Palliative Care, 23,* 404–411.

Sweeney, N., Glaser, D., & Tedeschi, C. (2007). The eating and physical activity habits of inner-city adolescents. *Journal of Pediatric Health Care, 21,* 13–21.

Tseng, C., Chen, C., Wu, S., & Lin, L. (2007). Effects of a range-of-motion exercise program. *Journal of Advanced Nursing, 57,* 181–191.

CHAPTER

4 Reading and Critiquing Research Reports

STUDENT OBJECTIVES

On completing this chapter, you will be able to:

➤ Name major types of research reports

➤ Identify and describe the major sections in a research journal article

➤ Characterize the style used in quantitative and qualitative research reports

➤ Read a research article and grasp key aspects of the "story"

➤ Describe aspects of a research critique

➤ Understand the many challenges researchers face and identify some tools for addressing methodologic challenges

➤ Define new terms in the chapter

Evidence from nursing studies is communicated through *research reports* that describe what was studied, how it was studied, and what was found. Research reports—especially those for quantitative studies—are often daunting to readers without research training. This chapter is designed to help make research reports more accessible early in your course. This chapter also provides preliminary guidance regarding critiques of research reports, and discusses some of the key challenges that researchers face in generating evidence that is valid and trustworthy.

TYPES OF RESEARCH REPORTS

Researchers communicate information about their studies in various ways. The most common types of research reports are theses and dissertations, books, conference presentations, and journal articles. Nurses are most likely to encounter research evidence at professional conferences or in journals.

Presentations at Professional Conferences

Research findings are presented at conferences as oral presentations or poster sessions.

➤ *Oral presentations* follow a format similar to that used in journal articles, which we discuss next. The presenter is typically allotted 10 to 20 minutes to describe key features of the study.

➤ In **poster sessions,** many researchers simultaneously present visual displays summarizing their studies, and conference attendees circulate around the room perusing these displays.

Conference presentations are an important avenue for communicating research information. Results are typically disseminated more quickly than in the case of journal publication. Conferences also offer an opportunity for dialogue between researchers and conference attendees. The attendees can ask questions to help them better understand how the study was conducted or what the findings mean; moreover, they can offer the researchers suggestions relating to clinical implications of the study. Thus, professional conferences offer a particularly valuable forum for a clinical audience.

Research Journal Articles

Research **journal articles** summarize studies in professional journals. Because competition for journal space is keen, the typical research article is brief—generally only 10 to 20 double-spaced manuscript pages. This means that researchers must condense a lot of information about the study into a short report.

Journals accept research reports on a competitive basis. Usually, manuscripts are reviewed by two or more **peer reviewers** (other researchers doing work in the field) who make recommendations about whether to accept or reject the manuscript, or to suggest revisions and re-review. These are usually **"blind" reviews**—reviewers are not told researchers' names, and authors are not told reviewers' names.

In major journals, the rate of acceptance is low—it can be as low as 5% of sub-mitted articles. Thus, consumers have some assurance that journal articles have already been scrutinized for their merit by other nurse researchers. Nevertheless, the publication of an article does not mean that the findings can be uncritically accepted. Research methods courses help nurses to evaluate the quality of evidence reported in research journal articles.

THE CONTENT OF RESEARCH JOURNAL ARTICLES

Quantitative journal articles—and many qualitative ones—typically follow a con-ventional organization called the **IMRAD format**. This format, which loosely follows the steps of quantitative studies, involves organizing material into four main sections—**I**ntroduction, **M**ethod, **R**esults, and **D**iscussion. The text of the report is usually preceded by a title and an abstract and is followed by references.

The Title and Abstract

Research reports begin with a title that succinctly conveys (typically in 15 or fewer words) the nature of the study. In qualitative studies, the title normally includes the central phenomenon and group under investigation; in quantitative studies, the title generally indicates the independent and dependent variables and the population.

The **abstract** is a brief description of the study placed at the beginning of the article. The abstract answers, in about 100 to 150 words, the following questions: What were the research questions? What methods did the researcher use to address those questions? What did the researcher find? and What are the implications for nursing practice? Readers can review an abstract to assess whether to read the full report. (Unfortunately, the strict word counts of some journals make it difficult for authors to include as much information in these abstracts as one would like.)

Some journals have moved from having traditional abstracts—which are single paragraphs summarizing the study's main features—to slightly longer, structured abstracts with headings. For example, abstracts in *Nursing Research* after 1997 present summaries organized under the following headings: Background, Objec-tives, Method, Results, and Conclusions. Beck's (2006) qualitative study in Appen-dix B of this book exemplifies this longer abstract style, whereas the abstract in Appendix A (Howell et al., 2007) illustrates the traditional one-paragraph format.

The Introduction

The introduction to a research article acquaints readers with the research problem and its context. This section usually describes the following:

❖ The central phenomena, concepts, or variables under study
❖ The study purpose and research questions, or hypotheses to be tested
❖ A review of the related literature

➤ The theoretical or conceptual framework

➤ The significance of and need for the study

Thus, the introduction sets the stage for a description of what the researcher did and what was learned. The introduction corresponds roughly to the conceptual phase (phase 1) of a study, as described in Chapter 3.

Example of an introductory paragraph:

Mutuality, or the positive quality of care relationship, is an important protective factor for family caregivers providing care to a frail older adult . . . , yet little is known about frail older adults' mutuality with their family caregiver, how their mutuality changes over time, and how it is affected by changes in the care situation . . . The purpose of the study reported in this article was to examine mutuality in care dyads over time, and the impact of health changes on the quality of the care relationship (Lyons et al., 2007).

In this paragraph, the researchers described the concepts of interest (mutuality among frail elders and their caregivers), the need for the study (the fact that little is known about aspects of mutuality), and the study purpose.

TIP

The introduction section of many reports are not specifically labeled "Introduction." The report's intro-duction immediately follows the abstract.

The Method Section

The method section describes the methods the researcher used to answer the research questions. It describes major methodologic decisions made in the design and planning phase of the study (phase 2), and may offer rationales for those deci-sions. In a quantitative study, the method section usually describes the following, which may be presented in labeled subsections:

➤ The research design

➤ The sampling plan and description of study participants

➤ Methods of operationalizing variables and collecting data, and specific instru-ments used

➤ Study procedures, including procedures to protect the rights of study partici-pants

➤ Analytic procedures and methods.

Qualitative researchers discuss many of the same issues, but with different emphases. For example, a qualitative study often provides more information about the research setting and the context of the study, and less information on sampling. Also, because formal instruments are not used to collect qualitative data, there is little discussion about specific methods, but there may be more information on data collection procedures. Increasingly, reports of qualitative studies are including descriptions of the researchers' efforts to enhance the integrity of the study.

In quantitative studies, the method section describes decisions made during the design and planning phase of the study and implemented during the empirical phase (see Chapter 3). In qualitative studies, the methodologic decisions are made during the planning stage and also during the course of fieldwork.

TIP

The method section is sometimes called "Method" and sometimes called "Methods" (plural). Either is acceptable, although the manual of style used by many nursing journals (from the American Psychological Association) says "Method."

The Results Section

The results section presents the **findings** that were obtained from an analysis of the study data. The text presents a narrative summary of key findings, often accompanied by more detailed tables. Virtually all results sections contain basic descriptive information, including a description of the participants (e.g., average age, percent male or female). In quantitative studies, the researcher provides basic descriptive information for the key variables, using simple statistics. For example, in a study of the effect of prenatal drug exposure on the birth outcomes of infants, the results section might begin by describing the infants' average birthweights or the percentage who were of low birth weight (under 2,500 g).

In quantitative studies, the results section also reports the following information relating to any statistical tests performed:

➤ *The names of statistical tests used.* A **statistical test** is a procedure for testing researchers' hypotheses and estimating the probability that the results are right. For example, if the percentage of low-birth-weight infants in the sample of drug-exposed infants is computed, how probable is it that the percentage is accurate? If the researcher finds that the average birth weight of drug-exposed infants in the sample is lower than the birth weight of infants not exposed to drugs, how probable is it that the same would be true for other infants not in the sample? A statistical test helps answer the question: Is the relationship between prenatal drug exposure and infant birth weight *real,* and would it likely be observed with a new sample of infants from the same population? Statistical tests are based on common principles; you do not have to know the names of all statistical tests (there are dozens of them) to comprehend the findings.

➤ *The value of the calculated statistic.* Computers are used to calculate a numeric value for the particular statistical test used. The value allows researchers to draw inferences about the accuracy of their hypotheses. The *actual* numeric value of the statistic, however, is not inherently meaningful and need not concern you.

➤ *The significance.* A critical piece of information is whether the results of the statistical tests were significant (not to be confused with important or clinically relevant). If a researcher reports that the results are **statistically significant,** it means the findings are probably true and replicable with a new sample. Research reports also indicate the **level of significance,** which is an index of how *probable* it is that the findings are reliable. For example, if a report indicates that a finding was significant at the .05 level, this means that only 5 times out of 100 (5 ÷ 100 = .05) would the obtained result be spurious. In other words, 95 times out of 100, similar results would be obtained with a new sample. Readers can therefore have a high degree of confidence—but not total assurance—that the findings are accurate.

➤ *The precision and magnitude of the effects.* Increasingly, there is an emphasis on reporting not only what the findings are and whether they are statistically reliable, but also the degree of precision around any estimated effects, and how sizeable the effects are. These two aspects, which correspond to the second and third question from Box 2.1 on "Appraising the Evidence" within an evidence-based practice (EBP) framework, have not been emphasized as much in the nursing literature as in the medical literature, but this situation is changing. These aspects will be briefly described in Chapter 15 on statistical analysis.

Example from the results section of a quantitative study:
Efe and Ozer (2007) examined the pain-relieving effect of breastfeeding during immunization injections in healthy neonates. Half the infants breastfed before, during, and after the injection, and the other half (the control group) did not breastfeed. Here is a sentence adapted from the reported results: Total crying durations were found to be significantly shorter in the breastfeeding group (average of 35.85 seconds) than in the control group (average of 76.24 seconds); $t = 3.64$, $p = .001$.

In this example, the researchers stated that crying was *significantly* shorter among infants who were being breastfed during immunizations than among those who did not breastfeed. The average group difference in crying time—more than 40 seconds—was not likely to have been a haphazard difference, and would probably be replicated with a new sample of infants. This finding is highly reliable: only 1 time in 1,000 ($p = 0.001$) could a difference this great have occurred as a fluke. Note that to comprehend this finding, you do not need to understand what a t statistic is, nor do you need to concern yourself with the actual value of the statistic, 3.64.

TIP

Be especially alert to the p values (probabilities) when reading statistical results. If a p value is greater than .05 (e.g., $p = .08$), the results are considered *not* to be statistically significant by conventional standards. Nonsignificant results are sometimes abbreviated NS. Also, be aware that the results are *more* reliable if the p value is smaller. For example, there is a higher probability that the results are accurate when $p = .01$ (only 1 chance in 100 of a spurious result) than when $p = .05$ (5 chances in 100 of a spurious result). Researchers sometimes report an exact probability estimate (e.g., $p = .03$) or a probability below conventional threshholds (e.g., $p < .05$—less than 5 in 100).

In qualitative reports, researchers often organize findings according to the major themes, processes, or categories that were identified in the data. The results section of qualitative reports sometimes has several subsections, the headings of which correspond to the researcher's labels for the themes. Excerpts from the *raw data* (the actual words of participants) are presented to support and provide a rich description of the thematic analysis. The results section of qualitative studies may also present the researcher's emerging theory about the phenomenon under study, although this may appear in the concluding section of the report.

Example from the results section of a qualitative study:
Polzer and Miles (2007) undertook a grounded theory study to explain how the spirituality of African Americans affects their self-management of diabetes. One biblical allusion made by several study participants was the body as the Temple of God: "Some of the men and women in this group stated that the body is the Temple of God. A consequence of not taking care of the body is a sin. According to Betty, age 70 and a Baptist: *It's wrong to eat a piece of cake. God knows that if you know it's wrong, you're sinning. It's a sin because you're defiling His body . . . You're defiling God's body if you don't take care of it."* (p. 183).

The Discussion

In the discussion section, the researcher draws conclusions about the meaning and implications of the findings. This section tries to unravel what the results mean, why things turned out the way they did, how the findings fit into the existing evidence base, and how the results can be used in practice. The discussion in both qualitative and quantitative reports may incorporate the following elements:

➤ An interpretation of the results

➤ Clinical and research implications

➤ Study limitations and ramifications for the believability of the results

The researcher is in the best position possible to point out sample deficiencies, design problems, weaknesses in data collection, and so forth. A discussion section that presents the researcher's understanding of the limitations demonstrates to readers that the author was aware of the limitations and probably took them into account in interpreting the findings.

References

Research articles conclude with a list of the books and journal articles that were referenced in the report. If you are interested in pursuing additional reading on a topic, the reference list of a recent study is an excellent place to begin.

THE STYLE OF RESEARCH JOURNAL ARTICLES

Research reports tell a story. However, the style in which many research journal articles are written—especially reports of quantitative studies—makes it difficult for some readers to figure out or become interested in the story.

Why Are Research Articles So Hard to Read?

To unaccustomed audiences, research reports may seem stuffy and bewildering. Four factors contribute to this impression:

1. *Compactness*. Journal space is limited, so authors compress a lot of information into a short space. Interesting, personalized aspects of the investigation cannot be reported, and, in qualitative studies, only a handful of supporting quotes can be included.

2. *Jargon*. The authors of both qualitative and quantitative reports use research terms that may seem esoteric.

3. *Objectivity*. Quantitative researchers tend to avoid any impression of subjectivity, and so they tell their research stories in a way that makes them sound impersonal. For example, most quantitative research reports are written in the passive voice (i.e., personal pronouns are avoided). Use of the passive voice tends to make a report less inviting and lively than the use of the active voice. (Qualitative reports, by contrast, are often written in a more conversational style.)

4. *Statistical information*. In quantitative reports, numbers and statistical symbols may intimidate readers who do not have strong mathematic interest or training.

A goal of this textbook is to assist you in understanding the content of research reports and in overcoming anxieties about jargon and statistical information.

HOW-TO-TELL TIP

How can you tell if the voice is active or passive? In the active voice, the article would say what the researchers *did* (e.g., "We used a mercury sphygmomameter to measure blood pressure"). In the passive voice, the article indicates that something *was done*, without indicating who did it, although it is implied that the researchers were the acting agents ("e.g., A mercury sphygmomameter *was used* to measure blood pressure").

Tips on Reading Research Articles

As you progress through this textbook, you will acquire skills for evaluating various aspects of research reports critically, but the skills involved in critical appraisal take time to develop. The first step in being able to use research findings in clinical practice is to comprehend research reports. Your first few attempts to read a research report might be overwhelming, and you may wonder whether being able to understand, let alone appraise, research reports is a realistic goal. Here are some preliminary hints on digesting research reports.

➣ Grow accustomed to the style of research reports by reading them frequently, even though you may not yet understand all the technical points.

➣ Read from a report that has been photocopied (or downloaded and printed) so that you use a highlighter, underline portions, write questions or notes in the margins, and so on.

➤ Read journal articles slowly. It may be useful to skim the article first to get the major points and then read the article more carefully a second time.

➤ On the second reading, train yourself to become an *active* reader. Reading actively means that you are constantly monitoring yourself to determine whether you understand what you are reading. If you have difficulty, go back and reread difficult passages or make notes about your confusion so that you can ask someone for clarification. In most cases, that "someone" will be your research instructor, but also consider contacting the researchers themselves. The postal and e-mail addresses of the lead author are usually noted in the journal article, and researchers are often quite willing to discuss their research with others.

➤ Keep this textbook with you as a reference while you are reading articles so that you can look up unfamiliar terms in the glossary or the index.

➤ Try not to get bogged down in (or scared away by) statistical information. Try to grasp the gist of the story without letting symbols and numbers frustrate you.

➤ Until you become accustomed to the style and jargon of research articles, you may want to "translate" them mentally or in writing. You can do this by expanding compact paragraphs into looser constructions, by translating jargon into more familiar terms, by recasting the report into an active voice, and by summarizing the findings with words rather than numbers. As an example, Box 4.1 presents a summary of a fictitious study about the psychological consequences of having an abortion, written in the style typically found in research journal articles. Terms that can be looked up in the glossary of this book are underlined, and bolded marginal notes indicate the type of information the author is communicating. Box 4.2 presents a "translation" of this summary, recasting the research information into more digestible language.

When you attain a reasonable level of comprehension, a useful next step is to write a one- to two-page synopsis of the article. A synopsis summarizes the study's purpose, research questions, methods, findings, interpretation of the findings, and implications. By preparing a synopsis, you will become more aware of aspects of the study that you did not understand.

CRITIQUING RESEARCH REPORTS

Although it is certainly important to read research reports with understanding, it is also important to read them critically. A critical reading involves a careful appraisal of the researcher's major conceptual and methodologic decisions. It will be difficult to criticize these decisions at this point, but your skills will get stronger as you progress through this book.

What Is a Research Critique?

A research **critique** is different from a research summary or synopsis. A research critique is a careful and objective appraisal of a study's strengths and limitations.

BOX 4.1   SUMMARY OF A FICTITIOUS STUDY FOR TRANSLATION

Purpose of the study	The potentially negative sequelae of having an abortion on the psychological adjustment of adolescents have not been adequately studied. The present study sought to determine whether alternative pregnancy resolution decisions have different long-term effects on the psychological functioning of young women.	**Need for the study**
Research design **Research instruments**	Three groups of low-income pregnant teenagers attending an inner-city clinic were the <u>subjects</u> in this study: those who delivered and kept the baby; those who delivered and relinquished the baby for adoption; and those who had an abortion. There were 25 subjects in each group. The study <u>instruments</u> included a self-administered <u>questionnaire</u> and a battery of psychological tests measuring depression, anxiety, and psychosomatic symptoms. The instruments were administered upon entry into the study (when the subjects first came to the clinic) and then 1 year after termination of the pregnancy.	**Study population** **Research sample**
Data analysis procedure	The <u>data</u> were analyzed using <u>analysis of variance (ANOVA)</u>. The ANOVA tests indicated that the three groups did not differ significantly in terms of depression, anxiety, or psychosomatic symptoms at the initial testing. At the <u>post-test</u>, however, the abortion group had significantly higher scores on the depression scale, and these girls were significantly more likely than the two delivery groups to report severe tension headaches. There were no <u>significant</u> differences on any of the <u>dependent variables</u> for the two delivery groups.	**Results**
Implications	The <u>results</u> of this study suggest that young women who elect to have an abortion may experience a number of long-term negative consequences. It would appear that appropriate efforts should be made to follow up abortion patients to determine their need for suitable treatment.	**Interpretation**

Critiques usually conclude with the reviewer's summary of the study's merits, recommendations regarding the value of the evidence, and suggestions about improving the study or the report itself.

Research critiques of individual studies are prepared for various reasons, and they differ in scope, depending on their purpose. Peer reviewers who are asked to prepare a written critique for a journal considering publication of a manuscript generally evaluate the strengths and weaknesses of the following aspects of the study:

➤ *Substantive*—Was the research problem significant to nursing? Can the study make an important contribution?

BOX 4.2 TRANSLATED VERSION OF FICTITIOUS RESEARCH STUDY

As researchers, we wondered whether young women who had an abortion had any emotional problems in the long run. It seemed to us that not enough research had been done to know whether any psychological harm resulted from an abortion.

We decided to study this question ourselves by comparing the experiences of three types of teenagers who became pregnant—first, girls who delivered and kept their babies; second, those who delivered the babies but gave them up for adoption; and third, those who elected to have an abortion. All teenagers in our sample were poor, and all were patients at an inner-city clinic. Altogether, we studied 75 girls—25 in each of the three groups. We evaluated the teenagers' emotional states by asking them to fill out a questionnaire and to take several psychological tests. These tests allowed us to assess things such as the girls' degree of depression and anxiety and whether they had any complaints of a psychosomatic nature. We asked them to fill out the forms twice: once when they came into the clinic, and then again a year after the abortion or the delivery.

We learned that the three groups of teenagers looked pretty much alike in terms of their emotional states when they first filled out the forms. But when we compared how the three groups looked a year later, we found that the teenagers who had abortions were more depressed and were more likely to say they had severe tension headaches than teenagers in the other two groups. The teenagers who kept their babies and those who gave their babies up for adoption looked pretty similar 1 year after their babies were born, at least in terms of depression, anxiety, and psychosomatic complaints.

Thus, it seems that we might be right in having some concerns about the emotional effects of having an abortion. Nurses should be aware of these long-term emotional effects, and it even may be advisable to institute some type of follow-up procedure to find out if these young women need additional help.

➤ *Theoretical*—Were the conceptual or theoretical underpinnings sound?

➤ *Methodologic*—Were the methods rigorous and appropriate? Are the findings sound?

➤ *Interpretive*—Did the researcher properly interpret data and make defensible inferences?

➤ *Ethical*—Were the rights of study participants protected?

➤ *Stylistic*—Is the report clearly written, grammatical, and well organized?

In short, peer reviewers do a comprehensive review to provide feedback to the researchers and to journal editors about the merit of both the study and the report, and typically offer suggestions for improvements.

Students taking a research methods course also may be asked to critique a study. Such critiques are usually expected to be comprehensive, encompassing the various dimensions just described. The purpose of such a thorough critique is to cultivate critical thinking, to induce students to use newly acquired skills in research methods, and to prepare students for a professional nursing career in which evaluating research will almost surely play a role. Writing research critiques is an important first step on the path to developing an evidence-based practice.

> **TIP**
>
> A critique that is designed to inform decisions about nursing practice is seldom comprehensive. For example, it is of little significance to practicing nurses whether a research report is ungrammatical. A critique on the clinical utility of a study focuses on whether the findings are accurate, believable, and clinically meaningful. If the findings cannot be trusted, it makes little sense to incorporate them into nursing practice.

Critiquing Support in This Textbook

We provide support for critiques of studies in several ways. First, detailed critiquing suggestions relating to chapter content are included at the end of most chapters. Second, we offer an abbreviated set of key critiquing guidelines for quantitative and qualitative reports in this chapter, in Tables 4.1 and 4.2, respectively. Finally, it is always illuminating to have a good model, and so we have prepared comprehensive research critiques of a quantitative and a qualitative study, which appear in Appendix C and D. These appendices are included in files on the accompanying CD-ROM, ☻ together with the studies themselves in their entirety.

The guidelines in Tables 4.1 and 4.2 are organized according to the IMRAD format. The second column lists some key critiquing questions that have broad applicability to research reports, and the third column gives cross-references to the more detailed guidelines in the various chapters of the book. We know that most of the critiquing questions are too difficult for you to answer at this point, but your methodologic and critiquing skills will develop as you progress through this book.

In these guidelines, the wording of the questions calls for a yes or no answer (although it may well be that the answer sometimes will be "Yes, *but* . . ."). In all cases, the desirable answer is *yes*, that is, a *no* suggests a possible limitation and a *yes* suggests a strength. Therefore, the more *yeses* a study gets, the stronger it is likely to be. Thus, these guidelines can cumulatively suggest a global assessment: a report with 25 *yeses* is likely to be superior to one with only 10. However, it is also important to realize that not all *yeses* and *nos* are equal. Some elements are more important in drawing conclusions about the rigor of a study than others. For example, the inadequacy of a literature review is far less damaging to the worth of the study's *evidence* than the use of a faulty design. In general, the questions addressing the researchers' methodologic decisions (i.e., the questions under "Method") are especially important in evaluating the quality of a study's evidence.

Although the questions in these guidelines elicit *yes* or *no* responses, a comprehensive written critique would obviously need to do more than point out what the study did and did not do. Each relevant issue would need to be discussed and your criticism justified. For example, if you answered *no* to the question about whether the hypotheses were appropriately worded, you would need to articulate your criticisms and perhaps suggest improvements.

	GUIDE TO AN OVERALL CRITIQUE OF A QUANTITATIVE	
TABLE 4.1	**RESEARCH REPORT**	

ASPECT OF THE REPORT	CRITIQUING QUESTIONS	DETAILED CRITIQUING GUIDELINES
Title	➤ Is the title a good one, succinctly suggesting key variables and the study population?	
Abstract	➤ Does the abstract clearly and concisely summarize the main features of the report (problem, methods, results, conclusions)?	
Introduction Statement of the problem	➤ Is the problem stated unambiguously, and is it easy to identify? ➤ Does the problem statement build a cogent and persuasive argument for the new study? ➤ Does the problem have significance for nursing? ➤ Is there a good match between the research problem and the paradigm and methods used? Is a quantitative approach appropriate?	Box 6.3, page 163
Hypotheses or research questions	➤ Are research questions and/or hypotheses explicitly stated? If not, is their absence justified? ➤ Are questions and hypotheses appropriately worded, with clear specification of key variables and the study population? ➤ Are the questions/hypotheses consistent with the literature review and the conceptual framework?	Box 6.3, page 163
Literature review	➤ Is the literature review up-to-date and based mainly on primary sources? ➤ Does the review provide a state-of-the-art synthesis of evidence on the research problem? ➤ Does the literature review provide a solid basis for the new study?	Box 7.1, page 188
Conceptual/ theoretical framework	➤ Are key concepts adequately defined conceptually? ➤ Is there a conceptual/theoretical framework, rationale, and/or map, and (if so) is it appropriate? If not, is the absence of one justified?	Box 8.1, page 210
Method Protection of participants' rights	➤ Were appropriate procedures used to safeguard the rights of study participants? Was the study subject to external review by an IRB/ethics review board? ➤ Was the study designed to minimize risks and maximize benefits to participants?	Box 5.2, page 135
Research design	➤ Was the most rigorous possible design used, given the purpose of the research? ➤ Were appropriate comparisons made to enhance interpretability of the findings?	Box 9.1, page 250

TABLE 4.1

GUIDE TO AN OVERALL CRITIQUE OF A QUANTITATIVE RESEARCH REPORT (continued)

ASPECT OF THE REPORT	CRITIQUING QUESTIONS	DETAILED CRITIQUING GUIDELINES
	➤ Was the number of data collection points appropriate? ➤ Did the design minimize biases and threats to the internal construct, and external validity of the study (e.g., was blinding used, was attrition minimized)?	
Population and sample	➤ Was the population identified and described? Was the sample described in sufficient detail? ➤ Was the best possible sampling design used to enhance the sample's representativeness? Were sample biases minimized? ➤ Was the sample size adequate? Was a power analysis used to estimate sample size needs?	Box 12.1, page 325
Data collection and measurement	➤ Are the operational and conceptual definitions congruent? ➤ Were key variables operationalized using the best possible method (e.g., interviews, observations, and so on) and with adequate justification? ➤ Are the specific instruments adequately described and were they good choices, given the study purpose and study population? ➤ Does the report provide evidence that the data collection methods yielded data that were high on reliability and validity?	Box 13.3, page 361 Box 14.1, page 383
Procedures	➤ If there was an intervention, is it adequately described, and was it properly implemented? Did most participants allocated to the intervention group actually receive the intervention? Was there evidence of intervention fidelity? ➤ Were data collected in a manner that minimized bias? Were the staff who collected data appropriately trained?	Box 9.1, page 250
Results Data analysis	➤ Were analyses undertaken to address each research question or test each hypothesis? ➤ Were appropriate statistical methods used, given the level of measurement of the variables, number of groups being compared, and so on? ➤ Was the most powerful analytic method used? (e.g., did the analysis help to control for confounding variables)? ➤ Were Type I and Type II errors avoided or minimized?	Box 15.1, page 431
Findings	➤ Was information about statistical significance presented? Was information about effect size and precision of estimates (confidence intervals) presented?	Box 15.1, page 431

TABLE 4.1 ➤	**GUIDE TO AN OVERALL CRITIQUE OF A QUANTITATIVE RESEARCH REPORT** (continued)	
ASPECT OF THE REPORT	CRITIQUING QUESTIONS	DETAILED CRITIQUING GUIDELINES
	➤ Are the findings adequately summarized, with good use of tables and figures? ➤ Are findings reported in a manner that facilitates a meta-analysis, and with sufficient information needed for EBP?	
Discussion Interpretation of the findings	➤ Are all major findings interpreted and discussed within the context of prior research and/or the study's conceptual framework? ➤ Were causal inferences, if any, justified? ➤ Are the interpretations consistent with the results and with the study's limitations? ➤ Does the report address the issue of the generalizability of the findings?	Box 16.1, page 457
Implications/ recommendations	➤ Do the researchers discuss the implications of the study for clinical practice or further research—and are those implications reasonable and complete?	Box 16.1, page 457
Global Issues Presentation	➤ Is the report well written, well organized, and sufficiently detailed for critical analysis? ➤ In intervention studies, was a CONSORT flow chart provided to show the flow of participants in the study? ➤ Was the report written in a manner that makes the findings accessible to practicing nurses?	
Researcher credibility	➤ Do the researchers' clinical, substantive, or methodologic qualifications and experience enhance confidence in the findings and their interpretation?	
Summary assessment	➤ Despite any identified limitations, do the study findings appear to be valid—do you have confidence in the *truth* value of the results? ➤ Does the study contribute any meaningful evidence that can be used in nursing practice or that is useful to the nursing discipline?	

We acknowledge that our simplified critiquing guidelines have some shortcomings. In particular, they are generic despite the fact that critiquing cannot use a one-size-fits-all list of questions. Critiquing questions that are relevant to certain types of studies (e.g., experiments) do not fit into a set of general questions for all quantitative studies. Furthermore, supplementary questions would be needed to thoroughly assess certain types of research—for example, grounded theory studies. Thus, you need to use some judgment about whether the guidelines are sufficiently comprehensive for the type of study you are critiquing.

ASPECT OF THE REPORT	CRITIQUING QUESTIONS	DETAILED CRITIQUING GUIDELINES

TABLE 4.2 ▶ **GUIDE TO AN OVERALL CRITIQUE OF A QUALITATIVE RESEARCH REPORT**

ASPECT OF THE REPORT	CRITIQUING QUESTIONS	DETAILED CRITIQUING GUIDELINES
Title	➤ Was the title a good one, suggesting the key phenomenon and the group or community under study?	
Abstract	➤ Does the abstract clearly and concisely summarize the main features of the report?	
Introduction Statement of the problem	➤ Is the problem stated unambiguously and is it easy to identify? ➤ Does the problem statement build a cogent and persuasive argument for the new study? ➤ Does the problem have significance for nursing? ➤ Is there a good match between the research problem on the one hand and the paradigm, tradition, and methods on the other?	Box 6.3, page 163
Research questions	➤ Are research questions explicitly stated? If not, is their absence justified? ➤ Are the questions consistent with the study's philosophical basis, underlying tradition, conceptual framework, or ideological orientation?	Box 6.3, page 163
Literature review	➤ Does the report adequately summarize the existing body of knowledge related to the problem or phenomenon of interest? ➤ Does the literature review provide a solid basis for the new study?	Box 7.1, page 188
Conceptual underpinnings	➤ Are key concepts adequately defined conceptually? ➤ Is the philosophical basis, underlying tradition, conceptual framework, or ideological orientation made explicit?	Box 8.1, page 210
Method Protection of participants' rights	➤ Were appropriate procedures used to safeguard the rights of study participants? Was the study subject to external review by an IRB/ethics review board? ➤ Was the study designed to minimize risks and maximize benefits to participants?	Box 5.2, page 135
Research design and research tradition	➤ Is the identified research tradition (if any) congruent with the methods used to collect and analyze data? ➤ Was an adequate amount of time spent in the field or with study participants? ➤ Did the design unfold in the field, giving researchers opportunities to capitalize on early understandings? ➤ Was there an adequate number of contacts with study participants?	Box 10.1, page 277

TABLE 4.2	GUIDE TO AN OVERALL CRITIQUE OF A QUALITATIVE RESEARCH REPORT (continued)	
ASPECT OF THE REPORT	CRITIQUING QUESTIONS	DETAILED CRITIQUING GUIDELINES
Sample and setting	➤ Was the group or population of interest adequately described? Were the setting and sample described in sufficient detail? ➤ Was the approach used to gain access to the site or to recruit participants appropriate? ➤ Was the best possible method of sampling used to enhance information richness and address the needs of the study? ➤ Was the sample size adequate? Was saturation achieved?	Box 12.2, page 326
Data collection	➤ Were the methods of gathering data appropriate? Were data gathered through two or more methods to achieve triangulation? ➤ Did the researcher ask the right questions or make the right observations, and were they recorded in an appropriate fashion? ➤ Was a sufficient amount of data gathered? Was the data of sufficient depth and richness?	Box 13.3, page 361
Procedures	➤ Were data collection and recording procedures adequately described and do they appear appropriate? ➤ Were data collected in a manner that minimized bias or behavioral distortions? Were the staff who collected data appropriately trained?	Box 13.3, page 361
Enhancement of trustworthiness	➤ Did the researchers use strategies to enhance the trustworthiness/integrity of the study, and was the description of those strategies adequate? ➤ Were the methods used to enhance trustworthiness appropriate and sufficient? ➤ Did the researcher document research procedures and decision processes sufficiently that findings are auditable and confirmable? ➤ Is there evidence of researcher reflexivity?	Box 18.1, page 508
Results Data analysis	➤ Were the data management and data analysis methods sufficiently described? ➤ Was the data analysis strategy compatible with the research tradition and with the nature and type of data gathered? ➤ Did the analysis yield an appropriate "product" (e.g., a theory, taxonomy, thematic pattern, etc.)? ➤ Did the analytic procedures suggest the possibility of biases?	Box 17.2, page 483
Findings	➤ Were the findings effectively summarized, with good use of excerpts and supporting arguments?	Box 17.2, page 483

	GUIDE TO AN OVERALL CRITIQUE OF A QUALITATIVE RESEARCH REPORT (continued)	
TABLE 4.2 ▶		
ASPECT OF THE REPORT	CRITIQUING QUESTIONS	DETAILED CRITIQUING GUIDELINES
	➤ Do the themes adequately capture the meaning of the data? Does it appear that the researcher satisfactorily conceptualized the themes or patterns in the data?	
	➤ Did the analysis yield an insightful, provocative, authentic, and meaningful picture of the phenomenon under investigation?	
Theoretical integration	➤ Are the themes or patterns logically connected to each other to form a convincing and integrated whole?	Box 8.1, page 210 Box 17.2, page 483
	➤ Were figures, maps, or models used effectively to summarize conceptualizations?	
	➤ If a conceptual framework or ideological orientation guided the study, are the themes or patterns linked to it in a cogent manner?	
Discussion Interpretation of the findings	➤ Are the findings interpreted within an appropriate social or cultural context?	Box 18.1, page 508
	➤ Are major findings interpreted and discussed within the context of prior studies?	
	➤ Are the interpretations consistent with the study's limitations?	
	➤ Does the report support transferability of the findings?	
Implications/ recommendations	➤ Do the researchers discuss the implications of the study for clinical practice or further inquiry—and are those implications reasonable and complete?	Box 18.1, page 508
Global Issues Presentation	➤ Was the report well written, well organized, and sufficiently detailed for critical analysis?	
	➤ Was the description of the methods, findings, and interpretations sufficiently rich and vivid?	
Researcher credibility	➤ Do the researchers' clinical, substantive, or methodologic qualifications and experience enhance confidence in the findings and their interpretation?	
Summary assessment	➤ Do the study findings appear to be trustworthy— do you have confidence in the *truth* value of the results?	
	➤ Does the study contribute any meaningful evidence that can be used in nursing practice or that is useful to the nursing discipline?	

Another word of caution is that we developed these guidelines based on our years of experience as research methodologists. They do not represent a formal, rigorously developed set of questions that can be used for a systematic review. They should, however, facilitate beginning efforts to critically appraise nursing studies.

We also note that there are questions in these guidelines for which there are no totally objective answers. Even experts sometimes disagree about methodologic strategies. You should not be afraid to "stick out your neck" to express an evaluative opinion—but your comments should have some basis in methodologic principles discussed in this book. The critiquing guidelines are available in the Toolkit section ⊗ of the accompanying CD-ROM ❷; the question list can be adapted, as appropriate.

Understanding Key Research Challenges

In approaching the task of critiquing a study, it is important to be cognizant of the numerous challenges that researchers face in conducting a study. For example, there are conceptual challenges (e.g., How should key concepts be defined?); financial challenges (How will the study be paid for?); ethical challenges (e.g., Can the study achieve its goals without infringing on human rights?); practical challenges (Will I be able to recruit enough study participants?), and methodologic challenges (Will the adopted methods yield results that can be trusted and applied to other settings?). Most of this book provides guidance relating to the last question, and this section highlights key methodologic challenges as a way of introducing important terms and concepts and further illustrating key differences between qualitative and quantitative research. In reading this section, it is important for you to remember that the worth of a study's evidence for EBP is based on how well researchers deal with these challenges and communicate their decisions.

Inference
Inference is an integral part of doing and critiquing research. An **inference** is a conclusion drawn from the study evidence based on the methods used to generate that evidence. Inference is the attempt to generalize or come to conclusions based on limited information, using logical reasoning processes.

Inference is necessary because researchers use proxies that are intended to "stand in" for the things that are fundamentally of interest. A sample of study participants is a proxy for an entire population. A study site is a proxy for all relevant sites in which the phenomena of interest could unfold. A measuring tool yields proxy information about constructs that can only be captured through fallible approximations. A control group that does not receive an intervention is a proxy for what would happen to the *same* people if they simultaneously received *and* did not receive the intervention.

Researchers face the challenge of using methods that yield good and persuasive evidence in support of inferences that they wish to make. Readers must draw their own inferences based on a critique of methodologic decisions.

Reliability, Validity, and Trustworthiness
Researchers want their inferences to correspond to the *truth*. Research cannot contribute evidence to guide clinical practice if the findings are inaccurate, biased, misinterpreted, or fail to represent the experiences of the target group.

Quantitative researchers use several criteria to assess the quality of a study, sometimes referred to as its **scientific merit.** Two especially important criteria are reliability and validity. **Reliability** refers to the accuracy and consistency of information obtained in a study. The term is most often associated with the methods used to measure research variables. For example, if a thermometer measured Alan's temperature as 98.1°F one minute and as 102.5°F the next minute, the reliability of the thermometer would be highly suspect. The concept of reliability is also important in interpreting the results of statistical analyses. *Statistical reliability* refers to the probability that the same results would be obtained with a completely new sample of subjects—that is, that the results are an accurate reflection of a wider group than just the particular people who participated in the study.

Validity is a more complex concept that broadly concerns the *soundness* of the study's evidence and the degree of inferential support the evidence yields. As with reliability, validity is an important criterion for evaluating methods to measure variables. In this context, the validity question is whether there is evidence to support the inference that the methods are really measuring the abstract concepts that they purport to measure. Is a paper-and-pencil measure of depression *really* measuring depression? Or, is it measuring something else, such as loneliness or stress? Researchers strive for solid conceptual definitions of research variables and valid methods to operationalize them.

Another aspect of validity concerns the quality of the researcher's evidence regarding the link between the independent variable and the dependent variable. Did a nursing intervention *really* bring about improvements in patients' outcomes— or were other factors responsible for patients' progress? Researchers make numerous methodologic decisions that can influence this type of study validity.

Qualitative researchers use somewhat different criteria (and different terminology) in evaluating a study's quality. In general, qualitative researchers discuss methods of enhancing the trustworthiness of the study's data and findings (Lincoln & Guba, 1985). **Trustworthiness** encompasses several different dimensions—credibility, transferability, confirmability, dependability, and authenticity. These and other criteria for evaluating qualitative studies are described in Chapter 18.

Credibility is an especially important aspect of trustworthiness. Credibility is achieved to the extent that the research methods engender confidence in the truth of the data and in the researchers' interpretations of (and inferences from) the data. Credibility in a qualitative study can be enhanced through various approaches, but one strategy in particular merits early discussion because it has implications for the design of all studies, including quantitative ones. **Triangulation** is the use of multiple sources or referents to draw conclusions about what constitutes the truth. In a quantitative study, this might mean having multiple operational definitions of a dependent variable to determine if predicted effects are consistent. In a qualitative study, triangulation might involve trying to understand the full complexity of a poorly understood phenomenon by using multiple means of data collection to converge on the truth (e.g., having in-depth discussions with study participants, as well as watching their behavior in natural settings). Or, it might involve triangulating the ideas and interpretations of multiple researchers working together as a team. Nurse researchers are also beginning to triangulate across paradigms—that is, to integrate both qualitative and quantitative data in a single study to offset the shortcomings of each approach and enhance the validity of the conclusions.

Example of triangulation:
Casey (2007) explored how nurses encourage health-promoting practices in acute settings. Casey triangulated information from observations of nurse–patient interactions with data from in-depth interviews with both the observed nurses and, separately, the observed patients.

Nurse researchers need to design their studies in such a way that threats to the reliability, validity, and trustworthiness of their studies are minimized, and users of research must evaluate the extent to which they were successful.

TIP
In reading and critiquing research reports, it is appropriate to assume a "show me" attitude—that is, to expect researchers to build and present a solid case for the merit of their inferences. They do this by presenting evidence that the findings are reliable and valid or trustworthy.

Bias

Bias is a major concern in research because it can threaten the study's validity and trustworthiness. In general, a **bias** is an influence that produces an error in an estimate or an inference. Biases can affect the quality of evidence in both qualitative and quantitative studies. Bias can result from a number of factors, including study participants' lack of candor or desire to please, researchers' preconceptions, or faulty methods of collecting data.

To some extent, bias can never be avoided totally because the potential for its occurrence is so pervasive. Some bias is haphazard and affects only small segments of the data. As an example of such *random bias*, a handful of study participants might fail to provide accurate information because they were tired at the time of data collection. *Systematic bias* results when the bias is consistent or uniform. For example, if a spring scale consistently measured people's weight as being 2 pounds heavier than their true weight, there would be systematic bias in the data on weight. Rigorous research methods aim to eliminate or minimize bias—or, at least, to detect its presence so it can be taken into account in interpreting the findings.

Researchers adopt a variety of strategies to address bias. Triangulation is one such approach, the idea being that multiple sources of information or points of view help to counterbalance biases and offer avenues to identify them. In quantitative research, methods to combat bias often entail research control.

Research Control

One of the central features of quantitative studies is that they usually involve efforts to tightly control various aspects of the research. **Research control** most typically involves holding constant influences on the dependent variable so that the true relationship between the independent and dependent variables can be understood. In other words, research control attempts to eliminate contaminating factors that might cloud the relationship between the variables that are of central interest.

The issue of contaminating factors—**confounding** (or **extraneous**) **variables**, as they are called—can best be illustrated with an example. Suppose we were interested in studying whether urinary incontinence (UI) is a risk factor for depression. There is some prior evidence that this is the case, but previous studies have failed to clarify whether it is UI per se or other factors that contribute to the risk of depression. The question is whether UI itself (the independent variable) contributes to higher levels of depression, or whether there are other factors that can account for the relationship between UI and depression. We need to design a study to control other determinants of the dependent variable—determinants that are also related to the independent variable, UI.

One confounding variable in this example is age. Levels of depression tend to be higher in older people; at the same time, people with UI tend to be older than those without this problem. In other words, perhaps age is the *real* cause of higher depression in people with UI. If age is not controlled, then any observed relationship between UI and depression could be caused by UI, or by age.

Three possible explanations might be portrayed schematically as follows:

1. UI→depression

2. Age→UI→depression

3.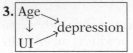

The arrows here symbolize a causal mechanism or an influence. In model 1, UI directly affects depression, independently of any other factors. In model 2, UI is a **mediating variable**—that is, the effect of age on depression is *mediated* by UI. In this model, age affects depression *through* its effect on UI. In model 3, both age and UI have effects on depression, but age also increases the risk of UI. Some research is specifically designed to test paths of mediation and multiple causation, but in the present example age is extraneous to the research question. Our task is to design a study so that the first explanation can be tested. Age must be controlled if our goal is to learn the validity of model 1, which posits that, no matter what a person's age, having UI makes a person more vulnerable to depression.

How can we impose such control? There are a number of ways, as we will discussed in Chapter 9, but the general principle underlying each alternative is that the confounding variables must be **held constant**. The confounding variable must somehow be handled so that, *in the context of the study*, it is not related to the independent or dependent variable. As an example, let us say we wanted to compare the average scores on a depression scale for those with and without UI. We must then design a study in such a way that the ages of the two groups are comparable, even though, in general, the two groups are not comparable in terms of age.

By exercising control over age in this example, we would be taking a step toward explaining the relationship between variables. The world is complex, and many variables are interrelated in complicated ways. When studying a particular problem within the positivist paradigm, it is difficult to study this complexity directly; researchers must usually analyze a couple of relationships at a time and put pieces together like a jigsaw puzzle. That is why even modest studies can contribute to knowledge. The extent of the contribution in a quantitative study, however, is often directly related to how well researchers control confounding influences.

Research rooted in the naturalistic paradigm does not impose controls. With their emphasis on holism and the individuality of human experience, qualitative researchers typically adhere to the view that to impose controls on a research setting is to remove irrevocably some of the meaning of reality.

Randomness

For quantitative researchers, a powerful tool for eliminating bias involves the concept of **randomness**—having certain features of the study established by chance rather than by design or researcher preference. When people are selected *at random* to participate in the study, for example, each person in the initial pool has an equal probability of being selected. This in turn means that there are no systematic biases in the make-up of the study group. Men and women have an equal chance of being selected, for example. Similarly, if study participants are allocated *at random* to groups that will be compared (e.g., an intervention and "usual care" group), then there can be no systematic biases in the composition of the groups. Randomness is a compelling method of controlling confounding variables and reducing bias.

Qualitative researchers do not consider randomness a desirable tool for understanding phenomena. Qualitative researchers tend to use information obtained early in the study in a purposive (nonrandom) fashion to guide their inquiry and to pursue information-rich sources that can help them expand or refine their conceptualizations. Researchers' judgments are viewed as indispensable vehicles for uncovering the complexities of the phenomena of interest.

Example of randomness:

Mok and colleagues (2007) evaluated the effectiveness and safety of three flush solutions for maintaining peripheral intravenous locks in children. A total of 123 children were randomly assigned to receive either normal saline, 1 unit/mL of heparin saline, or 10 units/mL of heparin saline.

Masking or Blinding

A rather charming (but problematic) quality of people is that they usually want things to turn out well. Researchers want their ideas to work and their hypotheses to be supported. Study participants want to be cooperative and helpful, and they also want to present themselves in the best light. These tendencies can affect what participants do and say (and what researchers ask and perceive) and can lead to biases.

A procedure known as **masking** is used in many quantitative studies to prevent biases stemming from *awareness*. Masking involves concealing information from participants, data collectors, care providers, or data analysts to enhance objectivity. For example, if study participants are not aware of whether they are getting an experimental drug or a sham drug (a **placebo**), then their outcomes cannot be influenced by their expectations of its efficacy. Masking involves disguising or withholding information about participants' status in the study (e.g., whether they are in a certain group) or about the study hypotheses.

The term **blinding** is widely used in lieu of *masking* to describe concealment strategies. This term has fallen into some disfavor, however, because of possible pejorative connotations. Medical researchers, however, appear to prefer *blinding* unless the people in the study have vision impairments.

When it proves to be unfeasible or undesirable to use masking, the study is sometimes called an *open study*, in contrast to a *closed study* that results from masking. When masking is used with only some of the people involved in the study (e.g., the study participants), it is often called a **single-blind study**, but when it is possible to mask with two groups (e.g., those delivering an intervention and those receiving it), it is called a **double-blind study.** The previously described study about children exposed to three different flush solutions (Mok et al., 2007) was double blind: neither the children nor the staff nurses (who collecting data about study outcomes such as intravenous complications) were aware of which solution had been used.

Reflexivity

Qualitative researchers do not use methods such as research control, randomness, or masking, but they are nevertheless as interested as quantitative researchers at discovering the true state of human experience. Qualitative researchers often rely on reflexivity to guard against personal bias in making judgments. **Reflexivity** is the process of reflecting critically on the self, and of analyzing and making note of personal values that could affect data collection and interpretation. Qualitative researchers are trained to explore these issues, to be reflexive about all decisions made during the inquiry, and to record their reflexive thoughts in personal diaries and memos.

Example of reflexivity:
Hordern and Street (2007) conducted an in-depth study focused on issues of intimacy and sexuality in the face of a diagnosis of cancer. The researchers were reflexive throughout the process of data collection and data analysis, making a "deliberate and systematic use" (p. E14) of their own responses to the evolving data analysis.

> **TIP**
> Reflexivity can be a useful tool in quantitative as well as qualitative research—self awareness and introspection can enhance the quality of any study.

Generalizability and Transferability

Nurses increasingly rely on evidence from disciplined research as a guide in their clinical practice. Evidence-based practice is based on the assumption that study findings are not unique to the people, places, or circumstances of the original research.

As noted in Chapter 1, **generalizability** is the criterion used in quantitative studies to assess the extent to which the findings can be applied to other groups and settings. How do researchers enhance the generalizability of a study? First and foremost, they must design studies strong in reliability and validity. There is little point in wondering whether results are generalizable if they are not accurate or valid. In selecting participants, researchers must also give thought to the types of people to whom results might be generalized—and then select subjects in such a way that a representative sample is obtained. If a study is intended to have implications for male and female patients, then men and women should be included as participants. If an intervention is intended to benefit poor and affluent patients, then perhaps a multisite study is warranted. Chapter 9 discusses generalizability at greater length.

Qualitative researchers do not specifically seek to make their findings generalizable. Nevertheless, qualitative researchers often seek information that might prove useful in other situations. Lincoln and Guba (1985), in their highly influential book on naturalistic inquiry, discuss the concept of **transferability**, the extent to which qualitative findings can be transferred to other settings, as another aspect of a study's trustworthiness. An important mechanism for promoting transferability is the amount of information qualitative researchers provide about the contexts of their studies. **Thick description**, a widely used term among qualitative researchers, refers to a rich and thorough description of the research setting and of observed transactions and processes. Quantitative researchers, like qualitative researchers, need to describe their study participants and their research settings thoroughly so that the utility of the evidence for others can be assessed.

⬤ RESEARCH EXAMPLES AND CRITICAL THINKING ACTIVITIES

Abstracts for a quantitative and a qualitative nursing study are presented below, followed by some questions to guide critical thinking. A review of the full journal articles would prove useful for learning more about the organization of the report and about study methods and findings.

EXAMPLE 1 ■ Quantitative Research

Study

Prevalence and variation of physical restraint use in acute care settings in the United States (Minnick et al., 2007).

Abstract

Purpose: To describe physical restraint (PR) rates and contexts in U. S. hospitals.

Design: This 2003–2005 descriptive study was done to measure PR prevalence and contexts (census, gender, age, ventilation status, PR type, and rationale) at 40 randomly selected acute care hospitals in six U.S. metropolitan areas. All units except psychiatric, emergency, operative, obstetric, and long-term care were included.

Methods: On 18 randomly selected days between 0500 and 0700 (5:00 am and 7:00 am), data collectors determined PR use and contexts via observation and nurse report.

Findings: PR prevalence was 50 per 1,000 patient days (based on 155,412 patient days). Preventing disruption of therapy was the chief reason cited. PR rates varied by unit type, with adult intensive care unit (ICU) rates the highest obtained. Intra- and interinstitutional variation was as high as 10-fold. Ventilator use was strongly associated with PR use. Elderly patients were over-represented among the physically restrained on some units (e.g., medical), but on many unit types (including most ICUs) their PR use was consistent with those of other adults.

Conclusions: Wide rate variation indicates the need to examine administratively mediated variables and the promotion of unit-based improvement efforts. Anesthetic and sedation practices have contributed to high variation in ICU PR rates. Determining the types of units to target to achieve improvements in care of older adults requires study of PR sequelae rate by unit type.

CRITICAL THINKING SUGGESTIONS*:

*See the Student Resource CD-ROM for a discussion of these questions.

1. "Translate" the abstract into a summary that is more consumer friendly. Underline any technical terms and look them up in the glossary. The Toolkit on the accompanying CD-ROM provides a worksheet that will allow you to enter your translation electronically.
2. Also, consider the following targeted questions, which may assist you in assessing aspects of the study's merit:
   a. Was this abstract an example of a traditional-style abstract?
   b. In which part of the full paper would the information relating to the study purpose be found? How about the information on the design? Where would the researcher's conclusions be located?
   c. What were the independent and dependent variables in this study?
   d. Is this study experimental or nonexperimental?
   e. How, if at all, was *randomness* used in this study?
   f. Comment on the possible generalizability of the study findings.
3. If the results of this study are valid and generalizable, what might be some of the uses to which the findings could be put in clinical practice?

EXAMPLE 2 ■ Qualitative Research

Study

Globalization and the cultural safety of an immigrant Muslim community (Baker, 2007).

Abstract

Aim: This paper reports a study the aim of which was to further understanding of cultural safety by focusing on the social health of a small immigrant community of Muslims in a relatively homogeneous region of Canada following the terrorist attacks on 11 September 2001 (9/11).

Background: The aftermath of 9/11 negatively affected Muslims living in many centers of western Europe and North America. Little is known about the social health of Muslims in smaller areas with little cultural diversity. Developed by Maori nurses, the cultural safety concept captures the negative health effects of inequities experienced by the indigenous people of New Zealand. Nurses in Canada have used the concept to understand the health of Aboriginal peoples. It has also been used to investigate the nursing care of immigrants in a Canadian metropolitan center. Findings indicated, however, that the dichotomy between culturally safe and unsafe groups was blurred.

Method: The methodology was qualitative, based on the constructivist paradigm. A purposive sample of 26 Muslims of Middle Eastern, Indian, or Pakistani origin residing in the province of New Brunswick, Canada were interviewed in 2002–2003.

Findings: Participants experienced a sudden transition from cultural safety to cultural risk following 9/11. Their experience of cultural safety included a sense of social integration in the community and invisibility as a minority. Cultural risk stemmed from being in the spotlight of an international media and becoming a visible minority.

Conclusion: Cultural risk is not necessarily rooted in historical events and may be generated by outside forces rather than by longstanding inequities in relationships between groups within the community. Nurses need to think about the cultural safety of their practices when caring for members of socially disadvantaged cultural minority groups because this may affect the health services delivered to them.

CRITICAL THINKING SUGGESTIONS:

1. "Translate" the abstract into a summary that is more consumer friendly. Underline any technical terms and look them up in the glossary. The Toolkit on the accompanying CD-ROM provides a worksheet that will allow you to enter your translation electronically. ✖
2. Also, consider the following targeted questions, which may assist you in assessing aspects of the study's merit:
   a. Was this abstract an example of a traditional-style abstract?
   b. In which part of the full paper would the information relating to the study aim and background be found? Where would the researcher's conclusions be located?
   c. On which qualitative research tradition, if any, was this study based?
   d. Is this study experimental or nonexperimental?
   e. How, if at all, was *randomness* used in this study?
   f. Is there any indication in the abstract that *triangulation* was used? *Reflexivity*?
   g. Comment on the possible transferability of the study findings.
3. If the results of this study are trustworthy and transferable, what might be some of the uses to which the findings could be put in clinical practice?

EXAMPLE 3 ■ Quantitative Research in Appendix A

1. Read the abstract for Howell and colleagues' (2007) study ("Anxiety, anger, and blood pressure in children") in Appendix A of this book. "Translate" the abstract into a summary that is more consumer friendly. Underline any technical terms and look them up in the glossary.
2. Also, consider the following targeted questions, which may assist you in assessing aspects of the study's merit:
   a. Was this abstract an example of a traditional-style abstract?
   b. How, if at all, was *randomness* used in this study?
   c. Comment on the possible generalizability of the study findings.

EXAMPLE 4 ■ Qualitative Research in Appendix B

1. Read the abstract for Beck's (2006) study ("Anniversary of birth trauma") in Appendix B of this book. "Translate" the abstract into a summary that is more consumer friendly. Underline any technical terms and look them up in the glossary.

2. Also, consider the following targeted questions, which may assist you in assessing aspects of the study's merit:

   a. Was this abstract an example of a traditional-style abstract?

   b. How, if at all, was *randomness* used in this study?

   c. Is there any indication in the abstract that *triangulation* was used? *Reflexivity*?

   d. Comment on the possible transferability of the study findings.

CHAPTER REVIEW

Key new terms introduced in the chapter, together with a summary of major points, are presented in this section. Chapter 4 of the *Study Guide for Essentials of Nursing Research,* 7th edition also offers exercises and study suggestions for reinforcing the concepts presented in this chapter. For additional review, see self-study questions on the CD-ROM provided with this book.

Key New Terms

Abstract	Inference	Research control
Bias	Journal article	Scientific merit
Blind review	Level of significance	Single blind study
Blinding	Masking	Statistical significance
Confounding variable	Mediating variable	Statistical test
Credibility	*p*	Thick description
Critique	Placebo	Transferability
Double-blind study	Poster session	Triangulation
Extraneous variable	Randomness	Trustworthiness
Findings	Reflexivity	Validity
IMRAD format	Reliability	

Summary Points

➤ Both qualitative and quantitative researchers disseminate their findings, most often by publishing reports of their research as **journal articles**, which concisely communicate what the researcher did and what was found.

➤ Journal articles often consist of an **abstract** (a brief synopsis of the study) and four major sections that typically follow the **IMRAD format**: an **I**ntroduction (explanation of the study problem and its context); **M**ethod section (the strategies used to address the problem); **R**esults section (study findings); and **D**iscussion (interpretation of the findings).

➤ Research reports are often difficult to read because they are dense, concise, and contain jargon. Quantitative research reports may be intimidating at first because, compared with qualitative reports, they are more impersonal and report on statistical tests.

➤ **Statistical tests** are used to test research hypotheses and to evaluate the believ-ability of the findings. Findings that are **statistically significant** are ones that have a high probability of being "real."

➤ The ultimate goal of this book is to help students to prepare a research **critique**, which is a careful, critical appraisal of the strengths and limitations of a piece of research, often for the purpose of considering the worth of its evidence for nursing practice.

➤ Researchers face numerous conceptual, ethical, and methodologic challenges that must be considered in critiquing a study. The manner in which method-ologic challenges are met affects the inferences that can be made.

➤ An **inference** is a conclusion drawn from the study evidence based on the meth-ods used to generate that evidence. Inference is the attempt to come to conclu-sions based on limited information. Researchers want their inferences to corre-spond to the *truth*.

➤ **Reliability** (a key challenge in quantitative research) refers to the accuracy and consistency of information obtained in a study. **Validity** is a more complex con-cept that broadly concerns the *soundness* of the study's evidence—that is, whether the findings are cogent, convincing, and well grounded.

➤ **Trustworthiness** in qualitative research encompasses several different dimen-sions, including credibility, dependability, confirmability, transferability, and authenticity.

➤ **Credibility** is achieved to the extent that the qualitative methods engender con-fidence in the truth of the data and in the researchers' interpretations of the data. **Triangulation**, the use of multiple sources or referents to draw conclusions about what constitutes the truth, is one approach to establishing credibility.

➤ A **bias** is an influence that produces a distortion in the study results. *Systematic bias* results when a bias is consistent across participants or situations.

➤ In quantitative studies, **research control** is used to *hold constant* outside influ-ences on the dependent variable so that the relationship between the independent and dependent variables can be better understood.

➤ Researchers seek to control **confounding** (or **extraneous**) **variables**—variables that are extraneous to the purpose of a specific study.

➤ For quantitative researchers, **randomness**—having certain features of the study established by chance rather than by design or personal preference—is a powerful tool to eliminate bias.

➤ **Masking** (or **blinding**) is sometimes used to avoid biases stemming from par-ticipants' or research agents' awareness of study hypotheses or research status. **Single-blind studies** involve masking for one group (e.g., participants) and **double-blind studies** involve masking for two groups.

➤ **Reflexivity,** the process of reflecting critically on the self and of scrutinizing per-sonal values that could affect data collection and interpretation, is an important tool in qualitative research.

➤ **Generalizability** in a quantitative study concerns the extent to which the findings can be applied to other groups and settings.

➤ A similar concept in qualitative studies is **transferability**, the extent to which qualitative findings can be transferred to other settings. One mechanism for promoting transferability is **thick description**, the rich and thorough description of the research setting or context so that others can make inferences about contextual similarities.

STUDIES CITED IN CHAPTER 4

Baker, C. (2007). Globalization and the cultural safety of an immigrant Muslim community. *Journal of Advanced Nursing, 57*, 296–305.

Casey, D. (2007). Findings from non-participant observational data concerning health promoting nursing practice in the acute hospital setting focusing on generalist nurses. *Journal of Clinical Nursing, 16*, 580–592.

Efe, E., & Özer, Z. (2007). The use of breastfeeding for pain relief during neonatal immunization injections. *Applied Nursing Research, 20*, 10–16.

Hordern, A., & Street, A. (2007). Issues of intimacy and sexuality in the face of cancer: The patient perspective. *Cancer Nursing, 30*, E11–18.

Lyons, K., Sayer, A., Archbold, P., Hornbrook, M., & Stewart, B. (2007). The enduring and contextual effects of physical health and depression on care-dyad mutuality. *Research in Nursing & Health, 30*, 84–98.

Minnick, A., Mion, L., Johnson, M., Catrambone, C., & Leipzig, R. (2007). Prevalence and variation of physical restraint use in acute care settings. *Journal of Nursing Scholarship, 39*, 30–37.

Mok, E., Kwong, T. K., & Chan, M. F. (2007). A randomized controlled trial for maintaining peripheral intravenous lock in children. *International Journal of Nursing Practice, 13*, 33–45.

Polzer, R., & Miles, M. (2007). Spirituality in African Americans with diabetes: Self-management through a relationship with God. *Qualitative Health Research, 17*, 176–188.

C H A P T E R

5 Ethics in Research

STUDENT OBJECTIVES

On completing this chapter, you will be able to:

➤ Discuss the historical background that led to the creation of various codes of ethics

➤ Understand the potential for ethical dilemmas stemming from conflicts between ethics and requirements for high-quality research evidence

➤ Identify the three primary ethical principles articulated in the *Belmont Report* and the important dimensions encompassed by each

➤ Identify procedures for adhering to ethical principles and protecting study participants

➤ Given sufficient information, evaluate the ethical dimension of a research report

➤ Define new terms in the chapter

ETHICS AND RESEARCH

In any discipline that involves research with human beings or animals, researchers must address ethical issues. Ethical concerns are especially prominent in nursing research because the line of demarcation between what constitutes the expected practice of nursing and the collection of research data can sometimes get blurred. Furthermore, ethics can create particular challenges because ethical requirements sometimes conflict with the need to produce high-quality evidence for practice. This chapter discusses major ethical principles that should be considered in reviewing studies.

Historical Background

As modern, civilized people, we might like to think that systematic violations of moral principles within a research context occurred centuries ago rather than recently, but this is not the case. The Nazi medical experiments of the 1930s and 1940s are the most famous examples of recent disregard for ethical conduct. The Nazi program of research involved the use of prisoners of war and racial "enemies" in numerous experiments designed to test the limits of human endurance and human reaction to diseases and untested drugs. The studies were unethical, not only because they exposed these people to physical harm and even death, but because subjects could not refuse participation.

There are more recent examples from the United States and other Western countries. For instance, between 1932 and 1972, a study known as the Tuskegee Syphilis Study, sponsored by the U.S. Public Health Service, investigated the effects of syphilis among 400 men from a poor African American community. Medical treatment was deliberately withheld to study the course of the untreated disease. A public health nurse, Eunice Rivers, was involved in carrying out that study and recruited most of the participants (Vessey & Gennaro, 1994). Similarly, Dr. Herbert Green of the National Women's Hospital in Auckland, New Zealand studied women with cervical cancer in the 1980s; patients with carcinoma in situ were not given treatment so that researchers could study the natural progression of the disease. Another well-known case of unethical research involved the injection of live cancer cells into elderly patients at the Jewish Chronic Disease Hospital in Brooklyn in the 1960s without the consent of those patients. At about the same time, Dr. Saul Krugman was conducting research at Willowbrook, an institution for the mentally retarded, where children were deliberately infected with the hepatitis virus. Even more recently, it was revealed in 1993 that U. S. federal agencies had sponsored radiation experiments since the 1940s on hundreds of people, many of them prisoners or elderly hospital patients. Many other examples of studies with ethical transgressions—often much more subtle than these examples—have emerged to give ethical concerns the visibility they have today.

Codes of Ethics

In response to human rights violations, various **codes of ethics** have been developed. One of the first international efforts to establish ethical standards was the

Nuremberg Code, developed in 1949 after the Nazi atrocities were made public. Several other international standards have subsequently been developed, the most notable of which is the Declaration of Helsinki, which was adopted in 1964 by the World Medical Association and most recently revised in 2000, with clarifications published in 2004.

Most disciplines have established their own code of ethics. For example, guidelines for psychologists were published by the American Psychological Association (2002) in *Ethical Principles of Psychologist and Code of Conduct*. The American Medical Association regularly updates its *Code of Medical Ethics*.

Nurses have developed their own ethical guidelines. In the United States, the American Nurses Association (ANA) issued *Ethical Guidelines in the Conduct, Dissemination, and Implementation of Nursing Research* in 1995 (Silva, 1995). ANA also published in 2001 a revised *Code of Ethics for Nurses with Interpretive Statements*, a document that covers primarily ethical issues for practicing nurses but that also includes principles that apply to nurse researchers. In Canada, the Canadian Nurses Association most recently published its *Ethical Research Guidelines for Registered Nurses* in 2002.

Some nurse ethicists have called for an international code of ethics for nursing research, but nurses in most countries have developed their own professional codes or follow codes established by their governments. The International Council of Nurses (ICN), however, has developed the *ICN Code of Ethics for Nurses*, which was most recently updated in 2006.

TIP

Many useful websites are devoted to ethical principles, several of which are listed in the "Useful Websites for Chapter 5" file on the accompanying CD-ROM, for you to click on directly.

Government Regulations for Protecting Study Participants

Governments throughout the world fund research and establish rules for adhering to ethical principles. For example, Health Canada specified the *Tri-Council Policy Statement: Ethical Conduct for Research Involving Humans* as the guidelines to protect human subjects in all types of research. In Australia, the National Health and Medical Research Council, issued the *National Statement on Ethical Conduct in Research Involving Humans* in 1999 and also issued a special statement on research with Aboriginal peoples in 2003.

In the United States, an important code of ethics was adopted by the National Commission for the Protection of Human Subjects of Biomedical and Behavioral Research. The commission issued a report in 1978, referred to as the ***Belmont Report***, which provided a model for many of the guidelines adopted by disciplinary organizations in the United States. The *Belmont Report* also served as the basis for regulations affecting research sponsored by the U.S. government, including studies supported by NINR. The U.S. Department of Health and Human Services (DHHS) has issued ethical regulations that have been codified at Title 45 Part 46 of the Code of Federal Regulations (45CFR46). These regulations, revised most recently in

2005, are among the most widely used guidelines in the United States for evaluating the ethical aspects of health-related studies.

Ethical Dilemmas in Conducting Research

Research that violates ethical principles is rarely done specifically to be cruel, but more typically occurs out of a conviction that knowledge is important and potentially life-saving or beneficial in the long run. There are research problems in which participants' rights and study demands are put in direct conflict, posing **ethical dilemmas** for researchers. Here are examples of research problems in which the desire for rigor conflicts with ethical considerations:

1. *Research question:* Are nurses equally empathic in their treatment of male and female patients in the ICU?

   Ethical dilemma: Ethics require that participants be made aware of their role in a study. Yet, if the researcher informs nurses participating in this study that their degree of empathy in treating male and female patients will be scrutinized, will their behavior be "normal?" If the nurses' usual behavior is altered because of the known presence of research observers, then the findings will not be valid.

2. *Research question:* What are the coping mechanisms of parents whose children have a terminal illness?

   Ethical dilemma: To answer this question, the researcher may need to probe into the psychological state of the parents at a vulnerable time; such probing could be painful and even traumatic. Yet knowledge of the parents' coping mechanisms might help to design more effective ways of dealing with parents' grief and stress.

3. *Research question:* Does a new medication prolong life in patients with cancer?

   Ethical dilemma: The best way to test the effectiveness of an intervention is to administer it to some participants but withhold it from others to see the groups have different outcomes. However, if the intervention is untested (e.g., a new drug), the group receiving the intervention may be exposed to harmful side effects. On the other hand, the group *not* receiving the drug may be denied a beneficial treatment.

4. *Research question:* What is the process by which adult children adapt to the day-to-day stresses of caring for a parent with Alzheimer's disease?

   Ethical dilemma: In a qualitative study, which would be appropriate for this question, a researcher may become so closely involved with participants that they become willing to share "secrets." Interviews can become confessions—sometimes of unseemly or even illegal behavior. In this example, suppose a woman admitted to physically abusing her mother—how can the researcher report such information to authorities without undermining a pledge of confidentiality? And, if the researcher divulges the information to appropriate authorities, how can a pledge of confidentiality be given in good faith to other participants?

As these examples suggest, researchers are sometimes in a bind. Their goal is to develop the highest-quality evidence for practice, using the best methods available—

but they must also adhere to rules for protecting human rights. Another type of dilemma may arise if nurse researchers face conflict-of-interest situations, in which their expected behavior as nurses conflicts with the standard behavior of researchers (e.g., deviating from a standard research protocol to give needed assistance to a patient). It is precisely because of such conflicts and dilemmas that codes of ethics have been developed to guide the efforts of researchers.

ETHICAL PRINCIPLES FOR PROTECTING STUDY PARTICIPANTS

The *Belmont Report* articulated three primary ethical principles on which standards of ethical conduct in research are based: beneficence, respect for human dignity, and justice. We briefly discuss these principles and then describe procedures researchers adopt to comply with these principles.

Beneficence

One of the most fundamental ethical principles in research is that of **beneficence,** which imposes a duty on researchers to minimize harm and to maximize benefits. Human research should be intended to produce benefits for participants themselves or—a situation that is more common—for other individuals or society as a whole. This principle covers multiple dimensions.

The Right to Freedom from Harm and Discomfort

Researchers have an obligation to avoid, prevent, or minimize harm (*nonmaleficence*) in studies with humans. Participants must not be subjected to unnecessary risks of harm or discomfort, and their participation in research must be essential to achieving scientifically and societally important aims that could not otherwise be realized. In research with humans, *harm* and *discomfort* can take many forms; they can be physical (e.g., injury), emotional (e.g., stress), social (e.g., loss of social support), or financial (e.g., loss of wages). Ethical researchers must use strategies to minimize all types of harm and discomfort, even ones that are temporary.

Exposing study participants to experiences that result in serious or permanent harm clearly is unacceptable. Ethical researchers must be prepared to terminate the research if there is reason to suspect that continuation would result in injury, death, or undue distress to study participants. Protecting human beings from physical harm is often straightforward, but it is not as easy to address the psychological consequences of participating in a study, which can be subtle. For example, participants may be asked questions about their personal views, weaknesses, or fears. Such queries might lead people to reveal sensitive personal information. The point is not that researchers should refrain from asking questions but rather that they need to be aware of the nature of the intrusion on people's psyches.

The need for sensitivity may be greater in qualitative studies, which often involve in-depth exploration into highly personal areas. In-depth probing may actually expose deep-seated fears and anxieties that study participants had previously repressed. Qualitative researchers, regardless of the underlying research tradition, must thus be especially vigilant in anticipating such problems.

The Right to Protection from Exploitation

Involvement in a study should not place participants at a disadvantage or expose them to situations for which they have not been prepared. Participants need to be assured that their participation, or information they might provide, will not be used against them in any way. For example, a person describing his or her economic circumstances to a researcher should not be exposed to the risk of losing public health benefits; a person reporting drug abuse should not fear exposure to criminal authorities.

Study participants enter into a special relationship with researchers, and it is crucial that this relationship not be exploited. Exploitation may be overt and malicious (e.g., sexual exploitation), but it might also be more subtle (e.g., getting participants to provide additional information in a 1-year follow-up interview, without having warned them of this possibility at the outset).

Because nurse researchers may have a nurse–patient (in addition to a researcher–participant) relationship, special care may need to be exercised to avoid exploiting that bond. Patients' consent to participate in a study may result from their understanding of the researcher's role as *nurse*, not as *researcher*.

In qualitative research, the risk of exploitation may become especially acute because the psychological distance between investigators and participants typically declines as the study progresses. The emergence of a pseudotherapeutic relationship is not uncommon, which imposes additional responsibilities on researchers— and additional risks that exploitation could inadvertently occur. On the other hand, qualitative researchers typically are in a better position than quantitative researchers to *do good*, rather than just to avoid doing harm, because of the close relationships they often develop with participants.

Example of therapeutic research experiences:

Participants in Beck's (2005) studies on birth trauma and post-traumatic stress disorder (PTSD) expressed a range of benefits they derived from e-mail exchanges with Beck. Here is what one informant voluntarily shared: "You thanked me for everything in your e-mail, and I want to THANK YOU for caring. For me, it means a lot that you have taken an interest in this subject and are taking the time and effort to find out more about PTSD. For someone to even acknowledge this condition means a lot for someone who has suffered from it" (p. 417).

Respect for Human Dignity

Respect for human dignity is the second ethical principle articulated in the *Belmont Report*. This principle includes the right to self-determination and the right to full disclosure.

The Right to Self-Determination

Researchers should treat participants as autonomous agents, capable of controlling their own activities. The principle of *self-determination* means that prospective participants have the right to decide voluntarily whether to participate in a study, without risking penalty or prejudicial treatment. It also means that people have the right to ask questions, to refuse to give information, and to withdraw from the study.

A person's right to self-determination includes freedom from coercion of any type. *Coercion* involves explicit or implicit threats of penalty from failing to participate in a study or excessive rewards from agreeing to participate. The obligation to protect people from coercion requires careful thought when researchers are in a position of authority, control, or influence over potential participants, as might be the case in a nurse–patient relationship. The issue of coercion may require scrutiny in other situations as well. For example, a generous monetary incentive (or **stipend**) offered to encourage the participation of an economically disadvantaged group (e.g., the homeless) might be considered mildly coercive because such incentives may place undue pressure on prospective participants.

The Right to Full Disclosure

The principle of respect for human dignity encompasses people's right to make informed, voluntary decisions about study participation, which requires full disclosure. **Full disclosure** means that the researcher has fully described the nature of the study, the person's right to refuse participation, the researcher's responsibilities, and likely risks and benefits. The right to self-determination and the right to full disclosure are the two major elements on which informed consent—discussed later in this chapter—is based.

Adherence to the guideline for full disclosure is not always straightforward. Full disclosure can sometimes create two types of bias: biases affecting the accuracy of the data and biases reflecting sample recruitment problems. Suppose we were testing the hypothesis that high school students with a high absentee rate are more likely to be substance abusers than students with good attendance. If we approached potential participants and fully explained the purpose of the study, some students likely would refuse to participate, and nonparticipation would be selective (biased); students who are substance abusers—the group of primary interest—might be least likely to participate. Moreover, by knowing the research question, those who do participate might not give candid responses. In such a situation, full disclosure could undermine the study.

One technique that researchers sometimes use in such situations is *covert data collection* or *concealment*—collecting data without participants' knowledge and thus without their consent. This might happen, for example, if a researcher wanted to observe people's behavior in a real-world setting and was concerned that doing so openly would result in changes in the very behavior of interest. Researchers might choose to obtain the information through concealed methods, such as by videotaping with hidden equipment or observing while pretending to be engaged in other activities.

A more controversial technique is the use of deception. **Deception** can involve deliberately withholding information about the study, or providing participants with false information. For example, in studying high school students' use of drugs, we might describe the research as a study of students' health practices, which is a mild form of misinformation.

Deception and concealment are problematic ethically because they interfere with participants' right to make truly informed decisions about personal costs and benefits of participation. Some people argue that deception is never justified. Others, however, believe that if the study involves minimal risk to subjects and if there are anticipated benefits to society, then deception may be justified to enhance the validity of the findings.

Full disclosure has emerged as a concern in connection with data collection over the Internet (e.g., analyzing the content of messages posted to chat rooms or on listserves). The issue is whether such messages can be used as data without the authors' consent. Some researchers believe that anything posted electronically is in the public domain and therefore can be used for research without formal consent. Others, however, feel that the same ethical standards must apply in cyberspace research and that electronic researchers must carefully protect the rights of individuals who are participants in "virtual" communities. Various protective strategies have been proposed—for example, that researchers negotiate their entry into an electronic community such as a chat room with the list owner before collecting data.

Justice

The third broad principle articulated in the *Belmont Report* concerns justice, which includes participants' right to fair treatment and their right to privacy.

The Right to Fair Treatment

One aspect of the justice principle concerns the equitable distribution of benefits and burdens of research. The selection of study participants should be based on research requirements and not on the vulnerability or compromised position of certain people. Historically, subject selection has been a key ethical concern, with many researchers selecting groups deemed to have lower social standing (e.g., poor people, prisoners, the mentally retarded) as study participants. The principle of justice imposes particular obligations toward individuals who are unable to protect their own interests (e.g., dying patients) to ensure that they are not exploited for the advancement of knowledge.

Distributive justice also imposes duties to neither neglect nor discriminate against individuals and groups who may benefit from advances in research. During the early 1990s, there was evidence that women and minorities were being unfairly *ex*cluded from many clinical studies in the United States. This led to the promulgation of regulations (updated in 2001) requiring that researchers who seek funding from the National Insitutes of Health (including NINR) include women and minorities as study participants. The regulations also require researchers to examine whether clinical interventions have differential effects (e.g., whether benefits are different for men than for women).

The right to fair treatment encompasses other obligations. It means that researchers must treat people who decline to participate in a study or who withdraw from it in a nonprejudicial manner; they must honor all agreements made with participants, including the payment of any promised stipends; demonstrate sensitivity to (and respect for) the beliefs, habits, and lifestyles of people from different backgrounds or cultures; and afford participants courteous and tactful treatment at all times.

The Right to Privacy

Virtually all research with humans involves intruding into personal lives. Researchers should ensure that their research is not more intrusive than it needs to be and that participants' privacy is maintained throughout the study. Participants have the right to expect that any data they provide will be kept in strictest confidence.

Privacy issues have become even more salient in the U.S. health care community since the passage of the Health Insurance Portability and Accountability Act of 1996 (HIPAA), which articulates federal standards to protect patients' medical records and other health information. In response to the HIPAA legislation, the U. S. Department of Health and Human Services issued the regulations *Standards for Privacy of Individually Identifiable Health Information*. For most covered entities (health care providers who transmit health information electronically), compliance with these regulations, known as the Privacy Rule, was required as of April 14, 2003.

> **TIP**
>
> Here are two websites that offer information about the implications of HIPAA for research: http://privacyruleandresearch.nih.gov/ and www.hhs.gov/ocr/hipaa/guidelines/research.pdf.

PROCEDURES FOR PROTECTING STUDY PARTICIPANTS

Now that you are familiar with fundamental ethical principles for conducting research, you need to understand the procedures researchers follow to adhere to them. It is these procedures that should be evaluated in critiquing the ethical aspects of a study.

> **TIP**
>
> When information about ethical considerations is presented in research reports, it almost always appears in the method section, typically in the subsection devoted to data collection procedures.

Risk–Benefit Assessments

One strategy that researchers use to protect participants is to conduct a **risk–benefit assessment.** Such an assessment is designed to determine whether the benefits of participating in a study are in line with the costs, be they financial, physical, emotional, or social (i.e., whether the *risk-to-benefit* ratio is acceptable). Box 5.1 summarizes major costs and benefits of research participation.

The risk-to-benefit ratio should also be considered in terms of whether the risks to participants are commensurate with the benefit to society and to nursing in terms of the quality of evidence produced. The general guideline is that the degree of risk to be taken by participants should never exceed the potential humanitarian benefits of the knowledge to be gained. Thus, the selection of a significant topic that

---

BOX 5.1 POTENTIAL BENEFITS AND RISKS OF RESEARCH TO PARTICIPANTS

▶

Major Potential Benefits to Participants

- Access to a potentially beneficial intervention that might otherwise be unavailable to them
- Comfort in being able to discuss their situation or problem with a friendly, objective person
- Increased knowledge about themselves or their conditions, either through opportunity for introspection and self-reflection or through direct interaction with researchers
- Escape from a normal routine, excitement of being part of a study
- Satisfaction that information they provide may help others with similar problems or conditions
- Direct monetary or material gain through stipends or other incentives

Major Potential Risks to Participants

- Physical harm, including unanticipated side effects
- Physical discomfort, fatigue, or boredom
- Psychological or emotional distress resulting from self-disclosure, introspection, fear of the unknown, discomfort with strangers, fear of eventual repercussions, anger or embarrassment at the type of questions being asked
- Social risks, such as the risk of stigma, adverse effects on personal relationships, loss of status
- Loss of privacy
- Loss of time
- Monetary costs (e.g., for transportation, child care, time lost from work)

---

has the potential to improve patient care is the first step in ensuring that research is ethical.

TIP

In evaluating the risk-to-benefit ratio of a study design, you might want to consider how comfortable *you* would have felt about being a study participant.

All research involves some risks, but in many cases, the risk is minimal. **Minimal risk** is defined as a risk expected to be no greater than those ordinarily encountered in daily life or during routine physical or psychological tests or procedures. When the risks are not minimal, researchers must proceed with caution, taking every step possible to reduce risks and maximize benefits.

In quantitative studies, most of the details of the study are usually spelled out in advance, and therefore a reasonably accurate risk–benefit assessment can be developed. Qualitative studies, however, usually evolve as data are gathered, and it may therefore be more difficult to assess all risks at the outset of a study. Qualitative researchers thus must remain sensitive to potential risks throughout the research process.

Example of ongoing risk-benefit assessment:

Carlsson and colleagues (2007) discussed methodologic and ethical issues relating to the conduct of interviews with people who have brain damage. The need for ongoing vigilance and attention to cues about risks and benefits was noted. The researchers stated that one interview had to be interrupted because the participant was displaying signs of distress. After the interview, however, the participant declined counseling, and expressed gratitude for having had the opportunity to discuss his experience.

Informed Consent

One particularly important procedure for safeguarding participants and protecting their right to self-determination involves obtaining their informed consent. **Informed consent** means that participants have adequate information regarding the research, comprehend the information, and have the power of free choice, enabling them to consent to or decline participation voluntarily.

Researchers usually document the informed consent process by having participants sign a **consent form**, an example of which is presented in Figure 5.1. This form includes information about the study purpose, specific expectations regarding participation (e.g., how much time will be required), the voluntary nature of participation, and potential costs and benefits.

Example of informed consent:

Esperat and co-researchers (2007) studied the health behaviors of low-income pregnant women in Texas. Consent forms were prepared in both English and Spanish. A bilingual research assistant explained the need for the consent form and determined the literacy levels of all participants. The research assistant provided any needed assistance in completing the form.

Researchers rarely obtain written informed consent when the primary means of data collection is through self-administered questionnaires. Researchers generally assume **implied consent** (i.e., that the return of the completed questionnaire reflects the respondent's voluntary consent to participate). This assumption may not always be warranted, however (e.g., if patients feel that their treatment might be affected by failure to cooperate).

In some qualitative studies, especially those requiring repeated contact with participants, it is difficult to obtain a meaningful informed consent at the outset. Qualitative researchers do not always know in advance how the study will evolve. Because the research design emerges during data collection and analysis, researchers may not know the exact nature of the data to be collected, what the risks and benefits will be, or how much of a time commitment will be required. Thus, in a qualitative study, consent may be viewed as an ongoing, transactional process, referred to as **process consent**. In process consent, researchers continuously renegotiate the consent, allowing participants to play a collaborative role in the decision-making process regarding their ongoing participation.

I understand that I am being asked to participate in a research study at Saint Francis Hospital and Medical Center. This research study will evaluate: What it is like being a mother of multiples during the first year of the infants' lives. If I agree to participate in the study, I will be interviewed for approximately 30 to 60 minutes about my experience as a mother of multiple infants. The interview will be tape-recorded and take place in a private office at St. Francis Hospital. No identifying information will be included when the interview is transcribed. I understand I will receive $25.00 for participating in the study. There are no known risks associated with this study.

I realize that I may not participate in the study if I am younger than 18 years of age or I cannot speak English.

I realize that the knowledge gained from this study may help either me or other mothers of multiple infants in the future.

I realize that my participation in this study is entirely voluntary, and I may withdraw from the study at any time I wish. If I decide to discontinue my participation in this study, I will continue to be treated in the usual and customary fashion.

I understand that all study data will be kept confidential. However, this information may be used in nursing publications or presentations.

I understand that if I sustain injuries from my participation in this research project, I will not be automatically compensated by Saint Francis Hospital and Medical Center.

If I need to, I can contact Dr. Cheryl Beck, University of Connecticut, School of Nursing, any time during the study.

The study has been explained to me. I have read and understand this consent form, all of my questions have been answered, and I agree to participate. I understand that I will be given a copy of this signed consent form.

_____   _____
Signature of Participant   Date

_____   _____
Signature of Witness   Date

_____   _____
Signature of Investigator   Date

FIGURE 5.1   Example of an informed consent form.

Example of process consent:
Treacy and colleagues (2007) conducted a three-round longitudinal study of children's emerging perspectives and experiences of cigarette smoking. Parents and children consented to the children's participation. At each round, consent to continue participating in the study was reconfirmed.

Confidentiality Procedures

Study participants have the right to expect that any data they provide will be kept in the strictest confidence. Participants' right to privacy is protected through various confidentiality procedures.

Anonymity

Anonymity, the most secure means of protecting confidentiality, occurs when even the researcher cannot link participants to their data. For example, if questionnaires were distributed to a group of nursing home residents and were returned without any identifying information on them, responses would be anonymous. As another example, if a researcher reviewed hospital records from which all identifying information (e.g., name, address, social security number, and so forth) had been expunged, anonymity would again protect participants' right to privacy.

Example of anonymity:
Houfek and colleagues (2008) distributed an anonymous questionnaire to learn about people's knowledge and beliefs about the relationship between genetics and smoking. Study participants, who were staff and visitors at a health care facility, returned completed questionnaires to a secure collection box at the facility or via postage-paid mail.

Confidentiality in the Absence of Anonymity

When anonymity is impossible, appropriate confidentiality procedures need to be implemented. A promise of **confidentiality** is a pledge that any information participants provide will not be publicly reported in a manner that identifies them and will not be made accessible to others.

Researchers generally develop elaborate confidentiality procedures. These include securing confidentiality assurances from everyone involved in collecting or analyzing research data; maintaining identifying information in locked files to which few people have access; substituting *identification (ID) numbers* for participants' names on study records and computer files to prevent any accidental breach of confidentiality; and reporting only aggregate data for groups of participants or taking steps to disguise a person's identity in a research report.

Anonymity is rarely possible in qualitative studies because qualitative researchers become thoroughly involved with participants. Confidentiality is especially salient in qualitative studies because, due to their in-depth nature, there may be a greater invasion of privacy than in quantitative research. Researchers who spend time in participants' homes may, for example, have difficulty segregating the public behavior participants are willing to share from the private behavior that unfolds unwittingly during data collection. A final issue many qualitative researchers face is adequately disguising participants in their reports to avoid a breach of confidentiality. Because the number of respondents is small and because rich descriptive information is presented, qualitative researchers need to take extra precautions to safeguard participants' identity. This may mean more than simply using a fictitious name—it may also mean withholding information about key characteristics of informants, such as age and occupation.

> **TIP**
>
> As a means of enhancing both individual and institutional privacy, research reports frequently avoid giving explicit information about the locale of the study. For example, a report might say that data were collected in a 200-bed, private nursing home, without mentioning its name or location.

It should be noted that there are situations in which confidentiality can create tensions between researchers and legal authorities, especially if study participants are involved in criminal activity (e.g., substance abuse). To avoid the possibility of forced, involuntary disclosure of sensitive research information (e.g., through a court order), researchers in the United States can apply for a **Certificate of Confidentiality** from the National Institutes of Health (NIH). A Certificate allows researchers to refuse to disclose identifying information on study participants in any civil, criminal, administrative, or legislative proceeding at the federal, state, or local level.

Example of confidentiality procedures:
Laughon (2007) conducted an in-depth study of the ways in which poor, urban African American women with a history of physical abuse stay healthy. The 15 participants signed informed consent forms that promised confidentially. The women were asked not to use real names during the interviews, which were tape recorded. Any names inadvertently included were deleted during transcription. Confidentiality was further protected through an NIH Certificate of Confidentiality.

Debriefings and Referrals

Researchers can show their respect for study participants—and proactively minimize emotional risks—by carefully attending to the nature of the interactions they have with them. For example, researchers should always be gracious and polite, phrase questions tactfully, and be sensitive to cultural and linguistic diversity.

There are also more formal strategies that researchers can use to communicate their respect and concern for participants' well-being. For example, it is sometimes advisable to offer **debriefing** sessions after data collection is completed to permit participants to ask questions or air complaints. Debriefing is especially important when the data collection has been stressful or when ethical guidelines had to be "bent" (e.g., if any deception was used).

Example of debriefing:
Sandgren and colleagues (2006) studied the strategies that palliative cancer nurses used to avoid being emotionally overloaded. They conducted in-depth interviews with 46 nurses, and after each interview, "we made sure that the participants were doing well, and we assessed possible needs for emotional support" (p. 81).

Researchers can also demonstrate their interest in participants by offering to share study findings with them once the data have been analyzed (e.g., by mailing them a summary). Finally, in some situations, researchers may need to assist study participants by making referrals to appropriate health, social, or psychological services.

Example of information sharing and referrals:
Baumgartner (2007) conducted a longitudinal study of how people incorporate an HIV/AIDS identity into their selves over time. Data were collected at three points over a 4-year period. Participants were told that if they experienced any psychological discomfort, they could terminate the interview and would be given a referral to a social service agency. Following each wave of data collection, participants were sent copies of published papers with the results.

Treatment of Vulnerable Groups

Adherence to ethical standards is often straightforward. The rights of special vulnerable groups, however, may need to be protected through additional procedures and heightened sensitivity. **Vulnerable subjects** (the term used in U.S. federal guidelines) may be incapable of giving fully informed consent (e.g., mentally retarded people) or may be at high risk of unintended side effects because of their circumstances (e.g., pregnant women). You should pay particular attention to the ethical dimensions of a study when people who are vulnerable are involved. Among the groups that should be considered as being vulnerable are the following:

➤ *Children.* Legally and ethically, children do not have the competence to give informed consent and so the consent of children's parents or guardians should be obtained. However, it is appropriate—especially if the child is at least 7 years of age—to obtain the child's assent as well. **Assent** refers to the child's affirmative agreement to participate. If the child is developmentally mature enough to understand the basics of informed consent (e.g., a 12-year-old), researchers should obtain written consent from the child as well, as evidence of respect for the child's right to self-determination.

➤ *Mentally or emotionally disabled people.* Individuals whose disability makes it impossible for them to weigh the risks and benefits of participation and make informed decisions (e.g., people affected by cognitive impairment, mental illness, coma, and so on) also cannot legally provide informed consent. In such cases, researchers should obtain the written consent of a legal guardian.

➤ *Severely ill or physically disabled people.* For patients who are very ill or undergoing certain treatments (e.g., mechanical ventilation), it might be necessary to assess their ability to make reasoned decisions about study participation. Another issue is that for certain disabilities, special procedures for obtaining consent may be required. For example, with people who cannot read and write or who have a physical impairment preventing them from writing, alternative procedures for documenting informed consent (e.g., videotaping the consent proceedings) should be used.

➤ *The terminally ill.* Terminally ill people can seldom expect to benefit personally from research, and thus the risk-to-benefit ratio needs to be carefully assessed. Researchers must also take steps to ensure that if the terminally ill do participate in a study, their health care and comfort are not compromised.

➤ *Institutionalized people.* Nurses often conduct studies with hospitalized or institutionalized people who might feel that their treatment would be jeopardized by failure to cooperate. Inmates of prisons and correctional facilities, who have lost their autonomy in many spheres of activity, may similarly feel constrained in their ability to give free consent. Researchers studying institutionalized groups need to emphasize the voluntary nature of participation.

➤ *Pregnant women.* The U.S. government has issued stringent additional requirements governing research with pregnant women and fetuses (Code of Federal Regulations, 2005, Subpart B). These requirements reflect a desire to safeguard both the pregnant woman, who may be at heightened physical and psychological risk, and the fetus, who cannot give informed consent. The regulations stipulate that a pregnant woman cannot be involved in a study unless the study purpose is to meet the woman's health needs and risks to her and the fetus are minimal.

Example of research with a vulnerable group:
Capezuti and colleagues (2007) evaluated the effectiveness of an advanced practice nurse's consultation intervention in reducing the use of restrictive side rails in nursing homes. Residents provided their own consent to participate if they were able to do so. For those who were not able, the resident's surrogate decision-maker provided consent.

External Reviews and the Protection of Human Rights

It is sometimes difficult for researchers to be objective in doing risk–benefit assessments or in developing procedures to protect participants' rights. Biases may arise as a result of researchers' commitment to an area of knowledge and their desire to conduct a valid study. Because of the risk of a biased evaluation, the ethical dimensions of a study are usually subjected to external review.

Most hospitals, universities, and other institutions where research is conducted have established formal committees for reviewing research plans. These committees are sometimes called *Human Subjects Committees* or (in Canada) *Research Ethics Boards*. In the United States, the committee is often called an **Institutional Review Board (IRB)**.

Studies supported with federal funds in the United States are subject to strict guidelines regarding the treatment of study participants, and the IRB's duty is to ensure that proposed procedures adhere to these guidelines. Before undertaking their study, researchers must submit research plans to the IRB, and must also undergo formal IRB training. An IRB can approve the proposed plans, require modifications, or disapprove them.

Not all research is subject to federal guidelines, and not all studies are reviewed by IRBs or other formal committees. Nevertheless, researchers have a responsibility to ensure that their research plans are ethically adequate, and it is a good practice for researchers to solicit external opinions even when they are not required to do so.

> **Example of IRB approval:**
> Taylor and McMullen (2008) explored the process of living kidney donation as experienced by the husbands of the donors. The procedures and protocols for the study were approved by the IRB of the researchers' university, and by the IRB of the university hospital where the transplants were performed.

OTHER ETHICAL ISSUES

In discussing ethical issues relating to the conduct of nursing research, we have given primary consideration to the protection of human study participants. Two other ethical issues also deserve mention: the treatment of animals in research and research misconduct.

Ethical Issues in Using Animals in Research

Some nurse researchers who focus on biophysiologic phenomena use animals rather than human beings as their subjects. Despite some opposition to animal research, it seems likely that researchers in health fields will continue to use animals to explore basic physiologic mechanisms and to test experimental interventions that could pose risks (as well as offer benefits) to humans.

Ethical considerations are clearly different for animals and humans; for example, the concept of *informed consent* is not relevant for animal subjects. In the United States, the Public Health Service has issued a policy statement on the humane care and use of animals, most recently amended in 2002. The guidelines articulate nine principles for the proper care and treatment of animals used in research. These principles cover such issues as the transport of research animals, alternatives to using animals, pain and distress in animal subjects, researcher qualifications, use of appropriate anesthesia, and euthanizing animals under certain conditions during or after the study.

Holtzclaw and Hanneman (2002), in discussing the use of animals in nursing research, noted several important considerations. For example, there must be a compelling reason to use an animal model—not simply convenience or novelty. Also, the study procedures should be humane, well planned, and well funded. They noted that animal studies are not necessarily less costly than those with human participants, and they require serious ethical and scientific consideration to justify their use.

Example of research with animals:
Briones and colleagues (2005) studied the effects of behavioral rehabilitation training following transient global cerebral ischemia on dentate gyrus neurogenesis using 72 adult male rats. They reported that "all efforts were made to minimize animal distress and to reduce the number of animals used" (p. 169). The experimental protocols were approved by an institutional animal care committee and were in accordance with federal guidelines on the use of animals in research.

Research Misconduct

Millions of movie-goers watched Dr. Richard Kimble (Harrison Ford) expose the fraudulent scheme of a medical researcher in the film *The Fugitive*. The film reminds us that ethics in research involves not only the protection of the rights of human and animal subjects, but also protection of the public trust.

The issue of **research misconduct** (also called *scientific misconduct)* has received increasing attention in recent years as incidents of researcher fraud and misrepresentation have come to light. Currently, the federal agency responsible for overseeing efforts to improve research integrity in the United States and for handling allegations of research misconduct is the Office of Research Integrity (ORI) within the Department of Health and Human Services.

Research misconduct, as defined by a U. S. Public Health Service regulation that was revised in 2005 (42 CFR Part 93, Subpart A), is fabrication, falsification, or plagiarism in proposing, conducting, or reviewing research, or in reporting results. Research misconduct does not include honest errors. *Fabrication* involves making up data or study results and reporting them. *Falsification* involves manipulating research materials, equipment, or processes; it also involves changing or omitting data, or distorting results such that the research is not accurately represented in reports. *Plagiarism* involves the appropriation of someone's ideas, results, or words without giving due credit, including information obtained through the confidential review of research proposals or manuscripts. Although the official definition focuses on only these three types of misconduct, there is widespread agreement that research misconduct covers many other issues including improprieties of authorship, poor data management, conflicts of interest, inappropriate financial arrangements, failure to comply with governmental regulations, and unauthorized use of confidential information.

Example of research misconduct:
In 1999, the U.S. Office of Research Integrity ruled that a nurse who had been the data manager for the National Surgical Adjuvant Breast and Bowel Project at a cancer center affiliated with Northwestern University engaged in scientific misconduct by intentionally falsifying or fabricating follow-up data on three patients enrolled in clinical trials for breast cancer (ORI Newsletter, March, 1999).

Although examples of publicly exposed misconduct by nurse researchers are not common, research dishonesty and fraud are major concerns in nursing. For example, Jeffers (2005) sought to identify and describe research environments that promote integrity. In a study that focused on ethical issues faced by editors of nursing journals, Freda and Kearney (2005) found that 64% of the 88 participating editors reported some type of ethical dilemma, such as duplicate publication, plagiarism, or conflicts of interest. And, since 2001, NINR and other institutes within NIH have teamed with ORI to offer grants for researchers to conduct "Research on Research Integrity"—that is, to study the factors that affect, both positively and negatively, integrity in research.

Example of research on research integrity:
In 2004, Sheila Santacroce of Yale University was awarded a 2-year grant through NINR under the Research on Research Integrity initiative. Her study is exploring *intervention fidelity* (the consistent delivery of an intervention according to a research plan and professional standards) in two federally funded nursing intervention studies. The premise is that lack of attention to fidelity can lead to misleading statements about the implementation and effects of an intervention.

CRITIQUING THE ETHICAL ASPECTS OF A STUDY

Guidelines for critiquing the ethical aspects of a study are presented in Box 5.2. Members of an IRB or human subjects committee should be provided with sufficient information to answer all these questions. Research articles, however, do not

---

BOX 5.2 GUIDELINES FOR CRITIQUING THE ETHICAL ASPECTS OF A STUDY

1. Was the study approved and monitored by an Institutional Review Board, Research Ethics Board, or other similar ethics review committee?
2. Were study participants subjected to any physical harm, discomfort, or psychological distress? Did the researchers take appropriate steps to remove or prevent harm?
3. Did the benefits to participants outweigh any potential risks or actual discomfort they experienced? Did the benefits to society outweigh the costs to participants?
4. Was any type of coercion or undue influence used to recruit participants? Did they have the right to refuse to participate or to withdraw without penalty?
5. Were participants deceived in any way? Were they fully aware of participating in a study and did they understand the purpose and nature of the research?
6. Were appropriate informed consent procedures used with all participants? If not, were there valid and justifiable reasons?
7. Were adequate steps taken to safeguard the privacy of participants? How were data kept anonymous or confidential? Were Privacy Rule procedures followed (if applicable)? Was a Certificate of Confidentiality obtained?
8. Were vulnerable groups involved in the research? If yes, were special precautions instituted because of their vulnerable status?
9. Were groups omitted from the inquiry without a justifiable rationale (e.g., women, minorities)?

always include detailed information about ethical procedures because of space constraints in journals. Thus, it may not always be possible to critique researchers' adherence to ethical guidelines. Nevertheless, we offer a few suggestions for considering ethical issues in a study.

Many research reports do acknowledge that the study procedures were reviewed by an IRB or human subjects committee of the institution with which the researchers are affiliated. When a report specifically mentions a formal external review, it is generally safe to assume that a panel of concerned people thoroughly reviewed the ethical issues raised by the study.

You can also come to some conclusions based on a description of the study methods. There may be sufficient information to judge, for example, whether study participants were subjected to physical or psychological harm or discomfort. Reports do not always specifically state whether informed consent was secured, but you should be alert to situations in which the data could not have been gathered as described if participation were purely voluntary (e.g., if data were gathered unobtrusively).

In thinking about the ethical aspects of a study, you should also consider who the study participants were. For example, if the study involves vulnerable groups, there should be more information about protective procedures. You might also need to attend to who the study participants were *not*. For example, there has been considerable concern about the omission of certain groups (e.g., minorities) from clinical research.

> ## RESEARCH EXAMPLES AND CRITICAL THINKING ACTIVITIES

Abstracts for a quantitative and a qualitative nursing study are presented below, followed by some questions to guide critical thinking about the ethical aspects of a study.

EXAMPLE 1 ■ Quantitative Research

Study

Health status in an invisible population: Carnival and migrant worker children (Kilanowski & Ryan-Wenger, 2007).

Study Purpose

The purpose of the study was to examine indicators of the health status of children of itinerant carnival workers and migrant farm workers in the United States.

Research Methods

A total of 97 boys and girls younger than 13 years were recruited into the study. Parents completed questionnaires about their children's health and health care, and most brought health records from which information about immunizations was obtained. All children received an oral health screening and were measured for height and weight.

Ethics-related Procedures

The families were recruited through the cooperation of gatekeepers at farms and carnival communities in seven states. Parents were asked to complete informed consent forms, which were available in both English and Spanish. Children who were older than 9 years were also asked whether they would like to participate, and they gave verbal assent. Confidentiality was a major concern to both the families and the gatekeepers, and the researchers needed to assure all parties that the data would be confidential and not used against families or facilities. Data were gathered in locations and time periods that had been suggested by the carnival managers and farm owners, so that parents did not need to forfeit work hours to participate in the study. Migrant farm workers were often eager to participate, and often waited in line to sign the consent forms. At the conclusion of the encounter, the researchers gave the parents a written report of the children's growth parameters and recommendations for follow-up. In appreciation of the parents' time, $10 was given to the parents, and the child was given an age-appropriate nonviolent toy (worth about $10) of their choice. Children were also given a new toothbrush. The IRB of the Ohio State University approved this study.

Key Findings

Carnival children were less likely than migrant children to have regularly scheduled well-child examinations and to have seen a dentist in the previous year. Among children ages 6 to 11, the itinerant children in both groups were substantially more likely to be overweight than same aged children nationally.

CRITICAL THINKING SUGGESTIONS*:

*See the Student Resource CD-ROM for a discussion of these questions. 💿

1. Answer the relevant questions from Box 5.2 regarding this study.
2. Also, consider the following targeted questions, which may further assist you in assessing the ethical aspects of the study:
   a. Could the data for this study have been collected anonymously?
   b. Why might a Certificate of Confidentiality have been helpful in this study?
3. If the results of this study are valid and generalizable, what might be some of the uses to which the findings could be put in clinical practice?

EXAMPLE 2 ■ Qualitative Research

Study

Perinatal violence assessment: Teenagers' rationale for denying violence when asked (Renker, 2006).

Study Purpose

The purpose of the study was to describe teenagers' experiences with violence assessments from health care and social service providers, and to explore their reasons for failing to disclose violence.

Study Methods

Renker recruited 20 teenagers (18 and 19 years of age) who were no longer pregnant but who had experienced physical or sexual abuse in the year before or during a pregnancy. All women were interviewed in person and asked in-depth questions about their experiences relating to violence.

Ethics-related Procedures

Renker recruited teenagers primarily at two outpatient gynecologic clinics. Teenagers who were deemed eligible for the study were invited to schedule an interview at a location of their choice. All but one of the young women who volunteered chose a public library or a university office rather than their own homes. Teens were offered a $50 stipend to partially compensate them for the time spent in the interview (30–90 minutes). Before beginning the interview, informed consent issues were discussed, including the researcher's responsibility to report child abuse and harm to third parties. Study participants were told that no specific questions would be asked about either of these reportable issues, but that the researcher would assist them in reporting any abuse situations if they so desired. To protect their confidentiality, Renker encouraged each teenager to make up a name for herself, the perpetrator, and other family members. Each interview was assigned an ID number, and the data files contained no information that could identify participants or the locale of their recruitment. Interviews were conducted in a private setting without the presence of the teenagers' partners, parents, or children aged 2 or older. At the end of the interview, Renker provided the teenagers with information designed to promote their safety (e.g., danger assessments, review of legal options, list of local community resources). Renker received IRB approval from her university and from the medical systems of the two clinics from which participants were recruited.

Key Findings

The teenagers reported a range of violent experiences from their current and previous intimate partners, their parents, and gangs. Their reasons for not disclosing violence to health care providers fell into categories that corresponded to four continua: Power/Powerlessness; Fear/Hope; Trust/Mistrust; and Action/Inertia.

CRITICAL THINKING SUGGESTIONS:

1. Answer the relevant questions from Box 5.2 regarding this study.
2. Also, consider the following targeted questions, which may further assist you in assessing the ethical aspects of the study:
   a. Renker paid participants a $50 stipend—was this ethically appropriate?
   b. What dilemma would Renker face if participants told her that they had abused their own children?
   c. What ethical principle(s) did Renker seek to address in providing participants with information to keep them safe?
   d. Did the teenagers' creation of a pseudonym result in anonymity?
   e. Might Renker have benefited from obtaining a Certificate of Confidentiality for this research?
   f. If you had a teenaged friend or family member who had been abused during pregnancy, how would you feel about her participating in the study?
3. If the results of this study are trustworthy and transferable, what might be some of the uses to which the findings could be put in clinical practice?

EXAMPLE 3 ■ Quantitative Study in Appendix A

1. Read the method section from Howell and colleagues' (2007) study ("Anxiety, anger, and blood pressure in children") in Appendix A of this book, and then answer relevant questions in Box 5.2.

2. Also consider the following targeted questions, which may further assist you in assessing the ethical aspects of the study:
   a. Where was information about ethical issues located in this report?
   b. What additional information regarding the ethical aspects of their study could the researchers have included in this article?
   c. If you had a school-aged sibling or child of your own, how would you feel about him or her participating in the study?

EXAMPLE 4 ■ Qualitative Study in Appendix B

1. Read the method section from Beck's (2006) study ("Anniversary of birth trauma") in Appendix B of this book and then answer relevant questions in Box 5.2.
2. Also, consider the following targeted questions, which may further assist you in assessing the ethical aspects of the study:
   a. Where was information about the ethical aspects of this study located in the report?
   b. What additional information regarding the ethical aspects of Beck's study could the researcher have included in this article?

CHAPTER REVIEW

Key new terms introduced in the chapter, together with a summary of major points, are presented in this section. Chapter 5 of the accompanying *Study Guide for Essentials of Nursing Research,* 7th edition also offers exercises and study suggestions for reinforcing the concepts presented in this chapter. For additional review, see self-study questions on the CD-ROM provided with this book. ●

Key New Terms

Anonymity	Confidentiality	Minimal risk
Assent	Debriefing	Process consent
Belmont Report	Ethical dilemma	Research misconduct
Beneficence	Full disclosure	Risk–benefit assessment
Certificate of	Implied consent	Stipend
Confidentiality	Informed consent	Vulnerable subjects
Code of ethics	Institutional Review	
Consent form	Board (IRB)	

Summary Points

➤ Because research has not always been conducted ethically, and because of genuine **ethical dilemmas** that researchers often face in designing studies that are both ethical and methodologically rigorous, **codes of ethics** have been developed to guide researchers.

➤ Three major ethical principles from the *Belmont Report* are incorporated into most guidelines: beneficence, respect for human dignity, and justice.

➤ **Beneficence** involves the performance of some good and the protection of participants from physical and psychological harm and exploitation (*nonmaleficence*).

➤ Respect for human dignity involves the participants' right to self-determination, which means participants have the freedom to control their own activities, including their voluntary participation in the study.

➤ **Full disclosure** means that researchers have fully described to prospective participants their rights and the costs and benefits of the study. When full disclosure poses the risk of biased results, researchers sometimes use *covert data collection* or *concealment* (the collection of information without the participants' knowledge or consent) or *deception* (either withholding information from participants or providing false information).

➤ Justice includes the right to fair equitable treatment and the right to privacy. In the United States, privacy has become a major issue because of the Privacy Rule regulations that resulted from the Health Insurance Portability and Accountability Act (HIPAA).

➤ Various procedures have been developed to safeguard study participants rights, including the performance of a risk–benefit assessment, the implementation of informed consent procedures, and taking steps to safeguard participants' confidentiality.

➤ In a **risk–benefit assessment,** the potential benefits of the study to individual participants and to society are weighed against the costs to individuals.

➤ **Informed consent** procedures, which provide prospective participants with information needed to make a reasoned decision about participation, normally involve signing a **consent form** to document voluntary and informed participation.

➤ In qualitative studies, consent may need to be continually renegotiated with participants as the study evolves, through **process consent** procedures.

➤ Privacy can be maintained through **anonymity** (wherein not even researchers know participants' identities) or through formal **confidentiality procedures** that safeguard the information participants provide.

➤ In some studies, it may be advantageous for U.S. researchers to obtain a **Certificate of Confidentiality** that protects them against the forced disclosure of confidential information through a court order or other administrative process.

➤ Researchers sometimes offer **debriefing** sessions after data collection to provide participants with more information or an opportunity to air complaints.

➤ **Vulnerable subjects** require additional protection. These people may be vulnerable because they are not able to make a truly informed decision about study participation (e.g., children), because of diminished autonomy (e.g., prisoners), or because their circumstances heighten the risk of physical or psychological harm (e.g., pregnant women, the terminally ill).

➤ External review of the ethical aspects of a study by a human subjects committee, Research Ethics Board (REB), or **Institutional Review Board (IRB)** is highly desirable and is often required by universities and organizations from which participants are recruited.

➤ Ethical conduct in research involves not only protecting the rights of human and animal subjects, but also efforts to maintain high standards of integrity and avoid such forms of **research misconduct** as plagiarism, fabrication of results, or falsification of data.

STUDIES CITED IN CHAPTER 5

Baumgartner, L. M. (2007). The incorporation of the HIV/AIDS identity into the self over time. *Qualitative Health Research, 17,* 919–931.

Beck, C. T. (2005). Benefits of participating in internet interviews: Women helping women. *Qualitative Health Research, 15,* 411–422.

Briones, T. L., Suh, E., Hattar, H., & Wadowska, M. (2005). Dentate gyrus neurogenesis after cerebral ischemia and behavioral training. *Biological Research for Nursing, 6,* 167–179.

Capezuti, E., Wagner, L., Brush, B., Boltz, M., Renz, S., Talerico, K. et al. (2007). Consequences of an intervention to reduce restrictive siderail use in nursing homes. *Journal of the American Geriatrics Society, 55,* 334–341.

Carlsson, E., Paterson, B., Scott-Findley, S., Ehnfors, M., & Ehrenberg, A. (2007). Methodological issues in interviews involving people with communication impairments after acquired brain damage. *Qualitative Health Research, 17,* 1361–1371.

Esperat, C., Feng, D., Zhang, Y., & Owen, D. (2007). Health behaviors of low-income pregnant minority women. *Western Journal of Nursing Research, 29,* 284–300.

Freda, M. C., & Kearney, M. (2005). Ethical issues faced by nursing editors. *Western Journal of Nursing Research, 27,* 487–499.

Houfek, J. F., Atwood, J., Wolfe, R., Agrawal, S., Reiser, G., Schaefer, G. B. et al. (2008). Knowledge and beliefs about genetics and smoking among visitors and staff at a health care facility. *Public Health Nursing, 25,* 77–87.

Kilanowski, J., & Ryan-Wenger, N. (2007). Health status in an invisible population: Carnival and migrant worker children. *Western Journal of Nursing Research, 29,* 100–120.

Laughon, K. (2007). Abused African American women's processes of staying healthy. *Western Journal of Nursing Research, 29,* 365–384.

Renker, P. R. (2006). Perinatal violence assessment: Teenagers' rationale for denying violence when asked. *Journal of Obstetric, Gynecologic, & Neonatal Nursing, 35,* 56–67.

Sandgren, A., Thulesius, H., Fridlund, B., & Petersson, K. (2006). Striving for emotional survival in palliative cancer nursing. *Qualitative Health Research, 16,* 79–96.

Taylor, L. A., & McMullen, P. (2008). Living kidney organ donation: Experiences of spousal support of donors. *Journal of Clinical Nursing, 17,* 232–241.

Treacy, M., Hyde, A., Boland, J., Whitaker, T., Abaunza, P. S., & Stewart-Knox, B. (2007). Children talking: Emerging perspectives and experiences of cigarette smoking. *Qualitative Health Research, 17,* 238–249.

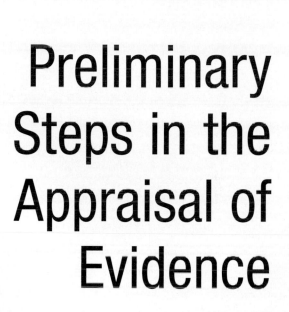

Preliminary Steps in the Appraisal of Evidence

6 Research Problems, Research Questions, and Hypotheses

STUDENT OBJECTIVES

On completing this chapter, you will be able to:

➤ Evaluate the compatibility of a research problem and a paradigm

➤ Describe the process of developing and refining a research problem

➤ Distinguish the functions and forms of statements of purpose and research questions for quantitative and qualitative studies

➤ Describe the function and characteristics of research hypotheses and distinguish different types of hypotheses (e.g., directional versus nondirectional, research versus null)

➤ Critique statements of purpose, research questions, and hypotheses in research reports with respect to their placement, clarity, wording, and significance

➤ Define new terms in the chapter

OVERVIEW OF RESEARCH PROBLEMS

Studies to generate new research evidence begin in much the same fashion as an evidence-based practice (EBP) effort—as problems that need to be solved or questions that need to be answered. This chapter discusses the formulation and evaluation of research problems. We begin by clarifying some relevant terms.

Basic Terminology

At the most general level, a researcher selects a **topic** or a phenomenon on which to focus. Examples of research topics are claustrophobia during magnetic resonance imaging (MRI) tests and pain management for sickle cell disease. Within these broad topic areas are many potential research problems. In this section, we illustrate various terms using the topic *side effects of chemotherapy*.

A **research problem** is an enigmatic, perplexing, or troubling condition. Both qualitative and quantitative researchers identify a research problem within a broad topic area of interest. The purpose of research is to "solve" the problem—or to contribute to its solution—by accumulating relevant information. A **problem statement** articulates the problem to be addressed and indicates the need for a study through the development of an *argument*. Table 6.1 presents a simplified problem statement related to the topic of side effects of chemotherapy.

Many reports include a **statement of purpose** (or purpose statement), which is the researcher's summary of the overall goal. A researcher might also identify several *aims* or *objectives*—the specific accomplishments the researcher hopes to achieve by conducting the study. The objectives include answering research questions or testing research hypotheses but may also encompass some broader aims (e.g., developing recommendations for changes to nursing practice based on the study results), as illustrated in Table 6.1.

Research questions are the specific queries researchers want to answer in addressing the research problem. Research questions guide the types of data to be collected in a study. Researchers who make specific predictions about answers to research questions pose **hypotheses** that are tested empirically.

These terms are not always consistently defined in research methods textbooks, and differences between the terms are often subtle. Table 6.1 illustrates the interrelationships among terms as we define them.

Research Problems and Paradigms

Some research problems are better suited to qualitative versus quantitative methods. Quantitative studies usually involve concepts that are fairly well developed, about which there is an existing body of literature, and for which reliable methods of measurement have been (or can be) developed. For example, a quantitative study might be undertaken to determine if people with chronic illness who continue working past age 62 are less (or more) depressed than those who retire. There are relatively accurate measures of depression that would yield quantitative

TABLE 6.1 ⊙ EXAMPLE OF TERMS RELATING TO RESEARCH PROBLEMS	
TERM	EXAMPLE
Topic	Side effects of chemotherapy
Research problem (Problem statement)	Nausea and vomiting are common side effects among patients on chemotherapy, and interventions to date have been only moderately successful in reducing these effects. New interventions that can reduce or prevent these side effects need to be identified.
Statement of purpose	The purpose of the study is to test an intervention to reduce chemotherapy-induced side effects—specifically, to compare the effectiveness of patient-controlled and nurse-administered antiemetic therapy for controlling nausea and vomiting in patients on chemotherapy.
Aims/objectives	This study has as its aim the following objectives: (1) to develop and implement two alternative procedures for administering antiemetic therapy for patients receiving moderate emetogenic chemotherapy (patient controlled versus nurse controlled); (2) to test three hypotheses concerning the relative effectiveness of the alternative procedures on medication consumption and control of side effects; and (3) to use the findings to develop recommendations for possible changes to clinical procedures.
Research question	What is the relative effectiveness of patient-controlled antiemetic therapy versus nurse-controlled antiemetic therapy with regard to (1) medication consumption and (2) control of nausea and vomiting in patients on chemotherapy?
Hypotheses	Subjects receiving antiemetic therapy by a patient-controlled pump will (1) be less nauseous (2) vomit less and (3) consume less medication than subjects receiving the therapy by nurse administration.

data about the level of depression in a sample of employed and retired chronically ill seniors.

Qualitative studies are often undertaken because a new phenomenon has emerged or some aspect of a phenomenon is poorly understood and the researcher wants to develop a rich, comprehensive, and context-bound understanding of it. Qualitative studies can be useful in heightening awareness and creating a dialogue about a phenomenon. Qualitative methods would not be well suited to comparing levels of depression among employed and retired seniors, but they would be ideal for exploring, for example, the *meaning* of depression among chronically ill retirees. In evaluating a research report, an important consideration is whether the research problem is suitable for the chosen paradigm and its associated methods.

Sources of Research Problems

Where do ideas for research problems come from? At the most basic level, research topics originate with researchers' interests. Because research is a time-consuming enterprise, curiosity about and interest in a topic are essential to a project's success.

Research reports rarely indicate the source of researchers' inspiration for a study, but a variety of explicit sources can fuel their curiosity, including the following:

➤ *Clinical experience.* Nurses' everyday experience is a rich source of ideas for research topics. Immediate problems that need a solution—analogous to problem-focused triggers discussed in Chapter 2—have high potential for clinical significance. Clinical fieldwork before a study may also help to identify clinical problems.

➤ *Nursing literature.* Ideas for studies often come from reading the nursing literature. Research reports may suggest problem areas indirectly by stimulating the reader's imagination and directly by explicitly stating what additional research is needed.

➤ *Social issues.* Topics are sometimes suggested by global social or political issues of relevance to the health care community. For example, the feminist movement has raised questions about such topics as gender equity in health care.

➤ *Theories.* Theories from nursing and other related disciplines are another source of research problems. Researchers ask, If this theory is correct, what would I predict about people's behaviors, states, or feelings? The predictions can then be tested through research.

➤ *Ideas from external sources.* External sources and direct suggestions can sometimes provide the impetus for a research idea. For example, ideas for studies may emerge by reviewing a funding agency's research priorities or from brainstorming with other nurses.

Additionally, researchers who have developed a *program of research* on a topic area may get inspiration for "next steps" from their own findings, or from a discussion of those findings with others.

Example of a problem source for a quantitative study:
Beck (one of this book's authors) has developed a strong research program on postpartum depression (PPD). In 2003, Beck was approached by Dr. Carol Lanni Keefe, a professor in nutritional sciences, who had been researching the effect of DHA (docosahexaemoic acid, a fat found in cold-water marine fish) on fetal brain development. The literature suggested that DHA might play a role in reducing the severity of PPD and so the two researchers collaborated in developing a proposal to rigorously test the effectiveness of dietary supplements of DHA on the incidence and severity of PPD. Their clinical trial, funded by the Donahue Medical Research Foundation, is currently underway.

Development and Refinement of Research Problems

The development of a research problem is a creative process. Researchers often begin with interests in a broad topic area, and then develop a more specific researchable problem. For example, suppose a nurse working on a medical unit begins to wonder why some patients complain about having to wait for pain medication when certain nurses are assigned to them. The general topic is discrepancy in patient complaints about pain medications administered by different nurses. The nurse might ask, What accounts for this discrepancy? This broad question may lead to other questions, such as, How do the two groups of nurses differ? or What characteristics do the complaining patients share? At this point, the nurse may observe that the ethnic background of the patients and nurses could be a relevant factor. This may direct the nurse to a review of the literature for studies concerning ethnic groups and their relationship to nursing behaviors, or it may provoke a discussion of these observations with peers. These efforts may result in several research questions, such as the following:

➤ What is the essence of patient complaints among patients of different ethnic backgrounds?

➤ How do complaints by patients of different ethnic backgrounds get expressed by patients and perceived by nurses?

➤ Is the ethnic background of nurses related to the frequency with which they dispense pain medication?

➤ Is the ethnic background of patients related to the frequency and intensity of their complaints of having to wait for pain medication?

➤ Does the number of patient complaints increase when the patients are of dissimilar ethnic backgrounds as opposed to when they are of the same ethnic background as the nurse?

➤ Do nurses' dispensing behaviors change as a function of the similarity between their own ethnic background and that of patients?

These questions stem from the same general problem, yet each would be studied differently; for example, some suggest a qualitative approach, and others suggest a quantitative one. A quantitative researcher might become curious about nurses' dispensing behaviors, based on some evidence in the literature regarding ethnic differences. Both ethnicity and nurses' dispensing behaviors are variables that can be reliably measured. A qualitative researcher who noticed differences in patient complaints would be more interested in understanding the *essence* of the complaints, the patients' *experience* of frustration, the *process* by which the problem got resolved, or the full *nature* of the nurse–patient interactions regarding the dispensing of medications. These are aspects of the research problem that would be difficult to measure quantitatively. Researchers choose a problem to study based on several factors, including its inherent interest to them and its fit with a paradigm of preference.

COMMUNICATING RESEARCH PROBLEMS AND QUESTIONS

Every study needs to have a problem statement—the articulation of what it is that is problematic and that is the impetus for the research. Most research reports also present either a statement of purpose, research questions, or hypotheses; often, combinations of these three elements are included.

Many students do not really understand problem statements and may even have trouble identifying them in a research article—not to mention developing one. A problem statement is presented early in a research report and often begins with the very first sentence after the abstract. Specific research questions, purposes, or hypotheses appear later in the introduction.

Problem Statements

Problem statements express the dilemma or disconcerting situation that needs investigation and incorporate a rationale for a new inquiry. A good problem statement is a well-structured formulation of what it is that is problematic, what it is that "needs fixing," or what it is that is poorly understood. Problem statements, especially for quantitative studies, often have most of the following six components:

1. *Problem identification*: What is wrong with the current situation?
2. *Background*: What is the nature of the problem, or the context of the situation, that readers need to understand?
3. *Scope of the problem*: How big a problem is it, how many people are affected?
4. *Consequences of the problem:* What is the cost of *not* fixing the problem?
5. *Knowledge gaps:* What information about the problem is lacking?
6. *Proposed solution*: How will the new study contribute to the solution of the problem?

Let us suppose that our topic was humor as a complementary therapy for reducing stress in hospitalized patients with cancer. One research question (which we discuss later in this section) might be, What is the effect of nurses' use of humor on stress and natural killer cell activity in hospitalized cancer patients? Box 6.1

BOX 6.1 DRAFT PROBLEM STATEMENT ON HUMOR AND STRESS

A diagnosis of cancer is associated with high levels of stress. Sizeable numbers of patients who receive a cancer diagnosis describe feelings of uncertainty, fear, anger, and loss of control. Interpersonal relationships, psychological functioning, and role performance have all been found to suffer following cancer diagnosis and treatment.

A variety of alternative/complementary therapies have been developed in an effort to decrease the harmful effects of stress on psychological and physiologic functioning, and resources devoted to these therapies (money and staff) have increased in recent years. However, many of these therapies have not been carefully evaluated to determine their efficacy, safety, or cost-effectiveness. For example, the use of humor has been recommended as a therapeutic device to improve quality of life, decrease stress, and perhaps improve immune functioning, but the evidence to justify its popularity is scant.

BOX 6.2   SOME POSSIBLE IMPROVEMENTS TO PROBLEM STATEMENT ON HUMOR AND STRESS

Each year, more than 1 million people are diagnosed with cancer, which remains one of the top causes of death among both men and women (reference citations). Numerous studies have documented that a diagnosis of cancer is associated with high levels of stress. Sizeable numbers of patients who receive a cancer diagnosis describe feelings of uncertainty, fear, anger, and loss of control (citations). Interpersonal relationships, psychological functioning, and role performance have all been found to suffer following cancer diagnosis and treatment (citations). These stressful outcomes can, in turn, adversely affect health, long-term prognosis, and medical costs among cancer survivors (citations).

A variety of alternative or complementary therapies have been developed in an effort to decrease the harmful effects of stress on psychological and physiologic functioning, and resources devoted to these therapies (money and staff) have increased in recent years (citations). However, many of these therapies have not been carefully evaluated to determine their efficacy, safety, or cost effectiveness. For example, the use of humor has been recommended as a therapeutic device to improve quality of life, decrease stress, and perhaps improve immune functioning (citations) but the evidence to justify its popularity is scant. Preliminary findings from a recent small-scale endocrinology study with a healthy sample exposed to a humorous intervention (citation), however, holds promise for further inquiry with immunocompromised populations.

presents a rough draft of a problem statement for such a study. This problem statement is a reasonable draft that has several of the six components, but it could be improved.

Box 6.2 illustrates how the problem statement could be made more powerful by adding information about scope (component 3), long-term consequences (component 4), and possible solutions (component 6). This second draft builds a stronger and more compelling *argument* for new research: millions of people are affected by cancer, and the disease has adverse consequences not only for those diagnosed and their families, but also for society. The revised problem statement also suggests a basis for the new study by describing a possible solution on which the new study might build.

HOW-TO-TELL TIP

How can you tell a problem statement? Problem statements are rarely explicitly labeled as such and, therefore, must be ferreted out. The first sentence of a research report is often the starting point of a problem statement. As this example suggests, the problem statement is usually interwoven with findings from the research literature (for convenience, we have omitted the actual references). Prior findings provide the evidence backing up assertions in the problem statement and suggest gaps in knowledge. In many research articles it is difficult to disentangle the problem statement from the literature review, unless there is a subsection specifically labeled "Literature Review" or something similar.

Problem statements for a qualitative study similarly express the nature of the problem, its context, its scope, and information needed to address it, as in the following example:

Example of a problem statement from a qualitative study:
Chantler and colleagues (2007) stated the following: "Little is known about why parents agree to engage in clinical research studies involving their children, yet this participation is essential for vaccine licensure and public health policy. In the United Kingdom, the incidence of meningococcal serogroup C disease in toddlers and teenagers dropped by 81% within 18 months of the introduction of the new meningococcal C conjugate vaccine (Miller et al., 2002). Licensure of this vaccine was possible only after a series of clinical trials in the pediatric population that provided the basis for vaccine licensure throughout Europe and in Canada. Further advances depend on parents' consenting to the participation of their children in vaccine research. Recruitment to this type of research is typically difficult, however, and many parents decline. An improved understanding of parental perceptions of the trials process might enhance the conduct of and recruitment to essential pediatric vaccine trials" (p. 311).

Qualitative studies that are embedded in a particular research tradition usually incorporate terms and concepts in their problem statements that foreshadow their tradition of inquiry. For example, the problem statement in a grounded theory study might refer to the need to generate a theory relating to social processes. A problem statement for a phenomenological study might note the need to know more about people's experiences or the meanings they attribute to those experiences. An ethnographer might indicate the desire to describe how cultural forces affect people's behavior.

Statements of Purpose

Many researchers articulate their research goals as a statement of purpose. The purpose statement establishes the general direction of the inquiry and captures—usually in one or two clear sentences—the substance of the study. It is usually easy to identify a purpose statement because the word *purpose* is explicitly stated: "The purpose of this study was . . ."—although sometimes the words *aim*, *goal*, *intent*, or *objective* are used instead, as in "The aim of this study was . . ."

In a quantitative study, a statement of purpose identifies the key study variables and their possible interrelationships, as well as the population of interest.

Example of a statement of purpose from a quantitative study:
The purpose of this study was to examine the impact of perceived prejudice in health care delivery (in relation to ethnicity, race, gender, homosexual orientation) on women's early cancer detection behavior and women's decisions to seek care for illness symptoms (Facione & Facione, 2007).

This purpose statement identifies the population of interest as women. The key study variables are women's perceptions about prejudice in the health care system (the independent variable), and decisions about seeking treatment and screening (the dependent variables).

In qualitative studies, the statement of purpose indicates the nature of the inquiry, the key concept or phenomenon, and the group, community, or setting under study.

Example of a statement of purpose from a qualitative study:
The purpose of this study was to describe satisfactory and unsatisfactory experiences of postpartum nursing care from the perspective of adolescent mothers (Peterson, Sword, Charles, & DiCenso, 2007).

This statement indicates that the central phenomenon of interest is patients' satisfaction with postpartum care and that the group under study is adolescent mothers.

The statement of purpose communicates more than just the nature of the problem. Researchers' selection of verbs in a purpose statement suggests the manner in which they sought to solve the problem, or the state of knowledge on the topic. A study whose purpose is to *explore* or *describe* some phenomenon is likely to be an investigation of a little-researched topic, often involving a qualitative approach such as a phenomenology or ethnography. A statement of purpose for a qualitative study—especially a grounded theory study—may also use verbs such as *understand*, *discover*, *develop*, or *generate*. The statements of purpose in qualitative studies often "encode" the tradition of inquiry not only through the researcher's choice of verbs but also through the use of certain terms or "buzz words" associated with those traditions, as follows:

➤ *Grounded theory*: Processes; social structures; social interactions
➤ *Phenomenological studies*: Experience; lived experience; meaning; essence
➤ *Ethnographic studies*: Culture; roles; lifeways; cultural behavior

Quantitative researchers also use verbs to communicate the nature of the inquiry. A statement indicating that the purpose of the study is to *test* or *evaluate* something (e.g., an intervention) suggests an experimental design, for example. A study whose purpose is to *examine* the relationship between two variables is more likely to involve a nonexperimental quantitative design. In some cases, the verb is ambiguous: a purpose statement indicating that the researcher's intent is to *compare* could be referring to a comparison of alternative treatments (using an experimental approach) or a comparison of two preexisting groups (using a nonexperimental approach). In any event, verbs such as *test*, *evaluate*, and *compare* suggest an existing knowledge base, quantifiable variables, and designs with scientific controls.

Note that the choice of verbs in a statement of purpose should connote objectivity. A statement of purpose indicating that the intent of the study was to *prove*, *demonstrate*, or *show* something suggests a bias.

Research Questions

Research questions, in some cases, are direct rewordings of statements of purpose, phrased interrogatively rather than declaratively, as in the following example:

➤ The purpose of this study is to assess the relationship between the dependency level of renal transplant recipients and their rate of recovery.

➤ What is the relationship between the dependency level of renal transplant recipients and their rate of recovery?

Questions that are simple and direct invite an answer and help to focus attention on the kinds of data needed to provide that answer. Some research reports thus omit a statement of purpose and state only research questions. Other researchers use a set of research questions to clarify or lend greater specificity to a global purpose statement.

Research Questions in Quantitative Studies

In Chapter 2, we discussed the framing of clinical "foreground" questions to guide an EBP inquiry. Many of the EBP question templates in Table 2.1 could yield questions to guide a research project as well, but *researchers* tend to conceptualize their questions in terms of their *variables*. Take, for example, the first question in Table 2.1, which states, "In (population), what is the effect of (intervention) on (outcome)?" A researcher would be more likely to think of the question in these terms: "In (population), what is the effect of (independent variable) on (dependent variable)?" The advantage of thinking in terms of variables is that researchers must consciously make decisions about how to operationalize their variables and design an analysis strategy with their variables. Thus, we can say that, in quantitative studies, research questions identify the key study variables, the relationships among them, and the population under study. The variables are all measurable concepts, and the questions suggest quantification.

Most research questions concern relationships among variables, and thus many quantitative research questions could be articulated using a general question template: "In (population), what is the relationship between (independent variable [IV]) and (dependent variable [DV])?" Examples of minor variations include the following:

➤ *Treatment, intervention:* In (population), what is the effect of (IV: intervention) on (DV)?

➤ *Prognosis:* In (population), does (IV: disease, condition) affect or influence (DV)?

➤ *Etiology/harm:* In (population), does (IV: exposure, characteristic) cause or increase risk of (DV)?

Thus, questions are sometimes phrased in terms of the *effects* of an independent variable on the dependent variable—but this still involves a *relationship* between the two.

Distinctions exist between the clinical foreground questions for an EBP-focused evidence search as described in Chapter 2 and a research question for an original study. As shown in Table 2.1, sometimes clinicians ask questions about explicit comparisons (e.g., they want to compare intervention A with intervention B) and sometimes they do not (e.g., they want to learn the effects of intervention A, compared with any other intervention that has been studied or with the absence of an intervention). In a research question, there is *always* a designated comparison, because the independent variable must be operationally defined; this definition would articulate exactly what is being studied. As we discuss in subsequent chapters, the nature of the comparison has implications for the strength of the study and the interpretability of the findings.

Another distinction between EBP and research questions is that research questions sometimes are more complex than clinical foreground questions. As an example, suppose that we began with an interest in nurses' use of humor with cancer patients, and the positive effects that humor has on these patients. One research question might be, "What is the effect of nurses' use of humor (the IV, versus absence of humor) on stress (the DV) in hospitalized cancer patients (the population)?" But we might also be interested in understanding a causal pathway, in which case we might ask a question that involves a mediating variable, as discussed in Chapter 4. For example, we might ask the following: "Does nurses' use of humor have a direct effect on the stress of hospitalized patients with cancer, or is the effect *mediated by* humor's effect on natural killer cell activity?" In questions involving mediators, researchers may be as interested in the mediator as they are in the independent variable, because mediators are key explanatory mechanisms.

Not all research questions are about relationships—some are primarily descriptive. As examples, here are some descriptive questions that could be answered in a quantitative study on nurses' use of humor:

❖ What is the frequency with which nurses use humor as a complementary therapy with hospitalized cancer patients?

❖ What are the characteristics of nurses who use humor as a complementary therapy with hospitalized cancer patients?

❖ Is my Use of Humor Scale an accurate and valid measure of nurses' use of humor with patients in clinical settings?

Answers to such questions might, if addressed in a methodologically sound study, be useful in developing effective strategies for reducing stress in patients with cancer.

Example of research questions from a quantitative study:
Taylor (2007) studied nurse requisites for spiritual care (i.e., what a client requires of a nurse before being receptive to spiritual care). Her questions included: "What characteristics does a client look for in a nurse before welcoming spiritual care?" and "What demographic or illness-related characteristics of the clients are related to nurse requisites for spiritual care?"

In this example, the first question is descriptive, and the second asks about the relationship between independent variables (client characteristics) and a dependent variable (nurse requisites for spiritual care).

Research Questions in Qualitative Studies
Research questions in qualitative statements include the phenomenon of interest and the group or population of interest. Researchers in the various qualitative traditions vary in their conceptualization of what types of questions are important. Grounded theory

researchers are likely to ask *process* questions, phenomenologists tend to ask *meaning* questions, and ethnographers generally ask *descriptive* questions about cultures. The terms associated with the various traditions, discussed previously in connection with purpose statements, are likely to be incorporated into the research questions.

Example of a research question from a phenomenological study:
What is the structure of the lived experience of feeling unsure? (Bunkers, 2007)

Not all qualitative studies are rooted in a specific research tradition. Many researchers use naturalistic methods to describe or explore phenomena without focusing on cultures, meaning, or social processes.

Example of a research question from a descriptive qualitative study:
Oliffe and Thorne (2007) explored patient–physician communication within the context of discussions about prostrate cancer. One of their research questions was "How do prostate cancer patients preserve a masculine self when communicating with male physicians about their prostrate cancer?"

In qualitative studies, research questions sometimes evolve over the course of the study. Researchers begin with a *focus* that defines the general boundaries of the inquiry, but the boundaries are not cast in stone—they "can be altered and, in the typical naturalistic inquiry, will be" (Lincoln & Guba, 1985, p. 228). Naturalists are often sufficiently flexible that the question can be modified as new information makes it relevant to do so.

> **TIP**
>
> Researchers most often state their purpose or research questions at the end of the introduction or immediately after the review of the literature. Sometimes, a separate section of a research report—typically located just before the method section—is devoted to stating the research problem formally and might be labeled "Purpose," "Statement of Purpose," "Research Questions," or, in quantitatve studies, "Hypotheses."

RESEARCH HYPOTHESES

Some quantitative researchers state explicit hypotheses in their reports. A hypothesis is a prediction, almost always involving the predicted relationship between two or more variables. Qualitative researchers do not begin with a hypothesis, in part because usually too little is known about the topic to justify a hypothesis, and in part because qualitative researchers want the inquiry to be guided by participants' viewpoints rather than by their own hunches. Thus, our discussion here focuses on hypotheses in quantitative research.

Function of Hypotheses in Quantitative Research

Many research questions, as we have seen, are queries about relationships between variables. Hypotheses are predicted answers to these queries. For instance, the research question might ask: "Does sexual abuse in childhood affect the development of irritable bowel syndrome in women?" The researcher might predict the following: Women who were sexually abused in childhood have a higher incidence of irritable bowel syndrome than women who were not.

Hypotheses sometimes emerge from a theory. Scientists reason from theories to hypotheses and test those hypotheses in the real world. The validity of a theory is never examined directly, but the soundness of a theory can be evaluated through hypothesis testing. For example, the theory of reinforcement posits that behavior that is positively reinforced (rewarded) tends to be learned (repeated). The theory is too abstract to test, but predictions based on it can be tested. For instance, the following hypothesis is deduced from reinforcement theory: Pediatric patients who are given a reward (e.g., a balloon or permission to watch television) when they cooperate during nursing procedures tend to be more cooperative during those procedures than nonrewarded peers. This proposition can be put to a test in the real world. The theory gains support if the hypotheses are confirmed.

Even in the absence of a theory, well-conceived hypotheses offer direction and suggest explanations. For example, suppose we hypothesized that the incidence of desaturation and bradycardia in low birth weight infants undergoing intubation and ventilation would be lower using the closed tracheal suction system (CTSS) than using the partially ventilated endotracheal suction method (PVETS). Our speculation might be based on earlier studies or clinical observations. *The development of predictions in and of itself forces researchers to think logically, to exercise critical judgment, and to tie together earlier findings.*

Now, let us suppose the preceding hypothesis is not confirmed; that is, we find that rates of bradycardia and desaturation are similar for both the PVETS and CTSS methods. *The failure of data to support a prediction forces researchers to analyze theory or previous research critically, to carefully review the limitations of the study's methods, and to explore alternative explanations for the findings.* The use of hypotheses in quantitative studies tends to induce critical thinking and to facilitate understanding and interpretation of the data.

To illustrate further the utility of hypotheses, suppose we conducted the study guided only by the research question, "Is there a relationship between suction method and rates of desaturation and bradycardia?" Without a hypothesis, the researcher is seemingly prepared to accept any results. The problem is that it is almost always possible to explain something superficially after the fact, no matter what the findings are. Hypotheses reduce the possibility that spurious results will be misconstrued.

TIP

Some quantitative research reports explicitly state the hypotheses that guided the study, but many do not. The absence of a hypothesis may be an indication that the researcher has failed to consider critically the implications of the existing knowledge base or has failed to disclose his or her hunches.

Characteristics of Testable Hypotheses

Testable research hypotheses state the expected relationship between the independent variable (the presumed cause or antecedent) and the dependent variable (the presumed effect or outcome) within a population.

Example of a research hypothesis:

Gungor and Beji (2007) tested the effect of fathers' attendance during labor and delivery on the childbirth experience in Turkey, where the prevailing culture has not supported a role for fathers during the birth process. They hypothesized that women whose partners attended labor and delivery would need less pain-relieving medication than women who were alone.

In this example, the population is women giving birth in Turkish hospitals; the independent variable is partners' presence or absence during labor and delivery; and the dependent variable is the mothers' need for pain medication. The hypothesis predicts that these two variables are related within the population—more medication is expected among mothers whose partners are not with them during labor and delivery.

Researchers occasionally present hypotheses that do not make a relational statement, as in the following example: *Pregnant women who receive prenatal instruction by a nurse regarding postpartum experiences are not likely to experience postpartum depression.* This statement expresses no anticipated relationship; in fact, there is only one variable (postpartum depression), and a relationship by definition requires at least two variables.

Without a prediction about an anticipated relationship, the hypothesis cannot be tested using standard statistical procedures. In our example, how would we know whether the hypothesis was supported—what standard would we use to decide whether to accept or reject the hypothesis? To illustrate the problem more concretely, suppose we asked a group of new mothers who had been given prenatal instruction the following question: "On the whole, how depressed have you been since you gave birth? Would you say (1) extremely depressed, (2) moderately depressed, (3) a little depressed, or (4) not at all depressed?"

Based on responses to this question, how could we compare the actual outcome with the predicted outcome? Would *all* the women have to say they were "not at all depressed?" Would the prediction be supported if 51% of the women said they were "not at all depressed" *or* "a little depressed?" It is difficult to test the accuracy of the prediction.

A test is simple, however, if we modify the prediction as follows: Pregnant women who receive prenatal instruction are less likely than those who do not to experience postpartum depression. Here, the dependent variable is the women's depression, and the independent variable is their receipt versus nonreceipt of prenatal instruction. The relational aspect of the prediction is embodied in the phrase *less...than*. If a hypothesis lacks a phrase such as *more than, less than, greater than, different from, related to, associated with*, or something similar, it is not readily testable. To test the revised hypothesis, we could ask two groups of women with different prenatal instruction experiences to respond to the question on depression and then compare the groups' responses. The absolute degree of depression of either group would not be at issue.

Hypotheses should be based on justifiable rationales. Hypotheses often follow from previous research findings or are deduced from a theory. When a relatively new area is being investigated, researchers may have to turn to logical reasoning or clinical experience to justify the predictions.

TIP

Hypotheses are typically fairly easy to identify because researchers make statements such as, "The study tested the hypothesis that . . ." or, "It was predicted that . . ."

Wording of Hypotheses

There are many ways to word hypotheses, but they should be worded in the present tense. Researchers make a prediction about a relationship in the population—not just about a relationship that will be revealed in a particular sample of study participants.

A hypothesis can predict the relationship between a single independent variable and a single dependent variable (a *simple hypothesis*) or it can predict a relationship between two or more independent variables or two or more dependent variables (a *complex hypothesis*). In the following examples, independent variables are indicated as IVs and dependent variables are identified as DVs:

Example of a complex hypothesis—multiple independent variables:
Schweitzer and colleagues (2007) hypothesized that, among patients with heart failure, depression (IV_1), anxiety (IV_2), and self-efficacy (IV_3) are independent predictors of adherence to medical treatment recommendations (DV).

Just as an outcome can be affected by more than one independent variable, so a single independent variable can affect or influence more than one outcome. A number of studies have found, for example, that cigarette smoking (the IV), can lead to both lung cancer (DV_1) and coronary disorders (DV_2). Complex hypotheses are common in studies that try to assess the impact of a nursing intervention on multiple outcomes.

Example of a complex hypothesis—multiple dependent variables:
McLeod and colleagues (2007) hypothesized that people with auditory hallucinations who participated in a cognitive behavioral intervention (IV) would, compared with nonparticipants, experience fewer hallucinations (DV_1), lower anxiety (DV_2), and fewer symptoms of distress (DV_3).

Hypotheses can be stated in various ways, as in the following example:

1. Older patients are more at risk of experiencing a fall than younger patients.
2. There is a relationship between a patient's age and the risk of falling.
3. The older the patient, the greater the risk that she or he will fall.
4. Older patients differ from younger ones with respect to their risk of falling.
5. Younger patients tend to be less at risk of a fall than older patients.
6. The risk of falling increases with the age of the patient.

In all of these examples, the hypotheses indicate the population (patients), the independent variable (patients' age), the dependent variables (risk of falling), and an anticipated relationship between them.

Hypotheses can be either directional or nondirectional. A **directional hypothesis** is one that specifies not only the existence but the expected direction of the relationship between variables. In the six versions of the hypothesis above, versions 1, 3, 5, and 6 are directional because there is an explicit prediction that older patients are at greater risk of falling than younger ones.

A **nondirectional hypothesis** does not stipulate the direction of the relationship, as illustrated in versions 2 and 4. These hypotheses state the prediction that a patient's age and the risk of falling are related, but they do not specify whether the researcher thinks that *older* patients or *younger* ones are at greater risk.

Hypotheses based on theory are almost always directional because theories explain phenomena and provide a rationale for explicit expectations. Existing studies also offer a basis for directional hypotheses. When no theory or related research exists, or when the findings of related studies are contradictory, nondirectional hypotheses may be appropriate. Some people argue, in fact, that nondirectional hypotheses are preferable because they suggest impartiality. According to this view, directional hypotheses imply that researchers are intellectually committed to certain outcomes, which might lead to bias. This argument fails to recognize that researchers typically *do* have hunches, whether they state them or not. We prefer directional hypotheses—when a reasonable basis for them exists—because they clarify the study's framework and demonstrate that researchers have thought critically about the concepts under study.

Another distinction is the difference between research and null hypotheses. **Research hypotheses** (also referred to as *substantive* or *scientific* hypotheses) are statements of expected relationships between variables. All the hypotheses presented thus far are research hypotheses that indicate actual expectations.

Statistical inference operates on a logic that may be somewhat confusing. This logic requires that hypotheses be expressed as an expected *absence* of a relationship. **Null hypotheses** (or *statistical hypotheses*) state that no relationship exists between the independent and dependent variables. The null form of the hypothesis used in our preceding example would be: "Older patients are just as likely as younger patients to fall." The null hypothesis might be compared with the assumption of innocence in English-based systems of criminal justice: The variables are assumed to be "innocent" of any relationship until they can be shown "guilty" through statistical procedures. The null hypothesis represents the formal statement of this assumption of innocence.

Research reports typically present research rather than null hypotheses. When statistical tests are performed, the underlying null hypotheses are assumed without being explicitly stated. If the researcher's *actual* research hypothesis is that no relationship among variables exists, the hypothesis cannot be adequately tested using traditional statistical procedures. This issue is explained in Chapter 15.

TIP

If a researcher uses any statistical tests (as is true in most quantitative studies), it means that there are underlying hypotheses—regardless of whether the researcher explicitly stated them—because statistical tests are designed to test hypotheses.

Hypothesis Testing and Proof

Hypotheses are formally tested through statistical analysis. Researchers seek to determine through statistics whether their hypotheses have a high probability of being correct. Statistical analysis does not provide proof, it only supports inferences that a hypothesis is *probably* correct (or not). Hypotheses are never *proved*; rather, they are *accepted* or *supported*. Findings are always tentative. Certainly, if the same results are replicated in numerous investigations, then greater confidence can be placed in the conclusions. Hypotheses come to be increasingly supported with mounting evidence.

To illustrate why this is so, suppose we hypothesized that height and weight are related. We predict that, on average, tall people weigh more than short people. We then obtain height and weight measurements from a sample and analyze the data. Now suppose we happened by chance to get a sample that consisted of short, heavy people, and tall, thin people. Our results might indicate that no relationship exists between a person's height and weight. Would we then be justified in stating that this study *proved* or *demonstrated* that height and weight are unrelated?

As another example, suppose we hypothesized that tall nurses are more effective than short ones. This hypothesis is used here only to illustrate a point because, in reality, we would expect no relationship between height and a nurse's job performance. Now suppose that, by chance again, we drew a sample of nurses in which tall nurses received better job evaluations than short ones. Could we conclude definitively that height is related to a nurse's performance? These two examples illustrate the difficulty of using observations from a sample to generalize to a population. Other issues, such as the accuracy of the measures, the effects of uncontrolled variables, and the validity of underlying assumptions, prevent researchers from concluding with finality that hypotheses are proved.

CRITIQUING RESEARCH PROBLEMS, RESEARCH QUESTIONS, AND HYPOTHESES

In critiquing research reports, you will need to evaluate whether researchers have adequately communicated their research problem. The delineation of the problem, statement of purpose, research questions, and hypotheses set the stage for the description of what was done and what was learned. Ideally, you should not have to dig too deeply to decipher the research problem or to discover the questions.

A critique of the research problem involves multiple dimensions. Substantively, you need to consider whether the problem has significance for nursing and has the potential to produce evidence to improve nursing practice. Studies that build on existing knowledge in a meaningful way are well-poised to make contributions to evidence-based nursing practice. Researchers who develop a systematic *program of research*, building on their own earlier findings, are especially likely to make significant contributions. For example, Beck's series of studies relating to postpartum depression (e.g., Beck, 1993, 1996, 2001; Beck & Gable, 2002, 2005) have influenced women's health care worldwide. Also, research problems stemming from established research priorities (see Chapter 1) have a high likelihood of yielding important new evidence for nurses because they reflect expert opinion about areas of needed research.

Another dimension in critiquing the research problem concerns methodologic issues—in particular, whether the research problem is compatible with the chosen research paradigm and its associated methods. You should also evaluate whether the statement of purpose or research questions have been properly worded and lend themselves to empirical inquiry.

In a quantitative study, if the research report does not contain explicit hypotheses, you need to consider whether their absence is justified. If there are hypotheses, you should evaluate whether the hypotheses are logically connected to the research problem and whether they are consistent with available knowledge or relevant theory. The wording of the hypothesis should also be assessed. The hypothesis is a valid guidepost to scientific inquiry only if it is testable. To be testable, the hypothesis must contain a prediction about the relationship between two or more measurable variables.

Specific guidelines for critiquing research problems, research questions, and hypotheses are presented in Box 6.3.

BOX 6.3 GUIDELINES FOR CRITIQUING RESEARCH PROBLEMS, RESEARCH QUESTIONS, AND HYPOTHESES

1. What is the research problem? Is the problem statement easy to locate and clearly stated? Does the problem statement build a cogent and persuasive argument for the new study?

2. Does the problem have significance for nursing? How might the research contribute to nursing practice, administration, education, or policy?

3. Is there a good fit between the research problem and the paradigm within which the research was conducted? Is there a good fit with the qualitative research tradition (if applicable)?

4. Does the report formally present a statement of purpose, research question, and/or hypotheses? Is this information communicated clearly and concisely, and is it placed in a logical and useful location?

5. Are purpose statements or questions worded appropriately? (e.g., are key concepts/variables identified and the population of interest specified? Are verbs used appropriately to suggest the nature of the inquiry and/or the research tradition?)

6. If there are no formal hypotheses, is their absence justified? Are statistical tests used in analyzing the data despite the absence of stated hypotheses?

7. Do hypotheses (if any) flow from a theory or previous research? Is there a justifiable basis for the predictions?

8. Are hypotheses (if any) properly worded—do they state a predicted relationship between two or more variables? Are they directional or nondirectional, and is there a rationale for how they were stated? Are they presented as research or as null hypotheses?

RESEARCH EXAMPLES AND CRITICAL THINKING ACTIVITIES

This section describes how the research problem and research questions were communicated in two nursing studies, one quantitative and one qualitative.

EXAMPLE 1 ■ Quantitative Research

Study

The effect of a multi-component smoking cessation intervention in African American women residing in public housing (Andrews et al., 2007).

Problem Statement

"Tobacco use is the leading cause of preventable death among all individuals in the United States (US), with widening gaps in health disparities occurring among ethnic minorities . . . African American women residing in urban subsidized housing developments report prevalence rates of 40–60% in some communities, which is at least twice the rate of women in the general population . . . African American women in subsidized housing developments indicate that cigarette smoking provides an alternate source of pleasure in the absence of other available resources, and that it is used to regulate mood and depression, manage stress, and cope with living conditions . . . Because of the limited research that has targeted African American women of low socioeconomic status who smoke, no evidence is available of the effectiveness of gender- and ethnic/racial-specific smoking cessation interventions…" (pp. 45–46) (Citations were omitted to streamline the presentation).

Statement of Purpose

The purpose of this study was to test the effectiveness of a community-partnered intervention (*Sister to Sister*) to promote smoking cessation among African American women in subsidized housing developments.

Hypotheses

Five hypotheses were tested in this study, including the following three: (1) Women who receive the *Sister to Sister* intervention will have higher 6-month continuous smoking abstinence than women who do not receive the intervention; (2) Women who receive the intervention will have higher 7-day abstinence at 6, 12, and 24 weeks than those who do not; and (3) Women who receive the intervention will have higher levels of social support, smoking cessation self-efficacy, and spiritual well-being at 6, 12, and 24 weeks than those who do not.

Intervention

A collaborative model involving a nurse researcher, community advisory board, and community members was used to plan, develop, and implement a culturally tailored, multicomponent intervention. The three major components were (1) a multiweek nurse-delivered, behavioral/empowerment counseling component in a group format; (2) nicotine replacement therapy; and (3) personal contact from a community health worker to enhance self-efficacy, social support and spiritual well-being.

Study Methods

Two of 16 subsidized housing developments in a county in Georgia were selected because of their similarity in size, level of poverty, and racial composition (99.5% African American). By coin toss, one community was selected to receive the intervention, and the other served as a comparison. The study participants were 103 women smokers who desired to quit—51 in the intervention group and 52 in the comparison group. Data were collected at the outset of the study and 6, 12, and 24 weeks later. Women in the comparison group received self-help written smoking cessation materials.

Key Findings

There was a 6-month continuous smoking abstinence rate of 27.5% in the intervention group and 5.7% in the comparison group, supporting hypothesis 1. Hypothesis 2 was also supported. For example, at 6 weeks, the 7-day prevalence rate was 49.0% for those who received the intervention and 7.6% for those who did not. Hypothesis 3 was only partially supported: there were significantly greater improvements for those in the intervention group on two of the three psychosocial outcomes (measures of social support and self-efficacy), but not at all three follow-up time periods.

CRITICAL THINKING SUGGESTIONS*:

*See the Student Resource CD-ROM for a discussion of these questions. 💿

1. Answer the relevant questions from Box 6.3 regarding this study.
2. Also consider the following targeted questions, which may further sharpen your critical thinking skills and assist you in understanding this study:
   a. Where in the research report do you think the researchers would have presented the hypotheses? Where in the report would the results of the hypothesis tests be placed?

    b. What clues does the summary give you that this study is quantitative?

    c. The report did not state research questions. What might some research questions be?

    d. Would it have been possible to state the three hypotheses as a single hypothesis? If yes, state what it would be.

    e. Develop a research question for a phenomenological and/or grounded theory study relating to the same general topic area as this study.

3. If the results of this study are valid and generalizable, what are some of the uses to which the findings might be put in clinical practice?

EXAMPLE 2 ■ Qualitative Research

Study

Family photographs: Expressions of parents raising children with disabilities (Lassetter, Mandleco, & Roper, 2007).

Problem Statement:

"The prevalence of disabilities in children is surprisingly high. In 2003, approximately 6.9% of children 18 years of age and younger in the United States had chronic conditions that limited their activities . . . The disabilities of these children influence not only their own lives but also the lives of their family members in a variety of ways . . . Raising a child with a disability can be a source of stress of parents . . . Specific sources of stress include learning to cope with the unanticipated event of having a child with a disability, the varying physical and psychological demands of child care, the likelihood of lifelong dependency, communication challenges, and an uncertain diagnosis . . . Much of the information concerning parents' experiences raising children with disabilities has been obtained through quantitative methods . . . Even though findings of quantitative studies are informative, the richness of parents' experiences can best be understood through qualitative research . . . In fact, several researchers have used qualitative methods to understand better the lives of parents with disabilities . . . However, there is still much to learn, and a different qualitative approach can help researchers discover some of the deep, unknown meanings of the phenomenon under study . . . " (p. 456) (Citations were omitted to streamline the presentation).

Statement of Purpose

The purpose of this descriptive study was to capture the perceptions of the everyday lives of parents raising a child with disabilities by using photography.

Research Questions

Two research questions were articulated in the report: (1) "How do parents raising children with disabilities perceive their everyday lives?" and (2) "Can information and meaning be distilled by using photography as a research tool with parents raising children with disabilities?"

Method

The study participants were 15 parental dyads raising a child with Down syndrome, developmental disabilities, visual impairments, or speech disorders. The parents were given a disposable camera and asked to photograph images of life that were important to them over a 2-week period. Then the researchers interviewed the parents, using the photographs as the focal point of the in-depth interviews.

Key Findings

Four themes emerged from the analysis of the photos (e.g., active activities, quiet activities). Six themes emerged when discussing photographs the parents would have liked to have taken but did not (e.g., normalcy, joys, struggles). The researchers concluded that photography was useful as a method of obtaining information from parents.

CRITICAL THINKING SUGGESTIONS:

1. Answer the relevant questions from Box 6.3 regarding this study.
2. Also, consider the following targeted questions, which may further sharpen your critical thinking skills and assist you in understanding this study:
   a. Where in the research report do you think the researchers would have presented the statement of purpose and research questions?
   b. Does it appear that this study was conducted within one of the three main qualitative traditions? If so, which one?
   c. What is a fundamental difference between the two research questions in this study?
   d. What clues does the summary give you that this study is qualitative?
3. If the results of this study are trustworthy, what are some of the uses to which the findings might be put in clinical practice?

EXAMPLE 3 ■ Quantitative Research in Appendix A

1. Read the abstract and the introduction from Howell and colleagues' (2007) study ("Anxiety, anger, and blood pressure in children") in Appendix A of this book, and then answer the relevant questions in Box 6.3.
2. Also, consider the following targeted questions, which may further sharpen your critical thinking skills and assist you in assessing aspects of the study's merit:
   a. Based on the review of the literature, it would be possible to state several research hypotheses. State one or two.
   b. If your hypothesis in exercise 2.a was a directional hypothesis, state it as a nondirectional hypothesis (or vice versa). Also state it as a null hypothesis.

EXAMPLE 4 ■ Qualitative Research in Appendix B

1. Read the abstract and introduction from Beck's (2006) study ("Anniversary of birth trauma") in Appendix B of this book and then answer the relevant questions in Box 6.3.
2. Also, consider the following targeted questions, which may further sharpen your critical thinking skills and assist you in assessing aspects of the study's merit:
   a. Do you think that Beck provided enough rationale for the significance of her research problem?
   b. Do you think that Beck needed to include research questions in her report, or was the purpose statement clear enough to stand alone?

CHAPTER REVIEW

Key new terms introduced in the chapter, together with a summary of major points, are presented in this section. In addition, Chapter 6 of the accompanying *Study Guide for Essentials of Nursing Research,* 7th edition offers various exercises and study suggestions for reinforcing the concepts presented in this chapter. For additional review, see the Student Self-Study Review Questions section of the Student Resource CD-ROM provided with this book.

Key New Terms

Directional hypothesis
Hypothesis
Nondirectional
    hypothesis

Null hypothesis
Problem statement
Research hypothesis
Research problem

Research question
Statement of purpose

Summary Points

➤ A **research problem** is a perplexing or troubling situation that a researcher wants to address through disciplined inquiry.

➤ Researchers usually identify a broad *topic*, narrow the scope of the problem, and then identify questions consistent with a paradigm of choice.

➤ The most common sources of ideas for nursing research problems are clinical experience, relevant literature, social issues, theory, and external suggestions.

➤ Researchers communicate their aims in research reports as problem statements, statements of purpose, research questions, or hypotheses.

➤ The **problem statement** articulates the nature, context, and significance of a problem to be studied. Problem statements typically include several components to develop an *argument*: problem identification; background; problem scope; consequences of the problem; knowledge gaps; and possible solutions to the problem.

➤ A **statement of purpose**, which summarizes the overall study goal, identifies the key concepts (variables) and the study group or population. Purpose statements often communicate, through the use of verbs and other key terms, the underlying research tradition of qualitative studies, or whether study is experimental or nonexperimental in quantitative ones.

➤ A **research question** is the specific query researchers want to answer in addressing the research problem. In quantitative studies, research questions usually are about the existence, nature, strength, and direction of relationships.

➤ A **hypothesis** is a statement of predicted relationships between two or more variables. A testable hypothesis in quantitative studies states the anticipated association between one or more independent and one or more dependent variables.

➤ **Directional hypotheses** predict the direction of a relationship; **nondirectional hypotheses** predict the existence of relationships, not their direction.

➤ **Research hypotheses** predict the existence of relationships; **null hypotheses** express the absence of a relationship.

➤ Hypotheses are never proved or disproved in an ultimate sense—they are accepted or rejected, supported or not supported by the data.

STUDIES CITED IN CHAPTER 6

Andrews, J., Felton, G., Wewers, M. E., Waller, J., & Tingen, M. (2007). The effect of a multi-component smoking cessation intervention in African American women residing in public housing. *Research in Nursing & Health, 30,* 45–60.

Beck, C. T. (1993). "Teetering on the edge": A substantive theory of postpartum depression. *Nursing Research, 42,* 42–48.

Beck, C. T. (1996). Postpartum depressed mothers' experiences interacting with their children. *Nursing Research, 45,* 98–104.

Beck, C. T. (2001). Predictors of postpartum depression: An update. *Nursing Research, 50,* 275–285.

Beck, C. T., & Gable, R. K. (2002). Postpartum depression screening scale manual. Los Angeles: Western Psychological Services.

Beck, C. Y., & Gable, R. K. (2005). Screening performance of the Postpartum Depression Screening Scale-Spanish Version. *Journal of Transcultural Nursing, 16,* 331–338.

Bunkers, S. (2007). The experience of feeling unsure for women at end-of-life. *Nursing Science Quarterly, 20,* 56–63.

Chantler, T., Lees, A., Moxon, E. R., Mant, D., Pollard, A., & Fitzpatrick, R. (2007). The role familiarity with science and medicine plays in parents' decision making about enrolling a child in vaccine research. *Qualitative Health Research, 17,* 311–322.

Facione, N., & Facione, P. (2007). Perceived prejudice in healthcare and women's health protective behavior. *Nursing Research, 56,* 175–184.

Gungor, I., & Beji, N. K. (2007). Effects of fathers' attendance to labor and delivery on the experience of childbirth in Turkey. *Western Journal of Nursing Research, 29,* 213–231.

Lasseter, J., Mandleco, B., & Roper, S. (2007). Family photographs: Expressions of parents raising children with disabilities. *Qualitative Health Research, 17,* 456–467.

McLeod, T., Morris, M., Birchwood, M., & Dovey, A. (2007). Cognitive behavioural therapy group work with voice hearers. *British Journal of Nursing, 16,* 248–252.

Oliffe, J., & Thorne, S. (2007). Men, masculinities, and prostrate cancer: Australian and Canadian patient perspectives of communication with male physicians. *Qualitative Health Research, 17,* 149–161.

Peterson, W., Sword, W., Charles, C., & DiCenso, A. (2007). Adolescents' perceptions of inpatient postpartum nursing care. *Qualitative Health Research, 17,* 201–212.

Schweitzer, R., Head, K., & Dwyer, J. (2007). Psychological factors and treatment adherence behavior in patients with chronic heart failure. *Journal of Cardiovascular Nursing, 22,* 76–83.

Taylor, E. J. (2007). Client perspectives about nurse requisites for spiritual caregiving. *Applied Nursing Research, 20,* 44–46.

7 Literature Reviews: Finding and Reviewing Research Evidence

STUDENT OBJECTIVES

On completing this chapter, you will be able to:

➤ Understand the steps involved in writing a literature review

➤ Identify appropriate information to include in a research literature review

➤ Identify bibliographic aids for retrieving nursing research reports, and locate references for a research topic

➤ Understand the process of screening, abstracting, critiquing, and organizing research evidence

➤ Evaluate the style, content, and organization of a literature review

➤ Define new terms in the chapter

Literature reviews can serve a number of important functions in the research process—and they also play a critical role for nurses seeking to develop an evidence-based practice (EBP). Thus, this chapter describes a range of activities associated with conducting a literature review, as well as critiquing reviews prepared by others. Many of the activities in conducting a literature review overlap with early steps in an EBP project, as described in Chapter 2.

BASIC ISSUES RELATING TO LITERATURE REVIEWS

Before discussing the activities involved in undertaking a research-based literature review, we briefly discuss some general issues. The first concerns the purposes of doing a literature review.

Purposes of Research Literature Reviews

Literature reviews can inspire new research ideas, and help to lay the foundation for studies. A literature review is a crucial early task for most quantitative researchers. For example, a literature review in a quantitative study can help to shape research questions, contribute to the argument about the need for a new study, suggest appropriate methods, and point to a conceptual or theoretical framework. By doing a thorough review, researchers can determine how best to contribute to the existing evidence base—for example, whether there are gaps in a body of research, or whether a replication with a new population is the right next step. A literature review also helps researchers to interpret their findings.

As previously noted, qualitative researchers have varying opinions about literature reviews, with some deliberately avoiding an in-depth literature search before entering the field. In grounded theory studies, researchers typically begin to collect data before examining the literature. As the data are analyzed and the grounded theory takes shape, researchers then turn to the literature, seeking to relate prior findings to the theory. Phenomenologists, by contrast, often undertake a search for relevant materials at the outset of a study. Ethnographers, although they often do not do a thorough up-front literature review, often familiarize themselves with the literature to help shape their choice of a cultural problem before going into the field.

Researchers usually summarize relevant literature in the introduction to their reports, regardless of when they perform the literature search. The literature review provides readers with a background for understanding current knowledge on a topic and illuminates the significance of the new study. Literature reviews are often intertwined with the argument for the study that is part of the statement of the problem.

Research reviews are not prepared solely in the context of doing a study. Nursing students and faculty, clinical nurses, and nurses in many other roles also need to review and synthesize evidence on a topic. As noted in earlier chapters, *systematic reviews* are carefully designed and executed integrations of a body of research, often conducted as a meta-analysis or metasynthesis. Thus, literature reviews are undertaken for many different purposes. Both consumers and producers of nursing research need to acquire skills for preparing and critiquing written summaries of knowledge on a problem.

Types of Information to Seek for a Research Review

Written materials vary in their quality, their intended audience, and the kind of information they contain. In performing a review of the research literature, you will have to decide what to read and what to include in the review.

Findings from prior studies are the most important type of information for a research review. If you are writing a literature review for a new study or preparing a review as a class assignment, you should rely mostly on **primary source** research reports, which are descriptions of studies written by the researchers who conducted them. **Secondary source** research documents are descriptions of studies prepared by someone other than the original researcher. Literature reviews, then, are secondary sources. Existing reviews, if they are recent, are often a good place to start because they provide a quick overview of the literature and a valuable bibliography. However, secondary descriptions of studies should not be considered substitutes for primary sources for a new literature review. Secondary sources typically fail to provide much detail about studies, and they are seldom completely objective.

TIP

For an EBP project, a recent, high-quality systematic review may be sufficient to provide the needed information about the evidence base, although it is usually wise to search for recent studies published after the review.

Examples of Primary and Secondary Sources

➤ Secondary source, a review of the literature on bladder training and voiding programs for managing urinary incontinence: Roe, B., Ostaszkiewicz, J., Milne, J., & Wallace, S. (2007). Systematic review of bladder training and voiding programmes in adults. *Journal of Advanced Nursing, 57,* 15–31.

➤ Primary source, an original experimental study of the effects of a nurse-initiated intervention for urinary incontinence: Zhang, A., Strauss, G., & Siminoff, L. (2007). Effects of combined pelvic muscle exercise and a support group on urinary incontinence and quality of life of postprostatectomy patients. *Oncology Nursing Forum, 34,* 47–53.

In addition to empirical references, a literature search may yield various non-research references, including opinion articles, case reports, and clinical anecdotes. Such materials may serve to broaden understanding of a research problem, illustrate a point, demonstrate a need for research, or describe aspects of clinical practice. These writings, however, usually have limited utility in written research reviews because they are subjective and do not address the central question of written reviews: What is the current state of *evidence* on this research problem?

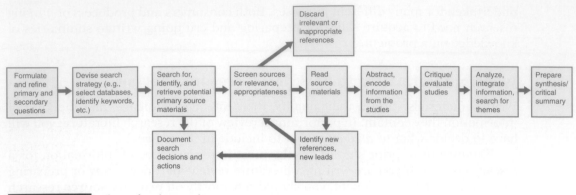

FIGURE 7.1 Flow of tasks in a literature review.

Major Steps and Strategies in Doing a Literature Review

Undertaking a literature review is a little bit like doing a full-fledged study, in the sense that a reviewer must start with a question (either an EBP question as discussed in Chapter 2, or a question for a new study, as described in Chapter 6), formulate and implement a plan for gathering information, and analyze and interpret the information. Then the "findings" are usually summarized in a written product. Figure 7.1 summarizes the literature review process. As the figure suggests, there are several potential feedback loops, with opportunities to go back to earlier steps in search of more information.

Conducting a high-quality literature review is not a mechanical exercise—it is an art and a science. Several qualities characterize a high-quality review. First, the review must be comprehensive and thorough, and must incorporate up-to-date references. Second, a high-quality review is systematic. Decision rules need to be clear, and the criteria for including or excluding a study need to be explicit. In part this is because a third characteristic of a good review is that it is reproducible. This means that another diligent reviewer would be able to apply the same decision rules and come to similar conclusions about the state of evidence on the topic. Another desirable attribute of a literature review is balance and the absence of bias.

> **TIP**
>
> Locating all relevant information on a research question is a bit like being a detective. The various literature retrieval tools we discuss in this chapter are a tremendous aid, but there inevitably needs to be some digging for (and a lot of sifting and sorting of) the clues to evidence on a topic. Be prepared for sleuthing!

A viewpoint that we recommend in doing a literature review is to think of it as doing a qualitative study. This means having a flexible approach to "data collection" and thinking creatively about opportunities for new sources of information. It also means that the analysis of the "data" typically involves a search for important themes.

LOCATING RELEVANT LITERATURE FOR A RESEARCH REVIEW

As shown in Figure 7.1, an early step in the literature review process is devising a strategy to locate relevant studies. The ability to locate documents on a research topic is an important skill that requires adaptability—rapid technological changes such as the Internet are making manual methods of finding information from print resources obsolete, and new methods of searching the literature are introduced continuously. We urge you to consult with librarians or faculty at your institution for updated suggestions.

Formulating a Search Strategy

There are many ways to go about searching for research evidence, and it is wise to begin a search with some strategies in mind. Cooper (1998) has identified several approaches, the first of which is one to which we devote considerable attention in this chapter: searching for references through the use of bibliographic databases. A second approach, called the *ancestry approach* (or "footnote chasing"), is to use the citations from relevant studies to track down earlier research on which the studies are based (the "ancestors"). A third method, called the *descendancy approach*, is to find a pivotal early study and to search forward in citation indexes to find more recent studies ("descendants") that cited the key study. For many practicing nurses, these strategies will usually suffice, but researchers may use other strategies for tracking down the *grey literature*—studies with more limited distribution, such as conference papers or unpublished reports.

TIP

You may be tempted to begin a literature search through an Internet search engine, such as Google or Yahoo. Such a search is likely to provide you with a lot of "hits" on your topic, including information about support groups, advocacy organizations, commercial products, and the like. However, such Internet searches are not likely to give you comprehensive bibliographic information on the *research* literature on your topic—and you might become frustrated with searching through the vast number of websites now available. Internet searches should be considered supplements, and not alternatives, to a search of bibliographic databases.

Another part of a search plan concerns decisions about delimiting the search. For example, many reviewers need to constrain their search to reports written in their own language. You may also want to limit your search to studies conducted within a certain time frame (e.g., within the past 15 years) or to certain operational definitions of key variables.

Searching Bibliographic Databases

Print-based bibliographic resources that must be searched manually are becoming outmoded. Reviewers typically begin by searching bibliographic databases that can be accessed by computer. Several commercial vendors (e.g., Ovid, EbscoHost, Pro-Quest) offer information retrieval services for bibliographic databases. Their programs are user friendly, offering menu-driven systems with on-screen support so that retrieval can usually proceed with minimal instruction. Some providers offer discount rates for students and trial services that allow you to test them before subscribing. In most cases, however, your university or hospital library is already a subscriber.

Getting Started with an Electronic Search

Before undertaking a search of a bibliographic database electronically, you should become familiar with the features of the software you are using to access the database. The software will give you options for restricting or expanding your search, for combining the results of two searches, for saving your search, and so on. Most programs have tutorials that offer useful information to improve the efficiency and effectiveness of your search.

An early task in doing an electronic search is to identify keywords to launch the search. A **keyword** is a word or phrase that captures the key concepts in your question. For quantitative studies, the keywords you begin with are usually the primary independent or dependent variables, and perhaps the population. For qualitative studies, they keywords would be the central phenomenon of interest and the population. If you have used the question templates for asking clinical questions that were included in Box 2.1, the words you entered in the blanks are likely to be good key words.

TIP

If you want to identify all major research reports on a topic, you need to be flexible and to think broadly about the keywords that could be related to your topic. For example, if you are interested in anorexia nervosa, you might look under *anorexia, eating disorders,* and *weight loss,* and perhaps under *appetite, eating behavior, food habits, bulimia,* and *body weight changes.*

For most bibliographic database searches, there are various types of search approaches. All citations included in a database have to be indexed so they can be retrieved, and databases and programs use their own system of categorizing the entries. The indexing systems have specific **subject headings** (subject codes) and a hierarchical organizational structure that permits various more specific subheadings.

You can undertake a *subject search* by entering a subject heading into the search field. You do not have to worry, however, if you are not familiar with the specific subject codes used in the program. Most software you are likely to use has mapping capabilities. *Mapping* is a feature that allows you to search for topics using your own keywords, rather than needing to enter a term that is exactly the same as a subject heading in the database. The software translates ("maps") the keywords you enter into the most plausible subject heading. Then it will retrieve all citations that have been coded with that subject heading.

Even when there are mapping capabilities, you should learn the relevant subject headings of the database you are using because keyword searches and subject heading searches yield overlapping but nonidentical search results. Subject headings for databases can be accessed in the database's thesaurus or other reference tools. Moreover, you may get additional suggestions for how to search if you learn something about the database's subject headings and structure.

When you enter a keyword into the search field, it is likely that the program will institute both a subject search, as just described, and a textword search. A *textword search* will search for your specific keyword in the text fields of the records in the database (e.g., the title or the abstract). Thus, if you searched for *lung cancer* in the MEDLINE database (which we describe in a subsequent section), the search would retrieve citations coded for the subject code of *lung neoplasms* (the MEDLINE subject heading used to code citations), and also any citations in which the phrase *lung cancer* appeared, even if it had not been coded for the *lung neoplasm* subject heading.

In addition to subject searches and textword searches, it is also possible to search for citations for a specific author. An *author search* might be productive if you are familiar with the names of leading researchers in a field, for example.

Although it is beyond the scope of this book to provide extensive guidance on doing an electronic bibliographic search, we can offer a few suggestions that could improve your search results. One tool available in most databases is wildcard characters. A **wildcard character**—which is a symbol such as "$" or "*", depending on the database and search program—can be used to search for multiple words that share the same root. To do this, the wildcard character is inserted immediately after the truncated root. For example, if we entered nurs* in the search field for a MEDLINE search, the computer would search for any word that begins with "nurs," such as *nurse*, *nurses*, and *nursing*. This can be very efficient, but note that the use of a wildcard character is likely to turn off the mapping feature, and result in a textword search exclusively.

Another way to force a textword search is to use quotation marks around a phrase, which will yield citations in which the exact phrase appears in text fields. In other words, *lung cancer* and "lung cancer" might yield different results. One strategy for a thorough search might be to do a search with and without wildcard characters and with and without quotation marks.

Boolean operators are another useful tool that can be used to expand or restrict a search. For example if you were interested in citations that concerned *lung cancer* and *smoking*, you could enter the following: *lung cancer AND smoking*. The Boolean operator "AND" would instruct the computer to restrict the search to citations that had both lung cancer and smoking as textwords or subject headings. The Boolean operator "OR" would expand the search—if you entered *lung cancer OR smoking*, you would get citations to all references with either term.

Two especially useful electronic databases for nurses are CINAHL (**C**umulative **I**ndex to **N**ursing and **A**llied **H**ealth **L**iterature) and MEDLINE (**Med**ical Literature

On-**Line**), which we discuss in greater detail in the next sections. Other potentially useful bibliographic databases for nurses include the Cochrane Database of Systematic Reviews, the Institute for Scientific Information (ISI)'s Web of Knowledge, and EMBASE (the Excerpta Medica database). The Web of Knowledge database is particularly effective for using the descendancy approach as a search strategy because of its strong citation indexes.

The CINAHL Database

The **CINAHL database** is an extremely important electronic database for nurses. It covers references to virtually all English-language nursing and allied health journals, as well as to books, book chapters, dissertations, and selected conference proceedings.

The CINAHL database includes materials dating from 1982 to the present and contains more than 1.3 million records. CINAHL provides bibliographic information for locating references (i.e., the author, title, journal, year of publication, volume, and page numbers), as well as abstracts of most citations. Supplementary information, such as names of data collection instruments, is available for many records in the database. Documents of interest can typically be ordered electronically. CINAHL can be accessed online or by CD-ROM, either directly through CINAHL (www.cinahl.com) or through a commercial vendor. We illustrate some of the features of the CINAHL database using Ovid software, but note that some of the features discussed may be unavailable or labeled differently if you are using different software to access CINAHL.

At the outset, you might begin with a "basic search" by simply entering keywords or phrases relevant to your primary question. You may want to restrict your search in a number of ways, for example, by limiting the records retrieved to a certain type of document (e.g., only research reports); to records with certain features (e.g., only ones with abstracts); to specific publication dates (e.g., only those after 1999); or to those written in English. A few simple clicks in the field labeled "Limits" can accomplish this, and clicking on "More Limits" offers more options.

To illustrate how searches can be delimited with a concrete example, suppose we were interested in recent nursing research on children's pain. Here is an example of how many "hits" there were on successive restrictions to the search, using one of many possible keyword search strategies, and using the CINAHL database through April 1, 2008:

SEARCH TOPIC/RESTRICTION	HITS
Pain	63,372
Pain AND child$	6,014
Limit to research reports	2,873
Limit to English	2,751
Limit to entries with abstracts	2,334
Limit to nursing journals	595
Limit to 2003 through 2008 publications	251

This narrowing of the search—from over 63,000 initial references on pain to 251 references for research reports published between 2003 and 2008 in nursing journals that has content on pain and children—took under 1 minute to perform. Note that we used the Boolean operator "AND" to search only for records that had *both* keywords in which we were interested. Also, we used a wildcard character, which in Ovid is "$." This instructed the computer to search for any word that begins with "child" such as children or childhood.

The 251 references from the search would be displayed on the monitor, and we could then print full information for ones that seemed promising. An example of an abridged CINAHL record entry for a report identified through this search on children's pain is presented in Figure 7.2. Each entry shows an accession number that is the unique identifier for each record in the database, as well as other identifying numbers. Then, the authors and title are displayed, followed by source information. The source indicates the following:

➤ Name of the journal (*Pain Management Nursing*)

➤ Year and month of publication (2007 Dec)

➤ Volume (8)

➤ Issue (4)

➤ Page numbers (156–65)

➤ Number of cited references (33)

Figure 7.2 also shows the CINAHL subject headings that were coded for this particular study. Any of these headings could have been used in the search to retrieve this reference. Note that the subject headings include substantive/topical headings such as *Comfort* and *Pain,* and also include methodologic headings (e.g., *Questionnaires, Diaries*) and sample characteristic headings (e.g., *Child*). Next, when formal instruments are used in a study, their names are printed under Instrumentation. The abstract for the study is then presented. Additional information, not shown here, includes any funding for the study and the full list of citations.

Based on the abstract, we would then decide whether this reference was pertinent to our inquiry. Documents referenced in the database usually can be ordered or directly downloaded, so it is not necessary for your library to subscribe to the referenced journal.

The MEDLINE Database

The MEDLINE database was developed by the U.S. National Library of Medicine (NLM), and is widely recognized as the premier source for bibliographic coverage of the biomedical literature. MEDLINE covers about 5,000 medical, nursing, and health journals published in about 70 countries and contains more than 16 million records dating back to the mid 1960s. Abstracts of reviews from the Cochrane Collaboration are also available through MEDLINE.

The MEDLINE database can be accessed online through a commercial vendor for a fee, but this database can be accessed for free on the Internet through the **PubMed** website (http://www.ncbi.nlm.nih.gov/PubMed). This means that anyone, anywhere in the world with Internet access can search for journal articles, and thus

ACCESSION NUMBER
2009743835 NLM Unique Identifier: 18036503.

AUTHOR
Wiggins SA, Foster RL

INSTITUTION
University of Nebraska Medical Center College of Nursing, Lincoln, Nebraska.

TITLE
Pain after tonsillectomy and adenoidectomy: "ouch it did hurt bad".

SOURCE
Pain Management Nursing. 2007 Dec; 8(4): 156-65. (33 ref)

ABBREVIATED SOURCE
PAIN MANAGE NURS. 2007 Dec; 8(4): 156-65. (33 ref)

CINAHL SUBJECT HEADINGS

*Adenoidectomy	Content Analysis	Midwestern United States
Adolescence	Convenience Sample	Nausea and Vomiting
Age Factors	Descriptive Research	*Pain Measurement
Analgesics/ad [Admin, Dosage]	Descriptive Statistics	Patient Attitudes/ev [Evaluation]
Analysis of Variance	Diaries	*Postoperative Pain
Art	Female	Purposive Sample
Audiorecording	Friedman Test	Questionnaires
Chi Square Test	Hospitals	Record Review
Child	Interviews	Repeated Measures
Comfort	Male	Thematic Analysis
Constant Comparative Method	Medical Records	*Tonsillectomy

INSTRUMENTATION
Hurt/Pain Diary. Body Outline for children aged 4–7 years (Van Cleve and Savedra). Poker Chip Tool (PCT) (Hester).

ABSTRACT
Severe pain experiences for children at home after tonsillectomy and adenoidectomy (T & A) have been described for more than a decade. Children and their parents are responsible for pain and symptom management during the postoperative home recovery. The purpose of this research was to more fully explore the pain experience and home management practices from the child's perspective. Diaries were used by 34 children (4–18 years of age) to document their pain and other symptoms. A home interview, stories, art work, and personal notes were also explored to fully capture the experience. From the evening of surgery through the second postoperative day, children reported mean pain intensity ratings of 3.1–3.3 out of a possible 4. Pain awakened 64.7% of the children from nighttime sleep and 52.9% reported vomiting associated with nausea. Children received an average of only 50% of the analgesic doses prescribed. Across the 3 postoperative days studied, pain remained severe and interventions offered minimal relief. Neither older children (chi(2) = 1.357, n = 13, df = 2, p = .259) nor younger children (chi(2) = 1.357, n = 12, df = 2, p = .507) reported significant differences in their mean pain intensity across the first 3 postoperative days. Results supported concerns for inadequate home pain management practices in the pediatric T & A population.

FIGURE 7.2 Example of a printout from a CINAHL (**C**umulative **I**ndex to **N**ursing and **A**llied **H**ealth **L**iterature) search.

PubMed is a lifelong resource regardless of your institutional affiliation. PubMed has an excellent tutorial.

MEDLINE/PubMed uses a controlled vocabulary called **MeSH** (Medical Subject Headings) to index articles. MeSH terminology provides a consistent way to retrieve information that may use different terminology for the same concepts. If you begin a search with your own keyword, you can click on the "Display" tab near the top right of the screen to see how the term you entered mapped onto MeSH terms, which might lead you to pursue other leads. You can also search for references using the MeSH database directly by clicking on "MeSH database" in the left blue panel of the PubMed home page, listed under PubMed services. Note that MeSH subject headings may overlap with, but are not identical to, the subject headings used in the CINAHL database

If we did a PubMed search of MEDLINE similar to the one we described earlier for CINAHL, this is what we would find:

SEARCH TOPIC/RESTRICTION	HITS
Pain	369,331
Pain AND child*	36,424
Limit to research reports	(NA)
Limit to English	29,353
Limit to entries with abstracts	24,588
Limit to nursing journals	1,103
Limit to 2003 through 2008 publications	390

This search yielded more references than the CINAHL search, but we were not able to limit the search to research reports because the publication types in this database are categorized differently than in CINAHL. For example, in PubMed we could limit the search to certain *types* of research (e.g., clinical trials), but it may be risky to use this restriction criterion. Note that in PubMed, the wildcard code used to extend truncated words is * rather than $.

Figure 7.3 shows the full citation for the same reference we located earlier in the CINAHL database (Figure 7.2). To get this full citation, you would need to use a pull-down menu near the top that offers alternative Displays—in this case, you would designate "Citation." The citation display presents all the MeSH terms that were used for this reference and, as you can see, the MeSH terms are different than the subject headings in CINAHL.

TIP

Many database search programs have an extremely useful feature that allows you to find references to other similar studies. That is, once you have found a study that is exemplar of what you are looking for, you can search for other similar studies. In PubMed, for example, after identifying a key study, you could click on "Related Articles" on the right of the screen to search for other similar studies. In CINAHL via Ovid, you would click on "Find Similar."

Screening and Gathering References

References that have been identified through the literature search need to be screened. One screen is totally practical—is the reference readily accessible? For

Pain Manag Nurs. 2007 Dec;8(4):156–65.

Pain after tonsillectomy and adenoidectomy: "ouch it did hurt bad".

Wiggins SA, Foster RL.

University of Nebraska Medical Center College of Nursing, Lincoln, Nebraska, USA. swiggins@unmc.edu

Severe pain experiences for children at home after tonsillectomy and adenoidectomy (T & A) have been described for more than a decade. Children and their parents are responsible for pain and symptom management during the postoperative home recovery. The purpose of this research was to more fully explore the pain experience and home management practices from the child's perspective. Diaries were used by 34 children (4–18 years of age) to document their pain and other symptoms. A home interview, stories, art work, and personal notes were also explored to fully capture the experience. From the evening of surgery through the second postoperative day, children reported mean pain intensity ratings of 3.1–3.3 out of a possible 4. Pain awakened 64.7% of the children from nighttime sleep and 52.9% reported vomiting associated with nausea. Children received an average of only 50% of the analgesic doses prescribed. Across the 3 postoperative days studied, pain remained severe and interventions offered minimal relief. Neither older children ($chi(2) = 1.357$, $n = 13$, $df = 2$, $p = .259$) nor younger children ($chi(2) = 1.357$, $n = 12$, $df = 2$, $p = .507$) reported significant differences in their mean pain intensity across the first 3 postoperative days. Results supported concerns for inadequate home pain management practices in the pediatric T & A population.

MeSH Terms:
- Adenoidectomy*
- Adolescent
- Adolescent Psychology
- Child
- Child Psychology
- Child, Preschool
- Female
- Humans
- Male
- Pain Measurement/nursing
- Pain, Postoperative/nursing*
- Pain, Postoperative/psychology*
- Pediatric Nursing*
- Tonsillectomy*

PMID: 18036503 [PubMed - indexed for MEDLINE]

FIGURE 7.3   Example of a printout from a PubMed search.

example, full dissertations may not be easy to retrieve. A second screen is the relevance of the reference, which you can usually (but not always) surmise by reading the abstract. A third criterion may include the study's methodologic quality—that is, the quality of evidence the study yields, a topic discussed in a later section.

We strongly urge you to obtain full copies of relevant studies rather than simply taking notes. It is often necessary to re-read a report or to get further details about an aspect of a study, which can easily be done if you have a copy of the article. Each obtained article should be stored in a manner that permits easy retrieval. Some authors advocate chronological filing (e.g., by date of publication), but we think that alphabetical filing (using last name of the first author) is easier.

Documentation in Literature Retrieval

If your goal is to do a thorough review, you will be using a variety of databases, keywords, and strategies. As you meander through the complex world of research information, you will likely lose track of your efforts if you do not document your actions.

It is wise to maintain a notebook (or computer database program) to record your search strategies and results. You should make note of information such as databases searched; limits put on your search; specific keywords, subject headings, and authors used to direct the search; studies used to inaugurate a "Related Articles" or "descendancy" search; websites visited; and any other information that would help you keep track of what you have done. Part of your strategy can be documented by printing your search history from the electronic databases.

By documenting your actions, you will be able to conduct a more efficient search—that is, you will not inadvertently duplicate a strategy you have already pursued. Documentation will also help you to assess what else needs to be tried—where to go next in your search.

Abstracting and Recording Information

Tracking down relevant research on a topic is only the beginning of doing a literature review. Once you have a stack of useful articles, you need to develop a strategy for making sense of the mass of information contained in the articles. If a literature review is fairly simple, it may be sufficient to jot down notes about key features of the studies under review, and to use these notes as the basis for your integration. However, literature reviews are often more elaborate—for example, there may be numerous studies in the review, or the studies may vary in how key constructs were operationalized. In such situations, it is helpful to use a formal system of recording information from each study. One such mechanism is to use a formal literature review protocol. Another—one that we recommend for complex reviews involving numerous primary studies—is to use a coding scheme and a set of matrices, a system that we have described in detail elsewhere (Polit & Beck, 2008).

Protocols are a means of recording various aspects of a study systematically, including the full citation, theoretical foundations, methodologic features, findings, and conclusions. Evaluative information (e.g., your assessment of the study's strengths and weaknesses) can also be noted. There is no fixed format for such a protocol. You must decide what elements are important to *consistently* record across studies to help you organize and analyze information. We present an example in Figure 7.4, which can be adapted to fit your needs. Although many of the terms on this protocol are probably not familiar to you at this point, you will learn their meaning in subsequent chapters. The Toolkit for this chapter includes this protocol as a Word document for your use or adaptation. ✷

Once you have developed a draft protocol, you should pilot test it with several studies to make sure it is sufficiently comprehensive and well-structured.

EVALUATING AND ANALYZING THE EVIDENCE

In drawing conclusions about a body of research, reviewers must make judgments about the worth of the studies' evidence. Within an EBP context, this corresponds

Citation:	Authors: _____
	Title: _____
	Journal: _____
	Year: _____ Volume: _____ Issue: _____ Pages: _____

| Type of Study: | ☐ Quantitative   ☐ Qualitative   ☐ Mixed Method |

Location/setting: _____

Key Concepts/	Concepts: _____
Variables:	Intervention/IndependentVariable: _____
	Dependent Variable: _____
	Controlled Variables: _____

Framework/Theory: _____

Design Type:	☐ Experimental ☐ Quasi-experimental ☐ Nonexperimental
	Specific Design: _____
	Blinding? ☐ None ☐ Single: _____ ☐ Double _____
	Descrip. of Intervention: _____
	_____
	Comparison group(s): _____
	☐ Cross-sectional ☐ Longitudinal/prospective No. of data collection points: ____

| Qual. Tradition: | ☐ Grounded theory ☐ Phenomenology   ☐ Ethnography   ☐ Other: _____ |

| Sample: | Size: _____   Sampling method: _____ |
| | Sample characteristics: _____ |

Data Sources:	Type: ☐ Self-report ☐ Observational ☐ Biophysiologic ☐ Other ____
	Description of measures: _____
	_____
	Data Quality: _____

| Statistical Tests: | Bivariate: ☐ T test ☐ ANOVA   ☐ Chi-square   ☐ Pearson's r ☐ Other: _____ |
| | Multivar:☐ Multiple regression ☐ MANOVA ☐ Logistic Regression ☐Other: __ |

Findings/	_____
Effect Sizes/	_____
Themes	_____
	_____
	_____
	_____

Recommendations:	_____
	_____
Strengths:	_____
	_____
Weaknesses:	_____
	_____

FIGURE 7.4   Example of a literature review protocol. ✺

to the first question in Box 2.1—how rigorous and reliable is the research evidence? Thus, an important part of a literature review is evaluating the body of completed studies and integrating the evidence across studies.

Evaluating Studies for a Review

In reviewing the literature, you typically would not undertake a comprehensive critique of each study such as the type we discussed in Chapter 4. Nevertheless, you would need to evaluate the quality of each study so that you could draw conclusions about the overall body of evidence and about gaps in the evidence base. Critiques for a literature review tend to focus on methodologic aspects.

In literature reviews undertaken by students and practicing nurses, methodologic features of the studies under review need to be assessed with an eye to answering a very broad question: To what extent do the findings, taken together, reflect the *truth* (the true state of affairs) or, conversely, to what extent do biases and flaws undermine the believability of the evidence? The "truth" is most likely to be discovered when researchers use powerful designs, good sampling plans, strong data collection instruments and procedures, and appropriate analyses.

In free-standing systematic reviews, methodologic quality often plays a role right at the outset of the review because studies judged to be of low quality may be screened out from further consideration. Using methodologic quality as a screening criterion is somewhat controversial, however. Systematic reviews are also especially likely to involve the use of a formal evaluation instrument that gives quantitative ratings to different aspects of the study, so that appraisals across studies ("scores") can be compared and summarized. Methodologic screening issues and formal scoring instruments are described in Chapter 19.

> **TIP**
>
> An important thing to remember is that it is appropriate to assume the posture of a skeptic when you are critiquing research reports. Just as a careful clinician seeks evidence from research findings that certain practices are or are not effective, you as a reviewer should demand evidence from reports that the researchers' methodologic decisions were sound.

Analyzing and Synthesizing Information

Once all the relevant studies have been retrieved, read, abstracted, and critiqued, the information has to be analyzed and synthesized. As previously noted, we find the analogy between performing a literature review and a qualitative study useful, and this is particularly true with respect to the analysis of the "data" (i.e., the information from the retrieved studies). In both, the focus is on the identification of important *themes*.

A thematic analysis essentially involves the detection of patterns and regularities—as well as inconsistencies. A number of different types of themes can be identified in a literature review analysis, including the following:

➤ *Substantive themes*: What is the pattern of evidence? How much evidence is there? How consistent is the body of evidence? How powerful are the observed effects? How persuasive is the evidence? What gaps are there in the body of evidence?

➤ *Methodologic themes*: What designs and methods have been used to address the question? What methodologic strategies have *not* been used? What are the predominant methodologic deficiencies and strengths? Do findings vary in relation to differences in methodologic approaches?

➤ *Generalizability/transferability themes*: To what types of people or settings do the findings apply? Do the findings vary for different types of people (e.g., men versus women) or setting (e.g., urban versus rural)?

➤ *Historical themes*: Have there been substantive, theoretical, or methodologic trends over time? Is the evidence getting better? When was most of the research conducted?

➤ *"Researcher" themes*: Who has been doing the research, in terms of discipline, specialty area, nationality, prominence, and so on? Has the research been developed within a systematic program of research?

Clearly, it is not possible—even in lengthy free-standing reviews—to analyze all the themes we have identified. Reviewers have to make decisions about which patterns to pursue. In preparing a review, you would need to determine which pattern is of greatest relevance for the purpose at hand.

PREPARING A WRITTEN LITERATURE REVIEW

Writing literature reviews can be challenging, especially when voluminous information and thematic analyses must be condensed into a small number of pages. We offer a few suggestions, but readily acknowledge that skills in writing literature reviews develop over time.

Organizing the Review

Organization is crucial in preparing a written review. When literature on a topic is extensive, it is useful to summarize information in a table. The table could include columns with headings such as Author, Sample Characteristics, Design, Data Collection Approach, and Key Findings. Such a table provides a quick overview that allows you to make sense of a mass of information. We provide a template for such a table in the Toolkit for this chapter. ✦

Most writers find it helpful to work from an outline—a written one if the review is lengthy or complex, a mental one for simpler reviews. The important point is to have a plan before starting to write so that the review has a meaningful and understandable flow. Lack of organization is a common weakness in first attempts at writing a research literature review. Although the specifics of the organization differ from topic to topic, the overall goal is to structure the review in such a way that the presentation is logical, demonstrates meaningful thematic integration, and leads to a conclusion about the state of evidence on the topic.

After an organizing structure has been decided, you should review your notes or protocols. This helps refresh your memory about material read earlier and lays the groundwork for decisions about where a particular reference fits in the outline. If some references do not seem to fit anywhere, they may need to be put aside. Remember that the number of references is less important than their relevance and the overall organization of the review.

Writing a Literature Review

Although it is beyond the scope of this textbook to offer detailed guidance on writing research reviews, we offer a few comments on their content and style. Additional assistance is provided in books such as those by Fink (2005), Galvan (2003), and Garrard (2004).

Content of the Written Literature Review

A written research review should provide readers with an objective, well-organized synthesis of the current state of evidence on a topic. A literature review should be neither a series of quotes nor a series of abstracts. The central tasks are to summarize and critically evaluate the overall evidence so as to reveal the current state of knowledge on a topic with regard to themes deemed to be important—not simply to describe what researchers have done.

Although key studies may be described in detail, it is not necessary to provide particulars for every reference. Studies with comparable findings often can be summarized together.

Example of grouped studies:
Bonner and colleagues (2008, p. 91) summarized several studies as follows: "Fatigue is prevalent in most chronic illnesses (Glaken et al., 2003; Jenkin et al., 2006)...Despite advances in renal replacement therapies, fatigue remains ranked as one of the most troublesome symptoms for people with ESRD (end-stage renal disease); physical fatigue is one of the most frequently experienced symptoms with >90% of patients reporting a lack of energy and feeling tired (Thomas-Hawkins, 2000; Braun Curtin et al., 2002)."

The literature should be summarized in your own words. The review should demonstrate that consideration has been given to the cumulative worth of the body of research. Stringing together quotes from various documents fails to show that previous research has been assimilated and understood.

The review should be objective, to the extent possible. Studies with findings that conflict with personal values or hunches should not be omitted. The review also should not ignore a study because its findings contradict other studies. Inconsistent results should be analyzed and the supporting evidence evaluated objectively.

A literature review typically concludes with a concise summary of current evidence on the topic. The summary should recap key findings, indicate how credible they are, and make note of gaps in the evidence. When the literature review is conducted as part of a new study, the critical summary should demonstrate the need for the research and should clarify the context within which any hypotheses were developed.

As you progress through this book, you will become increasingly proficient in critically evaluating the research literature. We hope you will understand the mechanics of doing a research review once you have completed this chapter, but we do not expect that you will be in a position to write a state-of-the-art review until you have acquired more skills in research methods.

Style of a Research Review

Students preparing written research reviews often have trouble figuring out an acceptable style for such reviews. In particular, students sometimes accept research results without criticism or skepticism. You should keep in mind that hypotheses cannot be proved or disproved by empirical testing, and no research question can be definitely answered in a single study. Every study has at least some methodologic limitations. The fact that hypotheses cannot be ultimately proved or disproved does not, of course, mean that we must disregard research evidence—especially if findings have been replicated. The problem is partly semantic: hypotheses are not proved, they are *supported* by research findings.

TIP

When describing study findings, you should generally use phrases indicating tentativeness of the results, such as the following:

➤ Several studies have *found* . . .
➤ Findings thus far *suggest* . . .
➤ The results *are consistent* with the conclusion that . . .
➤ Results from a landmark study *imply* that . . .
➤ There *appears* to be fairly strong evidence that . . .

A related stylistic problem is the interjection of opinions into the review. The review should include opinions sparingly, if at all, and should be explicit about their source. Reviewers' own opinions do not belong in a review, with the exception of assessments of study quality.

The left-hand column of Table 7.1 presents several examples of stylistic flaws. The right-hand column offers recommendations for rewording the sentences to conform to a more acceptable form for a research literature review. Many alternative wordings are possible.

Length of a Research Review

There are no formulas for how long a review should be. The length depends on several factors, including the complexity of the question, the extent of prior research, and the purpose for which the review is being prepared.

Because of space limitations in journal articles, literature reviews that appear within research reports are concise. Literature reviews in the introduction to research reports demonstrate the need for the new study and provide a context for the research questions. However, stand-alone research reviews in nursing journals are more extensive than those appearing in the introductions of research reports. If

TABLE 7.1 ▶ EXAMPLES OF STYLISTIC DIFFICULTIES	
PROBLEMATIC STYLE OR WORDING	IMPROVED STYLE OR WORDING
Women who do not participate in childbirth preparation classes manifest a high degree of anxiety during labor.	Studies have found that women who participate in childbirth preparation classes tend to manifest less anxiety than those who do not (Boyd, 2008; McTygue, 2008; Yepsen, 2009).
Studies have proved that doctors and nurses do not fully understand the psychobiologic dynamics of recovery from a myocardial infarction.	Studies by Fortune (2009) and Crampton (2008) suggest that many doctors and nurses do not fully understand the psychobiologic dynamics of recovery from a myocardial infarction.
Attitudes cannot be changed quickly.	Attitudes have been found to be relatively stable, enduring attributes that do not change quickly (Nicolet, 2007; Carroll, 2008).
It is known that uncertainty engenders stress.	According to Dr. A. Cassard (2008), an expert on stress and anxiety, uncertainty is a stressor.

you are preparing a comprehensive literature review as a classroom assignment, your instructor will likely suggest page length guidelines.

CRITIQUING RESEARCH LITERATURE REVIEWS

Some nurses never prepare a written research review, and perhaps you will never be required to do one. Most nurses, however, do *read* research reviews (including the literature review sections of research reports) and they should be prepared to evaluate such reviews critically.

You may find it difficult to critique a research review, because you are probably a lot less familiar with the topic than the writer. You may thus not be able to judge whether the author has included all relevant literature and has adequately summarized knowledge on that topic. Many aspects of a research review, however, are amenable to evaluation by readers who are not experts on the topic. Some suggestions for critiquing written research reviews are presented in Box 7.1. ✪ Additionally, when a review is published as a stand-alone article, it should include information to help readers evaluate its thoroughness, as discussed in the chapter on systematic reviews (Chapter 19).

In assessing a literature review, the overarching question is whether it summarizes the current state of research evidence. If the review is written as part of an original research report, an equally important question is whether the review lays a solid foundation for the new study.

BOX 7.1   GUIDELINES FOR CRITIQUING LITERATURE REVIEWS

1. Does the review seem thorough—does it include all or most of the major studies on the topic? Does it include recent research? Are studies from other related disciplines included, if appropriate?

2. Does the review rely on appropriate materials (e.g., mainly on research reports, using primary sources)?

3. Is the review merely a summary of existing work, or does it critically appraise and compare key studies? Does the review identify important gaps in the literature?

4. Is the review well organized? Is the development of ideas clear?

5. Does the review use appropriate language, suggesting the tentativeness of prior findings? Is the review objective? Does the author paraphrase, or is there an over-reliance on quotes from original sources?

6. If the review is part of a research report for a new study, does the review support the need for the study?

7. If it is a review designed to summarize evidence for clinical practice, does the review draw appropriate conclusions about practice implications?

RESEARCH EXAMPLES AND CRITICAL THINKING EXERCISES

The best way to learn about the style, content, and organization of a research literature review is to read reviews that appear in the nursing literature. We present excerpts from two reviews here and urge you to read other reviews on topics of interest to you.

EXAMPLE 1 ■ Literature Review from a Quantitative Study

Study

Complementary therapy and older rural women: Who uses it and who does not? (Shreffler-Grant, Hill, Weinert, Nichols, & Ide, 2007).

Statement of Purpose

The purpose of this study was to identify factors that predict the use of complementary therapy among older rural women.

Literature Review (Excerpt)

"Complementary or alternative therapy has become an important component of the U. S. healthcare system as healthcare consumers increasingly turn to these therapies and practices as adjuncts to or substitutes for conventional healthcare (Astin, 1998, Eisenberg et al., 1998; McFarland et al., 2002). In 2004, 62% of U.S. adults used some form of complementary care when prayer for health was included in the definition of complementary care, 36% when prayer was excluded from the definition (Barnes et al., 2004) . . .

Complementary or alternative care has been defined by the National Center for Complementary and Alternative Medicine (NCCAM) as a group of diverse healthcare systems, practices, and products that are not considered presently a part of conventional healthcare . . .

Complementary therapy implies care that complements or is used together with allopathic care, whereas *alternative* therapy implies that care is used as a substitute for allopathic care . . . For brevity, CAM (complementary and alternative medicine or healthcare) will be used in the remainder of this article.

Although national data regarding factors associated with the use of CAM are somewhat inconsistent, one common finding is that women are significantly more likely to use these therapies than are men (Barnes et al., 2004; Wolsko et al., 2000) . . . In a recent publication based on the 1999 National Health Interview Survey data, it was reported that 22.5% of American women used CAM in the prior 12 months (Upchurch & Chyu, 2005). Women who were older, more educated, in poorer health, and living in the west or Midwest were found to be more likely to use CAM, and the most commonly used therapies were spiritual healing or prayer and herbal medicine . . .

Most national studies on the use of CAM either do not report place of residence (rural or urban) of participants or focus only on urban samples (Astin, 1998; Eisenberg et al., 1993, 1998), despite the fact that one quarter of the U.S. population reside in rural areas (Eberhardt et al., 2001). One national study included limited rural versus urban comparisons, and the findings indicated that fewer rural than urban adults used CAM (Barnes et al., 2004). Studies that have focused specifically on rural dweller's use of CAM have had conflicting results: use has been found to be more prevalent in rural than urban areas (Harron & Glasser, 2003), less prevalent in rural areas (Vallerand et al., 2003), and equally prevalent in rural and urban areas (Shreffler-Grant et al., 2005). Many studies of CAM use by rural dwellers are characterized by sampling limitations, with samples drawn from physician practices, small geographic areas, rural subgroups, or a combination of these (Harron & Glasser, 2003; Trotter, 1981; Vallerand et al., 2003) . . .

With few exceptions, most research with rural samples has been focused on estimating the proportion of a population that uses CAM and the extent of use rather than identifying demographic or health-related factors associated with use . . . To address these gaps in the literature, a study on the use of CAM among older adults living in sparsely populated rural areas of Montana and North Dakota was conducted . . . The purpose of this presentation is to report a portion of a larger study that sought to answer the following research question: What factors predict use of complementary therapy among older rural women? The predictors were selected from the literature and clinical observations and included education, age, rurality, marital status, spirituality, number of chronic illnesses, and health status" (pp. 28–29).

CRITICAL THINKING SUGGESTIONS*:

*See the Student Resource CD-ROM for a discussion of these questions. 💿

1. Answer the relevant questions from Box 7.1 regarding this study.
2. Also, consider the following targeted questions, which may further sharpen your critical thinking skills and assist you in understanding this study:
   a. What were the independent variables in this study? Did the literature review cover findings from prior studies about these variables?
   b. What were the dependent variables in this study? Did the literature review cover findings from prior studies about these variables?
   c. In performing the literature review, what keywords might the researchers have used to search for prior studies?
   d. Using the keywords, perform a computerized search to see if you can find a recent relevant study to augment the review.

EXAMPLE 2 ■ Literature Review from a Qualitative Study

Study

The experiences and challenges of pregnant women coping with thrombophilia (Martens & Emed, 2007).

Statement of Purpose

This study explored the experiences, challenges, and coping strategies of pregnant women diagnosed with thrombophilia and who are on daily heparin injections.

Literature Review (Excerpt)

"Thrombophilia is a serious hypercoagulability disorder that contributes to maternal mortality and has been associated with significant pregnancy complications including intrauterine growth restriction, preeclampsia, and recurrent fetal loss. The incidence of thrombophilia is approximately 15% in the general population (Greer, 2003) and recurrent fetal loss occurs in as many as 65% of pregnant women with thrombophilia (Kovalesky et al., 2004; Kujovich, 2004; Rey et al., 2003). At this time, there are no screening protocols in place and thrombophilia often goes undiagnosed until several pregnancy complications have already occurred (Kujovich, 2004; Walker et al., 2001). This may lead to considerable emotional and psychological distress greatly impacting the experience of women with thrombophilia who desire to have children . . .

Intrauterine growth restriction, stillbirth, preeclampsia, and recurrent fetal loss have all been associated with thrombophilic disorders (Alfirevic et al., 2001; Kujovich, 2004) . . . The treatment of choice for women with known thrombophilia, thromboembolic episodes, previous unexplained fetal losses . . . or abruption who are or wish to become pregnant is prophylactic unfractionated heparin (UFH) or low-molecular-weight heparin (LMWH) (Bates et al., 2004; Gris et al., 2004). Unfractionated heparin and LMWH are administered as daily subcutaneous injections that may be prescribed as out-patient medication...The anxiety and fear related to daily self-injections may be an additional factor impacting the pregnancy experience (Mohr et al., 2002).

There remains a significant gap in the literature exploring the unique needs, experiences, and coping strategies of pregnant women diagnosed with thrombophilia. Studies that have explored the concerns of pregnant women with disabilities, inherited disorders, and pregnancy complications have identified topics such as loss of control, need for support from health professionals, feelings of despair, overpowering uncertainty, and increasing stress (Bachman & Lind, 1997; Berg & Dahlberg, 1998; Briscoe et al., 2002; Thomas, 1999, 2004) . . . Medical and nursing research highlights the seriousness of thrombophilia during pregnancy and suggests that pregnant women coping with thrombophilia will confront many difficult challenges" (pp. 55–56).

CRITICAL THINKING SUGGESTIONS:

1. Answer the relevant questions from Box 7.1 regarding this study.
2. Also, consider the following targeted questions, which may further sharpen your critical thinking skills and assist you in understanding this study:
   a. What was the central phenomenon that the researchers focused on in this study? Was that phenomenon adequately covered in the literature review?
   b. In performing the literature review, what keywords might the researchers have used to search for prior studies?
   c. Using the keywords, perform a computerized search to see if you can find a recent relevant study to augment the review.

EXAMPLE 3 ■ Quantitative Research in Appendix A

1. Read the abstract and the introduction from Howell and colleagues' (2007) study ("Anxiety, anger, and blood pressure in children") in Appendix A of this book, and then answer the relevant questions in Box 7.1.
2. Also, consider the following targeted questions, which may further sharpen your critical thinking skills and assist you in assessing aspects of the study's merit:
   a. What was the independent variable in this study? Did the literature review cover findings from prior studies about this variable?
   b. What were the dependent variables in this study? Did the literature review cover findings from prior studies about these variables and its relationship with the independent variable?
   c. In performing the literature review, what keywords might have been used to search for prior studies?

EXAMPLE 4 ■ Qualitative Research in Appendix B

1. Read the abstract and introduction from Beck's (2006) study ("Anniversary of birth trauma") in Appendix B of this book and then answer the relevant questions in Box 7.1.
2. Also, consider the following targeted questions, which may further sharpen your critical thinking skills and assist you in assessing aspects of the study's merit:
   a. What was the central phenomenon that Beck focused on in this study? Was that phenomenon adequately covered in the literature review?
   b. In what sections of the report did Beck discuss prior research?
   c. In performing her literature review, what keywords might Beck have used to search for prior studies?

CHAPTER REVIEW

Key new terms introduced in the chapter, together with a summary of major points, are presented in this section. In addition, Chapter 7 of the *Study Guide for Essentials of Nursing Research,* 7th edition offers various exercises and study suggestions for reinforcing the concepts presented in this chapter. For additional review, see the Student Self-Study Review Questions section of the Student Resource CD-ROM provided with this book.

Key New Terms

Bibliographic database	Literature review	PubMed
CINAHL database	MEDLINE database	Secondary source
Keyword	Primary source	Subject heading

Summary Points

●●●

➤ A research **literature review** is a written summary of the state of evidence on a research problem. An important type of review for EBP is a systematic review, typically a meta-analysis or metasynthesis.

➤ The major steps in preparing a written research review include formulating a question, devising a search strategy, conducting a search, retrieving relevant sources, abstracting and encoding information, critiquing studies, analyzing the information, and preparing a written synthesis.

➤ For a review of research evidence, study findings (usually published in journal articles) are paramount. Information in nonresearch references—including opinion articles, case reports, and clinical anecdotes—may serve to broaden the understanding of a problem, but in general has limited utility in written research reviews.

➤ A **primary source** in a research review is the original description of a study prepared by the researcher who conducted it; a **secondary source** is a description of the study by a person unconnected with it. Literature reviews should be based on primary source material.

➤ Strategies for finding studies on a topic include the use of bibliographic tools, but also include the *ancestry approach* (tracking down earlier studies cited in a reference list of a report) and the *descendancy approach* (using a pivotal study to search forward to subsequent studies that cited it).

➤ An important development for locating references for a research review is the widespread availability of various **bibliographic databases** that can be searched electronically. For nurses, the **CINAHL** and **MEDLINE** databases are especially useful.

➤ In searching a bibliographic database, users can perform a keyword search that looks for searcher-specified terms in *text fields* of a database record (or that *maps* keywords onto the database's subject codes) or can search according to the **subject heading** codes themselves. Author searches are also available.

➤ Retrieved references must be screened for relevance, and then pertinent information must be abstracted and encoded for subsequent analysis. Formal review protocols facilitate the encoding process.

➤ Studies must also be critiqued to assess the strength of evidence in existing research. Critiques for research reviews tend to focus on the methodologic aspects of a set of studies.

➤ The analysis of information from a literature search essentially involves the identification of important *themes*—regularities and patterns in the information.

➤ In preparing a written review, it is important to organize materials in a logical, coherent fashion. The preparation of an outline is recommended. The reviewers' role is to point out what has been studied, how adequate and dependable the studies are, what gaps exist in the body of research, and (in the context of a new study) what contribution the study would make.

STUDIES CITED IN CHAPTER 7

Bonner, A., Wellard, S., Caltabiano, M. (2008). Levels of fatigue in people with ESRD living in far North Queensland. *Journal of Clinical Nursing, 17,* 90–98.

Martens, T., & Emed, J. (2007). The experiences and challenges of pregnant women coping with thrombophilia. *Journal of Obstetric, Gynecologic, & Neonatal Nursing, 36,* 55–62.

Roe, B., Ostaszkiewicz, J., Milne, J., & Wallace, S. (2007). Systematic review of bladder training and voiding programmes in adults. *Journal of Advanced Nursing, 57,* 15–31.

Shreffler-Grant, J., Hill, W., Weinert, C., Nichols, E., & Ide, B. (2007). Complementary therapy and older rural women: Who uses it and who does not? *Nursing Research, 56,* 28–33.

Zhang, A., Strauss, G., & Siminoff, L. (2007). Effects of combined pelvic muscle exercise and a support group on urinary incontinence and quality of life of postprostatectomy patients. *Oncology Nursing Forum, 34,* 47–53.

8 Theoretical and Conceptual Frameworks

STUDENT OBJECTIVES

On completing this chapter, you will be able to:

➤ Identify the major characteristics of theories, conceptual models, and frameworks

➤ Identify several conceptual models of nursing and other conceptual models frequently used by nurse researchers

➤ Describe how theory and research are linked in quantitative and qualitative studies

➤ Critique the appropriateness of a theoretical framework—or its absence—in a study

➤ Define new terms in the chapter

High-quality studies typically achieve a high level of *conceptual integration*. This means, for example, that the research questions are appropriate for the chosen methods, that the questions are consistent with the existing evidence, and that there is a plausible conceptual rationale for expected outcomes—including a rationale for any hypotheses to be tested or for designing an intervention in a certain way. For example, suppose a researcher hypothesized that a nurse-led smoking cessation intervention would reduce rates of smoking among patients with cardiovascular disease. Why would he or she make this prediction—what is the "theory" about how the intervention might change people's behavior? Is it predicted that the intervention will change patients' knowledge? Attitudes? Motivation? Social supports? Sense of control over their own decision making? The researcher's view of how the intervention would "work" should drive the design of both the intervention and the study.

Design decisions and data collection strategies cannot be developed in a vacuum—there must be an underlying conceptualization of people's behaviors and characteristics, and how these affect and are affected by interpersonal and environmental forces. In some studies, the underlying conceptualization is fuzzy or unstated, but in good research, a clear and defensible conceptualization is made explicit. This chapter discusses theoretical and conceptual contexts for nursing research problems.

THEORIES, MODELS, AND FRAMEWORKS

Many terms have been used in connection with conceptual contexts for research, including theories, models, frameworks, schemes, and maps. There is some overlap in how these terms are used, partly because they are used differently by different writers, and partly because they are interrelated. We offer guidance in distinguishing these terms, but note that our definitions are not universal.

Theories

Nursing instructors and students frequently use the term *theory* to refer to the content covered in classrooms, as opposed to the actual practice of nursing. In both lay and scientific language, *theory* connotes an *abstraction*.

Classically, **theory** is defined in research circles as an abstract generalization that systematically explains how phenomena are interrelated. The traditional definition requires a theory to embody at least two concepts that are related in a manner that the theory purports to explain. As classically defined, theories consist of concepts and a set of propositions that form a logically interrelated system, providing a mechanism for logically deducing new statements from the original propositions. To illustrate, consider *reinforcement theory*, which posits that behavior that is reinforced (i.e., rewarded) tends to be repeated and learned. This theory consists of concepts (reinforcement and learning) and a proposition stating the relationship between them. The proposition lends itself to hypothesis generation. For example, if reinforcement theory is valid, we could deduce that hyperactive children who are praised or rewarded when they are engaged in quiet play will exhibit less acting-out behaviors than similar children who are not praised. This prediction, as well as many others based on the theory of reinforcement, could then be tested in a study.

Other researchers use the term *theory* less restrictively to refer to a broad characterization of a phenomenon. Some authors specifically refer to this type of theory as **descriptive theory**—a theory that accounts for and thoroughly describes a single phenomenon. Descriptive theories are inductive, empirically driven abstractions that "describe or classify specific dimensions or characteristics of individuals, groups, situations, or events by summarizing commonalities found in discrete observations" (Fawcett, 1999, p. 15). Such theories play an especially important role in qualitative studies.

Both classical and descriptive theories help to make research findings meaningful and interpretable. Theories allow researchers to knit together observations into an orderly system. Theories also serve to explain research findings: theory may guide researchers' understanding not only of the "what" of natural phenomena but also of the "why" of their occurrence. Finally, theories help to stimulate research and the extension of knowledge by providing both direction and impetus.

Theories are sometimes classified in terms of their level of generality. *Grand theories* (also called *macro-theories*) purport to explain large segments of the human experience. Some sociologists, such as Talcott Parsons, developed general theoretical systems to account for broad classes of behavior and social functioning. Within nursing, theories are more restricted in scope, focusing on a narrow range of phenomena. Theories that explain a portion of the human experience are sometimes called **middle-range theories**. For example, there are middle-range theories to explain such phenomena as decision-making, infant attachment, and stress. Smith and Liehr (2003) have described eight specific middle-range theories that are especially relevant in nursing.

Models

A **conceptual model** deals with abstractions (concepts) that are assembled because of their relevance to a common theme. Conceptual models provide a conceptual perspective regarding interrelated phenomena, but they are more loosely structured than theories and do not link concepts in a logically derived deductive system. A conceptual model broadly presents an understanding of the phenomenon of interest and reflects the assumptions and philosophical views of the model's designer. There are many conceptual models of nursing that offer broad explanations of the nursing process. Like theories, conceptual models can serve as springboards for generating hypotheses.

Some writers use the term **model** to designate a mechanism for representing phenomena with a minimal use of words. Words that define a concept can convey different meanings to different people; thus, a visual or symbolic representation of a phenomenon can sometimes help to express abstract ideas in a more understandable or precise form. Two types of models that are used in research contexts are schematic models and statistical models. *Statistical models*, not elaborated on here, are mathematic equations that express the nature and magnitude of relationships among a set of variables. These models are tested using sophisticated statistical methods.

Schematic models (also called **conceptual maps**) are visual representations of relationships among phenomena and are common in both qualitative and quantitative research. Concepts and the linkages between them are represented graphically through boxes, arrows, or other symbols. An example of a schematic model is presented in Figure 8.1. This model, known as **Pender's Health Promotion**

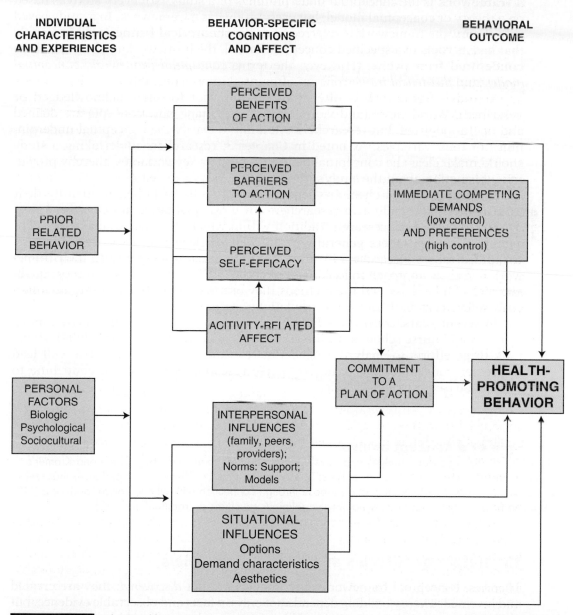

 FIGURE 8.1   The Health Promotion Model. (From Pender's website, www.nursing.umich.edu/faculty/pender/chart.gif. Retrieved January 13, 2006.)

Model, is a model for explaining and predicting the health-promotion component of lifestyle (Pender, Murdaugh, & Parsons, 2006). Schematic models of this type can be useful in clarifying and succinctly communicating linkages among concepts.

Frameworks

A **framework** is the conceptual underpinnings of a study. Not every study is based on a theory or conceptual model, but every study has a framework. In a study based on a theory, the framework is referred to as the **theoretical framework**; in a study that has its roots in a specified conceptual model, the framework is often called the **conceptual framework**. (However, the terms *conceptual framework, conceptual model,* and *theoretical framework* are often used interchangeably.)

A study's framework is often implicit (i.e., not formally acknowledged or described). World views (and views on nursing) shape how concepts are defined and operationalized, but researchers often fail to clarify the conceptual underpinnings of their variables. As noted in Chapter 3, researchers undertaking a study should make clear the conceptual definition of their key variables, thereby providing information about the study's framework.

Quantitative researchers are generally more guilty of failing to identify their frameworks than qualitative researchers. In most qualitative studies, the frameworks are part of the research tradition within which the study is embedded. For example, ethnographers generally begin their work within a theory of culture. Grounded theory researchers incorporate sociological principles into their framework and their approach to looking at phenomena. The questions that most qualitative researchers ask and the methods they use to address those questions inherently reflect certain theoretical formulations.

In recent years, *concept analysis* has become an important enterprise among students and nurse scholars (Chinn & Kramer, 2003; Walker & Avant, 2004). Hopefully these efforts to analyze concepts of relevance to nursing practice will lead to greater conceptual clarity among nurse researchers desiring to contribute to evidence-based nursing practice.

Example of a concept analysis:
Buck (2006) did a concept analysis and developed a model of *spirituality* using Chinn and Kramer's method. The concept was defined as follows: Spirituality is "that most human of experiences that seeks to transcend self and find meaning and purpose through connection with others, nature, and/or a Supreme Being, which may or may not involve religious structures or tradition" (p. 288).

The Nature of Theories and Conceptual Models

Theories, conceptual frameworks, and models are not *discovered*; they are created and invented. Theory building depends not only on facts and observable evidence, but also on the theorist's ingenuity in pulling facts together and making sense of them. Thus, theory construction is a creative enterprise that can be engaged in by anyone who is insightful, has a firm grounding in existing evidence, and has the ability to knit evidence together into an intelligible pattern. Because theories are not just "out there" waiting to be discovered, it follows that theories are tentative. A theory can never be proved—a theory simply represents a theorist's best efforts to describe and explain phenomena. Through research, theories evolve and are sometimes discarded. This may happen if new evidence or observations undermine a previously accepted theory. Or, a new theory might integrate new observations with an existing theory to yield a more parsimonious or accurate explanation of a phenomenon.

The relationship between theory and research is reciprocal. Theories and models are built inductively from observations, and an excellent source for those observations is prior research, including in-depth qualitative studies. Concepts and relationships that are validated empirically through research become the foundation for theory development. The theory, in turn, must be tested by subjecting deductions from it (hypotheses) to further systematic inquiry. Thus, research plays a dual and continuing role in theory building and testing. Theory guides and generates ideas for research; research assesses the worth of the theory and provides a foundation for new theories.

Example of theory development:
Jean Johnson (1999) developed a middle-range theory called the Self-Regulation Theory that explicates relationships between health care experiences, coping, and health outcomes. Here is how she described theory development: "The theory was developed in a cyclic process. Research was conducted using the self-regulation theory of coping with illness. Propositions supported by data were retained, other propositions were altered when they were not supported. And new theoretical propositions were added when research produced unexpected findings. This cycle has been repeated many times over three decades leading to the present stage of development of the theory" (pp. 435–436). As an example of related research, Allard (2007) developed and tested an intervention based on the Self-Regulation Theory to enhance physical and emotional well-being in women who underwent day surgery for breast cancer.

CONCEPTUAL MODELS AND THEORIES USED BY NURSE RESEARCHERS

Nurse researchers have used both nursing and non-nursing frameworks to provide a conceptual context for their studies. This section briefly discusses several frameworks that have been found useful by nurse researchers.

Conceptual Models of Nursing

In the past few decades, several nurses have formulated conceptual models of nursing practice. These models constitute formal explanations of what the nursing discipline is and what the nursing process entails, according to the model developer's point of view. As Fawcett (2005) has noted, four concepts are central to models of nursing: *human beings*, *environment*, *health*, and *nursing*. The various conceptual models, however, define these concepts differently, link them in diverse ways, and give different emphases to relationships among them. Moreover, different models emphasize different processes as being central to nursing. For example, Sister Calista Roy's Adaptation Model identifies adaptation of patients as a critical phenomenon (Roy & Andrews, 1999). Martha Rogers (1986), by contrast, emphasized the centrality of the individual as a unified whole, and her model views nursing as a process in which clients are aided in achieving maximum well-being within their potential.

The conceptual models were not developed primarily as a base for nursing research. Indeed, most models have had more impact on nursing education and clinical practice than on nursing research. Nevertheless, nurse researchers have turned to these conceptual frameworks for inspiration in formulating research questions and hypotheses. Table 8.1 lists 10 prominent conceptual models in nursing that have been used by researchers. The table briefly describes the model's key feature and identifies a study that has claimed the model as its framework.

Let us consider one conceptual model of nursing that has received considerable attention from nurse researchers, **Roy's Adaptation Model**. In this model, humans are viewed as biopsychosocial adaptive systems who cope with environmental change through the process of adaptation (Roy & Andrews, 1999). Within the human system, there are four subsystems: physiologic/physical, self-concept/group identity, role function, and interdependence. These subsystems constitute adaptive modes that provide mechanisms for coping with environmental stimuli and change. Health is viewed as both a state and a process of being and becoming integrated and whole that reflects the mutuality of persons and environment. The goal of nursing, according to this model, is to promote client adaptation; nursing also regulates stimuli affecting adaptation. Nursing interventions usually take the form of increasing, decreasing, modifying, removing, or maintaining internal and external stimuli that affect adaptation.

Example using Roy's Adaptation Model:
Flood and Scharer (2006) tested a creativity enhancement intervention designed to promote successful adaptation to aging within the context of the Roy Adaptation Model.

Other Models and Middle Range Theories Developed by Nurses

In addition to conceptual models that are designed to describe and characterize the entire nursing process, nurses have developed other middle-range theories and models that focus on more specific phenomena of interest to nurses. Examples of other middle-range theories developed by nurses that have been used in research include the Theory of Unpleasant Symptoms (Lenz et al., 1997), Kolcaba's (2003) Comfort Theory, Reed's Self-Transcendence Theory (1991), the Theory of Transitions (Meleis et al., 2000), the Symptom Management Model (Dodd et al., 2001),

Pender's Health Promotion Model, and Mishel's Uncertainty in Illness Theory (1990). The latter two are briefly described here.

Nola Pender's (2006) **Health Promotion Model (HPM)** focuses on explaining health-promoting behaviors, using a wellness orientation. According to the recently revised model (Figure 8.1), *health promotion* entails activities directed toward developing resources that maintain or enhance a person's well-being. The model embodies a number of propositions that can be used in developing and testing interventions and understanding health behaviors. For example, one HPM proposition is that people commit to engaging in behaviors from which they anticipate deriving valued benefits, and another is that perceived competence or self-efficacy relating to a given behavior increases the likelihood of commitment to action and actual performance of the behavior.

Example using the HPM:
Ronis and colleagues (2006) tested the revised HPM to explain the decisions of 703 construction workers to use hearing protection devices. Results supported the revised model and suggested the new model was more successful in predicting hearing protection than the original HPM.

Mishel's **Uncertainty in Illness Theory** (Mishel, 1990) focuses on the concept of uncertainty—the inability of a person to determine the meaning of illness-related events. According to this theory, people develop subjective appraisals to assist them in interpreting the experience of illness and treatment. Uncertainty occurs when people are unable to recognize and categorize stimuli. Uncertainty results in the inability to obtain a clear conception of the situation, but a situation appraised as uncertain will mobilize individuals to use their resources to adapt to the situation. Mishel's conceptualization of uncertainty (and her Uncertainty in Illness Scale) have been used in many nursing studies.

Example using Uncertainty in Illness Theory:
Clayton and colleagues (2006) tested a model of symptoms, communication with providers, and uncertainty in affecting the well-being of older breast cancer survivors. In their model, communication was conceptualized as a factor influencing uncertainty, which in turn was seen as influencing emotional and cognitive well-being.

Other Models Used by Nurse Researchers

Many concepts in which nurse researchers are interested are not unique to nursing, and therefore their studies are sometimes linked to frameworks that are not models from the nursing profession. Several of these alternative models have gained special prominence in the development of multifaceted nursing interventions to promote health-enhancing behaviors and life choices. Five non-nursing models or theories have frequently been used in nursing studies: Bandura's Social Cognitive Theory, Prochaska's Transtheoretical (Stages of Change) Model, the Health Belief

TABLE 8.1	CONCEPTUAL MODELS OF NURSING USED BY NURSE RESEARCHERS		
THEORIST AND REFERENCE	NAME OF MODEL/THEORY	KEY THESIS OF THE MODEL	RESEARCH EXAMPLE
F. Moyra Allen, 2002	McGill Model of Nursing	Nursing is the science of health-promoting interactions. The goal of nursing is to actively promote patient and family strengths and the achievement of life goals.	Cossette and colleagues (2002) used the McGill Model in their study to document nursing approaches associated with reductions in psychological distress among patients post-myocardial infarction.
Madeline Leininger, 2006	Theory of Culture Care Diversity and Universality	Caring is a universal phenomenon but its mani-festation and processes vary transculturally.	Guided by Leininger's theory, Polyakova & Pacquiao (2006) examined the cultural context of mental illness among elder immigrants from the former Soviet Union.
Myra Levine, 1973	Conservation Model	Conservation of integrity by nurses contributes to maintenance of a person's wholeness.	Gagner-Tjellesen et al. (2001) used concepts from Levine's model in studying the clinical use of music therapy in acute inpatient settings.
Betty Neuman, 2001	Health Care Systems Model	Each person is a complete system; the goal of nursing is to assist in maintaining client system stability.	Jones-Cannon and Davis (2005) used Neuman's model as the framework in their study of the coping strategies of African-American daughters who functioned as caregivers.
Margaret Newman, 1994	Health as Expanding Consciousness	Health is viewed as an expansion of consciousness with health and disease parts of the same whole; health is seen in an evolving pattern of the whole in time, space, and movement.	Rosa (2006) used Newman's theory to study patterns of healing and personal trans-formation among persons with chronic skin wounds.

	CONCEPTUAL MODELS OF NURSING USED BY NURSE RESEARCHERS		
TABLE 8.1	**(continued)**		
THEORIST AND REFERENCE	NAME OF MODEL/THEORY	KEY THESIS OF THE MODEL	RESEARCH EXAMPLE
Dorothea Orem, 2003	Self-Care Deficit Nursing Theory	Self-care activities are what people do on their own behalf to maintain health and well-being; the goal of nursing is to help people meet their own therapeutic self-care demands.	Tsai (2007) studied the self-care strategies for depressive symptoms among residents of public elder care homes in Taiwan using concepts from Orem's theory.
Rosemarie Rizzo Parse, 1999	Theory of Human Becoming	Health and meaning are co-created by indivisible humans and their environment; nursing involves having clients share views about meanings.	Kagan (2008) studied the universal lived experience of feeling listened to using Parse's methods and theory.
Martha Rogers, 1986	Science of Unitary Human Beings	The individual is a unified whole in constant interaction with the environment; nursing helps individuals achieve maximum well-being within their potential.	Shearer and colleagues (2007) tested the effect of a telephone-delivered empowerment intervention, guided by Rogers' theory, with patients diagnosed with heart failure.
Sr. Callista Roy, 1999	Adaptation Model	Humans are adaptive systems that cope with change through adaptation; nursing helps to promote client adaptation during health and illness.	Buckner and colleagues (2007) described adaptation (in the four adaptive modes of Roy's model) among adolescent campers attending a Young Teen Camp.
Jean Watson, 2005	Theory of Caring	Caring is the moral ideal, and entails mind–body–soul engagement with one another.	Watson's conceptual model of caring-healing underpinned a study of the culture of nursing care on a medical unit as perceived by staff and patients (Carter et al., 2008)

Model, the Theory of Planned Behavior, and Lazarus and Folkman's Theory of Stress and Coping.

➤ **Social Cognitive Theory** (Bandura, 1985) offers an explanation of human behavior using the concepts of self-efficacy, outcome expectations, and incentives. Self-efficacy expectations are focused on people's belief in their own capacity to carry out particular behaviors (e.g., smoking cessation). Self-efficacy expectations determine the behaviors a person chooses to perform, their degree of perseverance, and the quality of the performance. The role of self-efficacy has been studied in relation to numerous health behaviors. For example, Chang and colleagues (2007) tested a theory-based intervention, the Self-Care Self-Efficacy Enhancement Program, to improve self-care ability in Chinese nursing home elders.

> **TIP**
>
> Bandura's self-efficacy construct is a key mediating variable in several models and theories discussed in this chapter. Self-efficacy has repeatedly been found to explain a significant degree of variation in people's behaviors and to be amenable to change, and so self-efficacy enhancement is often a goal in interventions designed to change people's health-related actions and behaviors.

➤ The **Transtheoretical Model** (Prochaska et al., 2002) has been used in numerous interventions to change people's behavior. The core construct is *stages of change*, which conceptualizes a continuum of motivational readiness to change problem behavior. The five stages of change are precontemplation, contemplation, preparation, action, and maintenance. Studies have shown that successful self-changers use different processes at each particular stage, thus suggesting the desirability of interventions that are individualized to the person's stage of readiness for change. For example, Ham (2007) identified the stages and processes of change related to smoking cessation among high school students in Korea.

➤ Becker's **Health Belief Model** (HBM) is a framework for explaining people's health-related behavior, such as health care use and compliance with a medical regimen. According to the model, health-related behavior is influenced by a person's perception of a threat posed by a health problem as well as by the value associated with actions aimed at reducing the threat (Becker, 1976). A revised HBM (RHBM) has incorporated the concept of self-efficacy (Rosenstock et al., 1988). Nurse researchers have used the HBM extensively—for example, Ueland and colleagues (2006) developed and tested an HBM-based education intervention to promote awareness of colorectal cancer prevention and screening.

➤ The **Theory of Planned Behavior** (TPB; Ajzen, 2005), which is an extension of an earlier theory called the Theory of Reasoned Action, provides a framework for understanding people's behavior and its psychological determinants. According to the theory, behavior that is volitional is determined by people's intention to perform that behavior. Intentions, in turn, are affected by attitudes toward the behavior, subjective norms (i.e., perceived social pressure to perform or not perform the behavior), and perceived behavioral control (i.e., anticipated ease or difficulty of engaging in the behavior). Sauls (2007), for example, examined the utility of the TPB for explaining intrapartum nurses' intentions to provide professional labor support to parturient women.

➤ Lazarus and Folkman's (1984) **Theory of Stress and Coping** offers an explanation of people's methods of dealing with stress (i.e., environmental and internal demands that tax or exceed a person's resources and endanger his or her well-being). The theory posits that coping strategies are learned and deliberate responses to stressors, and are used to adapt to or change the stressors. According to this model, people's perception of mental and physical health is related to the ways they evaluate and cope with the stresses of living. As an example Côté-Arsenault (2007) studied stress and coping in pregnant women who had experienced perinatal loss.

The use of theories and conceptual models from other disciplines, such as psychology (*borrowed theories*), has not been without controversy; some commentators advocate the development of unique nursing theories. However, nursing research is likely to continue on its current path of conducting studies within a multidisciplinary and multitheoretical perspective. Moreover, when a borrowed theory is tested and found to be empirically adequate in health-relevant situations of interest to nurses, it becomes **shared theory**.

TIP

There are websites devoted to many of the theories and models mentioned in this chapter. Several specific websites are listed in the "Useful Websites for Chapter 8" file on the accompanying CD-ROM, for you to click on directly. ● An excellent Internet resource on nursing theory has been developed by the Hahn School of Nursing and Health Science at the University of San Diego: www.sandiego.edu/nursing/theory. Also, two good websites for dozens of theories relating to behavior change (a key construct in nursing intervention studies) are maintained by The Communication Initiative: http://www.comminit.com/changetheories.html and by the University of South Florida: http://hsc.usf.edu/~kmbrown/hlth_beh_models.htm.

USING A THEORY OR FRAMEWORK IN RESEARCH

The manner in which theory and conceptual frameworks are used by qualitative and quantitative researchers is elaborated on in this section. In the discussion, the term *theory* is used in its broadest sense to include conceptual models, formal theories, and frameworks.

Theories in Qualitative Research

Theory is almost always present in studies that are embedded in a qualitative research tradition such as ethnography or phenomenology. These research traditions inherently provide an overarching framework that gives qualitative studies a theoretical grounding. However, different traditions involve theory in different ways.

Sandelowski (1993) made a useful distinction between **substantive theory** (conceptualizations of the target phenomenon that is being studied) and theory that reflects a conceptualization of human inquiry. Some qualitative researchers insist on an atheoretical stance vis-à-vis the phenomenon of interest, with the goal of suspending *a priori* conceptualizations (substantive theories) that might bias their inquiry. For example, phenomenologists are in general committed to theoretical naiveté, and explicitly try to hold preconceived views of the phenomenon in check. Nevertheless, phenomenologists are guided by a framework or philosophy that focuses their analysis on certain aspects of a person's lifeworld. That framework is based on the premise that human experience is inherently part of the experience itself, not constructed by an outside observer.

Ethnographers typically bring a strong cultural perspective to their studies, and this perspective shapes their initial fieldwork. Fetterman (1997) has observed that most ethnographers adopt one of two cultural theories: *ideational theories*, which suggest that cultural conditions and adaptation stem from mental activity and ideas, or *materialistic theories*, which view material conditions (e.g., resources, money, production) as the source of cultural developments.

Grounded theory is a general inductive method that is not attached to a particular theoretical perspective (Glaser, 2005). Grounded theorists can use any theoretical perspective that fits with their data, such as systems theory or social organization theory. A popular theoretical underpinning of grounded theory used by nurse researchers is *symbolic interaction* (or *interactionism*), which has three underlying premises (Blumer, 1986). First, humans act toward things based on the meanings that the things have for them. Second, the meaning of things is derived from (or arises out of) the interaction humans have with other fellow humans. And third, meanings are handled in, and modified through, an interpretive process.

> **Example of a grounded theory study:**
> St. John and colleagues (2005) conducted a grounded theory study based on a symbolic interactionist framework to explore the social reality and symbolic meanings that words, gestures, activities, and experiences had for new fathers during the early weeks after childbirth as they interacted with their partners, the newborn, family, friends, and others.

Despite this theoretical perspective, grounded theory researchers, such as phenomenologists, attempt to hold prior substantive theory about specific phenomena in abeyance until their own substantive theory begins to emerge. Grounded theory methods are designed to facilitate the generation of theory that is *conceptually dense*, that is, with many conceptual patterns and relationships. The goal is to develop a conceptualization of a phenomenon that is *grounded* in actual observations—that is, to explicate an empirically based conceptualization for integrating and making sense of a process or phenomenon. The goal is to use the data, grounded in reality, to provide a description or an explanation of events as they occur in reality—not as they have been conceptualized in preexisting theories. Once the grounded theory starts to take shape, however, grounded theorists use previous literature for comparison with the emerging and developing categories of the theory.

In recent years, a growing number of qualitative nurse researchers have been adopting a perspective know as *critical theory* as a framework in their research. Critical theory is a paradigm that involves a critique of society and societal processes and structures, as we discuss in greater detail in Chapter 10.

Qualitative researchers sometimes use conceptual models of nursing or other formal theories as interpretive frameworks. For example, a number of qualitative nurse researchers acknowledge that the philosophic roots of their studies lie in conceptual models of nursing such as those developed by Newman, Parse, and Rogers.

Example of using nursing theory in a qualitative study:
Brown and colleagues (2007) conducted a qualitative study of the help-seeking process of older husbands caring for wives with dementia. They used relevant concepts from Margaret Newman's Theory of Health as Expanding Consciousness to interpret their data.

Finally, a systematic review of qualitative studies on a specific topic is another strategy that can lead to theory development. In such metasyntheses, qualitative studies are combined to identify their essential elements. The findings from different sources are then used for theory building. Paterson (2001), for example, used the results of 292 qualitative studies that described the experiences of adults with chronic illness to develop the shifting perspectives model of chronic illness. This model depicts living with chronic illness as an ongoing, constantly shifting process in which individuals' perspectives change in the degree to which illness is in the foreground or background in their lives.

Theories in Quantitative Research

Quantitative researchers also link research to theory or models in various ways. The classic approach is to test hypotheses deduced from a previously proposed theory. For example, a nurse might read about Pender's Health Promotion Model (Figure 8.1) and might conjecture the following: "If the HPM is valid, then I would expect that patients with osteoporosis who understood the benefit of a calcium-enriched diet would be more likely to alter their eating patterns than those who perceived no benefits." Such a conjecture, derived from a theory or conceptual framework, can serve as a starting point for testing the theory's adequacy.

In testing a theory, quantitative researchers deduce implications (as in the preceding example) and develop hypotheses, which are predictions about the manner in which variables would be interrelated if the theory were correct. Key variables in the theory would have to be measured, data would be collected from an appropriate sample, and then the hypotheses would be tested through statistical analysis. The focus of the testing process involves a comparison between observed outcomes with those predicted in the hypotheses.

> **TIP**
>
> When a quantitative study is based on a theory or conceptual model, the research report generally states this fact fairly early—often in the first paragraph, or even in the title. Many studies also have a subsection of the introduction called "Conceptual Framework" or "Theoretical Framework." The report usually includes a brief overview of the theory so that even readers with no theoretical background can understand, in a general way, the conceptual context of the study.

Tests of a theory increasingly are taking the form of testing theory-based interventions. If a theory is correct, it has implications for strategies to influence people's health-related attitudes or behavior, and hence their health outcomes. And, if an intervention is developed on the basis of an explicit conceptualization of human behavior and thought, then it likely has a greater chance of being effective than if it is developed in a conceptual vacuum. Interventions rarely affect outcomes directly—mediating factors play a role in the causal pathway between the intervention and the outcomes. For example, interventions based on Social Cognitive Theory posit that improvements to a person's self-efficacy will result in positive changes in health behavior. The impetus for a nursing intervention may be a formal theory such as the ones we described or a theory developed within the context of qualitative studies.

Example of theory testing in an intervention study:
Chung-Park (2008) developed a Contraceptive Behavior Change (CBC) Model within the framework of the Transtheoretical Model of Change. Based on concepts within the CBC Model, a pregnancy prevention program was developed for enlisted females in the U.S. Navy. The effects of the program on the enlisted women's knowledge, attitudes, self-efficacy, contraceptive behavior, and pregnancies were rigorously evaluated.

It should be noted that many researchers who cite a theory or model as their framework are not directly *testing* the theory. Silva (1986), in her analysis of 62 studies that claimed their roots in 5 nursing models, found that only 9 were direct and explicit tests of the models cited by the researchers. She found that the most common use of the nursing models was to provide an organizing structure for the studies. In such an approach, researchers begin with a broad conceptualization of nursing (or stress, health beliefs, and so on) that is consistent with that of the model developers. The researchers *assume* that the models they espouse are valid, and then use the models' constructs or proposed schemas to provide a broad organizational or interpretive context. Some use data collection instruments that are allied with the model. Silva pointed out that using models in this fashion can serve a valuable organizing purpose, but noted that such studies offer little evidence about the validity of the theory itself. To our knowledge, Silva's study has not been replicated with a more recent sample of studies—although Taylor and colleagues (2000) also found that most studies of Orem's Self-Care Deficit Theory were primarily descriptive rather than theory-testing. We suspect that, even today, a high percentage of quantitative studies that cite theories as their conceptual frameworks are using them primarily as organizational or interpretive tools.

Example of using a model as organizing structure:
Shin and colleagues (2006) studied the relationship between maternal sensitivity on the one hand and maternal identity, social support, and maternal-fetal attachment on the other. Their study used Roy's Adaptation Model as the organizing framework, but the model itself was not formally tested.

CRITIQUING FRAMEWORKS IN RESEARCH REPORTS

You will find references to theories and conceptual frameworks in some (but not all) of the studies you read. It is often challenging to critique the theoretical context of a published research report—or its absence—but we offer a few suggestions.

In a qualitative study in which a grounded theory is developed and presented, you probably will not be given sufficient information to refute the proposed descriptive theory because only evidence supporting the theory is presented. However, you can determine whether the theory seems logical, whether the conceptualization is truly insightful, and whether the evidence is solid and convincing. In a phenomenological study you should look to see if the researcher addresses the philosophical underpinnings of the study. The researcher should briefly discuss the philosophy of phenomenology on which the study was based.

Critiquing a theoretical framework in a quantitative report is also difficult, especially because you are not likely to be familiar with a full range of theories and models that might be relevant. Some suggestions for evaluating the conceptual basis of a quantitative study are offered in the following discussion and in Box 8.1. ✖

The first task is to determine whether the study does, in fact, have a conceptual framework. If a theory, model, or framework is not mentioned, you should consider whether the study's merit is diminished by the absence of an explicit conceptual context. Nursing research has been criticized for producing isolated findings that are difficult to integrate because of the absence of a theoretical foundation, but in some cases, a study may be so pragmatic that it does not need a theory to enhance its usefulness. For example, research designed to determine the optimal frequency of turning patients has a utilitarian goal; a theory might not enhance the value of the findings. If, however, the study involves the test of a complex intervention or hypotheses, the absence of a formally stated framework suggests conceptual fuzziness and perhaps ensuing methodologic problems.

TIP

In most quantitative nursing studies, the research problem is not linked to a specific theory or conceptual model. You may read many studies before finding one with an explicit theoretical underpinning.

BOX 8.1 GUIDELINES FOR CRITIQUING THEORETICAL AND CONCEPTUAL FRAMEWORKS

1. Does the report describe an explicit theoretical or conceptual framework for the study? If not, does the absence of a framework detract from the significance of the research or its conceptual integration?

2. Does the report adequately describe the major features of the theory or model so that readers can understand the conceptual basis of the study?

3. Is the theory or model appropriate for the research problem? Would a different framework have been more fitting? Does the purported link between the problem and the framework seem contrived?

4. If there is an intervention, was there a cogent theoretical basis or rationale for the intervention?

5. Is the theory or model used as the basis for generating hypotheses that were tested, or is it used as an organizational or interpretive framework? Was this appropriate?

6. Do the hypotheses (if any) naturally flow from the framework? Are deductions from the theory logical?

7. Are the concepts adequately defined in a way that is consistent with the theory? If there is an intervention, are intervention components consistent with the theory?

8. Is the framework based on a conceptual model of nursing or on a model developed by nurses? If it is borrowed from another discipline, is there adequate justification for its use?

9. Did the framework guide the study methods? For example, was the appropriate research tradition used if the study was qualitative? If quantitative, do the operational definitions correspond to the conceptual definitions? Were hypotheses tested statistically?

10. Does the researcher tie the findings of the study back to the framework at the end of the report? How do the findings support or undermine the framework? Are the findings interpreted within the context of the framework?

If the study does involve an explicit framework, you can then ask whether the particular framework is appropriate. You may not be in a position to challenge the researcher's use of a particular theory or model or to recommend an alternative, but you can evaluate the logic of using a particular framework and assess whether the link between the problem and the theory is genuine. Does the researcher present a convincing rationale for the framework used? Do the hypotheses flow from the theory? Will the findings contribute to the validation of the theory? Does the researcher interpret the findings within the context of the framework? If the answer to such questions is no, you may have grounds for criticizing the study's framework, even though you may not be able to articulate how the conceptual basis of the study could be improved.

TIP

Some studies claim theoretical linkages that are not justified. This is most likely to occur when researchers first formulate the research problem and then later find a theoretical context to fit it. An after-the-fact linkage of theory to a research question is usually problematic because the researcher will not have taken the nuances of the theory into consideration in designing the study. If a research problem is truly linked to a conceptual framework, then the design of the study, the measurement of key constructs, and the analysis and interpretation of data will flow from that conceptualization.

This section presents two detailed examples of studies that have a strong theoretical link. Read these summaries and then answer the critical thinking questions, referring to the full research report if necessary.

EXAMPLE 1 ■ The Health Belief Model in a Quantitative Study

Study

Structural model for osteoporosis preventing behavior in postmenopausal women (Estok, Sedlak, Doheny, & Hall, 2007).

Statement of Purpose

The purpose of the study was to evaluate the effects of an intervention involving access to personal knowledge about osteoporosis status through dual-energy X-ray absorptiometry (DXA) on calcium intake and weight-bearing exercise in postmenopausal women, and to examine relationships among theoretically relevant variables.

Theoretical Framework

The study was based on the revised Health Belief Model that incorporated a construct that has found its way into many health theories, namely self-efficacy. The RHBM is appropriate when a goal is to understand and predict why and under what conditions individuals take preventive health-related actions. According to the elements of the RHBM, the researchers reasoned that women would be more likely to engage in osteoporosis preventive behaviors (OPBs) if they (1) perceive themselves to be more susceptible to osteoporosis; (2) believe it is a serious threat; (3) believe they can modify the risks; (4) perceive fewer negative aspects to be associated with the preventive behaviors; and (5) have a concern and drive for their general health. The researchers hypothesized that women might be more likely to try to learn about osteoporosis, have a change in health beliefs, and participate in OPBs to prevent slow bone density loss if they had personal knowledge of their own bone density. The study tested whether personal knowledge via DXA screening adds to the effects of, and possibly influences, health beliefs and general knowledge about osteoporosis, and plays a role in altering OPBs. Their theoretical model is shown in Figure 8.2.

Method

A sample of 203 community-based women aged 50 to 65 years was randomly assigned to receive feedback from a DXA scan or not. Data were collected from study participants at three points in time: at baseline before DXA screening, and then 6 and 12 months later. All women in the intervention group received free DXA, and were then sent a letter that included a description and interpretation of normal bone density or osteoporosis, and highlighted the participants' own results. If the results were below normal, the women were urged to obtain follow-up advice from their own physician. Women in the control group were offered a free DXA following the 12-month follow-up data collection.

Key Findings

The DXA results had a direct positive effect on calcium intake at 6 months after screening, especially for those who learned they had osteoporosis or osteopenia. Providing DXA results did not affect the women's exercise behavior. The women's initial calcium intake and exercise levels were found to be correlated with their health beliefs, consistent with the RHBM.

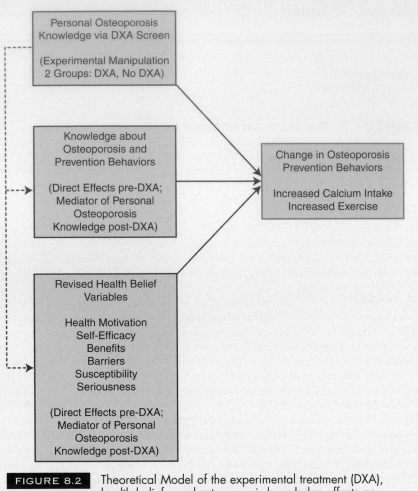

Theoretical Model of the experimental treatment (DXA), health beliefs, and osteoporosis knowledge effects on change in prevention behaviors. (From Estok, P., Sedlak, C., Doheny, M., & Hall, R. [2007]. Structural model for osteoporosis preventing behavior in postmenopausal women. *Nursing Research, 56,* 148–158, with permission.)

CRITICAL THINKING SUGGESTIONS*:

*See the Student Resource CD-ROM for a discussion of these questions.

1. Answer the relevant questions from Box 8.1 regarding this study.
2. Also, consider the following targeted questions, which may further sharpen your critical thinking skills and assist you in understanding this study:
   a. According to the model shown in Figure 8.2, which "box" corresponds to the intervention? And, according to this model, what did the researchers predict that the intervention would affect?

b. Is there another model or theory that was described in this chapter that could have been used to study the effect of this intervention on women's calcium intake or exercise behavior?

3. If the results of this study are valid and generalizable, what might be some of the uses to which the findings could be put in clinical practice?

EXAMPLE 2 ■ A Grounded Theory Study

Study

Persevering through postpartum fatigue (Runquist, 2007).

Statement of Purpose

The purpose of the study was to construct a substantive theory of postpartum fatigue (PPF) in the everyday lives of women after childbirth.

Method

Grounded theory methods were used. Data were collected through individual interviews with 13 women between 2 and 5 weeks postpartum from diverse ethnic, age, parity, obstetric, and financial contexts. All but one were interviewed in their own homes. Among the questions posed in the interviews were the following: "What is it like to have fatigue with a newborn baby?" and "How does being fatigued change you?" All interviews were audiotaped and transcribed for analysis. The investigator also made informal observations during the home visits, which were recorded in field notes.

Theoretical Framework

A grounded theory method was chosen "because this methodology offered the benefit of a process-oriented methodological approach that could accommodate and capture everyday complexities of phenomena" (p. 29). Runquist also noted that the literature had identified PPF as a process-oriented phenomenon and that the goal of the study was to use grounded theory methods to develop a substantive theory of the phenomenon.

Key Findings

Based on her in-depth interviews, Runquist identified a basic process that she labeled *Persevering through Postpartum Fatigue.* The process of *persevering* was explained through the relationships of various influencing factors—coping techniques, self-transcendence, and caregiving. PPF was characterized by four dimensions—mental, physical, stress-worry, and frustration—each of which had context-dependent manifestations. A schematic model for the substantive theory is presented in Figure 8.3.

CRITICAL THINKING SUGGESTIONS:

1. Answer the relevant questions from Box 8.1 regarding this study.
2. Also, consider the following targeted questions, which may further sharpen your critical thinking skills and assist you in understanding this study:
   a. In what way was the use of theory different in Runquist's study than in the previous study by Estok and colleagues?
   b. Comment on the utility of the schematic model shown in Figure 8.3.
3. If the results of this study are trustworthy, what might be some of the uses to which the findings could be put in clinical practice?

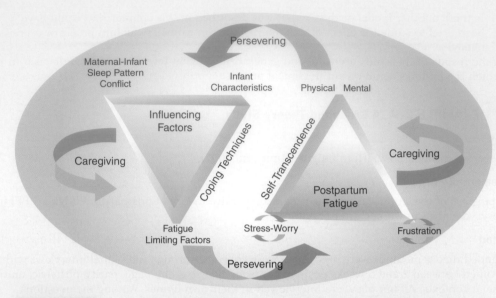

FIGURE 8.3 Model for a grounded theory, "Persevering through Postpartum Fatigue," (from Runquist, J. [2007]. Persevering through postpartum fatigue. *Journal of Obstetric, Gynecologic, & Neonatal Nursing, 36,* 28–37, with permission.)

EXAMPLE 3 ■ Quantitative Research in Appendix A

1. Read the abstract and the introduction from Howell and colleagues' (2007) study ("Anxiety, anger, and blood pressure in children") in Appendix A of this book, and then answer relevant questions from Box 8.1.
2. Also, consider the following targeted questions, which may further sharpen your critical thinking skills and assist you in assessing aspects of the study's merit:
   a. Develop a simple schematic model that captures the hypothesized relationships that were implied in this study.
   b. Would any of the theories or models described in this chapter have provided an appropriate conceptual context for this study?

EXAMPLE 4 ■ Qualitative Research in Appendix B

1. Read the abstract and introduction from Beck's (2006) study ("The anniversary of birth trauma") in Appendix B of this book and then answer relevant questions from Box 8.1.
2. Also, consider the following targeted questions, which may further sharpen your critical thinking skills and assist you in assessing aspects of the study's merit:
   a. Do you think that a schematic model would have helped to synthesize the findings in this report?
   b. Did Beck present convincing evidence to support her use of the philosophy of phenomenology?

CHAPTER REVIEW

Key new terms introduced in the chapter, together with a summary of major points, are presented in this section. In addition, Chapter 8 of the *Study Guide for Essentials of Nursing Research,* 7th edition offers various exercises and study suggestions for reinforcing the concepts presented in this chapter. For additional review, see the Student Self-Study Review Questions section of the Student Resource CD-ROM provided with this book.

Key New Terms

Conceptual framework	Framework	Shared theory
Conceptual map	Middle-range theory	Substantive theory
Conceptual model	Model	Theoretical framework
Descriptive theory	Schematic model	Theory

Summary Points

➤ High-quality research requires *conceptual integration,* one aspect of which is having a defensible theoretical rationale for undertaking the study in a given manner or for testing specific hypotheses. Researchers demonstrate their conceptual clarity through the delineation of a theory, model, or framework on which the study is based.

➤ A **theory** is a broad abstract characterization of phenomena. As classically defined, a theory is an abstract generalization that systematically explains relationships among phenomena. **Descriptive theory** thoroughly describes a phenomenon.

➤ The basic components of a theory are concepts; classically defined theories consist of a set of propositions about the interrelationships among concepts, arranged in a logically interrelated system that permits new statements to be derived from them.

➤ *Grand theories* (or *macro-theories*) attempt to describe large segments of the human experience. **Middle-range theories** are more specific to certain phenomena.

➤ Concepts are also the basic elements of **conceptual models**, but concepts are not linked in a logically ordered, deductive system. Conceptual models, like theories, provide context for nursing studies.

➤ In research, the overall objective of theories and models is to make findings meaningful, to summarize existing knowledge into coherent systems, to stimulate new research, and to explain phenomena and relationships among them.

➤ **Schematic models** (or **conceptual maps**) are graphic representations of phenomena and their interrelationships using symbols or diagrams and a minimal use of words.

➤ A **framework** is the conceptual underpinning of a study, including an overall rationale and conceptual definitions of key concepts. In qualitative studies, the framework usually springs from distinct research traditions.

➤ Several conceptual models of nursing have been used in nursing research. The concepts central to models of nursing are *human beings*, *environment*, *health*, and *nursing*. An example of a model of nursing used by nurse researchers is Roy's Adaptation Model.

➤ Non-nursing models used by nurse researchers (e.g., Bandura's Social Cognitive Theory) are referred to as *borrowed theories*; when the appropriateness of borrowed theories for nursing inquiry is confirmed, the theories become **shared theories**.

➤ In some qualitative research traditions (e.g., phenomenology), the researcher strives to suspend previously held **substantive theories** of the phenomena under study, but nevertheless there is a rich theoretical underpinning associated with the tradition itself.

➤ Some qualitative researchers specifically seek to develop *grounded theories*, data-driven explanations to account for phenomena under study through inductive processes.

➤ In the classical use of theory, quantitative researchers test hypotheses deduced from an existing theory. An emerging trend is the testing of theory-based interventions.

➤ In both qualitative and quantitative studies, researchers sometimes use a theory or model as an organizing framework, or as an interpretive tool.

STUDIES CITED IN CHAPTER 8

Allard, N. C. (2007). Day surgery for breast cancer: Effects of a psychoeducational telephone intervention on functional status and emotional distress. *Oncology Nursing Forum, 34*, 133–141.

Brown, J., Chen, S., Mitchell, C., & Province, A. (2007). Help-seeking by older husbands caring for wives with dementia. *Journal of Advanced Nursing, 59*, 352–360.

Buck, H. G. (2006). Spirituality: Concept analysis and model development. *Holistic Nursing Practice, 20*, 288–292.

Buckner, E., Simmons, S., Brakefield, J., Hawkins, A., Feeley, C., Kilgore, L. et al. (2007). Maturing responsibility in young teens participating in an asthma camp: Adaptive mechanisms and outcomes. *Journal for Specialists in Pediatric Nursing, 12*, 24–36.

Carter, L., Nelson, J., Sievers, B., Dukek, S., Pipe, T., & Holland, D. (2008). Exploring a culture of caring. *Nursing Administration Quarterly, 32*, 57–63.

Chang, S., Crogan, N., & Wung, S. (2007). The Self-Care Self-Efficacy Enhancement Program for Chinese nursing home elders. *Geriatric Nursing, 28*, 31–36.

Chung-Park, M. S. (2008). Evaluation of a pregnancy prevention programme using the Contraceptive Behavior Change model. *Journal of Advanced Nursing, 61*, 81–91.

Clayton, M. F., Mishel, M. H., & Belyea, M. (2006). Testing a model of symptoms, communication, uncertainty, and well-being in older breast cancer survivors. *Research in Nursing & Health, 29*, 18–29.

Cossette, S., Frasure-Smith, N., & Lespérance, F. (2002). Nursing approaches to reducing psychological distress in men and women recovering from myocardial infarction. *International Journal of Nursing Studies, 39,* 479–494.

Côté-Arsenault, D. (2007). Threat appraisal, coping, and emotions across pregnancy subsequent to perinatal loss. *Nursing Research, 56,* 108–116.

Estok, P., Sedlak, C., Doheny, M., & Hall, R. (2007). Structural model for osteoporosis preventing behavior in postmenopausal women. *Nursing Research, 56,* 148–158.

Flood, M., & Scharer, K. (2006). Creativity enhancement: Possibilities for successful aging. *Issues in Mental Health Nursing, 27,* 939–959.

Gagner-Tjellesen, D., Yurkovich, E. E., & Gragert, M. (2001). Use of music therapy and other ITNIs in acute care. *Journal of Psychosocial Nursing & Mental Health Services, 39,* 26–37.

Ham, O. K. (2007). Stages and processes of smoking cessation among adolescents. *Western Journal of Nursing Research, 29,* 301–315.

Jones-Cannon, S., & Davis, B.L. (2005). Coping among African-American daughters caring for aging parents. *The ABNF Journal, 16,* 118–123.

Kagan, P. N. (2008). Feeling listened to: A lived experience of human becoming. *Nursing Science Quarterly, 21,* 59–67.

Paterson, B. (2001). The shifting perspectives model of chronic illness. *Journal of Nursing Scholarship, 33,* 21–26.

Polyakova, S., & Pacquiao, D. (2006). Psychological and mental illness among older immigrants from the former Soviet Union. *Journal of Transcultural Nursing, 17,* 40–49.

Ronis, D., Hong, O., & Lusk, S. (2006). Comparison of the original and revised structures of the Health Promotion Model in predicting construction workers' use of hearing protection. *Research in Nursing & Health, 29,* 3–17.

Rosa, K. (2006). A process model of healing and personal transformation in persons with chronic skin wounds. *Nursing Science Quarterly, 19,* 349–358.

Runquist, J. (2007). Persevering through postpartum fatigue. *Journal of Obstetric, Gynecologic, & Neonatal Nursing, 36,* 28–37.

Sauls, D. (2007). Nurses' attitudes toward provision of care and related health outcomes. *Nursing Research, 56,* 117–123.

Shearer, N., Cisar, N., & Greenberg, E. (2007). A telephone-delivered empowerment intervention with patients diagnosed with heart failure. *Heart & Lung, 36,* 159–169.

Shin, H., Park, Y., & Kim, M. (2006). Predictors of maternal sensitivity during the early postpartum period. *Journal of Advanced Nursing, 55,* 425–434.

St. John, W., Cameron, C., & McVeigh, C. (2005). Meeting the challenge of new fatherhood during the early weeks. *Journal of Obstetric, Gynecologic, & Neonatal Nursing, 34,* 180–189.

Tsai, Y. (2007). Self-care management and risk factors for depressive symptoms among Taiwanese institutionalized older persons. *Nursing Research, 56,* 124–131.

Ueland, A., Hornung, P., & Greenwald, B. (2006). Colorectal cancer prevention and screening: A Health Belief Model-based research study to increase disease awareness. *Gastroenterology Nursing, 29,* 357–363.

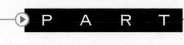 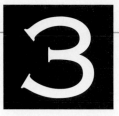

Designs for Nursing Research

9 Quantitative Research Design

STUDENT OBJECTIVES

On completing this chapter, you will be able to:

➤ Discuss decisions that are specified in a research design for a quantitative study

➤ Discuss the concepts of causality and counterfactuals, and identify criteria for causal relationships

➤ Describe and evaluate experimental, quasi-experimental, and nonexperimental designs

➤ Distinguish between and evaluate cross-sectional and longitudinal designs

➤ Identify and evaluate alternative methods of controlling confounding variables

➤ Understand various threats to the validity of quantitative studies

➤ Evaluate a quantitative study in terms of its overall research design and methods of controlling confounding variables

➤ Define new terms in the chapter

As we noted in Chapter 2, *best evidence* for nursing practice comes from research findings that are rigorous and methodologically appropriate for the research question. For quantitative studies, no aspect of a study's methods has a bigger impact on the validity and accuracy of the results than the research design—particularly if the inquiry is *cause probing*. Thus, the information in this chapter has great significance for making proper inferences from study results and drawing conclusions about the worth of the evidence in a quantitative study.

OVERVIEW OF RESEARCH DESIGN ISSUES

The research design of a study spells out the basic strategies that researchers adopt to answer their questions and test their hypotheses. This section describes some basic design features and also discusses the concept of causality.

Key Research Design Features

Table 9.1 describes seven key design features that typically need to be addressed in the design of a quantitative study. Many of these features are also pertinent in qualitative studies, as we will discuss in the next chapter. The design decisions that researchers must make include the following:

➤ *Will there be an intervention?* A basic design issue is whether or not researchers will actively introduce an intervention and examine its effects, or whether the researchers will more passively observe phenomena as they exist. As noted in Chapter 3, this is the distinction between experimental and nonexperimental research, and many specific designs exist for both types.

➤ *What types of comparisons will be made?* In most studies, especially quantitative ones, researchers incorporate comparisons into their designs to provide a context for interpreting results. Researchers can structure their studies to make various types of comparison. Sometimes, the *same* people are compared under multiple conditions or at different points in time (e.g., preoperative versus postoperatively); this is called a *within-subjects design*. Sometimes different people are compared (e.g., those getting versus not getting an intervention); this is called a *between-subjects design*.

➤ *How will confounding variables be controlled?* The complexity of relationships among variables makes it difficult to test hypotheses unambiguously unless efforts are made to control factors extraneous to the research question (i.e., confounding variables). This chapter discusses techniques for achieving such control.

➤ *Will masking be used?* Researchers must decide if information about the study—such as the study hypotheses or the allocation of interventions—should be (or can be) withheld from data collectors, study participants, analysts, or others to minimize the risk of **expectation bias** (i.e., the risk that such knowledge could influence the study outcomes).

TABLE 9.1	KEY DESIGN FEATURES	
FEATURE	KEY QUESTIONS	DESIGN OPTIONS
Intervention	Will there be an intervention? What specific design will be used?	Experimental (RCT)*, quasi-experimental (controlled trial), nonexperimental (observational) design
Comparisons	What type of comparisons will be made to illuminate key processes or relationships?	Within-subject design, between-subject design
Control over confounding variables	How will confounding variables be controlled? Which confounding variables will be controlled?	Randomization, crossover, homogeneity, matching, statistical control
Masking	From whom will critical information be withheld to avert bias?	Open versus closed study; single-blind, double-blind
Timeframes	How often will data be collected? When, relative to other events, will data be collected?	Cross-sectional, longitudinal design
Relative timing	When will information on independent and dependent variables be collected—looking backward or forward?	Retrospective, prospective design
Location	Where will the study take place?	Single site versus multi-site; in the field versus controlled setting

*RCT, randomized clinical (controlled) trial.

➤ *How often will data be collected?* In some studies, data are collected from participants at a single point in time *(cross-sectionally)*, but others involve multiple points of data collection *(longitudinally)*, for example, to determine how things have changed over time. The research design designates the frequency and timing of data collection.

➤ *When will "effects" be measured, relative to potential causes?* Some studies collect information about outcomes and then look back *retrospectively* for potential causes or antecedents. Other studies, however, begin with a potential cause or antecedent and then see what outcomes ensue, in a *prospective* fashion.

➤ *Where will the study take place?* Data for quantitative studies sometimes are collected in real-world settings, such as in clinics or people's homes. Other studies are conducted in highly controlled environments established for research purposes (e.g., laboratories). Another important design decision concerns how many different sites will be involved in the study—a decision that could affect the generalizability of the results.

There is no single typology of research designs, because designs can vary along a number of the dimensions identified in Table 9.1. Many of the dimensions are independent of the others. For example, an experimental design can be a between-subjects or within-subjects design; experiments can also be cross-sectional or longitudinal, and so on. This chapter describes the major dimensions and the implications of design decisions on the study's rigor.

> **TIP**
>
> Research reports typically present information about the research design early in the method section. Complete information about the design is not always provided, however, and some researchers use terminology that differs from that used in this book. (Occasionally, researchers even misidentify the study design.)

Causality

As we noted in early chapters of this book, many research questions and questions for evidence-based practice (EBP) are about *causes* and *effects*:

➤ Does a telephone therapy intervention for patients with prostate cancer *cause* improvements in their psychological distress and coping skills? (intervention question)

➤ Do birthweights under 1,500 g *cause* developmental delays in children? (prognosis question)

➤ Does cigarette smoking *cause* lung cancer? (etiology/harm question)

Although causality is a hotly debated philosophical issue, we all understand the general concept of a **cause**. For example, we understand that failure to sleep *causes* fatigue and that high caloric intake *causes* weight gain. Most phenomena are multiply determined. Weight gain, for example, can reflect high caloric intake, but other factors cause weight gain as well. Also, most causes are not *deterministic*, they only increase the probability that an effect will occur. For example, smoking is a cause of lung cancer, but not everyone who smokes develops lung cancer, and not everyone with lung cancer was a smoker.

Although it might be easy to grasp what researchers mean when they talk about a *cause*, what exactly is an **effect**? A good way to grasp the meaning of an effect is by conceptualizing a counterfactual (Shadish et al., 2002). A **counterfactual** is *what would have happened to the same people exposed to a causal factor if they simultaneously were not exposed to the causal factor*. An effect represents the difference between what actually did happen with the exposure and what would have happened without it. This counterfactual model clearly cannot ever be realized, but it is a good model to keep in mind in thinking about and critiquing research design.

Several writers have proposed criteria for establishing cause-and-effect relationships, among them three that are attributed to John Stuart Mill. The first criterion is *temporal*: a cause must precede an effect in time. If we tested the hypothesis that aspartame causes fetal abnormalities, we would need to demonstrate that abnormalities developed *after* the mothers' exposure to aspartame. Second, there must be an *empirical relationship* between the presumed cause and the presumed effect. In our example, we would have to demonstrate an association between aspartame consumption and fetal abnormalities—that is, that a higher percentage of aspartame users than nonusers had infants with fetal abnormalities. The third criterion for inferring a causal relationship is that the relationship cannot be explained as being *caused by a third variable*. Suppose that users of aspartame tended also to drink more coffee than nonusers. There would then be a possibility that the relationship between maternal aspartame use and fetal abnormalities reflects an underlying causal connection between coffee consumption and the abnormalities.

Additional criteria were proposed by Bradford-Hill (1971) as part of the discussion about the causal connection between smoking and lung cancer—these are sometimes referred to as the Surgeon General's criteria for that reason. Two of Bradford-Hill's criteria foreshadow the importance of meta-analyses. The criterion of *coherence* involves similar evidence from multiple sources, and the criterion of *consistency* involves having similar levels of statistical relationship in several studies. Another important criterion in health research is *biologic plausibility*, that is, evidence from basic physiologic studies that a causal pathway is credible.

Researchers investigating casual relationships must provide persuasive evidence regarding these criteria through their research design. Some designs are better at revealing cause-and-effect relationships than others, as suggested by the evidence hierarchy in Figure 2.1 in Chapter 2. Most of the next section is devoted to designs that have been used to illuminate causal relationships.

EXPERIMENTAL, QUASI-EXPERIMENTAL, AND NONEXPERIMENTAL DESIGNS

This section describes designs that differ with regard to whether or not there is an experimental intervention.

Experimental Design

Early physical scientists learned that complexities occurring in nature often made it difficult to understand important relationships through pure observation. This problem was handled by isolating phenomena in a laboratory and controlling the conditions under which they occurred. These procedures were profitably adopted by biologists in the 19th century, resulting in many achievements in physiology and medicine. The 20th century has witnessed the use of experimental methods by researchers interested in human behavior.

Characteristics of True Experiments
A true experimental design or randomized controlled trial (RCT) is characterized by the following properties:

➤ *Manipulation*—the experimenter *does* something to some subjects—that is, there is some type of intervention.

➤ *Control*—the experimenter introduces controls into the study, including devising a good approximation of a counterfactual—usually a control group that does not receive the intervention.

➤ *Randomization*—the experimenter assigns subjects to a control or experimental condition on a random basis.

Using *manipulation*, experimenters consciously vary the independent variable and then observe its effect on the dependent variable. Researchers manipulate the independent variable by administering an experimental *treatment* (or *intervention*) to some subjects while withholding it from others. To illustrate, suppose we were investigating the effect of physical exertion on mood in healthy young adults. One experimental design for this research problem is a **pretest–posttest design** (or **before–after design**). This design involves the observation of the dependent variable (mood) at two points in time: before and after the treatment. Participants in the experimental group are subjected to a physically demanding exercise routine, whereas those in the control group undertake a sedentary activity. This design permits us to examine what changes in mood were *caused* by the exertion because only some people were subjected to it, providing an important comparison. In this example, we met the first criterion of a true experiment by manipulating physical exertion, the independent variable.

This example also meets the second requirement for experiments, the use of a control group. Inferences about causality require a comparison, but not all comparisons provide equally persuasive evidence. For example, if we were to supplement the diet of premature neonates with special nutrients for 2 weeks, the infants' weight at the end of 2 weeks would tell us nothing about the treatment's effectiveness. At a minimum, we would need to compare their posttreatment weight with their pretreatment weight to determine whether, at least, their weights had increased. But suppose we find an average weight gain of half a pound. Does this finding support an inference of a causal relationship between the nutritional intervention (the independent variable) and weight gain (the dependent variable)? No, it does not. Infants normally gain weight as they mature. Without a control group—a group that does not receive the supplements—it is impossible to separate the effects of maturation from those of the treatment. The term **control group** refers to a group of participants whose performance on a dependent variable is used to evaluate the performance of the **experimental group** (the group receiving the intervention) on the same dependent variable. The control group condition used as a basis of comparison represents a proxy for the ideal counterfactual as previously described.

Experimental designs also involve placing subjects in groups at random. Through **randomization** (*random assignment*), every participant has an equal chance of being included in any group. If people are randomly assigned, there is no systematic bias in the groups with regard to attributes that may affect the dependent variable. *Randomly assigned groups are expected to be comparable, on average, with respect to an infinite number of biologic, psychological, and social traits at the outset of the study.* Group differences on outcomes observed after random assignment can therefore be inferred as being caused by the treatment.

Random assignment can be accomplished by flipping a coin or pulling names from a hat. Researchers typically either use computers to perform the randomization or rely on a *table of random numbers*, a table displaying hundreds of digits arranged in a random order.

TIP

There is considerable confusion about random assignment versus random sampling. Random assignment is a *signature* of an experimental design. If there is no random allocation of subjects to treatment conditions, then the design is not a true experiment. Random *sampling,* by contrast, refers to a method of selecting subjects for a study, as we discuss in Chapter 12. Random sampling is *not* a signature of an experimental design. In fact, most experiments or RCTs do *not* involve random sampling.

Experimental Designs
Basic Designs

The most basic experimental design involves randomizing subjects to different groups and then measuring the dependent variable. This design is sometimes called a **posttest-only** (or **after-only**) **design**. A more widely used design, discussed previously, is the pretest–posttest design, which involves collecting **pretest data** (also called **baseline data**) on the dependent variable before the intervention and **posttest** (outcome) **data** after it.

Example of a pretest–posttest design:

Beckham (2007) evaluated the effectiveness of motivational interviewing on hazardous drinking in a sample of rural people at risk for alcohol dependence. Data on alcohol use (as measured by both self-report and a liver function test) were collected both before and after the intervention among experimental and control group members.

TIP

Experimental designs can be depicted graphically using symbols to represent features of the design. In these diagrams, the convention is that R stands for randomization to treatment groups, X represents the receipt of the intervention, and O is the measurement of outcomes. So, for example, a pretest–posttest design would be depicted as follows:

$$R \; O_1 \; X \; O_2$$
$$R \; O_1 \quad\;\; O_2$$

Space does not permit us to present these diagrams in this book for all designs, but there are tables in the Toolkit on the accompanying CD-ROM that portray many designs.

Factorial Design

Researchers sometimes manipulate two or more independent variables simultaneously. Suppose we were interested in comparing two therapeutic strategies for premature infants: tactile stimulation versus auditory stimulation. We are also interested in learning whether the daily amount of stimulation affects infants' progress. Figure 9.1 illustrates the structure of this experiment. This factorial design allows us to address three questions: (1) Does auditory stimulation cause different effects on

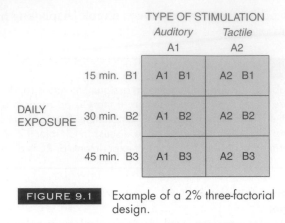

FIGURE 9.1   Example of a 2% three-factorial design.

infant development than tactile stimulation? (2) Does the amount of stimulation (independent of modality) affect infant development? and (3) Is auditory stimulation most effective when linked to a certain dose and tactile stimulation most effective when coupled with a different dose?

The third question demonstrates an important strength of factorial designs: they permit us to evaluate not only **main effects** (effects resulting from the manipulated variables, as exemplified in questions 1 and 2) but also **interaction effects** (effects resulting from combining the treatments). Our results may indicate, for example, that 15 minutes of tactile stimulation and 45 minutes of auditory stimulation are the most beneficial treatments. We could not have learned this by conducting two separate experiments that manipulated one independent variable at a time.

In factorial experiments, subjects are assigned at random to a combination of treatments. In our example, premature infants would be assigned randomly to one of the six cells. The term *cell* refers to a treatment condition and is represented in a diagram as a box. In this factorial design, type of stimulation is factor A and amount of exposure is factor B. Each factor must have two or more *levels*. Level one of factor A is *auditory*, and level two of factor A is *tactile*. The research design in Figure 9.1 would be described as a 2 × 3 factorial design: two levels of factor A times three levels of factor B.

Example of a factorial design:

Forsyth (2007) used a 2 × 2 × 2 factorial design to study the effects of two different mental health diagnoses (borderline personality disorder and major depressive disorder) and reasons for patients' noncompliance with therapy tasks (controllable versus uncontrollable and also stable versus unstable) on mental health workers' reactions. Case reports of noncompliant patients were identical except for the manipulated information. Study participants, who were randomly assigned to read one of the eight case reports, rated their own level of anger and empathy.

Crossover Design

Thus far, we have described experiments in which subjects who are randomly assigned to treatments are different people. For instance, the infants given 15 minutes of auditory stimulation in the factorial experiment are not the same infants as those exposed to other treatment conditions. This broad class of designs is called between-subjects designs because the comparisons are between different people. When the same subjects are compared, the designs are within-subjects designs.

A **crossover design** involves exposing participants to more than one treatment. Such studies are true experiments only if participants are randomly assigned to different orderings of treatment. For example, if a crossover design were used to compare the effects of auditory and tactile stimulation on infants, some would be randomly assigned to receive auditory stimulation first followed by tactile stimulation, and others would receive tactile stimulation first. In such a study, the three conditions for an experiment have been met: there is manipulation, randomization, and control—with *subjects serving as their own control group.*

A crossover design has the advantage of ensuring the highest possible equivalence among the subjects exposed to different conditions. Such designs are inappropriate for certain research questions, however, because of possible *carryover effects*. When subjects are exposed to two different treatments, they may be influenced in the second condition by their experience in the first. However, when carryover effects are implausible, as when treatment effects are immediate and short-lived, a crossover design is extremely powerful.

Example of a crossover design:
Voergaard and colleagues (2007) compared the performance and safety features of a new one-piece closed ostomy bag with those of an established bag. Patients with a colostomy tested each bag for 1 week in a randomized crossover study.

TIP

Research reports do not always identify the specific experimental design that was used by name; this may have to be inferred from information about the data collection plan (in the case of posttest-only and pretest–posttest designs) or from such statements as: "The subjects were used as their own controls (in the case of a crossover design)."

Experimental and Control Conditions

In designing experiments, researchers make many decisions about what the experimental and control conditions entail, and these decisions can affect the results.

To give an experimental intervention a fair test, researchers need to carefully design one that is appropriate to the problem and of sufficient intensity and duration that effects on the dependent variable might reasonably be expected. Researchers delineate the full nature of the intervention in formal *protocols* that stipulate exactly what the treatment is for those in the experimental group.

The control group condition (the counterfactual) must also be carefully conceptualized. Researchers have choices about what to use as the counterfactual, and the decision has implications for the interpretation of the findings. Among the possibilities for the counterfactual are the following:

➤ No intervention—the control group gets no treatment at all

➤ An alternative treatment (e.g., auditory versus tactile stimulation)

- ➤ A **placebo** or pseudo-intervention presumed to have no therapeutic value
- ➤ "Usual care"—standard or normal procedures used to treat patients
- ➤ An *attention control condition*—the control group gets researchers' attention but not the active ingredients of the intervention
- ➤ A lower dose or intensity of treatment, or only parts of the treatment
- ➤ **Delayed treatment** (i.e., control group members are *wait-listed* and exposed to the experimental treatment at a later point).

Example of a wait-listed control group:
Mastel-Smith and colleagues (2007) evaluated the effectiveness of a Life Story Workshop that involved life review, reflection, and story writing to improve depressive symptoms in community-dwelling older adults. Those who received the 10-week intervention were compared to wait-listed controls in terms of scores on a depression scale.

Methodologically, the best possible test is between two conditions that are as different as possible, as when the experimental group gets a strong treatment and the control group gets no treatment. Ethically, however, the most appealing counterfactual is probably the "delay of treatment" approach, which may be difficult to do pragmatically. Testing two alternative interventions is also appealing ethically, but the risk is that the results will be inconclusive because it may be difficult to detect differential effects.

Researchers constructing their control group strategy must also give thought to possibilities for masking. Many nursing interventions do not lend themselves easily to masking. For example, if the intervention were a smoking cessation program, the subjects would be aware that they were receiving the intervention, and the intervener would be aware of who was in the program. Certain control group strategies may, however, partially disguise treatment group condition, as in low-dose versus high-dose groups or wait-listed controls. It is often possible, and desirable, to at least mask the subjects' treatment status from the people collecting outcome data.

Example of a single-blind experiment:
Scott and colleagues (2005) compared the efficacy of two diets before bowel cleansing in preparation for a colonoscopy. The standard liquid diet was compared with a liberalized diet that included a normal breakfast and a low-residue lunch the day before the colonoscopy. Patients knew what group they were in, but the colonoscopists, who rated overall cleansing efficacy, did not.

Advantages and Disadvantages of Experiments

Experiments are the most powerful designs for testing hypotheses of cause-and-effect relationships. Experimental designs are considered the "gold standard" for intervention studies because they yield the highest quality evidence regarding the effects of an intervention. Through randomization and the use of a control group condition, experimenters come as close as possible to attaining the "ideal" counterfactual. Experiments offer greater corroboration than any other research approach that, *if* the independent variable (e.g., diet, drug dosage, teaching approach) is manipulated, *then* certain consequences in the dependent variable (e.g., weight loss, recovery of health, learning) may be expected to ensue.

The great strength of experiments, then, lies in the confidence with which causal relationships can be inferred. Through the controls imposed by manipulation, comparison, and—especially—randomization, alternative explanations to a causal interpretation can often be ruled out or discredited. This is especially likely to be the case if the intervention was developed on the basis of a sound theoretical rationale. It is because of these strengths that meta-analyses of RCTs, which integrate evidence from multiple studies that used an experimental design, are at the pinnacle of evidence hierarchies for questions relating to causes (Figure 2.1 of Chapter 2).

Despite the advantages of experiments, they have some limitations. First, a number of interesting variables simply are not amenable to manipulation. A large number of human characteristics, such as disease or health habits, cannot be randomly conferred on people.

Second, there are many variables that could technically—but not ethically—be manipulated. For example, to date there have been no experiments to study the effect of cigarette smoking on lung cancer. Such an experiment would require us to assign people randomly to a smoking group (people forced to smoke) or a non-smoking group (people prohibited from smoking). Experimentation with humans will always be subject to such ethical constraints.

In many health care settings, experimentation may not be feasible because it is impractical. It may, for instance, be impossible to secure the necessary cooperation from administrators or other key people to conduct an experiment.

Another potential problem is the *Hawthorne effect*, a term derived from a series of experiments conducted at the Hawthorne plant of the Western Electric Corporation in which various environmental conditions (e.g., light, working hours) were varied to determine their effect on worker productivity. Regardless of what change was introduced (i.e., whether the light was made better or worse), productivity increased. Thus, knowledge of being in a study may cause people to change their behavior, thereby obscuring the effect of the research variables.

In summary, experimental designs have some limitations that make them difficult to apply to real-world problems; nevertheless, experiments have a clear-cut superiority for testing causal hypotheses.

HOW-TO-TELL TIP

How can you tell if a study is experimental? Researchers usually indicate in the method section of their reports that they have used an experimental design, but they may also say they used a randomized design or an RCT. If such terms are missing, you can conclude that a study is experimental if the report says that the study purpose was to *test, evaluate,* or *examine the effectiveness of* an intervention, treatment, or innovation, AND if individual participants were put into groups (or exposed to different conditions) at random.

Quasi-Experiments

Quasi-experiments (called *controlled trials without randomization* in the medical literature), also involve an intervention; however, quasi-experimental designs lack randomization, the signature of a true experiment. Some quasi-experiments even lack a control group. The signature of a quasi-experimental design, then, is an intervention in the absence of randomization.

Quasi-Experimental Designs

There are several quasi-experimental designs, but only the most commonly used by nurse researchers are discussed here.

Nonequivalent Control Group Design

The most frequently used quasi-experimental design is the **nonequivalent control group before–after design,** which involves two or more groups of subjects observed before and after the implementation of an intervention. As an example, suppose we wished to study the effect of introducing a new hospital-wide model of care that involved having a patient care facilitator (PCF) to be the primary point person for all patients during their stay. Our main outcome is patient satisfaction. Because the new system is being implemented throughout the hospital, randomization to PCF versus "usual care" is not possible. Therefore, we decide to collect data in another similar hospital that is not instituting the PCF model. Data on patient satisfaction are collected in both hospitals, before the change is made (at baseline), and again after its implementation.

This quasi-experimental design is identical to the before–after experimental design discussed in the previous section, *except* subjects were not randomly assigned to the groups. The quasi-experimental design is weaker because, without randomization, *it cannot be assumed that the experimental and comparison groups are equivalent at the outset.* Quasi-experimental comparisons are much farther from an ideal counterfactual than experimental comparisons. The design is, nevertheless, a strong one because the collection of pretest data allows us to determine whether patients in the two hospitals had similar satisfaction before the change was made. If the comparison and experimental groups are similar at baseline, we could be relatively confident inferring that any posttest difference in satisfaction was the result of the new model of care. If patient satisfaction is different initially, however, it will be difficult to interpret any posttest differences. Note that in quasi-experiments, the term **comparison group** is sometimes used in lieu of *control group* to refer to the group against which outcomes in the treatment group are evaluated.

Now suppose we had been unable to collect baseline data. This design (*nonequivalent control group after-only*) has a flaw that is difficult to remedy. We no longer have information about the initial equivalence of the two hospitals. If we find that patient satisfaction in the experimental hospital is higher than that in the control hospital at the posttest, can we conclude that the new method of delivering care *caused* improved satisfaction? There could be alternative explanations for the posttest differences. In particular, it might be that patient satisfaction in the two hospitals differed initially. Even though quasi-experiments lack some of the controlling properties of experiments, the hallmark of strong quasi-experiments is the effort to introduce some controls, such as baseline measurements.

Example of a nonequivalent control group design:
Jones and colleagues (2007) used a nonequivalent control group before–after design to test the effectiveness of the Deaf Health Heart Intervention in increasing self-efficacy for heart health behaviors in deaf adults. Participants in Tucson, who received the intervention, were compared with similar adults from Phoenix who did not receive it.

Time–Series Design

In the designs just described, a control group was used but randomization was not, but some quasi-experiments have neither. Let us suppose that a hospital is adopting a new requirement that all its nurses accrue a certain number of continuing education units before being eligible for a promotion or raise. The nurse administrators want to assess the consequences of this mandate on turnover rate, absentee rate, and number of promotions awarded. Let us assume there is no other hospital that can serve as a reasonable comparison, and so the only kind of comparison that can be made is a before–after contrast. If the requirement were inaugurated in January, one could compare the turnover rate, for example, for the 3-month period before the new rule with the turnover rate for the subsequent 3-month period.

This **one-group, before–after design** seems logical, but it has problems. What if one of the 3-month periods is atypical, apart from the mandate? What about the effect of any other rules instituted during the same period? What about the effects of external factors, such as changes in the local economy? The design in question offers no way of controlling these factors.

The inability to obtain a meaningful control group, however, does not eliminate the possibility of conducting research with integrity. The previous design could be modified so that at least some alternative explanations for change in nurses' turnover rate could be ruled out. One such design is the **time–series design**, which involves collecting data over an extended time period, and introducing the treatment during that period. The present study could be designed with four observations before the new continuing education rule and four observations after it. For example, the first observation might be the number of resignations between January and March in the year before the new rule, the second observation might be the number of resignations between April and June, and so forth. After the rule is implemented, data on turnover similarly would be collected for four consecutive 3-month periods, giving us observations 5 through 8.

Although the time–series design does not eliminate all the problems of interpreting changes in turnover rate, the extended time perspective strengthens the ability to attribute change to the intervention. This is because the time–series design rules out the possibility that changes in resignations represent a random fluctuation of turnover measured at only two points.

Example of a time–series design:
Mastel-Smith and colleagues (2006) used a time series design to evaluate the effectiveness of an intervention—therapeutic life review—to reduce depression in home-dwelling older women. Depression scores were obtained for the participants for 10 weeks before the intervention and during the 6-week intervention period.

Advantages and Disadvantages of Quasi-Experiments

A strength of quasi-experiments is that they are practical—it is not always possible to conduct true experiments. Nursing research often occurs in natural settings, where it is difficult to deliver an innovative treatment randomly to some people but not to others. Strong quasi-experimental designs introduce some research control when full experimental rigor is not possible.

Another issue is that people are not always willing to be randomized in clinical trials. Quasi-experimental designs, because they do not involve random assignment, are likely to be acceptable to a broader group of people. This, in turn, has implications for the generalizability of the results—but the problem is that the results are usually less conclusive.

The major disadvantage of quasi-experiments is that causal inferences cannot be made as easily as with experiments. With quasi-experiments, there are alternative explanations for observed results. Take as an example the case in which we administer a certain diet to a group of frail nursing home residents to assess whether this treatment results in weight gain. If we use no comparison group or a nonequivalent control group and then observe a weight gain, we must ask: Is it *plausible* that some other factor caused the gain? Is it *plausible* that pretreatment differences between the experimental and comparison groups resulted in differential gain? Is it *plausible* that the elders on average gained weight simply because the most frail died or were transferred to a hospital? If the answer to any of these **rival hypotheses** is yes, then the inferences that can be made about the causal effect of the intervention are weakened. With quasi-experiments, there is almost always at least one plausible rival explanation.

HOW-TO-TELL TIP

How can you tell if a study is quasi-experimental? Researchers do not always identify their studies as quasi-experimental. If a study involves an intervention and if the report does not explicitly mention random assignment, it is probably safe to conclude that the design is quasi-experimental. Oddly, some researchers misidentify true experimental designs as quasi-experimental. If individual subjects are randomized to groups or conditions, the design is not quasi-experimental.

Nonexperimental Studies

Many research questions—including cause-probing ones—cannot be addressed with an experimental or quasi-experimental design. For example, earlier we posed this prognosis question: Do birthweights under 1,500 grams *cause* developmental delays in children? Clearly, we cannot manipulate birthweight, the independent variable. Babies' weights are neither random nor subject to research control. When researchers do not intervene by manipulating the independent variable, the study is *nonexperimental*, or, in the medical literature, *observational*.

There are various reasons for doing a nonexperimental study, including situations in which the independent variable inherently cannot be manipulated or in which it would be unethical to manipulate the independent variable. There are also research questions for which an experimental design is not appropriate, such as studies whose purpose is description.

Types of Nonexperimental Studies

When researchers study the effect of a potential *cause* that they cannot manipulate, they use designs that examine relationships between variables—often called **correlational designs**. A **correlation** is an interrelationship or association between two variables, that is, a tendency for variation in one variable to be related to variation in another (e.g., people's height and weight). Correlations can be detected through statistical analyses.

As noted earlier, one criterion for causality is that an empirical relationship between variables must exist. It is, however, risky to infer causal relationships in correlational research, not only because of the researchers' lack of control over the independent variable, but also because of the absence of an exemplary counterfactual. In experiments, investigators make a prediction that deliberate variation of *X*, the independent variable, will result in a change to *Y*, the dependent variable. In correlational research, on the other hand, investigators do not control the independent variable, which often has already occurred. A famous research dictum is relevant: *correlation does not prove causation*. That is, the mere existence of a relationship between variables is not sufficient to warrant the conclusion that one variable caused the other, even if the relationship is strong.

Although correlational studies are inherently weaker than experimental studies in elucidating causal relationships, different designs offer varying degrees of supportive evidence. Correlational studies with a **retrospective design** are ones in which a phenomenon observed in the present is linked to phenomena occurring in the past. For example, in retrospective lung cancer research, researchers begin with some people who have lung cancer and others who do not, and then look for differences in antecedent behaviors or conditions, such as smoking habits. Such a retrospective design is sometimes called a **case-control design**—that is, *cases* with a certain condition such as lung cancer are compared with *controls* without it. In designing a case-control study, researchers try to identify controls without the disease who are as similar as possible to the cases with regard to key confounding variables (e.g., age, gender). To the degree that researchers can demonstrate comparability between cases and controls with regard to extraneous traits, causal inferences are enhanced. The difficulty, however, is that the two groups are almost never comparable with respect to *all* potential factors influencing the outcome variable.

Example of a case-control design:

Menihan and co-researchers (2006) compared infants who died of sudden infant death syndrome (the cases) with control infants who did not. The two groups were matched by date of birth. The researchers examined group differences on a number of antecedent factors, including birthweight, maternal characteristics, fetal heart rate variability, and sleep–wake cycles before birth.

Correlational studies with a **prospective design** (called a *cohort design* by medical researchers) start with a presumed cause and then go forward to the presumed effect. For example, in prospective lung cancer studies, researchers start with samples of smokers and nonsmokers and later compare the two groups in terms of lung cancer incidence. Prospective studies are more costly, but much stronger, than retrospective studies. For one thing, any ambiguity about the temporal sequence of phenomena is resolved in prospective research (i.e., smoking is known to precede the lung cancer). In addition, samples are more likely to be representative of smokers and nonsmokers, and investigators may be better able to impose controls to rule out competing explanations for observed effects.

Example of a prospective design:
Parsons and colleagues (2006) used a prospective design to study the effect of pregnant women's natural eating behavior during the latent phase of labor on outcomes in active labor. Women who voluntarily ate food were compared with women who consumed only clear fluids in terms of duration of labor, need for medical intervention, vomiting, and adverse birth outcomes.

> **TIP**
> All experimental studies are inherently prospective, because the researcher institutes the intervention (manipulates the independent variable) and subsequently determines its effect. Thus, it is not necessary to describe an RCT as prospective.

A second broad class of nonexperimental studies is **descriptive research.** The purpose of descriptive studies is to observe, describe, and document aspects of a situation. For example, an investigator may wish to determine the percentage of teenagers who engage in risky behavior (e.g., drug use, unsafe sex)—i.e., the *prevalence* of such behaviors. Or, sometimes a study design is **descriptive correlational**, meaning that researchers seek to describe relationships among variables, without attempting to infer causal connections. For example, researchers might be interested in describing the relationship between fatigue and psychological distress in patients with HIV. Because the intent in these situations is not to explain or to understand the underlying causes of the variables of interest, a descriptive nonexperimental design is appropriate.

Example of a descriptive correlational study:
Fox and colleagues (2007) studied relationships among co-occurring symptoms (depression, fatigue, pain, sleep disturbance, and cognitive impairment) and functional status in patients with high-grade glioma.

Advantages and Disadvantages of Nonexperimental Research
The major disadvantage of nonexperimental research is its inability to illuminate causal relationships with assurance. Although this is not a problem when the aim is purely descriptive, correlational studies are often undertaken with an underlying desire to discover causes. Yet correlational studies are susceptible to faulty interpretation because researchers work with preexisting groups that have formed through **self-selection** (also called *selection bias*). A researcher doing a correlational study, unlike an experimental study, cannot assume that the groups being compared are similar before the occurrence of the independent variable—the

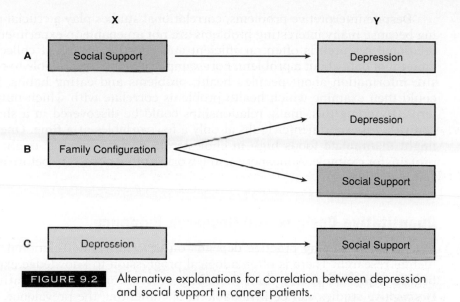

FIGURE 9.2 Alternative explanations for correlation between depression and social support in cancer patients.

hypothesized cause. Thus, preexisting differences may be a plausible alternative explanation for any group differences in outcomes.

As an example of such interpretive problems, suppose we studied differences in depression levels of cancer patients who do or do not have adequate social support (i.e., emotional sustenance through a social network). The independent variable is social support, and the dependent variable is depression. Suppose we found a correlation—that is, we found that patients without social support were more depressed than patients with adequate social support. We could interpret this to mean that people's emotional state is influenced by the adequacy of their social support, as diagrammed in Figure 9.2*A*. There are, however, alternative explanations for the findings. Perhaps a third variable influences *both* social support and depression, such as patients' family structure (e.g., whether they are married). It may be that the availability of a "significant other" affects how depressed cancer patients feel *and* the quality of their social support. These relationships are diagrammed in Figure 9.2*B*. A third possibility may be reversed causality, as shown in Figure 9.2*C*. Depressed cancer patients may find it more difficult to elicit social support than patients who are more cheerful. In this interpretation, it is the person's emotional state that causes the amount of received social support, and not the other way around. The point here is that correlational results should be interpreted cautiously, especially if the research has no theoretical basis.

TIP

Be prepared to think critically when a researcher claims to be studying the "effects" of one variable on another in a nonexperimental study. For example, if a report title were "The Effects of Dieting on Depression," the study would likely be nonexperimental (i.e., subjects were not randomly assigned to dieting or not dieting). In such a situation, you might ask, Did dieting have an effect on depression—or did depression have an effect on dieting? or, Did a third variable (e.g., being overweight) have an effect on both?

Despite interpretive problems, correlational studies play a crucial role in nursing because many interesting problems are not amenable to experimentation. Correlational research is often an efficient and effective means of collecting a large amount of data about a problem. For example, it would be possible to collect extensive information about people's health problems and eating habits. Researchers could then examine which health problems correlate with which nutritional patterns. By doing this, many relationships could be discovered in a short time. By contrast, an experimenter looks at only a few variables at a time. One experiment might manipulate foods high in cholesterol, whereas another might manipulate protein, for example. Nonexperimental work is often necessary before interventions can be justified.

Quantitative Designs and Research Evidence

Evidence for nursing practice depends on descriptive, correlational, and experimental research. There is often a logical progression to knowledge expansion that begins with rich description, including description from qualitative research. Descriptive studies can be invaluable in documenting the prevalence, nature, and intensity of health-related conditions and behaviors.

Correlational studies are often undertaken in the next phase of developing an evidence base. Exploratory retrospective or case-control studies may pave the way for more rigorous prospective studies. As the evidence base builds, conceptual models may be developed and tested using nonexperimental theory-testing strategies. These studies can provide hints about how to structure an intervention, who can most profit from it, and when it can best be instituted. Thus, the next important phase is to develop interventions to improve health outcomes. Evidence regarding the effectiveness of interventions and health strategies is strongest when it comes from RCTs.

Many important research questions, however, will never be answered using information from level I (meta-analyses of RCTs) or level II studies (RCTs) on the evidence hierarchy shown in Figure 2.1 (see Chapter 2). An important example is the question of whether smoking causes lung cancer. Despite the absence of any RCTs with humans, few people doubt that this causal connection exists. Thinking about the criteria for causality discussed earlier, there is ample evidence of a correlation between smoking and developing lung cancer and, through prospective studies, that smoking precedes lung cancer. Through repeated replications, researchers have been able to control for, and thus rule out, other possible "causes" of lung cancer. There has been a great deal of consistency and coherence in the findings. And, the criterion of biologic plausibility has been met through basic physiologic research.

Thus, it is appropriate to think of alternative evidence hierarchies. For questions about the effects of an intervention, experimental designs are the "gold standard" and meta-analyses of multiple RCTs are at the pinnacle of the hierarchy. For questions about prognosis or etiology/harm; however, strong prospective (cohort) studies are usually the best design available for studying causal relationships. Systematic reviews of multiple prospective studies, together with support from theories or biophysiologic studies, provide the strongest evidence for these types of question.

THE TIME DIMENSION IN RESEARCH DESIGN

The research design incorporates decisions about when and how often data will be collected in a study. In many nursing studies, data are collected just once but other studies involve data collection on multiple occasions. Indeed, we have already discussed several designs involving more than one point of data collection, such as pretest–posttest experimental designs, time–series designs, and prospective designs.

Studies are often categorized in terms of how they deal with time. The major distinction is between cross-sectional and longitudinal designs.

Cross-Sectional Designs

Cross-sectional designs involve the collection of data at one point in time (or multiple times in a short time period, such as 2 hours and 4 hours postoperatively). All phenomena under study are captured during one data collection period. Cross-sectional designs are especially appropriate for describing the status of phenomena or relationships among phenomena at a fixed point. For example, a researcher might study whether psychological symptoms in menopausal women are correlated contemporaneously with physiologic symptoms. Retrospective studies are usually cross-sectional: data on the independent and dependent variables are collected concurrently (e.g., the lung cancer status of respondents and their smoking habits), but the independent variable usually captures events or behaviors occurring in the past.

Cross-sectional designs are sometimes used to study time-related phenomena, but the designs are less persuasive than longitudinal ones. Suppose, for example, we were studying changes in children's health promotion activities between ages 7 and 10. One way to investigate this would be to interview the children at age 7 and then 3 years later at age 10—a longitudinal design. On the other hand, we could use a cross-sectional design by interviewing children ages 7 and 10 at one point in time and then comparing their responses. If 10-year-olds engaged in more health-promoting activities than the 7-year-olds, it might be inferred that children became more conscious of making good health choices as they age. To make this kind of inference, we would have to assume that the older children would have responded as the younger ones did had they been questioned 3 years earlier, or, conversely, that 7-year-olds would report more health-promoting activities if they were questioned again 3 years later.

The main advantage of cross-sectional designs is that they are economical and easy to manage. There are, however, problems in inferring changes and trends over time using a cross-sectional design. The amount of social and technological change that characterizes our society makes it questionable to assume that differences in the behaviors, attitudes, or characteristics of different age groups are the result of the passage through time rather than cohort or generational differences. In the previous example, 7- and 10-year-old children may have different attitudes toward health and health promotion independent of maturational factors. In such cross-sectional studies, there are often alternative explanations for observed differences.

Example of a cross-sectional study:
Dilorio and colleagues (2007) examined the relationship between age, on the one hand, and intimate behaviors, mother-adolescent discussions about sex, and adolescent-friend discussions about sex, on the other, in a cross-sectional study of African American youth aged 12, 13, 14, and 15. Intimate behavior and peer discussions increased with age, but discussions with mothers did not.

Longitudinal Designs

Researchers who collect data at more than one point in time over an extended period use a **longitudinal design**. Longitudinal designs are useful for studying changes over time and for ascertaining the temporal sequencing of phenomena, which is an essential criterion for establishing causality. Multiple points of data collection can also strengthen inferences in quasi-experimental studies, such as in a nonequivalent control group design in which the collection of pretreatment data offers evidence about the initial comparability of groups.

Sometimes longitudinal studies involve collecting data from different people in a population to examine trends over time. For example, Edwards and colleagues (2005) conducted a *trend study* to determine if gender differences associated with coronary artery revascularization changed over time from 1993 to 2003.

In a more typical longitudinal study, the same people provide data at two or more points in time. Longitudinal studies of general (nonclinical) populations are sometimes called *panel studies*. Panel studies typically yield more information than trend studies because researchers can examine correlates of change. That is, researchers can identify individuals who did and did not change (e.g., ones who did and did not become obese) and then explore characteristics that differentiate the two groups. Panel studies are appealing as a method of studying change but are difficult and expensive to manage.

Example of a panel study:
The U.S. government sponsors numerous large-scale panel studies, and many nurse researchers have analyzed data from these studies. For example, Atkins (2007) analyzed data from two waves of a national panel study of children, examining the relationship between the child's personality type at age 6, and the child's violent behavior at age 12.

Follow-up studies are undertaken to determine the subsequent status of subjects with a specified condition or those who received a specified intervention. For example, patients who have received a particular nursing intervention or clinical treatment may be followed up to ascertain the long-term effects of the treatment. To take a nonexperimental example, samples of premature infants may be followed up to assess their subsequent motor development.

Example of a follow-up study:
Lauver and colleagues (2007) did a follow-up study of cancer survivors at 4 weeks and 3 to 4 months after radiation or chemotherapy treatment to examine patterns of stress and coping.

In longitudinal studies, the number of data collection points and the time intervals between them depend on the nature of the study. When change or development is rapid, numerous data collection points at relatively short intervals may be required to document the pattern and to make accurate forecasts. By convention, however, the term *longitudinal* implies multiple data collection points over an extended period of time.

The most serious challenge in longitudinal studies is the loss of participants (**attrition**) over time. Subject attrition is problematic because those who drop out of the study often differ in important respects from those who continue to participate, resulting in potential biases, the risk of faulty inferences, and concerns about the generalizability of the findings.

> **TIP**
> Not all longitudinal studies are prospective, because sometimes the independent variable occurred even before the initial wave of data collection. And not all prospective studies are longitudinal in the classic sense. For example, an experimental study that collects data at 2, 4, and 6 hours after an intervention would be considered prospective but not longitudinal (i.e., data are not collected over a long time period.)

TECHNIQUES OF RESEARCH CONTROL

A major purpose of research design in quantitative studies is to maximize researchers' control over potentially confounding variables. There are two broad categories of confounders that need to be controlled—those that are intrinsic to study participants and those that are external, stemming from the research situation.

Controlling the Study Context

Various external factors, such as the research environment, can affect study outcomes. In carefully controlled quantitative research, steps are taken to minimize situational contaminants (i.e., to achieve **constancy of conditions** for the collection of data) so that researchers can be confident that outcomes reflect the influence of the independent variable and not the study context.

Although researchers cannot totally control the environment in studies that occur in natural settings, many opportunities exist. For example, in interview studies, researchers can restrict data collection to a specific *type* of setting (e.g., respondents' homes). Researchers can also control *when* data are collected. If an investigator were studying fatigue, for example, it would matter whether the data were gathered in the morning, afternoon, or evening, and so data from all subjects should be collected at the same time of day. Most quantitative studies also standardize communications to subjects. Formal scripts are often prepared to inform subjects about the study purpose, the use that will be made of the data, and so forth.

In research involving interventions, formal intervention protocols, or specifications for the interventions, are developed. For example, in an experiment to test the effectiveness of a new medication, care would be needed to ensure that the subjects in the experimental group received the same chemical substance and the same dosage, that the substance was administered in the same way, and so forth. There has been a recent surge in interest among nurse researchers in **intervention fidelity** (or *treatment fidelity*)—that is, in taking steps to ensure that an intervention is faithfully delivered in accordance with its plan and that the intended treatment was actually received. Intervention fidelity helps to avert biases and gives potential benefits a full opportunity to be realized.

Example of attention to intervention fidelity:
Spillane and co-researchers (2007) described their efforts to ensure treatment fidelity in implementing and testing the SPHERE program (Secondary Prevention of Heart Disease in General Practice). Their procedures included standardizing training sessions, observing intervention consultations, and using written practice and patient care plans. The research nurse in this RCT played a critical role in monitoring intervention implementation.

Controlling Intrinsic Factors

Control of study participants' characteristics is especially important and challenging. The outcomes in which nurse researchers are interested are affected by dozens of attributes, and most are irrelevant to the research question. For example, suppose we were investigating the effects of an innovative physical training program on the cardiovascular functioning of nursing home residents. In this study, variables such as the subjects' age, gender, and smoking history would be extraneous variables; each is likely to be related to the outcome variable (cardiovascular functioning), independent of the physical training program. In other words, the effects that these variables have on the dependent variable are extraneous to the study. In this section, we review methods of controlling confounding subject characteristics.

Randomization

We have already discussed the most effective method of controlling subject characteristics: randomization. The purpose of randomization is to secure a close approximation to an ideal counterfactual, that is, to have groups that are equal with respect to confounding variables. A distinct advantage of randomization, compared with other methods of control, is that it controls *all* possible sources of extraneous variation, without any conscious decision by researchers about which variables need to be controlled. In our example of a physical training intervention, random assignment of subjects to an intervention or control group would yield groups presumably comparable in terms of age, gender, smoking history, and thousands of other preintervention characteristics. Randomization to different treatment order-ings in a crossover design is especially powerful: participants serve as their own controls, thereby totally controlling all confounding characteristics.

Example of randomization:
Bennett and colleagues (2008) tested the effectiveness of a motivational interviewing (MI) intervention designed to increase physical activity in physically inactive rural adults. Participants were randomly assigned to an experimental group that received monthly MI telephone calls from a counselor over a 6-month period. Control group participants received an equal number of telephone calls, but without MI content.

Homogeneity

When randomization is not feasible, other methods of controlling extraneous sub-ject characteristics and achieving a counterfactual approximation can be used. One alternative is **homogeneity,** in which only subjects who are homogeneous with respect to confounding variables are included in the study. Confounding variables, in this case, are not allowed to vary. In the physical training example, if gender were a confounding variable, we might recruit only men (or women) as participants. If we were concerned about age as a confounding influence, participation could be limited to those within a specified age range.

This strategy of using a homogeneous sample is easy, but one problem is lim-ited generalizability. If the physical training program is found to have beneficial cardiovascular effects for men aged 65 to 75 years, its efficacy for women in their 80s would need to be tested in a separate study. Indeed, one noteworthy criticism of this approach is that researchers sometimes exclude subjects who are extremely ill or incapacitated, which means that the findings cannot be generalized to the very people who perhaps are most in need of interventions.

Example of control through homogeneity:
Gaillard and colleagues (2007) studied the relationship between level of aerobic fitness and risk for cardiovascular disease, as measured by postprandial serum glucose, insulin, and C-peptide levels. Sev-eral variables were controlled through homogeneity, including gender (only women were included), race (all were African American), weight (all were overweight or obese), and health status (all were healthy and nondiabetic).

Matching

A third method of controlling confounding variables is **matching**, which involves using information about subject characteristics to form comparable groups. For example, suppose we began with a sample of nursing home residents set to partic-ipate in the physical training program. A comparison group of nonparticipating residents could be created by matching subjects, one-by-one, on the basis of impor-tant confounding variables (e.g., age and gender). This procedure results in groups known to be similar in terms of the confounding variables of concern. Matching is the technique used to form comparable groups in case-control designs.

Matching has some drawbacks as a control method. To match effectively, researchers must know in advance what the relevant confounders are. Also, after two or three variables, it becomes difficult to match. Suppose we wanted to control the age, gender, race, and length of nursing home stays of the participants. In this situation, if participant 1 in the physical training program were an African American woman, aged 80 years, whose length of stay was 5 years, we would have to seek another woman with these same characteristics as a comparison group counterpart. With more than three variables, matching becomes cumbersome. Thus, matching as a control method is usually used only when more powerful procedures are not feasible.

Example of control through matching:
Talashek and colleagues (2006) compared inner-city teenagers who were pregnant or never-pregnant to examine factors that might predict pregnancy status. Although homogeneity controlled participants' area of residence (living in an inner city), matching was used to control the teenagers' age and ethnicity.

Statistical Control
Researchers can also control confounding variables statistically. You may be unfamiliar at this point with basic statistical procedures, let alone sophisticated techniques such as those referred to here. Therefore, a detailed description of powerful statistical control mechanisms, such as *analysis of covariance*, will not be attempted. You should recognize, however, that nurse researchers are increasingly using powerful statistical techniques to control extraneous variables. A brief description of methods of statistical control is presented in Chapter 15.

Example of statistical control:
McConkey and colleagues (2008) conducted a cross-cultural study of the impact on mothers of raising a child with intellectual disabilities. Women from three countries (Ireland, Taiwan, and Jordan) were compared with regard to stress, coping, and family functioning. To make the groups as comparable as possible, the researchers statistically controlled demographic characteristics on which the groups differed, such as mothers' age and education.

Evaluation of Control Methods
Overall, random assignment is the most effective approach to controlling confounding variables because randomization tends to cancel out individual variation on all possible confounders. Crossover designs are especially powerful, but they cannot be applied to all nursing research problems because of the possibility of carryover effects. The three remaining alternatives described here have two disadvantages in common. First, researchers must know which variables to control in advance. To select homogeneous samples, match, or use statistical controls,

researchers must decide which variables to control. Second, these three methods control only for identified characteristics, possibly leaving others uncontrolled.

Although randomization is the best mechanism for controlling subject characteristics, randomization is not always possible. If the independent variable cannot be manipulated, other techniques should be used. It is far better to use matching or analysis of covariance than simply to ignore the problem of confounding variables.

CHARACTERISTICS OF GOOD DESIGN

In evaluating the merits of a quantitative study, one overarching question is whether the research design did the best possible job of providing valid and reliable evidence. Shadish and colleagues (2002), who elaborated on an earlier classic treatise on research design, described four important considerations for evaluating research design in studies that focus on relationships among variables—particularly cause-probing studies. The questions that must be addressed by researchers (and evaluated by consumers) regarding research design are as follows:

1. What is the strength of the evidence that a relationship exists between two variables?

2. If a relationship exists, what is the strength of the evidence that the independent variable of interest (e.g., an intervention), rather than other factors, *caused* the outcome?

3. What is the strength of evidence that observed relationships are generalizable across people, settings, and time?

4. What are the theoretical constructs underlying the related variables and are those constructs adequately captured?

These questions, respectively, correspond to four aspects of a study's **validity**: (1) statistical conclusion validity; (2) internal validity; (3) external validity; and (4) construct validity. In this section we briefly discuss some aspects of validity. Validity issues are elaborated on in later chapters.

Statistical Conclusion Validity

As noted earlier in this chapter, the key criterion for establishing causality is demonstrating that there is an empirical relationship between the independent and dependent variables. Statistical tests are used to support inferences about whether or not such a relationship exists. Design decisions can influence whether statistical tests will actually detect true relationships, and so researchers need to make decisions that protect against reaching false statistical conclusions. Although we cannot discuss all aspects of **statistical conclusion validity**, we can describe a few design issues that can affect it.

One issue concerns **statistical power**, which is the ability of the design to detect true relationships among variables. Statistical power can be achieved in various ways, the most straightforward of which is to use a sufficiently large sample.

With small samples, statistical power tends to be low, and the analyses may fail to show that the independent and dependent variables are related—*even when they are*. Power and sample size are discussed in Chapter 12.

Another aspect of a powerful design concerns the construction or definition of the independent variable and the counterfactual. Both statistically and substantively, results are clearer when differences between the groups (treatment conditions) being compared are large. Researchers should maximize group differences on the independent variables (i.e., make the *cause* powerful) so as to maximize differences on the dependent variable (i.e., the effect). If the groups or treatments are not very different, the statistical analysis might not be sufficiently sensitive to detect outcome effects that actually exist. Intervention fidelity can enhance the power of an intervention.

Thus, if you are critiquing a study that indicates that the groups being compared were not statistically different with respect to outcomes, one possibility is that the study had low statistical conclusion validity. The report might give clues about this possibility (e.g., too small a sample or substantial subject attrition) that should be taken into consideration in drawing inferences about what the results mean.

Internal Validity

Internal validity refers to the extent to which it is possible to make an inference that the independent variable is truly causing or influencing the dependent variable. Experiments tend to have a high degree of internal validity because randomization to different groups enables researchers to rule out competing explanations. With quasi-experiments and correlational studies, investigators must contend with rival hypotheses. Competing explanations, sometimes called **threats to internal validity**, have been grouped into several classes.

Threats to Internal Validity
Temporal Ambiguity
As we discussed earlier, one criterion for inferring a causal relationship is that the cause must precede the effect. In RCTs, researchers create the independent variable and then observe performance on an outcome variable, so establishing a temporal sequence is never a problem. In correlational studies, however—especially ones using a cross-sectional design—it may be unclear whether the independent variable preceded the dependent variable, or vice versa.

Selection
The **selection threat** encompasses biases resulting from preexisting differences between groups. When people are not assigned randomly to groups, the possibility always exists that groups being compared are not equivalent. In such a situation, researchers contend with the possibility that any difference in the dependent variable is caused by extraneous factors rather than by the independent variable. Selection bias is the most challenging threat to the internal validity of studies not using an experimental design (e.g., nonequivalent control group designs, case-control designs), but can be partially addressed using the control mechanisms described in the previous section. Selection can also enter into experimental designs if many subjects elect not to receive the treatment; these subjects essentially select themselves into the control condition.

History

The **history threat** is the occurrence of events concurrent with the independent variable that can affect the dependent variable. For example, suppose we were studying the effectiveness of a program to encourage flu shots among community-dwelling elderly using a time–series design. Let us further suppose that, at about the same time the program was launched, there was a public media campaign focusing on the flu. Our dependent variable, number of flu shots administered, is subject to the influence of at least two forces, and it would be hard to disentangle the two effects. (This type of threat is sometimes referred to as *co-intervention bias*). In experiments, history is not typically a threat because external events are as likely to affect one randomized group as another. The designs most likely to be affected by the history threat are one-group before–after designs and time–series designs.

Maturation

The **maturation threat** arises from processes occurring as a result of time (e.g., growth, fatigue) rather than the independent variable. For example, if we wanted to study the effect of a special intervention for developmentally delayed children, we would have to address the fact that progress would occur even without the intervention. The term *maturation* does not refer to developmental changes exclusively, but rather to any kind of change that occurs as a function of time. Phenomena such as wound healing, postoperative recovery, and other bodily changes can occur with little nursing intervention, and thus maturation may be a rival explanation for positive posttreatment outcomes in the absence of a nontreated group. One-group before–after designs are especially vulnerable to the maturation threat.

Mortality/Attrition

Mortality is the threat that arises from attrition in groups being compared. If different kinds of people remain in the study in one group versus another, then these differences, rather than the independent variable, could account for observed differences on the outcome variables at the end of the study. The most severely ill patients might drop out of an experimental condition because it is too demanding, or they might drop out of the comparison group because they see no personal advantage to staying in the study. In a prospective cohort study, there may be differential attrition between groups being compared because of death, illness, or geographic relocation. Attrition bias essentially is a selection bias that occurs after the unfolding of the study: groups initially equivalent can lose comparability because of subject loss, and it could be that the differential composition, rather than the independent variable, is the "cause" of any group differences on the dependent variables.

TIP

If attrition is random (i.e., those dropping out of a study are similar to those remaining in it), then there would not be bias. However, attrition is rarely totally random. In general, the higher the rate of attrition, the greater the risk of bias. Biases are usually of concern if the rate exceeds 20%.

Internal Validity and Research Design

Quasi-experimental and correlational studies are especially susceptible to threats to internal validity. These threats represent alternative explanations (rival hypotheses) that compete with the independent variable as a cause of the dependent variable. *The aim of a good quantitative research design is to rule out these competing explanations.* The control mechanisms previously reviewed are strategies for improving the internal validity of studies—and thus for strengthening the quality of evidence they yield.

An experimental design often, but not always, eliminates competing explanations. For example, if constancy of conditions is not maintained for experimental and control groups, history might be a rival explanation for obtained results. Experimental mortality is, in particular, a salient threat. Because the experimenter does different things with the experimental and control groups, members of the two groups may drop out of the study differentially. This is particularly likely to happen if the experimental treatment is stressful, inconvenient, or time-consuming or if the control condition is boring or aggravating. When this happens, participants remaining in the study may differ from those who left, thereby nullifying the initial equivalence of the groups.

You should carefully consider possible rival explanations for study results, especially in studies not using an experimental design. When researchers do not have control over critical confounding variables, caution in interpreting results and drawing conclusions about the evidence is appropriate.

External Validity

External validity concerns inferences about the extent to which relationships observed in a study hold true for different people, conditions, and settings. External validity has emerged as a major concern in an EBP world in which it is important to generalize evidence from controlled research settings to real-world practice settings.

As Shadish and colleagues (2002) have noted, external validity questions may take on several different forms. For example, we may wish to ask whether relationships observed with a study sample can be generalized to a larger population—for example, whether results from a smoking cessation program found effective with teenagers in Boston can be generalized to teenagers throughout the United States. Thus, one aspect of a study's external validity concerns the adequacy of the sampling plan. If the characteristics of the sample are representative of those of the population, the generalizability of the results to the population is enhanced. Sampling is discussed in Chapter 12.

Many EBP questions, however, are about going from a broad study group to a *particular* client—for example, whether the pelvic muscle exercises found to be effective in alleviating urinary incontinence in one study are an effective strategy for Ann Smith. Other external validity questions are about generalizing to somewhat different types of people, settings, situations, or treatments. For example, can findings about a pain reduction treatment in Canada be generalized to people in the United States? Or, would a 6-week intervention to promote dietary changes in patients with diabetes be equally effective if the content were condensed into a 3-week program? Sometimes new studies are needed to answer questions about external validity, but sometimes external validity can be enhanced by decisions researchers make in designing a study.

An important concept relevant to external validity is that of *replication*. Multisite studies are powerful because more confidence in the generalizability of the results can be attained if the results have been replicated in several sites—particularly if the sites are different on dimensions considered important (e.g., size, location). Studies involving a diverse sample of participants can test whether study results are replicated for various subgroups—for example, whether an intervention benefits men *and* women, or older *and* younger patients. Systematic reviews represent a crucial aid to external validity precisely because they focus on replications across time, space, people, and settings to explore consistencies.

Sometimes the demands for internal and external validity conflict. If a researcher exercises tight control in a study to maximize internal validity, the setting may become too artificial to generalize to a more naturalistic environment. Therefore, compromises must sometimes be reached.

Construct Validity

Research cannot be undertaken without using constructs. When researchers conduct a study with specific exemplars of treatments, outcomes, settings, and people, these are all stand-ins for general constructs. **Construct validity** involves inferences from the particulars of the study to the higher-order constructs they are intended to represent. Construct validity is important because constructs are the means for linking the operations used in a study to a relevant conceptualization and to mechanisms for translating the resulting evidence into practice. If studies contain construct errors, there is a risk that the evidence will be misleading. One aspect of construct validity concerns the degree to which an intervention is a good representation of the underlying construct that was theorized as having the potential to cause beneficial outcomes. Another concerns whether the measures of the dependent variable are good operationalizations of the constructs for which they are intended. This aspect will be discussed more fully in Chapter 14.

CRITIQUING QUANTITATIVE RESEARCH DESIGNS

The overriding consideration in evaluating a research design is whether the design enables the researcher to answer the research question conclusively. This must be determined in terms of both substantive and methodologic issues.

Substantively, the issue is whether the researcher selected a design that matches the aims of the research. If the research purpose is descriptive or exploratory, an experimental design is not appropriate. If the researcher is searching to understand the full nature of a phenomenon about which little is known, a highly structured design that allows little flexibility might block insights (flexible designs are discussed in Chapter 10). We have discussed research control as a mechanism for reducing bias, but in certain situations, too much control can introduce bias—for example, when the researcher tightly controls the ways in which the phenomena under study can be manifested and thereby obscures their true nature.

Methodologically, the main design issue in quantitative studies is whether the research design provides the most accurate, unbiased, interpretable, and replicable evidence possible. Indeed, there usually is no other aspect of a quantitative study that affects the quality of evidence as much as the research design. Box 9.1 provides questions to assist you in evaluating the methodologic aspects of quantitative research designs; these questions are key to a meaningful critique of a quantitative study.

From an EBP perspective, it is important to remember that drawing inferences about causal relationships relies not only on how high up on the evidence hierarchy a study is (see Figure 2.1), but also, for any given level of the hierarchy, how successful the researcher was in enhancing study validity.

BOX 9.1 **GUIDELINES FOR CRITIQUING RESEARCH DESIGNS IN QUANTITATIVE STUDIES**

1. Does the study involve an intervention? If yes, was the design experimental or quasi-experimental? Given potential constraints, was this an appropriate design?

2. In intervention studies, was the intervention adequately described? Was the control or comparison condition adequately described? Is there evidence that attention was paid to intervention fidelity? Was masking/blinding used at all? If yes, who was blinded—and was this adequate? If not, is there an adequate rationale for failure to mask?

3. If the study was nonexperimental, why did the researcher not manipulate the independent variable? Was the decision regarding manipulation appropriate? Was this a cause-probing study? What criteria for inferring causality were potentially compromised? Was a retrospective or prospective design used—and was such a design appropriate?

4. Was the study longitudinal or cross-sectional? Was the number of data collection points appropriate, given the research question?

5. What types of comparisons were called for in the research design (e.g., was the study design within-subjects or between-subjects)? Was the comparison strategy effective in illuminating the relationship between the independent and dependent variables?

6. What did the researcher do to control confounding external factors and intrinsic subject characteristics? Were the procedures effective?

7. What steps did the researcher take in designing the study to enhance statistical conclusion validity? Were these steps adequate?

8. What steps did the researcher take to enhance the internal validity of the study? To what extent were those steps successful? What types of alternative explanations must be considered—what are the threats to internal validity? Does the design enable the researcher to draw causal inferences about the relationship between the independent and dependent variables?

9. To what extent is the study externally valid? What did the researchers do, if anything, to enhance generalizability?

10. What are the major limitations of the design used? Are these limitations acknowledged by the researcher and taken into account in interpreting results?

⏵   RESEARCH EXAMPLES AND CRITICAL THINKING ACTIVITIES

This section presents examples of studies with different research designs. Read these summaries and then answer the critical thinking questions, referring to the full research report if necessary.

EXAMPLE 1 ■ Experimental Design

Study

Acupressure for chemotherapy-induced nausea and vomiting (Dibble et al., 2007).

Statement of Purpose

The purpose of the study was to evaluate the efficacy of acupressure in reducing nausea and vomiting among women undergoing chemotherapy treatment for breast cancer.

Treatment Groups

Three groups of women were compared: (1) an intervention group trained in digital acupressure to P6 point in their forearm; (2) a placebo group trained to administer acupressure to an inactive pressure point, SI3; and (3) a control group that got usual care only.

Method

A sample of 160 women who were in their second or third cycle of chemotherapy at 19 different sites throughout the United States was randomly assigned to one of the three treatment groups. Women receiving specific chemotherapy treatments and whose score on a nausea intensity scale at the previous round of chemotherapy was at least moderate were invited to participate. Women in the intervention group received instruction from trained clinical staff in how to apply the acupressure treatment to one of the *nei guan* points (P6) in both forearms, and when to apply it. Women in the placebo group received the same instruction, but were trained to apply pressure to the *hou xi* point (SI3, a point on the ulnar side of the hand). The researchers chose this point because it was close to the active P6 point but was not expected to affect nausea treatment. Research assistants who trained women in the two acupressure groups were unaware of the active acupressure point. Women in all groups completed questionnaires at baseline when they came in for their scheduled chemotherapy treatment and 3 weeks later at their next cycle of chemotherapy. They also maintained daily logs for 10 days after their chemotherapy in which they recorded levels of nausea, episodes of vomiting, use of prescribed antiemetic therapy, and use of any other interventions to control nausea/vomiting, including (in the acupressure groups) how often acupressure was used. A comparison of patients in the three study groups at baseline indicated that the three groups were comparable in terms of demographic characteristics (e.g., age, marital status, education) and disease and treatment variables (e.g., type of breast surgery, number of positive nodes). There was some attrition during the study (about 8%), but attrition was similar across groups.

Key Findings

There were no significant differences among the three groups in terms of acute nausea or vomiting on the day of chemotherapy. Women in the treatment group did, however, have significantly less delayed nausea and vomiting than those in the placebo or control groups, leading the researchers to conclude that acupressure at the P6 point is a safe and effective value-added tool for managing delayed chemotherapy-induced nausea and vomiting.

CRITICAL THINKING SUGGESTIONS*:

*See the Student Resource CD-ROM for a discussion of these questions. 🔵

1. Answer the relevant questions from Box 9.1 regarding this study.
2. Also, consider the following targeted questions, which may further sharpen your critical thinking skills and assist you in understanding this study:
   a. What specific experimental design was used in this study? Was this appropriate?
   b. What was the purpose of the placebo group in this study?
   c. Could a crossover design have been used? Could a factorial design have been used?
   d. Was randomization successful?
3. If the results of this study are valid, what are some of the uses to which the findings might be put in clinical practice?

EXAMPLE 2 ■ Quasi-Experimental Design

Study

A quasi-experimental trial on individualized, developmentally supportive family-centered care (Byers, et al., 2006).

Statement of Purpose

The purpose of the study was to evaluate the impact of individualized, developmentally supportive family-centered care for premature infants on a range of infant outcomes (e.g., growth, behavioral stress cues, physiologic variables) and parental satisfaction.

Treatment Groups

The intervention group was cared for in a developmental nursery within the neonatal intensive care unit (NICU). The intervention involved individualized developmental assessments of the infants and the creation and implementation of individualized plans of care. In this model of care, the families were incorporated early and actively into the care of their high-risk infants. There was open visitation in the intervention nursery. All staff who interacted with the infants received 5 consecutive days of training on developmentally supportive care. Infants in the control nursery, which was also in the NICU of the same hospital, received traditional standards of care. The control NICU nursery had limited visitation.

Method

A sample of 114 premature infants born at a tertiary medical center in southeastern United States participated in the study. Infants were included if they were admitted to one of the two NICUs and if their gestational age was under 33 weeks. Those in the intervention nursery had to have English-speaking parents and an expected stay of at least 3 weeks. The control nursery was similar to the intervention nursery in terms of size, equipment, floor plan, staffing ratios, and infant acuity levels. Some background and outcome variables were retrieved from the infant's hospital records. Physiologic variables (e.g., heart rate, respiratory rate, oxygen saturation) were obtained at baseline, during caregiver activity, and postactivity over a 4-week period via a monitor. Behavioral stress cues were measured multiple times via observation by development specialists. Parental satisfaction was measured using a self-report scale.

Key Findings

- The intervention and comparison group infants did not differ significantly at baseline in terms of a wide range of risk factors, including Apgar scores, gestational age, birthweight, congenital anomalies, gender, ethnicity, and maternal age.
- There were no differences between the groups in terms of most outcomes—days to medical or developmental milestones, length of hospital stay, complications, or direct cost per case. There were also no group differences in parental satisfaction.
- At every point of data collection, stress cues were lower in the developmentally supported group. Infants in the intervention group had 8% less sedatives or narcotics and 15% lower vasopressors costs than those in the comparison group.

CRITICAL THINKING SUGGESTIONS:

1. Answer the relevant questions from Box 9.1 regarding this study.
2. Also, consider the following targeted questions, which may further sharpen your critical thinking skills and assist you in understanding this study:
   a. What specific quasi-experimental design was used in this study? Was this appropriate?
   b. Comment on the issue of constancy of conditions in this study.
   c. Is this study prospective or retrospective?
3. If the results of this study are valid, what are some of the uses to which the findings might be put in clinical practice?

EXAMPLE 3 ■ Nonexperimental Study in Appendix A

1. Read the method section from Howell and colleagues' (2007) study ("Anxiety, anger, and blood pressure in children") in Appendix A of this book, and then answer the relevant questions in Box 9.1.
2. Also, consider the following targeted questions, which may further sharpen your critical thinking skills and assist you in assessing aspects of the study's merit:
   a. Could Howell and colleagues have used an experimental or quasi-experimental design to address the research questions?
   b. If the design was retrospective, how could the study have been done prospectively (or vice versa)?

CHAPTER REVIEW

Key new terms introduced in the chapter, together with a summary of major points, are presented in this section. In addition, Chapter 9 of the *Study Guide for Essentials of Nursing Research,* 7th edition offers various exercises and study suggestions for reinforcing the concepts presented in this chapter. For additional review, see the Student Self-Study Review Questions section of the Student Resource CD-ROM provided with this book. ☻

Key New Terms

Attrition
Baseline data
Between-subjects design
Blinding
Case-control design
Comparison group
Control group
Correlational research
Crossover design
Cross-sectional design
Counterfactual
Experiment
External validity

Factorial design
History threat
Homogeneity
Internal validity
Intervention fidelity
Longitudinal design
Masking
Manipulation
Matching
Maturation threat
Mortality threat
Nonequivalent control
group design

Nonexperimental
study
Posttest-only design
Pretest–posttest design
Prospective design
Quasi-experiment
Random assignment
(randomization)
Retrospective design
Selection threat (self-
selection)
Time–series design
Within-subjects design

Summary Points

✻ The **research design** is the researcher's overall plan for answering research questions. In quantitative studies, the design indicates whether there is an intervention, the nature of any comparisons, the methods used to control confounding variables, whether there will be **masking (blinding)**, and the timing and location of data collection.

✻ Causality is a key issue in quantitative design. Various criteria have been proposed for inferring causality, the most tricky of which is to rule out the possibility that an observed relationship between the presumed cause (the independent variable) and the effect (dependent variable) does not reflect the influence of a third (confounding) variable.

✻ In an idealized counterfactual model, a counterfactual is what would have happened to the same people simultaneously exposed *and* not exposed to the causal factor. The *effect* represents the difference between the two. Good research design entails finding a good approximation to the idealized counterfactual.

✻ **Experiments** (or randomized controlled trials [RCTs]) involve **manipulation** (the researcher manipulates the independent variable by introducing a **treatment** or **intervention**); control (including the use of a **control group** that is not given the intervention and represents the comparative counterfactual); and **randomization** or **random assignment** (with subjects allocated to experimental and control groups at random to make the groups comparable at the outset).

✻ Experimental designs are considered by many to be the gold standard because they come closer than any other design in meeting the criteria for inferring causal relationships.

✻ **Posttest-only** (or *after-only*) **designs** involve collecting data only once—after random assignment and the introduction of the treatment; in **pretest–posttest** (or *before–after*) designs, data are collected both before introducing the intervention (at **baseline)** and after it.

❧ **Factorial designs**, in which two or more variables are manipulated simultaneously, allow researchers to test both **main effects** (effects from the experimentally manipulated variables) and **interaction effects** (effects resulting from combining the treatments).

❧ In **crossover designs**, subjects are exposed to more than one experimental condition in random order and serve as their own controls; such designs are **within-subjects designs**.

❧ Experimenters can expose the control group to various conditions, including no treatment; an alternative treatment; a **placebo** or pseudointervention; standard treatment ("usual care"); different doses of the treatment; and a wait-list (**delayed treatment**) condition.

❧ **Quasi-experiments** (controlled trials without randomization) involve manipulation but lack a comparison group or randomization. Strong quasi-experimental designs introduce controls to compensate for these missing components.

❧ **The nonequivalent control-group before–after design** involves the use of a **comparison group** that was not created through random assignment, and the collection of pretreatment data that permits an assessment of initial group equivalence.

❧ In a **time–series design**, there is no comparison group; information on the dependent variable is collected over a period of time before and after the treatment.

❧ **Nonexperimental** (*observational*) **research** includes **descriptive research**—studies that summarize the status of phenomena—and **correlational studies** that examine relationships among variables but involve no manipulation of the independent variable.

❧ There are two major correlational designs. **Retrospective designs** involve collecting data about an outcome in the present and then looking back in time for possible causes or antecedents (e.g., a **case-control design**). In **prospective designs,** researchers begin with a possible cause, and then subsequently collect data about outcomes.

❧ Making causal inferences in correlational studies is risky; a primary weakness is that correlational studies can harbor biases owing to **self-selection** into groups being compared.

❧ **Cross-sectional designs** involve the collection of data at one time period, whereas **longitudinal designs** involve data collection at two or more times over an extended period. Three types of longitudinal studies, which are used to study changes or development over time, are **trend studies, panel studies,** and **follow-up studies.**

❧ Longitudinal studies are typically expensive, time-consuming, and subject to the risk of **attrition** (loss of participants over time), but yield valuable information about time-related phenomena.

➤ Quantitative researchers strive to control external factors that could affect the study outcomes (e.g., the environment or the intervention) and subject characteristics that are extraneous to the research question.

➤ Researchers delineate the intervention in formal *protocols* that stipulate exactly what the treatment is. Researchers must also attend to **intervention fidelity** (*treatment fidelity*)—whether the intervention was properly implemented and actually received.

➤ Techniques for controlling subject characteristics include **homogeneity** (restricting the selection of subjects to eliminate variability on the confounding variable); **matching** (matching subjects on a one-to-one basis to make groups comparable on the extraneous variables); statistical procedures, such as *analysis of covariance*; and randomization—the most effective control procedure because it controls all possible confounding variables without researchers having to identify or measure them.

➤ Study **validity** concerns the extent to which appropriate inferences can be made. **Threats to validity** are reasons that an inference could be wrong. A key function of quantitative research design is to rule out validity threats by exercising various types of control.

➤ **Statistical conclusion validity** concerns the strength of evidence that a relationship exists between two variables. Threats to statistical conclusion validity include low **statistical power** (the ability to detect true relationships among variables) and factors that undermine a strong treatment.

➤ **Internal validity** concerns inferences that the outcomes of interest were caused by the independent variable, rather than by other factors extraneous to the research. Threats to internal validity include temporal ambiguity (lack of clarity about whether the presumed cause occurred before the outcome); **selection** (preexisting group differences); **history** (the occurrence of events external to an independent variable that could affect outcomes); **maturation** (changes resulting from the passage of time); and **mortality** (effects attributable to subject attrition).

➤ **External validity** concerns inferences about generalizability (i.e., about whether observed relationships hold true over variations in people, conditions, settings, and operationalizations of variables).

STUDIES CITED IN CHAPTER 9

Atkins, R. (2007). The association of personality type in childhood with violence in adolescence. *Research in Nursing & Health, 30,* 308–319.

Beckham, N. (2007). Motivational interviewing with hazardous drinkers. *Journal of the American Academy of Nurse Practitioners, 19,* 103–110.

Bennett, J., Young, H., Nail, L., Winters-Stone, K., & Hanson, G. (2008). A telephone-only motivational intervention to increase physical activity in rural adults: A randomized controlled trial. *Nursing Research, 57,* 24–32.

Byers, J., Lowman, L., Francis, J., Kaigle, L., Lutz, N., Waddell, T. et al. (2006). A quasi-experimental trial on individualized, developmentally supportive family-centered care. *Journal of Obstetric, Gynecologic, & Neonatal Nursing, 35,* 105–115.

Dibble, S., Luce, J., Cooper, B., Israel, J., Cohen, M., Nussey, B. et al. (2007). Acupressure for chemotherapy-induced nausea and vomiting: A randomized clinical trial. *Oncology Nursing Forum, 34,* 813–820.

DiIorio, C., McCarty, F., Denzmore, P., & Landis, A. (2007). The moderating influence of mother-adolescent discussion on early and middle African American adolescent sexual behavior. *Research in Nursing & Health, 30,* 193–202.

Edwards, M. L., Albert, N. M., Wang, C., & Apperson-Hansen, C. (2005). 1993–2003 gender differences in coronary revascularization: Has anything changed? *Journal of Cardiovascular Nursing, 20,* 461–467.

Fox, S., Lyon, D., & Farace, E. (2007). Symptom clusters in patients with high-grade glioma. *Journal of Nursing Scholarship, 39,* 61–67.

Gaillard, T., Sherman, W., M., Devor, S., Kirby, T., & Osei, K. (2007). Importance of aerobic fitness in cardiovascular risks in sedentary overweight and obese African American women. *Nursing Research, 56,* 407–415.

Jones, E., Renger, R., & Kang, Y. (2007). Self-efficacy for health related behaviors among deaf adults. *Research in Nursing & Health, 30,* 185–192.

Lauver, D., Connolly-Nelson, K., & Vang, P. (2007). Stressors and coping strategies among female cancer survivors after treatments. *Cancer Nursing, 30,* 101–111.

Mastel-Smith, B., Binder, B., Malecha, A., Hersch, G., Symes, L., & McFarlane, J. (2006). Testing therapeutic life review offered by home care workers to decrease depression among home-dwelling older women. *Issues in Mental Health Nursing, 27,* 1037–1049.

Mastel-Smith, B., McFarlane, J., Sierpina, M., Malecha, A., & Haile, B. (2007). Improving depressive symptoms in community-dwelling older adults: A psychosocial intervention using life review and writing. *Journal of Gerontological Nursing, 33,* 13–19.

McConkey, R., Truesdale-Kennedy, M., Chang, M., Jarrah, S., & Shukri, R. (2008). The impact on mothers of bringing up a child with intellectual disabilities: A cross-cultural study. *International Journal of Nursing Studies, 45,* 65–74.

Menihan, C. A., Phipps, M., & Weitzen, S. (2006). Fetal heart rate patterns and sudden infant death syndrome. *Journal of Obstetric, Gynecologic, & Nenonatal Nursing, 35,* 116–122.

Parsons, M., Bidewell, J., & Nagy, S. (2006). Natural eating behavior in latent labor and its effect on outcomes in active labor. *Journal of Midwifery & Women's Health, 51,* 1–6.

Spillane, V., Byrne, M., Byrne, M., Leathem, C., O'Malley, M., & Cupples, M. (2007). Monitoring treatment fidelity in a randomized controlled trial of a complex intervention. *Journal of Advanced Nursing, 60,* 343–352.

Scott, S., Raymond, P., Thompson, W., & Galt, D. (2005). Efficacy and tolerance of sodium phosphates oral solution after diet liberalization. *Gastroenterology Nursing, 28,* 133–139.

Talashek, M. L., Alba, M. L., & Patel, A. (2006). Untangling health disparities of teen pregnancy. *Journal for Specialists in Pediatric Nursing, 11,* 14–27.

Voergaard, L., Vendelbo, G., Carlsen, B., Jacobsen, L., Nissen, B., Moretensen, J. et al. (2007). Ostomy bag management: Comparative study of a new one-piece closed bag *British Journal of Nursing, 16,* 98–101.

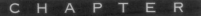

CHAPTER

10 Qualitative Designs and Approaches

THE DESIGN OF QUALITATIVE STUDIES
Characteristics of Qualitative Research Design
Qualitative Design and Planning
Qualitative Design Features
Causality in Qualitative Research

QUALITATIVE RESEARCH TRADITIONS
Overview of Qualitative Traditions
Ethnography
Phenomenology
Grounded Theory

OTHER TYPES OF QUALITATIVE RESEARCH
Case Studies
Narrative Analysis
Descriptive Qualitative Studies

RESEARCH WITH IDEOLOGIC PERSPECTIVES
Critical Theory
Feminist Research
Participatory Action Research

CRITIQUING QUALITATIVE DESIGNS

RESEARCH EXAMPLES AND CRITICAL THINKING ACTIVITIES

CHAPTER REVIEW
Key New Terms
Summary Points

STUDIES CITED IN CHAPTER 10

STUDENT OBJECTIVES

On completing this chapter, you will be able to:

➤ Discuss the rationale for an emergent design in qualitative research and describe qualitative design features

➤ Identify the major research traditions for qualitative research and describe the domain of inquiry of each

➤ Describe the main features of ethnographic, phenomenological and grounded theory studies

➤ Discuss the goals and methods of various types of research with an ideologic perspective

➤ Define new terms in the chapter

THE DESIGN OF QUALITATIVE STUDIES

Quantitative researchers carefully specify a research design before collecting even one piece of data, and rarely depart from that design once the study is underway. They design and *then* they do. In qualitative research, by contrast, the study design typically evolves over the course of the project. Qualitative researchers design *as* they do. Decisions about how best to obtain data, from whom to obtain data, how to schedule data collection, and how long each data collection session should last are made as the study unfolds. Qualitative studies use an **emergent design**—a design that emerges as researchers make ongoing decisions reflecting what has already been learned. An emergent design in qualitative studies is not the result of laziness on the part of researchers, but rather a reflection of their desire to have the inquiry based on the realities and viewpoints of those under study—realities and viewpoints that are not known or understood at the outset.

Characteristics of Qualitative Research Design

Qualitative inquiry has been guided by different disciplines, and each has developed methods for addressing questions of particular interest. However, some general characteristics of qualitative research design tend to apply across disciplines. In general, qualitative design:

➤ Is flexible and elastic, capable of adjusting to what is being learned during the course of data collection

➤ Often involves a merging together of various data collection strategies (i.e., triangulation)

➤ Tends to be holistic, striving for an understanding of the whole

➤ Requires researchers to become intensely involved, often remaining in the field for lengthy periods of time

➤ Requires ongoing analysis of the data to formulate subsequent strategies and to determine when field work is done

Qualitative researchers tend to put together a complex array of data, derived from a variety of sources and using a variety of methods. A qualitative researcher has been referred to as a **bricoleur**, a person who "is adept at performing a large number of diverse tasks, ranging from interviewing to intensive reflection and introspection" (Denzin & Lincoln, 2000, p. 6).

Qualitative Design and Planning

Although design decisions are not specified in advance, qualitative researchers typically do considerable advance planning that supports their flexibility. In the total absence of planning, design choices might actually be constrained. For example, researchers initially might anticipate a 6-month period for data collection, but may need to be prepared (financially and emotionally) to spend even longer periods of time in the field to pursue data collection opportunities that could not have been foreseen. In other words, qualitative researchers plan for broad contingencies that may be expected to pose decision opportunities once the study has begun. Advanced planning is especially useful with regard to the following:

➤ Selecting a broad framework or tradition to guide certain design decisions

➤ Determining the maximum amount of time for the study, given costs and other constraints

➤ Developing a broad data collection strategy (e.g., will interviews be conducted?)

➤ Selecting the study site and identifying appropriate settings

➤ Taking steps to gain entrée into the site through negotiations with key "gate-keepers"

➤ Identifying the types of equipment that could aid in the collection and analysis of data in the field (e.g., recording equipment, laptop computers)

➤ Identifying personal biases, views, and presuppositions vis-à-vis the phenomenon or the study site (reflexivity)

Thus, qualitative researchers need to plan for a variety of circumstances, but decisions about how to deal with them must be resolved when the social context of time, place, and human interactions are better understood. By both allowing for and anticipating an evolution of strategies, qualitative researchers seek to make their research design responsive to the situation and to the phenomenon under study.

Qualitative Design Features

Some of the design features discussed in Chapter 9 apply to qualitative studies. However, qualitative design features are often *post hoc* characterizations of what happened in the field rather than features specifically planned in advance. To further contrast qualitative and quantitative research design, we refer you to the design elements identified in Table 9.1.

Intervention, Control, and Masking

Qualitative research is almost always nonexperimental—although a qualitative sub-study may be embedded in an experiment. Qualitative researchers do not conceptualize their studies as having independent and dependent variables, and they rarely control or manipulate any aspect of the people or environment under study. Masking is also not a strategy used by qualitative researchers because there is no intervention or hypotheses to conceal. The goal is to develop a rich understanding of a phenomenon as it exists and as it is constructed by individuals within their own context.

Comparisons

Qualitative researchers typically do not plan in advance to make group comparisons because the intent is to describe and explain a phenomenon thoroughly. Nevertheless, patterns emerging in the data sometimes suggest comparisons that are illuminating. Indeed, as Morse (2004) noted in an editorial in *Qualitative Health Research*, "All description requires comparisons" (p. 1323). In analyzing qualitative data and in determining whether categories are saturated, there is a need to compare "this" to "that."

Example of qualitative comparisons:
Hilden and Honkasalo (2006) explored how nurses interpret patient autonomy in end-of-life decision-making. Based on interviews with 17 nurses, they discovered three distinct patterns, which they called the "supporter," the "analyst," and the "practical," each of which involved a certain position for patients and relatives and a certain identity for nurses in end-of-life decision making.

Research Settings

Qualitative researchers usually collect their data in real-world, naturalistic settings. And, whereas a quantitative researcher usually strives to collect data in one type of setting to maintain control over the environment (e.g., conducting all interviews in study participants' homes), qualitative researchers may deliberately strive to study phenomena in a variety of natural contexts.

Example of variation in settings and sites:
Hughes and colleagues (2007) conducted a qualitative study of the everyday experiences of the urban poor living with advanced cancer and their struggle to survive. Interview data were collected multiple times with 14 patients in various community, residential, and clinical settings.

Timeframes

Qualitative research, like quantitative research, can be either cross-sectional, with one data collection point, or longitudinal, with multiple data collection points over an extended period, to observe the evolution of a phenomenon. Sometimes qualitative researchers plan in advance for a longitudinal design, but, in other cases, the decision to study a phenomenon longitudinally may be made in the field after preliminary data have been collected and analyzed.

Examples of the time dimension in qualitative studies:
➤ *Cross-sectional:* Haynes and Watt (2008) studied the experience of engaging in healthy behaviors among individuals with a debilitating illness. The data were gathered at a fixed point in time, relying on participants' retrospective accounts of adaptation processes, rather than gathering data over time as adaptation occurred.
➤ *Longitudinal:* Smithbattle (2007) conducted a longitudinal study of the experiences of teen mothers and their children. Sixteen families participated in five waves of interviews between 1988 and 2005. The teen mothers' life trajectories reflected legacies of unequal life chances that began in childhood and persisted into their 30s.

Causality in Qualitative Research

In evidence hierarchies that rank evidence in terms of its ability to support causal inferences (e.g., the one in Figure 2.1), qualitative inquiry is usually near the base—a fact that has led some to criticize the current evidence-based practice environment. The issue of causality, which has been a controversial topic throughout the history of science, is especially contentious in qualitative research.

Some qualitative researchers think that causality is not an appropriate construct within the naturalistic paradigm. For example, Lincoln and Guba (1985) devoted an entire chapter of their book to a critique of causality and argued that it should be replaced with a concept that they called *mutual shaping*. According to their view of mutual and simultaneous shaping, "Everything influences everything else, in the here and now. Many elements are implicated in any given action, and each element interacts with all of the others in ways that change them all while simultaneously resulting in something that we . . . label as outcomes or effects" (p. 151).

There are others, however, who believe that causal explanation is not only a legitimate pursuit in qualitative research, but also that qualitative methods are particularly well suited to understanding causal relationships. For example, Huberman and Miles (1994) argued that qualitative studies "can look directly and longitudinally at the local processes underlying a temporal series of events and states, showing how these led to specific outcomes, and ruling out rival hypotheses" (p. 434).

In attempting to not only describe, but to explain phenomena, qualitative researchers who undertake in-depth studies will inevitably reveal patterns and processes suggesting causal interpretations. These interpretations can be (and often are) subjected to more systematic testing using more controlled methods of inquiry.

QUALITATIVE RESEARCH TRADITIONS

Despite the fact that there are some features common to many qualitative research designs, there is nevertheless a wide variety of overall approaches. There is no readily agreed-on taxonomy, but one useful system is to describe qualitative research according to disciplinary traditions. These traditions vary in their conceptualization of what types of questions are important to ask and in the methods they consider appropriate for answering those questions. The section that follows provides an overview of several qualitative traditions (some of which we have previously introduced), and subsequent sections describe in greater detail traditions that have been especially prominent in nursing research.

Overview of Qualitative Traditions

The research traditions that have provided a theoretical underpinning for qualitative studies come primarily from the disciplines of anthropology, psychology, and sociology. As shown in Table 10.1, each discipline focuses on one or two broad domains of inquiry.

The discipline of anthropology is concerned with human cultures. **Ethnography** (discussed more fully later) is the primary research tradition in anthropology. Ethnographers study cultural patterns and experiences in a holistic fashion. *Ethnoscience* focuses on the cognitive world of a culture, with particular emphasis on the semantic rules and shared meanings that shape behavior. Cognitive anthropologists assume that a group's cultural knowledge is reflected in its language.

TABLE 10.1 ▸ OVERVIEW OF QUALITATIVE RESEARCH TRADITIONS

DISCIPLINE	DOMAIN	RESEARCH TRADITION	AREA OF INQUIRY
Anthropology	Culture	Ethnography Ethnoscience	Holistic view of a culture Mapping of the cognitive world of a culture; a culture's shared meanings
Philosophy	Lived experience	Phenomenology Hermeneutics	Experiences of individuals within their lifeworld Interpretations and meanings of individuals' experiences
Psychology	Behavior and events	Ethology Ecologic psychology	Behavior observed over time in natural context Behavior as influenced by the environment
Sociology	Social settings	Grounded theory Ethnomethodology	Social, psychological, and structural processes within a social setting Manner by which shared agreement is achieved in social settings
Sociolinguistics	Human communication	Discourse analysis	Forms and rules of conversation
History	Past behavior, events, and conditions	Historical analysis	Description and interpretation of historical events

Phenomenology has its disciplinary roots in philosophy. As noted in Chapter 3, phenomenology focuses on the meaning of lived experiences of humans. A closely related research tradition is **hermeneutics**, which uses lived experiences as a tool for better understanding the social, cultural, political, or historical context in which those experiences occur. Hermeneutic inquiry focuses on meaning and interpretation—how individuals interpret their world within their given context.

The discipline of psychology has several qualitative research traditions that focus on behavior. Human *ethology*, which has been described as the biology of human behavior, studies behavior as it evolves in its natural context. Human ethologists use primarily observational methods in an attempt to discover universal behavioral structures.

Example of an ethologic study:
Spiers (2006) used ethologic methods to study pain-related interactions between patients and home-care nurses. Spiers analyzed micropatterns of videotaped communication in the patients' homes over multiple home-nurse visits.

Ecologic psychology focuses more specifically on the influence of the environment on human behavior, and attempts to identify principles that explain the interdependence of humans and their environmental context. Viewed from an ecologic context, people are affected by (and affect) a multilayered set of systems, including family, peer group, and neighborhood as well as the more indirect effects of health care and social services systems, and the larger cultural belief and value systems of the society in which individuals live.

Example of an ecologic study:

Robertson and colleagues (2007) used an ecologic framework to study Latino construction workers' experiences with occupational noise and hearing protection. Their risk perceptions were examined with regard to environmental and personal factors.

Sociologists study the social world in which we live and have developed several research traditions of importance to qualitative researchers. The **grounded theory** tradition (elaborated on later in this chapter) seeks to describe and understand key social psychologic and structural processes in social settings.

Ethnomethodology seeks to discover how people make sense of their everyday activities and interpret their social worlds so as to behave in socially acceptable ways. Within this tradition, researchers attempt to understand a social group's norms and assumptions that are so deeply ingrained that the members no longer think about the underlying reasons for their behaviors.

Example of an ethnomethodologic study:

Lloyd's (2007) ethnomethodologic study explored the practice of 10 mental health nurses working in an acute admissions unit. The nurses were asked to discuss the taken-for-granted methods of empowerment they used with clients, their families, and colleagues.

The domain of inquiry for sociolinguists is human communication. **Discourse analysis** (sometimes called *conversation analysis*) seeks to understand the rules, mechanisms, and structure of conversations. Discourse analysts are interested in understanding the action that a given kind of talk "performs." Typically, the data are from transcripts of naturally occurring conversations, such as those between nurses and their patients. In discourse analysis, the texts are situated in their social, cultural, political, and historical context.

Example of a discourse analysis:

Hayter (2007) analyzed the discourse between nurses and women during contraceptive consultations in sexual health clinics.

Finally, **historical research**—the systematic collection and critical evaluation of data relating to past occurrences—is also a tradition that relies primarily on qualitative data. Nurses have used historical research methods to examine a wide range of phenomena in both the recent and more distant past.

Example of historical research:
Manocchio (2008) conducted a social historical analysis of nursing in the culturally diverse frontier setting of California in the mid 1900s. Manocchio concluded that primary source accounts tended to give secondary attention to the multiple roles midwives played in the communities they served.

TIP

Sometimes, a research report identifies more than one tradition as having provided the framework for a qualitative inquiry (e.g., a phenomenological study using the grounded theory method). However, such "method slurring" has been criticized because each tradition has different intellectual assumptions and methodologic prescriptions.

Ethnography

Ethnography is a type of qualitative inquiry that involves the description and interpretation of a culture and cultural behavior. *Culture* refers to the way a group of people live—the patterns of human activity and the symbolic structures (e.g., the values and norms) that give such activity significance. Ethnographies are a blend of a process and a product, field work and a written text. **Field work** is the process by which the ethnographer inevitably comes to understand a culture, and the ethnographic text is how that culture is communicated and portrayed. Because culture is, in itself, not visible or tangible, it must be constructed through ethnographic writing. Culture is inferred from the words, actions, and products of members of a group.

Ethnographic research, in some cases, is concerned with broadly defined cultures (e.g., the Maori culture of New Zealand) in what is sometimes referred to as a *macroethnography*. However, ethnographies sometimes focus on more narrowly defined cultures in a *microethnography* or focused ethnography. Focused ethnographies are exhaustive, fine-grained studies of small units in a group or culture (e.g., the culture of an intensive care unit). An underlying assumption of the ethnographer is that every human group eventually evolves a culture that guides the members' view of the world and the way they structure their experiences.

Example of a focused ethnography:
Johansson and colleagues (2007) used a focused ethnographic approach to describe encounters between people on a locked psychiatric ward for patients with affective and eating disorders.

Ethnographers seek to learn from (rather than to study) members of a cultural group—to understand their world view. Ethnographic researchers sometimes refer to "emic" and "etic" perspectives. An **emic perspective** refers to the way the members of the culture regard their world—it is the insiders' view. The emic is the local language, concepts, or means of expression that are used by the members of the group under study to name and characterize their experiences. The **etic perspective**, by contrast, is the outsiders' interpretation of the experiences of that culture—

the words and concepts they use to refer to the same phenomena. Ethnographers strive to acquire an emic perspective of a culture under study. Moreover, they strive to reveal what has been referred to as **tacit knowledge**, information about the culture that is so deeply embedded in cultural experiences that members do not talk about it or may not even be consciously aware of it.

Three broad types of information are usually sought by ethnographers: cultural behavior (what members of the culture do), cultural artifacts (what members of the culture make and use), and cultural speech (what people say). This implies that ethnographers rely on a wide variety of data sources, including observations, in-depth interviews, records, and other types of physical evidence (e.g., photographs, diaries). Ethnographers typically use a strategy known as **participant observation** in which they make observations of the culture under study while participating in its activities. Ethnographers observe people day after day in their natural environments to observe behavior in a wide array of circumstances. Ethnographers also enlist the help of **key informants** to help them understand and interpret the events and activities being observed.

Ethnographic research typically is a labor-intensive and time-consuming endeavor—months and even years of fieldwork may be required to learn about the cultural group of interest. The study of a culture requires a certain level of intimacy with members of the cultural group, and such intimacy can be developed only over time and by working directly with those members as active participants.

The product of ethnographic research usually is a rich and holistic description of the culture under study. Ethnographers also interpret the culture, describing normative behavioral and social patterns. Among health care researchers, ethnography provides access to the health beliefs and health practices of a culture or subculture. Ethnographic inquiry can thus help to facilitate understanding of behaviors affecting health and illness. Indeed, Leininger has coined the phrase **ethnonursing research**, which she defined as "the study and analysis of the local or indigenous people's viewpoints, beliefs, and practices about nursing care behavior and processes of designated cultures" (1985, p. 38).

Example of an ethnonursing study:
Martin and colleagues (2007) explored the culture of three tertiary care mental health facilities as the staff implemented a new intervention, the Transitional Discharge Model. Leininger's ethnonursing model and theory of culture care were used as the framework for the research. The findings revealed that clinical staff experienced numerous challenges, including ones involving relationships with others, values and beliefs of clients, and processes of care.

Ethnographers are often, but not always, "outsiders" to the culture under study. A type of ethnography that involves self-scrutiny (including scrutiny of groups or cultures to which researchers themselves belong) usually is referred to as **autoethnography**, but other terms such as *insider research* or *peer research* also have been used. There are numerous advantages to performing an autoethnography, the most obvious being ease of access, ease of recruitment, and the ability to get particularly candid, in-depth data based on pre-established trust. The drawback is that an "insider" may have developed biases about certain issues or may be so entrenched in the culture that valuable pieces of data get overlooked. Insider research demands that researchers maintain a high level of consciousness about their role and monitor their internal state and interactions with others.

Example of an autoethnography:

Schneider (2005) described an autoethnography that explored how mothers of adults with schizophrenia talk about their children. Schneider herself was the mother of a schizophrenic person.

Phenomenology

Phenomenology, rooted in a philosophic tradition developed by Husserl and Heidegger, is an approach to exploring and understanding people's everyday life experiences.

Phenomenological researchers ask: What is the *essence* of this phenomenon as experienced by these people and what does it *mean*? Phenomenologists assume there is an *essence*—an essential invariant structure—that can be understood, in much the same way that ethnographers assume that cultures exist. Essence is what makes a phenomenon what it is, and without which it would not be what it is. Phenomenologists investigate subjective phenomena in the belief that critical truths about reality are grounded in people's lived experiences. The phenomenological approach is especially useful when a phenomenon has been poorly defined or conceptualized. The topics appropriate to phenomenology are ones that are fundamental to the life experiences of humans; for health researchers, these include such topics as the meaning of suffering, the experience of domestic violence, and the quality of life with chronic pain.

Phenomenologists believe that lived experience gives meaning to each person's perception of a particular phenomenon. The goal of phenomenological inquiry is to understand fully lived experience and the perceptions to which it gives rise. Four aspects of lived experience that are of interest to phenomenologists are *lived space*, or spatiality; *lived body*, or corporeality; *lived time*, or temporality; and *lived human relation*, or relationality.

Phenomenologists view human existence as meaningful and interesting because of people's consciousness of that existence. The phrase **being-in-the-world** (or *embodiment*) is a concept that acknowledges people's physical ties to their world—they think, see, hear, feel, and are conscious through their bodies' interaction with the world.

In phenomenological studies, the main data source typically is in-depth conversations, with researchers and informants as co-participants. Researchers help informants to describe lived experiences without leading the discussion. Through in-depth conversations, researchers strive to gain entrance into the informants' world, to have full access to their experiences as lived. Typically, phenomenological studies involve a small number of study participants—often 10 or fewer. For some phenomenological researchers, the inquiry includes not only gathering information from informants but also efforts to experience the phenomenon in the same way, typically through participation, observation, and introspective reflection. Phenomenologists share their insights in rich, vivid reports. A phenomenological text that describes the results of a study should help the readers "see" something in a different way that enriches their understanding of experiences.

There are a number of variants and methodologic interpretations of phenomenology. The two main schools of thought are descriptive phenomenology and interpretive phenomenology (hermeneutics).

Descriptive Phenomenology

Descriptive phenomenology was developed first by Husserl, who was primarily interested in the question: *What do we know as persons?* His philosophy emphasized descriptions of human experience. Descriptive phenomenologists insist on the careful portrayal of ordinary conscious experience of everyday life—a depiction of "things" as people experience them. These "things" include hearing, seeing, believing, feeling, remembering, deciding, and evaluating.

Descriptive phenomenological studies often involve the following four steps: bracketing, intuiting, analyzing, and describing. **Bracketing** refers to the process of identifying and holding in abeyance preconceived beliefs and opinions about the phenomenon under study. Although bracketing can never be achieved totally, researchers strive to bracket out any presuppositions in an effort to confront the data in pure form. Bracketing is an iterative process that involves preparing, evaluating, and providing systematic ongoing feedback about the effectiveness of the bracketing. Phenomenological researchers (as well as other qualitative researchers) often maintain a **reflexive journal** in their efforts to bracket.

Intuiting, the second step in descriptive phenomenology, occurs when researchers remain open to the meanings attributed to the phenomenon by those who have experienced it. Phenomenological researchers then proceed to the analysis phase (i.e., extracting significant statements, categorizing, and making sense of the essential meanings of the phenomenon). Chapter 17 provides further information regarding the analysis of data collected in phenomenological studies. Finally, the descriptive phase occurs when researchers come to understand and define the phenomenon.

Example of a descriptive phenomenological study:

Porter (2007) used descriptive phenomenological methods to describe the day-to-day experiences of frail older women and the problems they faced preparing food.

Interpretive Phenomenology

Heidegger, a student of Husserl, moved away from his professor's philosophy into **interpretive phenomenology** or hermeneutics. To Heidegger, the critical question is: *What is being?* He stressed interpreting and understanding—not just describing—human experience. His premise is that lived experience is inherently an interpretive process. Heidegger argued that hermeneutics ("understanding") is a basic characteristic of human existence. Indeed, the term hermeneutics refers to the art and philosophy of interpreting the meaning of an object (e.g., a *text*, work of art, and so on). The goals of interpretive phenomenological research are to enter another's world and to discover the wisdom, possibilities, and understandings found there.

Gadamer, another influential interpretive phenomenologist, described the interpretive process as a circular relationship known as the **hermeneutic circle** where one understands the whole of a text (e.g., a transcribed interview) in terms of its parts and the parts in terms of the whole. In his view, researchers enter into a dialogue with the text, in which the researcher continually questions its meaning.

In an interpretive phenomenological study, bracketing does not occur. For Heidegger, it was not possible to bracket one's being-in-the-world. Hermeneutics presupposes prior understanding on the part of the researcher. Interpretive phenomenologists ideally approach each interview text with openness—they must be open to hearing what it is the text is saying.

Interpretive phenomenologists, like descriptive phenomenologists, rely primarily on in-depth interviews with individuals who have experienced the phenomenon of interest, but they may go beyond a traditional approach to gathering and analyzing data. For example, interpretive phenomenologists sometimes augment their understandings of the phenomenon through an analysis of supplementary texts, such as novels, poetry, or other artistic expressions—or they use such materials in their conversations with study participants.

Example of an interpretive phenomenological study:
Frid and co-researchers (2007) used a hermeneutic approach to explore close relatives' use of imagery to describe the experience of confronting the brain death of a loved one.

HOW-TO-TELL TIP

How can you tell if a phenomenological study is descriptive or interpretive? Phenomenologists often use key terms in their report that can help you make this determination. In a descriptive phenomenological study such terms may be bracketing, description, essence, Husserl, phenomenological reduction. The names of Colaizzi, Van Kaam, and Giorgi may be found in the methods section. In an interpretive phenomenological study, key terms can include being-in-the-world, shared interpretations, hermeneutics, understanding, and Heidegger. The names van Manen, Benner, and Diekelmann may appear in the method section. These names will be discussed in the chapter on qualitative data analysis.

Grounded Theory

Grounded theory has become an important research method for nurse researchers and has contributed to the development of many middle-range theories of phenomena relevant to nurses. Grounded theory was developed in the 1960s by two sociologists, Glaser and Strauss (1967), whose theoretic roots were in *symbolic interaction*, which focuses on the manner in which people make sense of social interactions and the interpretations they attach to social symbols (e.g., language).

Grounded theory tries to account for people's actions from the perspective of those involved. Grounded theory researchers seek to understand the actions by first discovering the main concern or problem and then the individuals' behavior that is designed to resolve it. The manner in which people resolve this main concern is called the **core variable**. One type of core variable is called a **basic social process (BSP)**. The goal of grounded theory is to discover this main concern and the basic social process that explains how people resolve it. The main concern or problem must be discovered from the data. Grounded theory researchers generate emergent conceptual categories and their properties and integrate them into a substantive theory grounded in the data.

Grounded Theory Methods

Grounded theory methods constitute an entire approach to the conduct of field research. For example, a study that truly follows Glaser and Strauss's precepts does not begin with a highly focused research problem; the problem emerges from the data. In grounded theory, both the research problem and the process used to resolve it are discovered during the study. A fundamental feature of grounded theory research is that data collection, data analysis, and sampling of participants occur simultaneously. The grounded theory process is recursive: researchers collect data, categorize them, describe the emerging central phenomenon, and then recycle earlier steps.

A procedure referred to as **constant comparison** is used to develop and refine theoretically relevant concepts and categories. Categories elicited from the data are constantly compared with data obtained earlier in the data collection process so that commonalities and variations can be determined. As data collection proceeds, the inquiry becomes increasingly focused on emerging theoretical concerns. Data analysis in a grounded theory framework is described in greater depth in Chapter 17.

In-depth interviews and participant observation are the most common data source in grounded theory studies, but existing documents and other data sources may also be used. Typically, a grounded theory study involves interviews with a sample of about 20 to 40 informants.

Example of a grounded theory study:
Griffiths and Jasper (2008) used grounded theory methods to explore military nurses' ability to reconcile the dichotomy between their caring role and being in an organization associated with conflict during a period of war. The core category they identified was "Caring for war: Transition to warrior."

Alternate Views of Grounded Theory

In 1990, Strauss and Corbin published what was to become a controversial book, *Basics of Qualitative Research: Grounded Theory Procedures and Techniques*. Strauss and Corbin stated that the purpose of the book was to provide beginning grounded theory researchers with basic knowledge and procedures involved in building theory at the substantive level.

Glaser, however, disagreed with some of the procedures advocated by Strauss (his original coauthor) and Corbin (a nurse researcher). Glaser published a rebuttal in 1992, *Emergence Versus Forcing: Basics of Grounded Theory Analysis*. Glaser believed that Strauss and Corbin developed a method that is not grounded theory but rather what he calls "full conceptual description." According to Glaser, the purpose of grounded theory is to generate concepts and theories about their relationships that explain, account for, and interpret variation in behavior in the substantive area under study. *Conceptual description*, in contrast, aims at describing the full range of behavior of what is occurring in the substantive area, "irrespective of relevance and accounting for variation in behavior" (Glaser, 1992, p. 19).

Nurse researchers have conducted grounded theory studies using both the original Glaser and Strauss and the Strauss and Corbin (1998) approaches.

OTHER TYPES OF QUALITATIVE RESEARCH

Qualitative studies often can be characterized and described in terms of the disciplinary research traditions discussed in the previous section. However, several other important types of qualitative research also deserve mention. This section discusses qualitative research that is not associated with any particular discipline.

Case Studies

Case studies are in-depth investigations of a single entity or a small number of entities. The entity may be an individual, family, institution, community, or other social unit. In a case study, researchers obtain a wealth of descriptive information and may examine relationships among different phenomena, or may examine trends over time. Case study researchers attempt to analyze and understand issues that are important to the history, development, or circumstances of the entity under study.

One way to think of a case study is to consider what is at center stage. In most studies, whether qualitative or quantitative, certain phenomena or variables are the core of the inquiry. In a case study, the *case* itself is central. The focus of case studies is typically on determining the dynamics of *why* an individual thinks, behaves, or develops in a particular manner rather than on *what* his or her status, progress, or actions are. It is not unusual for probing research of this type to require detailed study over a considerable period. Data are often collected that relate not only to the person's present state but also to past experiences and situational factors relevant to the problem being examined.

Case studies are sometimes a useful way to explore phenomena that have not been rigorously researched. Information obtained in case studies can be used to develop hypotheses to be tested more rigorously in subsequent research. The intensive probing that characterizes case studies often leads to insights about previously unsuspected relationships. Case studies also may serve the important role of clarifying concepts or of elucidating ways to capture them.

The greatest strength of case studies is the depth that is possible when a limited number of individuals, institutions, or groups is being investigated. Case studies provide researchers with opportunities of having an intimate knowledge of a person's condition, feelings, actions (past and present), intentions, and environment. On the other hand, this same strength is a potential weakness because researchers' familiarity with the person or group may make objectivity more difficult—especially if the data are collected by observational techniques for which the researchers are the main (or only) observers. Another criticism of case studies concerns generalizability: If researchers discover important relationships, it is difficult to know whether the same relationships would occur with others. However, case studies can often play a critical role in challenging generalizations based on other types of research.

Example of a case study:
James and colleagues (2007) conducted an in-depth case study of a family facing a member's death through cancer. Data were collected over a 10-month period through interviews, diary notations, and conversations with all family members.

TIP

Although most case studies involve the collection of in-depth qualitative information, some case studies are quantitative by design or use statistical methods to analyze data. As an example, Normann and colleagues (2005) did a case study to explore the presence of lucidity in a woman with severe dementia. Data from more than 20 hours of conversation with the woman and her daughter were analyzed statistically.

Narrative Analyses

Narrative analysis focuses on *story* as the object of inquiry, to determine how individuals make sense of events in their lives. Narratives are viewed as a type of "cultural envelope" into which people pour their experiences and relate their importance to others. What distinguishes narrative analysis from other types of qualitative research designs is its focus on the broad contours of a narrative; stories are not fractured and dissected. The broad underlying premise of narrative research is that people most effectively make sense of their world—and communicate these meanings—by constructing, reconstructing, and narrating stories. Individuals construct stories when they wish to understand specific events and situations that require linking an inner world of desire and motive to an external world of observable actions. Analyzing stories opens up *forms* of telling about experience, and is more than just content. Narrative analysts ask, "Why was the story told that way?" (Riessman, 1993, p. 2).

There are a number of structural approaches that researchers can use to analyze stories. For example, Gee (1996) offers a linguistic approach to narrative analysis that moves from the part to the whole. His method draws on oral rather than text-based tradition and attends to how the story is told. First he pays attention to changes in pitch, loudness, stress, and length of various syllables, as well as to hesitations and pauses. He also examines the cohesion of each sentence or line, and how these elements form larger units (stanzas) and, ultimately, themes.

Burke's (1969) **pentadic dramatism** is another approach for analysis of narratives. For Burke there are five key elements of a story: act, scene, agent, agency, and purpose. The five terms of Burke's pentad are meant to be understood paired together as ratios such as, act:agent, agent:agency, and purpose:agent. The analysis focuses on the internal relationships and tensions of these five terms to each other. Each pairing of terms in the pentad provides a different way of directing the researcher's attention. What drives the narrative analysis is not just the interaction of the pentadic terms but an imbalance between two or more of these terms.

Example of a narrative analysis using Burke's approach:
Beck (2006) used a narrative analysis to explore birth trauma. Eleven mothers sent their stories of traumatic childbirth to Beck via the Internet. Burke's pentad of terms was used to analyze these narratives. The most problematic and prominent ratio imbalance was between act and agency. Frequently in the mothers' narratives it was the "how" an act was carried out by the labor and delivery staff that led to the women perceiving their childbirth as traumatic.

Descriptive Qualitative Studies

Many qualitative studies acknowledge a link to one of the research traditions or types of research discussed in this chapter. Many other qualitative studies, however, claim no particular disciplinary or methodologic roots. The researchers may simply indicate that they have conducted a qualitative study or a naturalistic inquiry, or they may say that they have done a *content analysis* of their qualitative data (i.e., an analysis of themes and patterns that emerge in the narrative content). Thus, some qualitative studies do not have a formal name or do not fit into the typology presented in this chapter. We refer to these as **descriptive qualitative studies**.

In doing such descriptive qualitative studies, researchers tend not to penetrate their data in any interpretive depth. These studies present comprehensive summaries of a phenomenon or of events in everyday language. Qualitative descriptive designs tend to be eclectic and are based on the general premises of naturalistic inquiry.

Example of a descriptive qualitative study:
A descriptive qualitative study by Zehle and colleagues (2007) explored childhood obesity through mothers' perceptions, beliefs, and behaviors. In-depth interviews with 16 primiparous mothers with children under age 3 were conducted, and five themes were identified.

RESEARCH WITH IDEOLOGIC PERSPECTIVES

Some qualitative researchers conduct inquiries within an ideologic framework, typically to draw attention to certain social problems or the needs of certain groups and to bring about change. These approaches represent important investigative avenues and are briefly described in this section.

Critical Theory

Critical theory originated with a group of Marxist-oriented German scholars in the 1920s, collectively referred to as the "Frankfurt School." Variants of critical theory abound in the social sciences. Essentially, a critical researcher is concerned with a critique of society and with envisioning new possibilities.

Critical social science is typically action oriented. Its broad aim is to integrate theory and practice such that people become aware of contradictions and disparities in their beliefs and social practices, and become inspired to change them. Critical researchers reject the idea of an objective and disinterested inquirer and are oriented toward a transformation process. Critical theory calls for inquiries that foster enlightened self-knowledge and sociopolitical action. Moreover, critical theory involves a self-reflective aspect. To prevent a critical theory of society from becoming yet another self-serving ideology, critical theorists must account for their own transformative effects.

The design of research in critical theory often begins with a thorough analysis of certain aspects of the problem. For example, critical researchers might analyze and critique taken-for-granted assumptions that underlie the problem, the language used to depict the situation, and the biases of prior researchers investigating the problem. Critical researchers often triangulate multiple methodologies and emphasize multiple perspectives (e.g., alternative racial or social class perspectives) on problems. Critical researchers typically interact with study participants in ways that emphasize participants' expertise. Some of the features that distinguish more traditional qualitative research and critical research are summarized in Table 10.2.

Critical theory, which has been applied in a number of disciplines, has played an especially important role in ethnography. **Critical ethnography** focuses on raising consciousness and aiding emancipatory goals in the hope of effecting social change.

TABLE 10.2	COMPARISON OF TRADITIONAL QUALITATIVE RESEARCH AND CRITICAL RESEARCH	
ISSUE	TRADITIONAL QUALITATIVE RESEARCH	CRITICAL RESEARCH
Research aims	Understanding; reconstruction of multiple constructions	Critique; transformation; consciousness-raising; advocacy
View of knowledge	Transactional/subjective; knowledge is created in interaction between investigator and participants	Transactional/subjective; value-mediated and value-dependent; importance of historical insights
Methods	Dialectic: truth arrived at logically through conversations	Dialectic and didactic: dialogue designed to transform naivety and misinformation
Evaluative criteria for inquiry quality	Authenticity; trustworthiness	Historical situatedness of the inquiry; erosion of ignorance; stimulus for change
Researcher's role	Facilitator of multivoice reconstruction	Transformative agent; advocate; activist

Critical ethnographers address the historical, social, political, and economic dimensions of cultures and their value-laden agendas. An assumption in critical ethnographic research is that actions and thoughts are mediated by power relationships. Critical ethnographers attempt to increase the political dimensions of cultural research and undermine oppressive systems—there is always an explicit political purpose. Cook (2005) has argued that critical ethnography is especially well suited to health promotion research because both are concerned with enabling people to take control over their own situation.

Example of a critical ethnography:
Kalwinsky (2008) used a critical ethnographic approach to study the ways in which the Chamorro (a disenfranchised population of the U.S. territory Guam) with HIV/AIDS interact and negotiate with Western health care staff.

Feminist Research

Feminist research is similar to critical theory research, but the focus is sharply on gender domination and discrimination within patriarchal societies. Similar to critical researchers, feminist researchers seek to establish collaborative and nonexploitative relationships with their informants, to place themselves within the study to avoid objectification, and to conduct research that is transformative.

Gender is the organizing principle in feminist research, and investigators seek to understand how gender and a gendered social order have shaped women's lives and their consciousness. The aim is to facilitate change in ways relevant to ending women's unequal social position.

The scope of feminist research ranges from studies of the subjective views of individual women, to studies of social movements, structures, and broad policies that affect (and often exclude) women. Olesen (2000), a sociologist who studied nurses' career patterns and definitions of success, has noted that some of the best feminist research on women's subjective experiences has been done in the area of women's health.

Feminist research methods typically include in-depth, interactive, and collaborative individual interviews or group interviews that offer the possibility of reciprocally educational encounters. Feminists usually seek to negotiate the meanings of the results with those participating in the study and to be self-reflective about what they themselves are experiencing and learning. Feminist research, like other research that has an ideologic perspective, has raised the bar for the conduct of ethical research. With the emphasis on trust, empathy, and nonexploitative relationships, proponents of these newer modes of inquiry view any type of deception or manipulation as abhorrent.

Example of feminist research:
Ismail and colleagues (2007) used a feminist framework to examine the experience of dating violence from young women's perspectives, to investigate how contextual factors shape their experiences, and to explore ways that dating violence is perpetuated and normalized in young women's lives.

Participatory Action Research

A type of research known as participatory action research is closely allied to both critical research and feminist research. **Participatory action research (PAR)**, one of several types of *action research* that originated in the 1940s with social psychologist Kurt Lewin, is based on a recognition that the production of knowledge can be political and can be used to exert power. Researchers in this approach typically work with groups or communities that are vulnerable to the control or oppression of a dominant group or culture.

Participatory action research is, as the name implies, participatory. There is collaboration between researchers and study participants in the definition of the problem, the selection of an approach and research methods, the analysis of the data, and the use to which findings are put. The aim of PAR is to produce not only knowledge, but action and consciousness-raising as well. Researchers specifically seek to empower people through the process of constructing and using knowledge. The PAR tradition has as its starting point a concern for the powerlessness of the group under study. Thus, a key objective is to produce an impetus that is directly used to make improvements through education and sociopolitical action.

In PAR, the research methods are designed to facilitate emergent processes of collaboration and dialogue that can motivate, increase self-esteem, and generate community solidarity. Thus, "data-gathering" strategies used are not only the traditional methods of interview and observation (including both qualitative and quantitative approaches), but may include storytelling, sociodrama, drawing, plays and skits, and other activities designed to encourage people to find creative ways to explore their lives, tell their stories, and recognize their own strengths. Useful resources for learning more about PAR include Whyte (1990) and Morrison and Lilford (2001).

Example of PAR:
Etowa and colleagues (2007) conducted a PAR project to investigate the health status and use of health services among African-Canadian women living in rural and remote regions of Nova Scotia. Using a variety of data collection strategies, the project resulted in the generation of a database, community action, and interdisciplinary analysis of inequities in health care.

CRITIQUING QUALITATIVE DESIGNS

Evaluating a qualitative design is often difficult. Qualitative researchers do not always document design decisions and are even less likely to describe the process by which such decisions were made. Researchers often do, however, indicate whether the study was conducted within a specific qualitative tradition. This information can be used to come to some conclusions about the study design. For example, if a report indicated that the researcher conducted 1 month of field work for an ethnographic study, you might well suspect that insufficient time had been spent in the field to obtain a true emic perspective of the culture under study.

Ethnographic studies may also be critiqued if their only source of information was from interviews, rather than from a broader range of data sources, particularly observations.

In a grounded theory study, you might also be concerned if the researcher relied exclusively on data from interviews; a stronger design might have been obtained by including participant observations. Also, look for evidence about when the data were collected and analyzed. If the researcher collected all the data before analyzing any of it, you might question whether the constant comparative method was used correctly.

In critiquing a phenomenological study, you should first determine if the study is descriptive or interpretive. This will help you to assess how closely the researcher kept to the basic tenets of that qualitative research tradition. For example, in a descriptive phenomenological study, did the researcher bracket? When critiquing a phenomenological study, in addition to critiquing the methodology, you should also look at its power in capturing the meaning of the phenomena being studied.

No matter what qualitative design is identified in a study, look to see if the researchers stayed true to a single qualitative tradition throughout the study or if they mixed qualitative traditions. For example, did the researchers state that a grounded theory design was used, but then present results that described themes instead of generating a substantive theory?

The guidelines in Box 10.1 are designed to assist you in critiquing the designs of qualitative studies.

BOX 10.1 GUIDELINES FOR CRITIQUING QUALITATIVE DESIGNS

1. Is the research tradition for the qualitative study identified? If none was identified, can one be inferred? If more than one was identified, is this justifiable or does it suggest "method slurring"?

2. Is the research question congruent with a qualitative approach and with the specific research tradition (i.e., is the domain of inquiry for the study congruent with the domain encompassed by the tradition)? Are the data sources, research methods, and analytic approach congruent with the research tradition?

3. How well is the research design described? Are design decisions explained and justified? Does it appear that the researcher made all design decisions up-front, or did the design emerge during data collection, allowing researchers to capitalize on early information?

4. Is the design appropriate, given the research question? Does the design lend itself to a thorough, in-depth, intensive examination of the phenomenon of interest? What design elements might have strengthened the study (e.g., a longitudinal perspective rather than a cross-sectional one)?

5. Was there appropriate evidence of reflexivity in the design?

6. Was the study undertaken with an ideological perspective? If so, is there evidence that ideological methods and goals were achieved? (e.g., Was there evidence of full collaboration between researchers and participants? Did the research have the power to be transformative, or is there evidence that a transformative process occurred?)

This section presents examples of different types of qualitative studies. Read these summaries and then answer the critical thinking questions, referring to the full research report if necessary.

EXAMPLE 1 ■ A Critical Ethnography

Study

Betwixt and between: A critical ethnography of comfort in New Zealand residential aged care (Bland, 2007).

Statement of Purpose

The purpose of the study was to explore the nature of comfort within the context of nursing homes in New Zealand, and to examine how nursing actions contribute to residents' comfort.

Setting and Context

The research was completed in three nursing homes that ranged in size from 20 to 70 residents. Two were operated by not-for-profit organizations and provided three levels of care. The third was privately owned and offered intermediate care only. Bland wrote that New Zealand nursing homes have been increasingly subjected to audits from funding or licensing bodies using a range of evaluative indicators. As a nursing home manager, Bland questioned the relevance of some indicators and wondered if a primary care objective—residents' comfort—was being achieved.

Method

The fieldwork for this study was done over an 18-month period. Bland completed and tape-recorded 70 interviews with 27 nursing home residents and 28 staff, including 3 nursing home managers, 12 other RNs, and 13 other types of staff. Residents, most of whom had lived in their nursing homes for at least 1 year, were interviewed in the privacy of their bedrooms. They were asked to recount their experiences of living in the residence, and to contrast their current lives with their lives before admission. Staff interviews focused on their perceptions of nursing home life from a resident's perspective. Interviews were supplemented with extensive observations of life in the nursing homes. Initially, attention was directed to observations of daily life, with Bland participating in activities organized for the residents. As the study progressed, more focused and selective observations were undertaken to help understand care delivery practices and their rationales. For example, an emerging interest in staff communication led Bland to focus observations on end-of-shift handovers. Bland also extensively examined documents in the nursing homes, including medical and nursing notes, medication records, staff communications, and policy manuals. In her analysis, Bland concentrated on "intersecting cultural borderlines" (p. 939) that juxtaposed the different worlds of management, nursing staff, and residents.

Key Findings

The analysis suggested that *comfort* in these nursing homes was a multidimensional, idiosyncratic, and context-dependent phenomenon—and not simply the absence of discomfort. Although most residents could not find the words to define what comfort meant to them, five key dimensions of comfort were evident in their narratives: physical comfort, service availability, relationships with staff, continuing as a family member, and self-comforting. Residents could be "betwixt and between" comfort and discomfort simultaneously; because of the multidimensional nature of comfort, they could be comfortable in one dimension but uncomfortable in others. Nursing staff were also "betwixt and between," as they attempted to balance regulatory compliance with professional imperatives. Bland concluded that "Staff working in nursing homes must re-examine their care delivery practices to ensure these do not disempower residents" (p. 937).

CRITICAL THINKING SUGGESTIONS*

*See the Student Resource CD-ROM for a discussion of these questions.

1. Answer the relevant questions from Box 10.1 regarding this study.
2. Also consider the following targeted questions, which may further sharpen your critical thinking skills and assist you in understanding this study:
   a. Is this an example of an autoethnography? If yes, what might be some of the challenges the researcher faced—and what might be some of the advantages?
   b. Is this study a macroethnography or a microethnography?
   c. Could this study have been undertaken as a phenomenological study? As a grounded theory study? Why or why not?
3. If the results of this study are trustworthy, what are some of the uses to which the findings might be put in clinical practice?

EXAMPLE 2 ■ A Grounded Theory Study

Study

Relationships and their potential for change developed in difficult type 1 diabetes (Zoffman & Kirkevold, 2007).

Statement of Purpose

The purpose of this study was to develop a substantive theory that interprets how relationships between patients and nurses might change problem-solving in difficult diabetes care.

Method

Adult diabetic patients and nurses from an inpatient or day clinic at a Danish university hospital were invited to participate. Patients were included if they had had diabetes for at least 1 year and had been admitted because of poor glycemic control. Nurses all had at least 1 year of experience in a specialized diabetes unit. Altogether, there were dyads of 11 patients and 8 nurses. Two nurse–patient conversations were taped from each dyad, at the beginning and end of the patients' hospital stay. Each nurse also taped a discussion with a doctor, dietician, or another nurse that she considered important in assessing the patient. After listening to the three conversations, the researchers interviewed both the patients after discharge and the nurses. Finally, each patient was interviewed 6 months later to discuss how he or she assessed the outcome of the hospital stay. Constant comparison was used in the analysis of the data.

Key Findings

The researchers discovered that the core category was Relational Potential for Change, which encompassed three types of patient–provider relationships. Professionals mostly shifted between less effective relationships, characterized by *"I-you-distant provider dominance"* and *"I-you-blurred sympathy."* A third relationship—*"I-you-sorted mutuality"*—was rarely observed, but proved more effective than the others in exploiting the Relational Potential for Change.

The three types of relationships differed in terms of scope of problem-solving, roles played out by the patients and professionals, use of different points of view, and quality of knowledge achieved as the basis for problem-solving and decision-making.

CRITICAL THINKING SUGGESTIONS:

1. Answers the relevant questions from Box 10.1 regarding this study.
2. Also consider the following targeted questions, which may further sharpen your critical thinking skills and assist you in understanding this study:
   a. Was this study cross-sectional or longitudinal?
   b. Comment on the issue of *causality* within the context of this study.
   c. Could this study have been undertaken as an ethnography? A phenomenological inquiry? Could a critical or action framework have been used?
3. If the results of this study are trustworthy, what are some of the uses to which the findings might be put in clinical practice?

EXAMPLE 3 ■ Phenomenological Study in Appendix B

1. Read the method section from Beck's (2006) study ("The anniversary of birth trauma") in Appendix B of this book, and then answer the relevant questions in Box 10.1.
2. Also consider the following targeted questions, which may further sharpen your critical thinking skills and assist you in assessing aspects of the study's merit:
   a. Was this study a descriptive or interpretive phenomenology?
   b. Could this study have been conducted as a grounded theory study? As an ethnographic study? Why or why not?
   c. Could this study have been conducted as a feminist inquiry? If yes, what might Beck have done differently?

CHAPTER REVIEW

Key new terms introduced in the chapter, together with a summary of major points, are presented in this section. In addition, Chapter 10 of the accompanying *Study Guide for Essentials of Nursing Research,* 7th edition offers various exercises and study suggestions for reinforcing concepts presented in this chapter. For additional review, see the Student Self-Study Review Questions section of the Student Resource CD-ROM provided with this book. ●

Key New Terms

Autoethnography	Critical ethnography	Hermeneutics
Basic social process (BSP)	Critical theory	Interpretive phenomenology
Bracketing	Descriptive phenomenology	Narrative analysis
Case study	Emergent design	Participant observation
Constant comparison	Ethnonursing research	Participatory action research (PAR)
Core variable	Feminist research	

Summary Points

● ●

➤ Qualitative research involves an **emergent design**—a design that emerges in the field as the study unfolds.

➤ As **bricoleurs**, qualitative researchers tend to be creative and intuitive, putting together an array of data drawn from many sources to arrive at a holistic understanding of a phenomenon.

➤ Although qualitative design is elastic and flexible, qualitative researchers nevertheless plan for broad contingencies that can be expected to pose decision opportunities for study design in the field.

➤ Qualitative research traditions have their roots in anthropology (e.g., **ethnography** and **ethnoscience**); philosophy (**phenomenology** and **hermeneutics**); psychology (**ethology** and **ecologic** psychology); sociology (**grounded theory** and **ethnomethodology**); sociolinguistics (**discourse analysis**); and history (**historical research**).

➤ Ethnography focuses on the culture of a group of people and relies on extensive field work that usually includes **participant observation** and in-depth interviews with **key informants**. Ethnographers strive to acquire an **emic** (insider's) perspective of a culture rather than an **etic** (outsider's) perspective.

➤ The concept of **researcher as instrument** is frequently used by ethnographers to describe the significant role researchers play in analyzing and interpreting a culture. The product of ethnographic research is typically a rich, holistic description of the culture.

➤ Nurses sometimes refer to their ethnographic studies as **ethnonursing research**. **Autoethnographies** or *insider research* are ethnographies of a group or culture to which the researcher belongs.

➤ Phenomenology seeks to discover the *essence* and *meaning* of a phenomenon as it is experienced by people, mainly through in-depth interviews with people who have had the relevant experience.

➤ In **descriptive phenomenology**, which seeks to describe lived experiences, researchers strive to **bracket** out preconceived views and to **intuit** the essence of the phenomenon by remaining open to meanings attributed to it by those who have experienced it.

➤ **Interpretive phenomenology (hermeneutics)** focuses on interpreting the meaning of experiences, rather than just describing them.

➤ **Grounded theory** aims to discover theoretical precepts grounded in the data. Grounded theory researchers try to account for people's actions by focusing on the main concern that an individual's behavior is designed to resolve. The manner in which people resolve this main concern is the **core variable**. The goal of grounded theory is to discover this main concern and the **basic social process (BSP)** that explains how people resolve it.

➤ Grounded theory uses **constant comparison**: categories elicited from the data are constantly compared with data obtained earlier.

➤ A major controversy among grounded theory researchers concerns whether to follow the original Glaser and Strauss procedures or to use the adapted procedures of Strauss and Corbin; Glaser has argued that the latter approach does not result in *grounded theories* but rather in *conceptual descriptions*.

➤ **Case studies** are intensive investigations of a single entity or a small number of entities, such as individuals, groups, families, or communities; such studies usually involve collecting data over an extended period.

➤ **Narrative analysis** focuses on *story* in studies in which the purpose is to determine how individuals make sense of events in their lives. Several different structural approaches can be used to analyze narrative data (e.g., Burke's **pentadic dramatism**).

➤ **Descriptive qualitative studies** have no formal name and are not embedded in a disciplinary tradition. Such studies may simply be referred to as qualitative studies, naturalistic inquiries, or as qualitative content analyses.

➤ Research is sometimes conducted within an ideologic perspective, and such research tends to rely primarily on qualitative research.

➤ **Critical theory** is concerned with a critique of existing social structures. Critical researchers conduct inquiries that involve collaboration with participants and that foster enlightened self-knowledge and transformation. **Critical ethnography** uses the principles of critical theory in the study of cultures.

➤ **Feminist research,** like critical research, is designed to be transformative, but the focus is sharply on how gender domination and discrimination shape women's lives and their consciousness.

➤ **Participatory action research (PAR)** produces knowledge through close collaboration with groups that are vulnerable to control or oppression by a dominant culture; in PAR research, methods take second place to emergent processes that can motivate people and generate community solidarity.

STUDIES CITED IN CHAPTER 10

Beck, C. T. (2006). Pentadic cartography: Mapping birth trauma narratives. *Qualitative Health Research,16,* 453–466.

Bland, M. (2007). Betwixt and between: A critical ethnography of comfort in New Zealand residential aged care. *Journal of Clinical Nursing, 16,* 937–944.

Etowa, J., Bernard, W., Oyinsan, B., & Clow, B. (2007). Participatory action research (PAR): An approach for improving black women's health in rural and remote communities. *Journal of Transcultural Nursing, 18,* 349–357.

Frid, I., Haljamäe, H., Ohlén, J., & Bergbom, I. (2007). Brain death: Close relatives' use of imagery as a descriptor of the experience. *Journal of Advanced Nursing, 58,* 63–71.

Griffiths, L., & Jasper, M. (2008). Warrior nurse: Duality and complementarity of role in the operational environment. *Journal of Advanced Nursing, 61,* 92–99.

Haynes, D., & Watt, J. (2008). The lived experience of health behaviors in people with debilitating illness. *Holistic Nursing Practice, 22,* 44–53.

Hayter, M. (2007). Nurses' discourse in contraceptive prescribing. *Journal of Advanced Nursing, 58,* 358–367.

Hilden, H. M., & Honkasalo, M. L. (2006). Finnish nurses' interpretations of patient autonomy in the context of end-of-life decision making. *Nursing Ethics, 13,* 41–51.

Hughes, A., Gudmundsdottir, M., & Davies, B. (2007). Everyday struggling to survive: Experience of the urban poor living with advanced cancer. *Oncology Nursing Forum, 34,* 1113–1118,

Ismail, F., Berman, H., & Ward-Griffin, C. (2007). Dating violence and the health of young women: A feminist narrative study. *Health Care for Women International, 28,* 453–477.

James, I., Andershed, B., & Ternestedt, B. (2007). A family's belief about cancer, dying, and death in the end of life. *Journal of Family Nursing, 13,* 226–253.

Johansson, I., Skärsäter, I., & Danielson, E. (2007). Encounters in a locked psychiatric ward environment. *Journal of Psychiatric & Mental Health Nursing, 14,* 366–372.

Kalwinsky, R. (2008). Western wormel Explication of aspects of health care behavior among Chamorro with HIV/AIDS. *Journal of Transcultural Nursing, 19,* 55–63.

Lloyd, M. (2007). Empowerment in the interpersonal field: Discourses of acute mental health nurses. *Journal of Psychiatric & Mental Health Nursing, 14,* 485–494.

Manocchio, R. T. (2008). Tending communities, crossing cultures: Midwives in 19th century California. *Journal of Midwifery & Women's Health, 53,* 75–81.

Martin, M., Jensen, E., Coatsworth-Puspoky, R., Forchuk, C., Lysiak-Globe, T., & Beal, G. (2007). Integrating an evidence-based research intervention in the discharge of mental health clients. *Archives of Psychiatric Nursing, 21,* 101–111.

Normann, H. K., Henriksen, N., Norberg, A., & Asplund, K. (2005). Lucidity in a woman with severe dementia: A case study. *Journal of Clinical Nursing, 14,* 891–896.

Porter, E. J. (2007). Problems with preparing food reported by frail older women living alone. *Advances in Nursing Science, 30,* 159–174.

Robertson, C., Kerr, M., Garcia, C., & Halterman, E. (2007). Noise and hearing protection: Latino construction workers' experiences. *American Association of Occupational Health Nurses Journal, 55,* 153–160.

Schneider, B. (2005). Mothers talk about their children with schizophrenia: A performance autoethnography. *Journal of Psychiatric & Mental Health Nursing, 12,* 333–340.

Smithbattle, L. (2007). Legacies of advantage and disadvantage: The case of teen mothers. *Public Health Nursing, 24,* 409–420.

Spiers, J. (2006). Expressing and responding to pain and stoicism in home-care nurse–patient interactions. *Scandinavian Journal of Caring Science, 20,* 293–301.

Zehle, K., Wen, L., Orr, N., & Rissel, C. (2007). "It's not an issue at the moment": A qualitative study of mothers about childhood obesity. *MCN: The American Journal of Maternal/Child Nursing, 32,* 36–41.

Zoffman, V., & Kirkevold, M. (2007). Relationships and their potential for change developed in difficult type 1 diabetes. *Qualitative Health Research, 17,* 625–638.

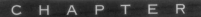

11 Specific Types of Research

MIXED METHOD RESEARCH
Rationale for Mixed Method Research
Applications of Mixed Method Research
Mixed Method Designs and Strategies

RESEARCH THAT INVOLVES INTERVENTIONS
Clinical Trials
Evaluation Research
Nursing Intervention Research

RESEARCH THAT DOES NOT INVOLVE INTERVENTIONS
Outcomes Research
Survey Research

Secondary Analysis
Methodologic Research

CRITIQUING STUDIES DESCRIBED IN THIS CHAPTER

RESEARCH EXAMPLES AND CRITICAL THINKING ACTIVITIES

CHAPTER REVIEW
Key New Terms
Summary Points

STUDIES CITED IN CHAPTER 11

STUDENT OBJECTIVES

On completing this chapter, you will be able to:

➤ Identify several advantages of mixed-method research and describe specific applications

➤ Identify the purposes and some of the distinguishing features of specific types of research (e.g., clinical trials, evaluations, surveys)

➤ Define new terms in the chapter

All quantitative studies can be categorized as experimental, quasi-experimental, or nonexperimental in design, as discussed in Chapter 9. And, most qualitative studies lie within one of the research traditions or typologies described in Chapter 10. This chapter describes types of research that vary according to study purpose rather than according to research design or tradition. Several of the types discussed in this chapter involve combining both qualitative and quantitative approaches, and so we begin by first discussing such mixed method research.

MIXED METHOD RESEARCH

A growing trend in nursing research is the planned integration of qualitative and quantitative data within single studies or coordinated clusters of studies. This section discusses the rationale for such **mixed method research** and presents a few applications.

Rationale for Mixed Method Research

The dichotomy between quantitative and qualitative data represents a key methodologic distinction in the social, behavioral, and health sciences. Some argue that the paradigms that underpin qualitative and quantitative research are fundamentally incompatible. Others, however, believe that many areas of inquiry can be enriched and the evidence base enhanced through the judicious triangulation of qualitative and quantitative data. The advantages of a mixed method design include the following:

➤ *Complementarity.* Qualitative and quantitative approaches are complementary they represent words and numbers, the two fundamental languages of human communication. By using mixed methods, researchers can allow each to do what it does best, possibly avoiding the limitations of a single approach.

➤ *Incrementality.* Progress on a topic tends to be incremental, relying on feedback loops. Qualitative findings can generate hypotheses to be tested quantitatively, and quantitative findings sometimes need clarification through in-depth probing. It can be productive to build such a loop into the design of a study.

➤ *Enhanced validity.* When a hypothesis or model is supported by multiple and complementary types of data, researchers can be more confident about their inferences and the validity of their results. The triangulation of methods can provide opportunities for testing alternative interpretations of the data, and for examining the extent to which the context helped to shape the results.

Perhaps the strongest argument for mixed methods research, however, is that certain questions *require* a mixed methods approach. **Pragmatism**, a paradigm often associated with mixed methods research, provides a basis for a position that has been stated as the "dictatorship of the research question" (Tashakkori & Teddlie, 2003, p. 21). Pragmatist researchers consider that it is the research question that should drive the inquiry, and its design and methods. They reject a forced choice between the traditional postpositivists' and naturalists' modes of inquiry.

Applications of Mixed Method Research

Mixed method research can be used to address various research goals. We illustrate a few applications here, and others will be discussed later in this chapter.

Instrumentation

Researchers sometimes collect qualitative data that are used in the development of formal, quantitative instruments used in research or clinical applications. The questions for a formal instrument are sometimes derived from clinical experience or prior research. When a construct is new, however, these mechanisms may be inadequate to capture its full complexity and dimensionality. Thus, nurse researchers sometimes gather qualitative data as the basis for generating and wording the questions on quantitative scales that are subsequently subjected to rigorous testing.

Example of instrumentation:
Choi and colleagues (2008) developed a scale to measure Korean women's intolerance to physical abuse by their husbands. In-depth interviews with Korean women living in abusive marriages revealed five themes, which formed the basis for developing a scale to tap each dimension. The scale was then tested using statistical procedures.

Hypothesis Generation and Testing

In-depth qualitative studies are often fertile with insights about constructs or relationships among them. These insights then can be tested and confirmed with larger samples in quantitative studies. This most often happens in the context of discrete investigations. One problem, however, is that it usually takes years to do a study and publish the results, which means that considerable time may elapse between the qualitative insights and the formal quantitative testing of hypotheses based on those insights. A research team interested in a phenomenon might wish to collaborate in a project that has hypothesis generation and testing as an explicit goal.

Example of hypothesis generation:
Judith Wuest has developed a strong program of qualitative research focusing on women's caregiving. Her grounded theory research, which gave rise to a *theory of precarious ordering*, revealed that the basic social problem for caregiving women is multiple competing, and changing demands. On the basis of her grounded theory, Wuest and colleagues (2007) developed hypotheses about how the nature and quality of the relationship between the caregiver and a care recipient can predict health consequences for women caregivers. The hypotheses received support in a quantitative study of 236 women caregivers of adult family members.

Explication

Qualitative data are sometimes used to explicate the *meaning* of quantitative descriptions or relationships. Quantitative methods can demonstrate that variables are systematically related but may fail to provide insights about *why* they are related. Such explications help to clarify important concepts and to corroborate the findings from the statistical analysis; they also help to illuminate the analysis and give guidance to the interpretation of results. Qualitative materials can be used to explicate specific statistical findings and to provide more global and dynamic views of the phenomena under study, sometimes in the form of illustrative case studies.

Example of explicating relationships with qualitative data:
Manuel and colleagues (2007) undertook a mixed method study of younger women's perceptions of coping with breast cancer. Results from the quantitative portion revealed that the most frequently used coping strategies were wishful thinking, making changes, and cognitive restructuring. Qualitative data suggested that the young women found different strategies particularly useful depending on the specific stressor.

Theory Building, Testing, and Refinement

A particularly ambitious application of mixed method research is in the area of theory construction. A theory gains acceptance as it escapes disconfirmation, and the use of multiple methods provides great opportunity for potential disconfirmation of a theory. If the theory can survive these assaults, it can provide a stronger context for the organization of clinical and intellectual work.

Example of theory building:
Riley and co-researchers (2008) examined the process of engaging in healthy behaviors, with particular emphasis on stress management, among HIV-infected low-income women. The quantitative measures were selected to represent concepts in the Transtheoretical Model of Behavior Change. A subsample of 8 of the 42 women in the overall study were interviewed in depth at a later point to gain further insights. Qualitative analysis suggested several processes of adopting healthy behaviors that were adequately reflected in the Transtheoretical Model, but a few emerged as additional processes that could suggest modifications for the theory.

Intervention Development

Qualitative research is beginning to play an increasingly important role in the development of promising nursing interventions and in efforts to test their efficacy and effectiveness. Morse (2006) has written a very useful discussion about qualitatively derived clinical interventions. There is also a growing recognition that the development of effective interventions must be based on some understanding of why people might not adhere to intervention protocols, or of the barriers they face in participating in a treatment. Intervention research is increasingly likely to be mixed method research.

Example of developmental research:
Svensson, Barclay, and Cooke (2006, in press) developed an antenatal education program based on extensive qualitative and quantitative data about the needs of expectant and new parents. Educational needs were explored through in-depth interviews, group interviews, and a series of longitudinal questionnaires. An innovative education program was then developed and rigorously tested.

Mixed Method Designs and Strategies

The growth in interest in mixed methods research in recent years has given rise to numerous typologies of mixed methods designs. For example, one typology contrasts *component designs* and *integrated designs*. In studies with a *component design*, the qualitative and quantitative aspects are implemented as discrete components of the overall inquiry, and remain distinct during data collection and analysis. The instrument development project by Choi and colleagues (2008) exemplifies a sequential component design.

In mixed method studies with an *integrated design*, there is greater integration of the method types at all phases of the project, from the development of research questions, through data collection and analysis, to the interpretation of the results. The blending of data occurs in ways that integrate the elements from the different paradigms and offers the possibility of yielding more insightful understandings of the phenomenon under study.

Sandelowski (2000) offered an alternative typology of mixed method designs. The scheme focuses on two key design dimensions for a mixed methods study: (1) which approach (qualitative or quantitative) has priority, and (2) how the approaches are sequenced in a study. In some cases (especially in component studies), data collection for the two approaches occurs more or less concurrently. In others, however, there are important advantages to a sequential approach, so that the second phase builds on knowledge gained in the first.

Although mixed method approaches can be used in a variety of contexts, they are becoming increasingly valuable in research involving interventions, which we discuss next.

RESEARCH THAT INVOLVES INTERVENTIONS

Interventions are developed and tested in many practice disciplines, and evidence from intervention research is increasingly being used to guide decisions in real-world applications. Different disciplines have developed their own methods and terminology in connection with intervention efforts. Nurse researchers, who have been doctorally trained in various disciplines, have used a rich assortment of approaches. There is overlap among these approaches, but to acquaint you with relevant terms, we discuss each separately. Clinical trials are associated with medical research, evaluation research is linked to the fields of education, social work, and public policy, and nurses are developing their own tradition of intervention research.

Clinical Trials

Clinical trials are studies designed to assess clinical interventions. Methods associated with clinical trials were developed primarily in the context of medical research, but the vocabulary is being used by many nurse researchers.

Clinical trials undertaken to test a new drug or an innovative therapy are often designed in a series of four phases, as described by the U. S. National Institutes of Health, as follows:

⮞ *Phase I* of the trial occurs after the initial development of the drug or therapy and is designed primarily to establish safety and tolerance, and to determine optimal dose or strength of the therapy. This phase typically involves small-scale studies using simple designs (e.g., before–after with no control group). The focus is not on efficacy, but on developing the best possible (and safest) treatment.

⮞ *Phase II* of the trial involves seeking preliminary evidence of controlled effectiveness. During this phase, researchers ascertain the feasibility of launching a more rigorous test, seek evidence that the treatment holds promise, look for signs of possible side effects, and identify refinements to improve the intervention. This phase is sometimes considered a pilot test of the treatment, and may be designed either as a small-scale experiment or as a quasi-experiment.

⮞ *Phase III* is a full experimental test of the treatment—a randomized controlled trial (RCT) involving random assignment to treatment conditions under tightly controlled conditions. The objective of this phase is to develop evidence about the treatment's *efficacy* (i.e., whether the innovation is more efficacious than the standard treatment or an alternative counterfactual). Adverse effects are also monitored. When the term *clinical trial* is used in the nursing literature, it most often is referring to a phase III trial, which may also be called an **efficacy study**. Phase III RCTs often involve the use of a large sample of subjects, sometimes selected from multiple sites to ensure that findings are not unique to a single setting, and to increase the sample size and hence the power of the statistical tests.

⮞ *Phase IV* of clinical trials involves studies of the *effectiveness* of an intervention in the general population. The emphasis in these **effectiveness studies** is on the external validity of an intervention that has shown promise of efficacy under controlled (but often artificial) conditions. Phase IV efforts often examine the cost-effectiveness and clinical utility of the new treatment. In pharmaceutical research, phase IV trials typically focus on postapproval safety surveillance and on long-term consequences over a larger population and timescale than was possible during earlier phases.

Example of a multisite phase III RCT:
Keefe and colleagues (2006) developed the REST intervention (reassurance, empathy, support, and time-out) for parents of irritable infants, based on a theory of infant colic that Keefe herself had previously developed. The trial to test the efficacy of REST involved randomly assigning infants in two sites to either the treatment or a control group.

The recent emphasis on evidence-based practice (EBP) has underscored the importance of research evidence that can be used in real-world clinical situations. One problem with traditional phase III RCTs is that, in an effort to enhance internal validity and the ability to infer causal pathways, the designs are so tightly controlled that their relevance to real-life applications comes into question. Concern about this situation has led to a call for **practical** (or **pragmatic**) **clinical trials** (i.e., trials for which the study design is formulated based on information needed to make a decision). Pragmatic trials address practical questions about the benefits and risks of an intervention—as well as its costs—as they would unfold in routine clinical practice.

Evaluation Research

Evaluation research focuses on developing useful information about a program, practice, procedure, or policy—information that decision-makers need on whether to adopt, modify, or abandon a practice or program. Usually (but not always), the evaluation is of a new intervention.

The term *evaluation research* is most often used when researchers want to assess the effectiveness of a complex program, rather than when they are evaluating a specific entity (e.g., alternative sterilizing solutions). Evaluation researchers tend to evaluate a program, practice, or intervention that is embedded in a political or organizational context. Evaluations often try to answer broader questions than simply whether an intervention is more effective than care as usual—for example, they often seek ways to improve the program (as in phase II of a clinical trial) or to learn how the program actually "works" in practice.

Evaluations are undertaken to answer a variety of questions. Some questions involve the use of an experimental (or quasi-experimental) design, but others do not. Because of the complexity of evaluations and the programs on which they typically focus, many evaluations are mixed method studies using a component design.

A **process** or **implementation analysis** is undertaken when a need exists for descriptive information about the process by which a program gets implemented and how it actually functions. A process analysis is typically designed to address such questions as the following: "Does the program operate the way its designers intended?" "What are the strongest and weakest aspects of the program?" "What exactly *is* the treatment, and how does it differ (if at all) from traditional practices?" "What were the barriers to implementing the program successfully?" "How do staff and clients feel about the intervention?"

Example of a process analysis:
Nicolaides-Bouman and colleagues (2007) performed a process evaluation of a home visiting program for older people with health problems. The evaluation examined patient compliance, the content of the intervention as it was actually delivered, and patients' experiences.

Many evaluations focus on whether a program or policy is meeting its objectives, and evaluation researchers sometimes distinguish between an outcome analysis and an impact analysis. An **outcome analysis** tends to be descriptive and does not use a rigorous experimental design. Such an analysis simply documents the extent to which the goals of the program are attained—the extent to which positive outcomes occur—without rigorous comparisons. Before-and-after designs without a control group are especially common.

Example of an outcome analysis:
Kyung and Chin (2008) studied the outcomes of a 4-week pulmonary rehabilitation program for older patients with chronic obstructive pulmonary disease (COPD). The program was associated with improvement in exercise performance and reduced dyspnea.

An **impact analysis** attempts to identify the *net impacts* of a program, that is, the impacts that can be attributed to the program, over and above the effects of the counterfactual (e.g., usual care). Impact analyses use an experimental or strong quasi-experimental design because the aim is to make a causal inference about the benefits of the special program. Many nursing evaluations are impact analyses, although they are not necessarily labeled as such.

Example of an impact analysis:
Hepburn and colleagues (2007) studied the impact of the Savvy Caregiver program, a psychoeducation program for dementia caregivers that was delivered to a group of caregivers in three states. There were significant beneficial effects on caregiver mastery and distress 6 months after the intervention for those in the experimental group.

In the current situation of spiraling health care costs, program evaluations may also include an **economic (cost) analysis** to determine whether the benefits of the program outweigh the monetary costs. Administrators and public policy officials make decisions about resource allocations for health services not only on the basis of whether something "works," but also on the basis of whether it is economically viable. Cost analyses are typically done in conjunction with impact analyses (or phase III clinical trials), that is, when researchers establish persuasive evidence regarding program efficacy

Example of an economic analysis:
Au and colleagues (2007) did an economic analysis that evaluated the effects of a program of supplementary prenatal care and home visitation, compared with standard care. The researchers compared the two groups in terms of costs of the health care services the parents accessed in the 12 months after the baby's birth.

Nursing Intervention Research

Both clinical trials and evaluations involve *interventions*. However, the term **intervention research** is increasingly being used by nurse researchers to describe a research approach distinguished not so much by a particular research methodology as by a distinctive *process* of planning, developing, testing, and disseminating interventions (e.g., Sidani & Braden, 1998; Whittemore & Grey, 2002). Proponents of the process are critical of the rather simplistic and atheoretic approach that is often used to design and evaluate interventions. The recommended process involves an in-depth understanding of the problem and the people for whom the intervention is being developed; careful, collaborative planning with a diverse team; and the development of an intervention theory to guide the inquiry.

Similar to clinical trials, nursing intervention research ideally involves several phases: (1) basic developmental research; (2) pilot research; (3) efficacy research; and (4) effectiveness research. Whittemore and Grey (2002) have proposed a fifth phase involving widespread implementation and efforts to document effects on public health.

Conceptualization, a major focus of the development phase, is supported through collaborative discussions, consultations with experts, critical literature reviews, and in-depth qualitative research to understand the problem. The construct validity of the emerging intervention is enhanced through efforts to develop an **intervention theory** that clearly articulates what must be done to achieve desired outcomes. The intervention design, which flows from the intervention theory, specifies what the clinical inputs would be, and also such aspects as duration and intensity of the intervention. A conceptual map (Chapter 8) is often a useful visual tool for articulating the intervention theory and for guiding the design of the intervention. During the developmental phase, key *stakeholders*—people who have a stake in the intervention—ideally are identified and "brought on board," which may involve participatory research. Stakeholders include potential beneficiaries of the intervention and their families, advocates and community leaders, and agents of the intervention.

The second phase of nursing intervention research is a pilot test of the intervention, typically using simple quasi-experimental designs. The central activities during the pilot test are to secure preliminary evidence of the intervention's benefits, to refine the intervention theory and intervention protocols, and to assess the feasibility of a rigorous test. The feasibility assessment should involve an analysis of factors that affected implementation during the pilot test (e.g., recruitment, retention, and adherence problems). Qualitative research can play an important role in gaining insight into the feasibility of a larger-scale RCT.

As in a classic clinical trial, the third phase involves a full experimental test of the intervention, and the final phase focuses on effectiveness and utility in real-world clinical settings. This full model of intervention research is, at this point, more of an ideal than an actuality. For example, effectiveness studies in nursing research are rare. A few research teams have begun to implement portions of the model, and efforts are likely to expand.

Example of nursing intervention research:
Duffy and colleagues (2005, 2008) described the developmental work that was undertaken in designing a caring-based nursing intervention for older adults with advanced heart failure discharged from acute care. A team of nurse researchers with complementary skills systematically developed the intervention. The intervention was based on pilot work, findings from recent research, clinical practice guidelines, and a modification of a theoretic framework that Duffy and others had developed in earlier research. The intervention is being tested using an experimental design.

RESEARCH THAT DOES NOT INVOLVE INTERVENTIONS

The studies described in the previous section often have a nonexperimental component, but, because they involve an intervention, almost always involve an experimental or quasi-experimental design as well. In this section, we look at types of research that do not involve interventions and thus rely on nonexperimental designs.

Outcomes Research

Outcomes research is designed to document the effectiveness of health care services. Whereas evaluation research typically focuses on an appraisal of a specific (and often local) program or policy, outcomes research represents a more global assessment of nursing and health care services. The impetus for outcomes research comes from quality assessment and quality assurance functions that grew out of the professional standards review organizations (PSROs) in the 1970s. Outcomes research represents a response to the increasing demand from policy makers, insurers, and the public to justify care practices and systems in terms of improved patient outcomes and costs. The original focus of outcomes research was on patient health status and costs associated with medical care, but there is a growing interest in studying broader patient outcomes in relation to nursing care.

Although many nursing studies evaluate patient outcomes, specific efforts to appraise and document the quality of nursing care—as distinct from the care provided by the overall health care system—are not numerous. A major obstacle is attribution—that is, linking patient outcomes to specific nursing actions or interventions, distinct from the actions of other members of the health care team. It is also difficult in some cases to determine a causal connection between outcomes and health care interventions because factors outside the health care system (e.g., patient characteristics) affect outcomes in complex ways.

Donabedian (1987), whose pioneering efforts created a framework for outcomes research, emphasized three factors in appraising quality in health care services: structure, process, and outcomes. The *structure* of care refers to broad organizational and administrative features (e.g., size, range of services). Nursing skill mix and nursing autonomy in decision-making are two structural variables that have been found to be related to patient outcomes. *Processes* involve aspects of clinical management, decision making, and clinical interventions. *Outcomes* refer to the specific clinical end results of patient care. There have been several suggested modifications to Donabedian's framework for appraising health care quality, the most noteworthy of which is the Quality Health Outcomes Model developed by the American Academy of Nursing (Mitchell et al., 1998). This model is less linear and more dynamic than Donabedian's original framework, and takes client and system characteristics into account.

Example of outcomes research:
Rafferty and colleagues (2007) examined the effect of hospital-wide nurse staffing levels on patient mortality, failure to rescue, and nurse-rated quality of care in the United Kingdom and found, similar to results in the United States, that high patient-to-nurse ratios are associated with worse patient outcomes.

Outcomes research usually concentrates on various linkages within such models, rather than on testing the overall model. Some studies have examined the effect of health care structures on various health care processes and outcomes, for example. Most outcomes research in nursing, however, has focused on the process/patient/ outcomes nexus, often using large-scale datasets. Examples of nursing process variables include nursing actions such as nurses' problem-solving skills, clinical decision making, clinical competence and leadership, and specific activities or interventions (e.g., communication, touch).

The work that nurses do is increasingly being documented in terms of established classification systems and taxonomies. Indeed, in the United States, the standard use of electronic health records to record all health care events, and the submission of the records to national data banks, are imminent. A number of research-based classification systems of nursing interventions are being developed, refined, and tested. Among the most prominent are the nursing diagnosis taxonomy and classification of the North American Nursing Diagnosis Association International (NANDA International, 2008), the Nursing Intervention Classification or NIC, developed at the University of Iowa (Bulecheck et al., 2007), and the Nursing-Sensitive Outcomes Classification (NOC), also developed by nurses at the University of Iowa College of Nursing (Moorhead et al., 2007).

Example of classification system research:
Lunney (2006) examined the effects of implementing NANDA diagnoses, interventions from NIC, and outcomes from the NOC on nurses' power and children's health outcomes, using nurses' reports of health visits with New York City children in six schools.

Survey Research

A **survey** obtains information about the prevalence, distribution, and interrelations of variables within a population. Political opinion polls, such as those conducted by Gallup or Harris, are examples of surveys. Survey data are used primarily in non-experimental correlational studies.

Surveys obtain information about people's actions, knowledge, intentions, opinions, and attitudes by means of **self-report**—that is, study participants respond to a set of questions. Surveys, which yield quantitative data primarily, may be cross-sectional or longitudinal (e.g., panel studies). Any information that can reliably be obtained by direct questioning can be gathered in a survey, although surveys include mostly questions that require brief responses (e.g., yes/no, always/ sometimes/never).

Survey data can be collected in a number of ways, but the most respected method is through **personal interviews** (or *face-to-face interviews*), in which interviewers meet in person with respondents to ask them questions. Personal interviews are expensive because they involve a lot of personnel time. Nevertheless, personal interviews are considered the best method of doing a survey because the quality of data is higher than with other methods and because the refusal rate tends to be low. **Telephone interviews** are a less costly method, but when the interviewer is unknown, respondents may be uncooperative on the phone. Telephoning can be a convenient method of collecting data if the interview is short and not too personal, or if researchers have had prior personal contact with respondents.

Questionnaires differ from interviews in that they are self-administered. Respondents read the questions on a form and give their answers in writing. Because respondents differ in their reading levels and in their writing skills, questionnaires are *not* merely a printed form of an interview schedule. Self-administered questionnaires are economical but are not appropriate for surveying certain populations (e.g., the elderly, children). Survey questionnaires are often distributed through the mail, but increasingly are being distributed over the Internet.

The greatest advantage of surveys is their flexibility and broadness of scope. Surveys can be used with many populations; they can focus on a wide range of topics and can be used for many purposes. The information obtained in most surveys, however, tends to be relatively superficial: surveys rarely probe deeply into such complexities as contradictions of human behavior and feelings. Survey research is better suited to extensive rather than intensive analysis.

Example of a survey:

Kulig and co-researchers (2008) conducted a survey of nurses practicing in rural and remote regions of Canada to learn about their experiences and perceptions. Questionnaires were mailed to more than 5,700 nurses, using postal codes from RN registration data to locate nurses in all Canadian provinces and in northern territories.

Secondary Analysis

Secondary analysis involves the use of data gathered in a previous study to test new hypotheses or address new questions. In most studies, researchers collect far more data than are actually analyzed. Secondary analysis of existing data is efficient and economical because data collection is typically the most time-consuming and expensive part of a research project. Nurse researchers have used secondary analysis with both large national data sets and smaller localized sets, and with both qualitative and quantitative data. Outcomes research frequently involves secondary analyses of clinical datasets.

A number of avenues are available for making use of an existing set of quantitative data. For example, variables and relationships among variables that were previously unanalyzed can be examined (e.g., a dependent variable in the original study could become the independent variable in the secondary analysis). In other cases, a secondary analysis focuses on a particular subgroup of the full original sample (e.g., survey data about health habits from a national sample of adults could be analyzed to study smoking among rural men).

Qualitative researchers also typically collect far more data than are analyzed originally. Secondary analyses of qualitative data provide opportunities to exploit rich data sets, although there may be difficulty in identifying a suitable data set. The availability of large quantitative data sets, especially from government-sponsored surveys, is widely publicized, but there are few repositories of qualitative data sets. Thorne (1994) identified several types of qualitative secondary analysis. In one type, called *analytic expansion*, researchers use their own data to answer new questions as the theory base increases or as they pursue questions at a higher level of analysis. A second, *retrospective interpretation*, involves using an original database to examine new questions that were not thoroughly assessed in the original study.

The use of available data from other studies makes it possible to bypass time-consuming and costly steps in the research process, but there are some noteworthy disadvantages in working with existing data. In particular, if researchers do not play a role in collecting the data, the chances are high that the data set will be deficient in one or more ways, such as in the sample used, the variables measured, and so forth. Secondary analysts may continuously face "if only" problems: if only an additional question had been asked, or if only a variable had been measured differently. Nevertheless, existing data sets present exciting opportunities for expanding the base of evidence in an economical way.

Example of a quantitative secondary analysis:
Schmalenberg and Kramer (2008) tested the hypothesis that staff nurses in Magnet hospitals would rate the quality of their work environment more highly than nurses in comparison hospitals. They used data that had been gathered previously from 10,514 nurses in 34 hospitals.

Example of a qualitative secondary analysis:
Malbasa and colleagues (2007) analyzed previously collected qualitative data from adolescents with acute lymphoblastic leukemia. The aim of the new study was to develop an understanding of the role of adolescent development in the participants' suboptimal adherence to 6-mercaptopurine therapy.

Methodologic Research

Methodologic research entails investigations of the methods of obtaining and organizing data and conducting rigorous research. Methodologic studies address the development, validation, and evaluation of research tools or methods. The growing demands for sound and reliable outcome measures, for rigorous tests of interventions, and for sophisticated procedures for obtaining data have led to an increased interest in methodologic research by nurse researchers.

Most methodologic studies are nonexperimental, often focusing on the development of new instruments. Instrument development research often involves complex and sophisticated research methods, including the use of mixed method designs. Occasionally, researchers use an experimental design to test competing methodologic strategies, for example, to test the effect of monetary incentives on response rates.

Example of a quantitative methodologic study:
Kelly and co-researchers (2007) sought to ascertain the cost implications and predictors of success of gathering follow-up data from a cohort of high-risk adolescent girls who had been part of a reproductive health promotion intervention. The study also examined which approaches were particularly effective in completing a follow-up interview.

In qualitative research, methodologic issues often arise within the context of a substantive study, rather than having a study originate as a purely methodologic endeavor. In such instances, however, the researcher typically performs separate analyses designed to highlight a methodologic issue and to generate strategies for solving a methodologic problem.

Example of a qualitative methodologic study:
Hadley and colleagues (2008) explored parents' perspectives on having their children interviewed for research. The researchers interviewed 142 parents about their perceptions, with the goal of gaining insights about how to work collaboratively with parents in research with children.

Methodologic research may appear less compelling than substantive clinical research, but it is virtually impossible to conduct rigorous and useful research on a substantive topic with inadequate research methods.

CRITIQUING STUDIES DESCRIBED IN THIS CHAPTER

It is difficult to provide guidance on critiquing the types of studies described in this chapter, because they are so varied and because many of the fundamental methodologic issues that require a critique concern the overall design. Guidelines for critiquing design-related issues were presented in the previous chapters.

You should, however, consider whether researchers took appropriate advantage of the possibilities of a mixed method design. Collecting both qualitative and quantitative data is not always necessary or practical, but in critiquing studies you can consider whether the study would have been strengthened by triangulating different types of data. In studies in which mixed methods were used, you should carefully consider whether the inclusion of both types of data was justified and whether the researcher really made use of both types of data to enhance knowledge on the research topic. Table 11.1 provides some examples of possibilities for mixed method studies. Box 11.1 offers a few specific questions for critiquing the types of studies included in this chapter. ✪

TABLE 11.1 ▸ EXAMPLES OF POSSIBILITIES FOR QUALITATIVE-QUANTITATIVE INTEGRATION

TYPE	EXAMPLE OF QUESTION FOR QUANTITATIVE COMPONENT	EXAMPLE OF QUESTION FOR QUALITATIVE COMPONENT
Clinical trial	Are boomerang pillows more effective than straight pillows in improving the respiratory capacity of hospitalized patients?	Why did some patients complain about the boomerang pillows? How did the pillows feel?
Evaluation	How effective is a nurse-managed special care unit compared with traditional intensive care units?	How accepting were other health care workers of the special unit, and what problems of implementation ensued?
Outcomes research	What effect do alternative levels of nursing intensity have on the functional ability of elderly residents in long-term care facilities?	How do elderly long-term care residents interact with nurses in environments with different nursing intensity?
Survey	How prevalent is asthma among inner-city children, and how is it treated?	How is asthma experienced by inner-city children and their parents?
Methodologic research	How accurate is a new measure of loneliness for hospitalized psychiatric patients?	Does the new measure adequately capture the dimensions of loneliness of psychiatric patients?
Ethnography	What percentage of women in rural Appalachia obtain prenatal care?	How do women in rural Appalachia view their pregnancies and prepare for childbirth?
Case study	What percentage of cases at St. Jude's Homeless Shelter are HIV positive or have AIDS?	How are health, nutrition, social, and psychological services integrated in St. Jude's Homeless Shelter?

▸ RESEARCH EXAMPLES AND CRITICAL THINKING ACTIVITIES

Drs. Barbara Given and Charles Given have devoted their careers to research on patients with cancer. Their extensive program of research includes several of the types of studies described in this chapter.

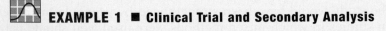 EXAMPLE 1 ■ Clinical Trial and Secondary Analysis

Studies

Effect of a cognitive behavioral intervention on reducing symptom severity during chemotherapy (Given et al., 2004); Physical functioning: effect of behavioral intervention for symptoms among individuals with cancer (Doorenbos et al., 2006).

BOX 11.1   GUIDELINES FOR CRITIQUING STUDIES DESCRIBED IN CHAPTER 11

1. Does the study purpose match the study design? Was the best possible design (or research tradition) used to address the study purpose?

2. Is the study exclusively qualitative or exclusively quantitative? If so, could the study have been strengthened by incorporating both approaches?

3. If the study used a mixed methods design, how did the inclusion of both approaches contribute to enhanced theoretical insights or enhanced validity? In what other ways (if any) did the inclusion of both types of data strengthen the study and further the aims of the research?

4. If the study used a mixed method design, would the design be described as a component design or an integrated design? Was this approach appropriate? Comment on the timing of collecting the various types of data.

5. If the study was a clinical trial or intervention study, was adequate attention paid to developing an appropriate intervention? Was there a well-conceived intervention theory that guided the endeavor? Was the intervention adequately pilot tested?

6. If the study was a clinical trial, evaluation, or intervention study, was there an effort to understand how the intervention was implemented (i.e., a process-type analysis)? Were the financial costs and benefits assessed? If not, should they have been?

7. If the study was outcomes research, which segments of the structure-process-outcomes model were examined? Would it have been desirable (and feasible) to expand the study to include other aspects? Do the findings suggest possible improvements to structures or processes that would be beneficial to patient outcomes?

8. If the study was a survey, was the most appropriate method used to collect the data (i.e., in-person interviews, telephone interviews, mail or Internet questionnaries)?

9. If the study was a secondary analysis, to what extent was the chosen dataset appropriate for addressing the research questions? What were the limitations of the dataset, and were these limitations acknowledged and taken into account in interpreting the results?

Background and Purpose

Drs. Barbara and Charles Given noted that patients who receive chemotherapy suffer many limitations caused by symptoms of the disease and its treatment. The purpose of the phase III research was to assess the efficacy of a nurse-led intervention designed to reduce emotional distress in cancer patients diagnosed with solid tumors and undergoing a first course of chemotherapy.

Intervention

In earlier research that helped to form the basis for this clinical trial (see Example 2), the Givens had found that a number of cancer symptoms, such as pain, insomnia, and fatigue, co-occurred, and that these co-occurring symptoms were associated with higher levels of depression (e.g., Given et al., 2001). They and colleagues undertook systematic reviews and consulted with experts in formulating an effective intervention for managing symptoms and reducing emotional distress (e.g., Smith et al., 2003). They identified cognitive–behavioral therapy (based on Social Cognitive Theory) as a promising approach, and developed specific evidence-based strategies for enhancing self-efficacy and building adaptive strategies that patients could use to address everyday problems. The intervention was delivered by trained nurses and entailed 10 contacts over a 20-week period.

Research Design

A sample of more than 200 patients and their caregivers in several cancer centers were randomly assigned to either the intervention or conventional care. Study participants were interviewed in person at baseline, and again 10 and 20 weeks later. Symptom severity and depression were the key outcomes measured at all three points in time.

Clinical Trial Findings

Given and colleagues (2004) found that at 20 weeks post-baseline, subjects in the experimental group were less depressed than those in the control group. They also found that the effect of the intervention on symptom severity was influenced by the patients' initial symptomatology. That is, patients in the experimental group who entered the trial with higher symptom severity were especially likely to benefit from the intervention.

Secondary Analysis

Doorenbos and colleagues (2006) used the data from the clinical trial to address a separate question that had not yet been explored. The primary outcome variable for the secondary analysis was physical functioning, and the focus was on whether the effect of the intervention on this outcome was moderated by patients' characteristics, such as their age, stage of cancer, gender, and comorbidities. The analysis suggested that the special intervention affected physical function trajectories differently for people with different health and personal characteristics. For example, the intervention benefited the rates of change in physical functioning among patients with high numbers of chronic health conditions to a greater extent than those with lower numbers of chronic problems.

CRITICAL THINKING SUGGESTIONS*:

*See the Student Resource CD-ROM for a discussion of these questions. 💿

1. Answer the relevant questions from Box 11.1 regarding this study.
2. Also. consider the following targeted questions, which may further sharpen your critical thinking skills and assist you in understanding this study:
    a. Was the clinical trial prospective or retrospective?
    b. In language associated with evaluation research, could any part of this study be described as a process analysis? Outcome analysis? Impact analysis? Cost analysis?
    c. Comment on the issue of *causality* within the context of this study.
    d. Suggest a qualitative component for this research and describe its potential utility in enhancing the study.
3. If the results of this study are valid, what are some of the uses to which the findings might be put in clinical practice?

📐 EXAMPLE 2 ■ A Survey, Methodologic Research, and Secondary Analysis

Studies

Research design and subject characteristics predicting nonparticipation in a panel survey of older families with cancer (Neumark, Stommel, Given, & Given, 2001); The influence of end-of-life cancer care on caregivers (Doorenbos et al., 2007).

The Survey

During the mid- to late-1990s, Drs. Given conducted a survey with more than 1,000 older patients who were newly diagnosed with lung, colon, breast, or prostate cancer. The panel study involved four rounds of telephone interviews (at 6–8 weeks, 12–16 weeks, 24–30 weeks, and 52 weeks after diagnosis) and self-administered questionnaires with study participants and their caregivers, who were recruited in multiple hospitals and treatment centers. The purpose of the original study was to examine physical, emotional, and financial outcomes for patients and family members over the first year following cancer diagnosis. Key findings from the original research were presented in several journal articles (e.g., Given et al., 2000, 2001).

Methodologic Research

Neumark and colleagues (2001) sought to identify factors that could account for loss of subjects in the earliest phases of sample accrual for a panel study. They compared three groups: eligible patients who declined to participate (nonconsenters), patients who originally consented to participate but then later declined (early dropouts), and subjects who actually took part in the study (participants). The researchers examined two broad types of factors that might help to explain nonparticipation: subject characteristics and research design characteristics. The aim was to obtain information that would benefit others in designing panel studies and recruiting subjects. They found, for example, that the most powerful design factor was whether a family caregiver was approached to participate. Patients were more likely to give consent and less likely to drop out early when caregivers were also approached.

Substantive Secondary Analysis

The survey data set has been used in several secondary analyses. For example, Doorenbos, Givens, and other colleagues (2007) used data from 619 caregivers who either completed the year-long study or whose family member died. The analysis focused on whether those caring for family members who ultimately died reported different caregiver depressive symptoms and burden than caregivers whose family survived throughout the study period. The findings suggested that caregiver depressive symptomatology improved over time for both groups, but symptoms were greater among caregivers whose relative died. Among spousal caregivers, those whose spouse died reported greater burden than caregivers whose spouse survived.

CRITICAL THINKING SUGGESTIONS:

1. Answer the relevant questions from Box 11.1 regarding this study.
2. Also, consider the following targeted questions, which may further sharpen your critical thinking skills and assist you in understanding this study:
   a. Is this study longitudinal or cross-sectional?
   b. In the Neumark et al. and Doorenbos et al. studies, what are the independent and dependent variables?
   c. Comment on the issue of causality within the context of the Doorenbos et al. study.
3. What are some of the uses to which the findings from these studies might be put in clinical practice?

CHAPTER REVIEW
• •

Key new terms introduced in the chapter, together with a summary of major points, are presented in this section. In addition, Chapter 11 of the accompanying *Study Guide for Essentials of Nursing Research*, 7th edition offers various exercises and study suggestions for reinforcing concepts presented in this chapter. For additional review, see the Student Self-Study Review Questions section of the Student Resource CD-ROM provided with this book. 🔘

Key New Terms

Clinical trial
Economic (cost) analysis
Effectiveness study
Efficacy study

Evaluation research
Intervention theory
Methodologic research
Mixed method research

Outcomes research
Secondary analysis
Survey research

Summary Points

➤ Studies vary according to purpose as well as design or research tradition. For many purposes, mixed method studies are advantageous. **Mixed method research** involves the triangulation of qualitative and quantitative data in a single project.

➤ Mixed method studies are used for many purposes, including the development and testing of high-quality instruments, the generation and testing of hypotheses, theory building, and intervention development.

➤ In mixed method studies with a *component design*, the qualitative and quantitative aspects of the study are implemented as discrete components, and are distinct during data collection and data analysis. The second broad category is *integrated designs*, in which there is greater integration of methods throughout the research process.

➤ **Clinical trials**, which are studies designed to assess the effectiveness of clinical interventions, often involve a series of phases. *Phase I* is designed to finalize the features of the intervention. *Phase II* involves seeking preliminary evidence of efficacy and opportunities for refinements. *Phase III* is a full experimental test of treatment **efficacy**. In *phase IV*, the researcher focuses primarily on generalized **effectiveness** and evidence about costs and benefits.

➤ **Practical** (or **pragmatic**) **clinical trials** are studies designed to provide information to clinical decision-makers, and involve designs aimed at reducing the gap between efficacy and effectiveness studies (i.e., between internal and external validity).

➤ **Evaluation research** assesses the effectiveness of a program, policy, or procedure to assist decision-makers in choosing a course of action. Evaluations can answer a variety of questions. **Process** or **implementation analyses** describe the process by which a program gets implemented and how it functions in practice. **Outcome analyses** *describe* the status of some condition after the introduction of an intervention. **Impact analyses** test whether an intervention caused any **net impacts** relative to the counterfactual. **Economic (cost) analyses** seek to determine whether the monetary costs of a program are outweighed by benefits.

➤ **Nursing intervention research** is a term sometimes used to refer to a distinctive *process* of planning, developing, testing, and disseminating interventions. A key feature of this process is the development of an **intervention theory** from which the design and evaluation of an intervention flow. Intervention research proceeds in several phases, and an especially important phase is early developmental work (phase I) that frequently involves mixed method research.

➤ **Outcomes research** is undertaken to document the quality and effectiveness of health care and nursing services. A model of health care quality encompasses several broad concepts, including *structure* (factors such as accessibility, range of services, facilities, and organizational climate); *process* (nursing interventions and actions); client risk factors (e.g., severity of illness and caseload mix); and *outcomes* (the specific end-results of patient care in terms of patient functioning).

➤ **Survey research** examines people's characteristics, behaviors, intentions, and opinions by asking them to answer questions. The preferred survey method is through **personal interviews**, in which interviewers meet respondents face-to-face and question them. **Telephone interviews** are less costly, but are inadvisable if the interview is long or if the questions are sensitive. **Questionnaires** are self-administered (i.e., questions are read by respondents, who then give written responses).

➤ **Secondary analysis** refers to studies in which researchers analyze previously collected data—either quantitative or qualitative. Secondary analyses are economical, but it is sometimes difficult to identify an appropriate existing dataset.

➤ In **methodologic research,** the investigator is concerned with the development, validation, and assessment of methodologic tools or strategies.

STUDIES CITED IN CHAPTER 11

Au, F., Shiell, A., van der Pol, M., Johnston, D., & Tough, S. (2007). Does supplementary prenatal nursing and home visitation reduce healthcare costs in the year after childbirth? *Journal of Advanced Nursing, 56,* 657–668.

Choi, M., Phillips, L., Figueredo, A., Insei, K., & Min, S. (2008). Construct validity of the Korean Women's Abuse Intolerance Scale. *Nursing Research, 57,* 40–50.

Doorenbos, A., Given, B., Given, C., & Verbitsky, N. (2006). Physical functioning: Effect of behavioral intervention for symptoms among individuals with cancer. *Nursing Research, 55,* 161–171.

Doorenbos, A., Given, B., Given, C., Wyatt, G., Gift, A., Rahbar, M. et al. (2007). The influence of end-of-life cancer care on caregivers. *Research in Nursing & Health, 30,* 270–281.

Duffy, J., Hoskins, L., & Dudley-Brown, S. (2005). Development and testing of a caring-based intervention for older adults with heart failure. *Journal of Cardiovascular Nursing, 20,* 325–333.

Duffy, J., & Hoskins, L. (2008). Research challenges and lessons learned from a heart failure telehome-care study. *Home Healthcare Nurse, 26,* 58–65.

Given, C., Given, B., Azzouz, F., Stommel, M., & Kozachik, S. (2000). Comparison of changes in physical functioning of elderly patients with new diagnoses of cancer. *Medical Care, 38,* 482–493.

Given, C., Given, B. Azzouz, F., Kozachik, S., & Stommel, M. (2001). Predictors of pain and fatigue in the year following diagnosis among elderly cancer patients. *Journal of Pain and Symptom Management, 21,* 456–466.

Given, C., Given, B., Rahbar, M., Jeon, S., McCorkle, R., Cimprich, B. et al. (2004). Effect of a cognitive behavioral intervention on reducing symptom severity during chemotherapy. *Journal of Clinical Oncology, 22,* 507–516.

Hadley, E., Smith, C., Gallo, A., Angst, D., & Knafl, K. (2008). Parents' perspectives on having their children interviewed for research. *Research in Nursing & Health, 31,* 4–11.

Hepburn, K., Lewis, M., Tornatore, J., Sherman, C., & Bremer, K. (2007). The Savvy Caregiver program: The demonstrated effectiveness of a transportable dementia caregiver psychoeducation program. *Journal of Gerontological Nursing, 33,* 30–36.

Keefe, M., Karlsen, K., Lobo, M., Kotzer, A., & Dudley, W. (2006). Reducing parenting stress in families with irritable infants, *Nursing Research, 55,* 198–205.

Kelly, P., Ahmed, A., Martinez, E., & Peralez-Dieckmann, E. (2007). Cost analysis of obtaining postintervention results in a cohort of high-risk adolescents. *Nursing Research, 56,* 269–274.

Kulig, J., Andrews, M., Stewart, N., Pitblado, R., MacLeod, M., Bentham, D. et al. (2008). How do registered nurses define rurality? *Australian Journal of Rural Health, 16,* 28–32.

Kyung, K., & Chin, P. (2008). The effect of a pulmonary rehabilitation programme on older patients with chronic pulmonary disease. *Journal of Clinical Nursing, 17,* 118–125.

Lunney, M. (2006). NANDA diagnoses, NIC interventions, and NOC outcomes used in an electronic health record with elementary school children. *Journal of School Nursing, 22,* 94–101.

Malbasa, T., Kodish, E., & Santacroce, S. (2007). Adolescent adherence to oral therapy for leukemia. *Journal of Pediatric Oncology Nursing, 24,* 139–151.

Manuel, J., Burwell, S., Crawford, S., Lawrence, R., Farmer, D., Hege, A. et al. (2007). Younger women's perceptions of coping with breast cancer. *Cancer Nursing, 30,* 85–94.

Neumark, D. E., Stommel, M., Given, C. W., & Given, B. A. (2001). Research design and subject characteristics predicting nonparticipation in a panel survey of older families with cancer. *Nursing Research, 50,* 363–368.

Nicolaides-Bouman, A., van Rossum, E., Habets, H., Kempen, G., & Knipschild, P. (2007). Home visiting programme for older people with health problems: Process evaluation. *Journal of Advanced Nursing, 58,* 425–435.

Rafferty, A., Clarke, S., Coles, J., Ball, J., James, P., McKee, M. et al. (2007). Outcomes of variation in hospital nurse staffing in English hospitals. *International Journal of Nursing Studies, 44,* 175–182.

Riley, T., Lewis, B., Lewis, M. P., & Fava, J. (2008). Low-income HIV-infected women and the process of engaging in health behavior. *Journal of the Association of Nurses in AIDS Care, 19,* 3–15.

Schmalenberg, C., & Kramer, M. (2008). Essentials of a productive nurse work environment. *Nursing Research, 57,* 2–13.

Smith, R., Lein, C., Collins, C., Lyles, J., Given, B., Dwamena, F. et al. (2003). Treating patients with medically unexplained symptoms in primary care. *Journal of General Internal Medicine, 18,* 478–489.

Svensson, J., Barclay, L., & Cooke, M. (2006). The concerns and interests of expectant and new parents: Assessing learning needs. *Journal of Perinatal Education, 15,* 18–27.

Svensson, J., Barclay, L., & Cooke, M. (in press). Randomised-controlled trial of two antenatal education programmes. *Midwifery.*

Wuest, J., Hodgins, M., Malcolm, J., Merritt-Gray, M., & Seamon, P. (2007). The effects of past relationship and obligation on health and health promotion in women caregivers of adult family members. *Advances in Nursing Science, 30,* 206–220.

CHAPTER

12 Sampling Plans

STUDENT OBJECTIVES

On completing this chapter, you will be able to:

➤ Identify differences in the logic of sampling for quantitative versus qualitative studies

➤ Distinguish between nonprobability and probability samples and compare their advantages and disadvantages in both qualitative and quantitative studies

➤ Identify several types of sampling in qualitative and quantitative studies and describe their main characteristics

➤ Evaluate the appropriateness of the sampling method and sample size used in a study

➤ Define new terms in the chapter

Sampling is a process familiar to all of us—we make decisions and form opinions about phenomena based on contact with only a sample of them. Researchers, too, derive knowledge and draw conclusions from samples. In testing the efficacy of a nursing intervention for patients with cancer, nurse researchers reach conclusions without testing the intervention with every victim of the disease. However, the consequences of drawing erroneous inferences are more momentous when evaluating evidence for nursing practice than in private decision making.

Quantitative and qualitative researchers have different approaches to sampling. Quantitative researchers desire samples that will allow them to achieve statistical conclusion validity and to generalize their results. They develop a **sampling plan** that specifies in advance how participants are to be selected and how many to include. Qualitative researchers are interested in developing a rich, holistic understanding of a phenomenon. They make sampling decisions during the course of the study based on informational and theoretical needs, and typically do not develop a formal sampling plan in advance. This chapter discusses sampling issues for both quantitative and qualitative research.

BASIC SAMPLING CONCEPTS

Sampling is a critical part of the design of quantitative research. Let us first consider some terms associated with sampling—terms that are used primarily (but not exclusively) with quantitative studies.

Populations

A **population** is the entire aggregation of cases in which a researcher is interested. For instance, if a researcher were studying American nurses with doctoral degrees, the population could be defined as all U.S. citizens who are RNs and who have acquired a PhD, DNSc, or other doctoral-level degree. Other possible populations might be all male patients who underwent cardiac surgery in St. Peter's Hospital in 2009 or all Australian children under age 10 with cystic fibrosis. A population may be broadly defined, involving thousands of individuals, or may be narrowly specified to include only hundreds.

Populations are not restricted to human subjects. A population might consist of all the hospital records on file in a particular hospital or all the high schools in the United States with clinics that dispense contraceptives. Whatever the basic unit, the population comprises the entire aggregate of elements in which the researcher is interested.

Researchers (especially quantitative researchers) specify the characteristics that delimit the study population through the **eligibility criteria** (or *inclusion criteria*). For example, consider the population of American nursing students. Would this population include part-time students? Would RNs returning to school for a bachelor's degree be included? Researchers establish criteria to determine whether a person qualifies as a member of the population—although populations sometimes are defined in terms of characteristics that people must *not* possess through *exclusion criteria* (e.g., excluding people who do not speak English).

Example of inclusion and exclusion criteria:
Lindgren and colleagues (2008) studied how elderly patients with ischemic coronary heart disease cluster based on presenting symptoms in the week before hospitalization. Patients from five medical centers were eligible for the study if they were unpartnered adults aged 65 or older; had positive enzyme tests considered diagnostic for myocardial infarction or coronary artery bypass surgery; read and spoke English; had a telephone; and lived within 50 miles of the medical center.

Quantitative researchers sample from an accessible population in the hope of generalizing to a target population. The **target population** is the entire population in which a researcher is interested. The **accessible population** is composed of cases from the target population that are accessible to the researcher as study participants. For example, the researcher's target population might be all diabetic patients in the United States, but, in reality, the population that is accessible might be diabetic patients in a particular clinic.

> **TIP**
>
> A key issue for the development of an evidence-based practice is information about the populations on whom research has been conducted. Many quantitative researchers fail to identify their target population, or discuss the issue of the generalizability of the results. Researchers should carefully communicate their populations so that users will know whether the findings are relevant to groups with whom they work.

Samples and Sampling

Sampling is the process of selecting a portion of the population to represent the entire population (Figure 12.1). A **sample** is a subset of population elements. In nursing research, the *elements* (basic units) are usually humans. Researchers work with samples rather than with populations because it is more economical and practical to do so.

Information from samples can, however, lead to erroneous conclusions, and this is especially a concern in quantitative studies. In quantitative studies, a key criterion of adequacy is a sample's representativeness. A **representative sample** is one whose main characteristics closely approximate those of the population. Unfortunately, there is no method for ensuring that a sample is representative. Some sampling plans are less likely to result in biased samples than others, but there is never a guarantee of a representative sample. Researchers operate under conditions in which error is possible, but quantitative researchers strive to minimize or control those errors. Consumers must assess their success in having done so—their success in minimizing sampling bias.

Sampling bias is the systematic overrepresentation or underrepresentation of some segment of the population in terms of a characteristic relevant to the research question. Sampling bias is affected by many things, including the homogeneity of the population. If the elements in a population were all identical on the critical attribute, any sample would be as good as any other. Indeed, if the population were

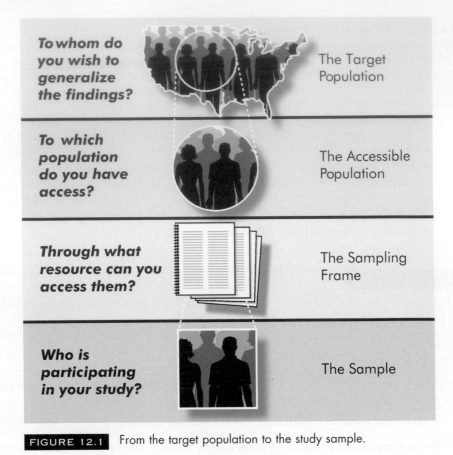

To whom do you wish to generalize the findings?	The Target Population
To which population do you have access?	The Accessible Population
Through what resource can you access them?	The Sampling Frame
Who is participating in your study?	The Sample

FIGURE 12.1 From the target population to the study sample.

completely homogeneous (i.e., exhibited no variability at all), a single element would be a sufficient sample for drawing conclusions about the population. For many physical or physiologic attributes, it may be safe to assume a reasonable degree of homogeneity. For example, the blood in a person's veins is relatively homogeneous, and so a single blood sample chosen haphazardly from a patient is adequate for clinical purposes. Most human attributes, however, are not homogeneous. Variables, after all, derive their name from the fact that traits vary from one person to the next. Age, blood pressure, and stress level are all attributes that reflect the heterogeneity of humans.

Strata

Populations consist of subpopulations, or **strata**. Strata are mutually exclusive segments of a population based on a specific characteristic. For instance, a population consisting of all RNs in the United States could be divided into two strata based on gender. Alternatively, we could specify three strata consisting of nurses younger than 30 years of age, nurses aged 30 to 45 years, and nurses 46 years or older. Strata are often used in sample selection to enhance the sample's representativeness.

> **TIP**
>
> The sampling plan is usually discussed in a report's Method section, sometimes in a subsection called "Sample" or "Study participants." Sample characteristics, however, may be described in the "Results" section. If researchers have performed an analysis of sample biases, these may be described in either the "Method" or "Results" section. For example, researchers might compare the characteristics of patients who were invited to participate in the study but who declined to do so with those of patients who actually became subjects.

SAMPLING DESIGNS IN QUANTITATIVE STUDIES

The two main sampling design issues in quantitative studies are how the sample is selected and how many elements are included. The two broad types of sampling designs in quantitative research are (1) probability sampling and (2) nonprobability sampling.

Nonprobability Sampling

In **nonprobability sampling**, researchers select elements by nonrandom methods. There is no way to estimate the probability of including each element in a nonprobability sample, and every element usually does not have a chance for inclusion. Nonprobability sampling is less likely than probability sampling to produce representative samples, yet most research samples in nursing and other disciplines are nonprobability samples. Four primary methods of nonprobability sampling in quantitative studies are convenience, quota, consecutive and purposive.

Convenience Sampling

Convenience sampling entails using the most conveniently available people as participants. A nurse who distributes questionnaires about vitamin use to the first 100 available community-dwelling elders is sampling by convenience. The problem with convenience sampling is that available subjects might be atypical of the population, and so the price of convenience is the risk of bias.

Snowball sampling (also called *network sampling* or *chain sampling*) is a variant of convenience sampling. With this approach, early sample members are asked to refer other people who meet the eligibility criteria. This method is most often used when the population is people with characteristics who might be difficult to identify (e.g., people who are afraid of hospitals).

Convenience sampling is the weakest form of sampling. It is also the most commonly used sampling method in many disciplines. In heterogeneous populations, there is no other sampling approach in which the risk of sampling bias is greater.

Example of a convenience sample:
Fraser and Polito (2007) compared the self-efficacy of men versus women with multiple sclerosis (MS). They used a convenience sample of 556 individuals with MS.

Quota Sampling

In **quota sampling**, researchers identify population strata and determine how many participants are needed from each stratum. By using information about population characteristics, researchers can ensure that diverse segments are adequately represented in the sample.

As an example, suppose we were interested in studying the attitudes of undergraduate nursing students toward working on an acquired immunodeficiency syndrome (AIDS) unit. The accessible population is a nursing school with an enrollment of 500 undergraduates; a sample size of 100 students is desired. With a convenience sample, we could distribute questionnaires to 100 students as they entered the nursing school library. Suppose, however, that we suspect that male and female students have different attitudes toward working with AIDS victims. A convenience sample might result in too many men, or too few. Table 12.1 presents some fictitious data showing the gender distribution for the population and for a convenience sample (second and third columns). In this example, the convenience sample seriously overrepresents women and underrepresents men. In a quota sample, researchers can guide the selection of subjects so that the sample includes an appropriate number of cases from both strata. The far-right panel of Table 12.1 shows the number of men and women required for a quota sample for this example.

If we pursue this same example a bit further, you may better appreciate the dangers of a biased sample. Suppose the key question in this study was, "Would you be willing to work on a unit that cared exclusively for AIDS patients?" The percentage of students in the population who would respond "yes" to this inquiry is shown in the second column of Table 12.2. Of course, we would not know these values; they are displayed to illustrate a point. Within the population, men were more likely than women to be willing to work on a unit with AIDS patients, yet men were not well represented in the convenience sample. As a result, there is a notable discrepancy between the population and sample values on the outcome variable: Nearly twice as many students in the population were favorable toward working with AIDS victims (20%) than we would conclude based on results from the convenience sample (11%). The quota sample, on the other hand, did a better job of reflecting the viewpoint of the population (19%). In actual research situations, the distortions from a convenience sample may be smaller than in this example, but could be larger as well.

TABLE 12.1	NUMBERS AND PERCENTAGES OF STUDENTS IN STRATA OF A POPULATION, CONVENIENCE SAMPLE, AND QUOTA SAMPLE		
STRATA	POPULATION	CONVENIENCE SAMPLE	QUOTA SAMPLE
Male	100 (20%)	5 (5%)	20 (20%)
Female	400 (80%)	95 (95%)	80 (80%)
Total	500 (100%)	100 (100%)	100 (100%)

	POPULATION	CONVENIENCE SAMPLE	QUOTA SAMPLE
TABLE 12.2 STUDENTS WILLING TO WORK ON AIDS UNIT, IN THE POPULATION, CONVENIENCE SAMPLE, AND QUOTA SAMPLE			
Males (Number)	28	2	6
Females (Number)	72	9	13
Total number of willing students	100	11	19
Total number of all students	500	100	100
Percentage willing	20%	11%	19%

Except for identifying key strata, quota sampling is procedurally similar to convenience sampling: subjects are a convenience sample from each population stratum. Because of this fact, quota sampling shares many of the weaknesses of convenience sampling. For instance, if we were required by the quota sampling plan to interview 20 male nursing students, a trip to the dormitories might be a convenient method of recruiting those subjects. Yet, this approach would fail to give any representation to male students living off campus, who may have distinctive views about working with AIDS patients. Despite its problems, however, quota sampling is an important improvement over convenience sampling for quantitative studies. Quota sampling is a relatively easy way to enhance the representativeness of a nonprobability sample, and does not require sophisticated skills or a lot of effort. Surprisingly, few researchers use this strategy.

Example of a quota sample:
Pieper and colleagues (2006) used quota sampling in their study of chronic venous insufficiency (CVI) in person who were HIV positive and the extent to which neuropathy increased the risk of CVI. They stratified their sample on the basis of whether or not the person had a history of injection drug use, and enrolled participants until the quotas were filled.

Consecutive Sampling
Consecutive sampling involves recruiting *all* of the people from an accessible population who meet the eligibility criteria over a specific time interval, or for a specified sample size. For example, in a study of ventilated-associated pneumonia in ICU patients, if the accessible population were patients in an ICU of a specific hospital, a consecutive sample might consist of all eligible patients who were admitted to that ICU over a 6-month period. Or it might be the first 250 eligible patients admitted to the ICU, if 250 were the targeted sample size.

Consecutive sampling is a far better approach than sampling by convenience, especially if the sampling period is sufficiently long to deal with potential biases that reflect seasonal or other time-related fluctuations. When all members of an accessible population are invited to participate in a study over a fixed time period, the risk of bias is greatly reduced. Consecutive sampling is often the best possible choice when there is "rolling enrollment" into an accessible population.

Example of a consecutive sample:
O'Meara and colleagues (2008) conducted a study to evaluate factors associated with interruptions in enteral nutrition in mechanically ventilated critically ill patients. A consecutive sample of 59 ICU patients who required mechanical ventilation and were receiving enteral nutrition participated in the study.

Purposive Sampling

Purposive sampling or *judgmental sampling* is based on the belief that researchers' knowledge about the population can be used to hand-pick sample members. Researchers might decide purposely to select subjects who are judged to be typical of the population or particularly knowledgeable about the issues under study. Sampling in this subjective manner, however, provides no external, objective method for assessing the typicalness of the selected subjects. Nevertheless, this method can be used to advantage in certain situations. For example, purposive sampling is often used when researchers want a sample of experts. Also, as discussed later in this chapter, purposive sampling is often used productively by qualitative researchers.

Example of purposive sampling:
Van den Heede and colleagues (2007) assessed the views of an international panel of experts regarding the state of nurse staffing and patient outcomes research. Two rounds of surveys were conducted with a purposively selected sample of researchers and nurse administrators from 10 countries.

Evaluation of Nonprobability Sampling

Nonprobability samples are rarely representative of the population. When every element in the population does not have a chance of being included in the sample, it is likely that some segment of it will be systematically underrepresented. And, when there is sampling bias, there is always a chance that the results could be misleading. Why, then, are nonprobability samples used in most nursing studies? Clearly, the advantages of these sampling designs lie in their convenience and economy. Probability sampling requires skill and resources. There is often no option but to use a nonprobability approach. Quantitative researchers using nonprobability samples must be cautious about the inferences and conclusions drawn from the data, and you as a reader should be alert to the possibility of sampling bias.

> **HOW-TO-TELL TIP**
>
> How can you tell what type of sampling design was used in a quantitative study? Researchers who have made efforts to achieve a representative sample usually describe their sampling design at some length in the method section. If the report is not explicit about the sampling method, it is usually safe to assume that a convenience sample was used.

Probability Sampling

Probability sampling involves the random selection of elements from a population. Random selection should not be (although it often is) confused with random assignment, which was described in connection with experimental designs in Chapter 9. Random assignment refers to the process of allocating subjects to different treatment conditions at random. Random *assignment* has no bearing on how subjects in an experiment were selected in the first place. A **random selection** process is one in which each element in the population has an equal, independent chance of being selected. The four most commonly used probability sampling designs are simple random, stratified random, cluster, and systematic sampling.

Simple Random Sampling

Simple random sampling is the most basic probability sampling design. Because more complex probability sampling designs incorporate features of simple random sampling, the procedures involved are briefly described here so you can understand what is involved.

In simple random sampling, researchers establish a **sampling frame**, the technical name for the list of population elements. If nursing students at the University of Connecticut were the accessible population, then a roster of those students would be the sampling frame. If the population were 500-bed or larger hospitals in Florida, then a list of all such hospitals would be the sampling frame. In practice, a population may be defined in terms of an existing sampling frame. For example, a researcher might use a telephone directory as a sampling frame. In such a case, the population would be defined as community residents with a listed telephone number. After a list of population elements has been developed, the elements are numbered consecutively. A table of random numbers or a computer program is then used to draw, at random, a sample of the desired size.

Samples selected randomly in such a fashion are not subject to researcher biases. There is no *guarantee* that the sample will be representative of the population, but random selection does guarantee that differences between the sample and the population are purely a function of chance. The probability of selecting a markedly deviant sample through random sampling is low, and this probability decreases as the sample size increases.

Simple random sampling is a laborious process. Developing the sampling frame, enumerating all the elements, and selecting the sample elements are time-consuming chores, particularly with a large population. Moreover, it is rarely possible to get a complete listing of population elements; hence, other methods are often used.

Stratified Random Sampling

In **stratified random sampling**, the population is first divided into two or more strata. As with quota sampling, the aim of stratified sampling is to enhance representativeness. Stratified sampling designs subdivide the population into subsets from which elements are selected at random. Stratification is often based on such demographic attributes as age or gender.

Stratifying variables usually divide the population into unequal subpopulations. Researchers may sample either proportionately (in relation to the size of the stratum) or disproportionately. If a population of students in a nursing school in the United States consisted of 10% African Americans, 5% Hispanics, 5% Asians, and 80% whites, a *proportionate sample* of 100 students, stratified on race or ethnicity, would consist of 10, 5, 5, and 80 students from the respective strata. Researchers often use a *disproportionate sample* whenever comparisons between strata of unequal size are desired. In our example, the researcher might select 20 African Americans, 10 Hispanics, 10 Asians, and 60 whites to ensure a more adequate representation of the viewpoints of the racial minorities.

By using stratified random sampling, researchers can sharpen the representativeness of their samples. Stratified sampling may, however, be impossible if information on the stratifying variables is unavailable (e.g., student rosters rarely include information on race and ethnicity). Furthermore, a stratified sample requires even more work than simple random sampling because the sample must be drawn from multiple enumerated listings.

Cluster Sampling

For many populations, it is impossible to get a listing of all elements. For example, the population of full-time nursing students in the United States would be difficult to list and enumerate for the purpose of drawing a simple or stratified random sample. Large-scale surveys almost never use simple or stratified random sampling; they usually rely on cluster sampling.

In **cluster sampling**, there is a successive random sampling of units. The first unit is large groupings, or clusters. In drawing a sample of nursing students, we might first draw a random sample of nursing schools and then draw a random sample of students from those schools. The usual procedure for selecting samples from a general population is to sample successively such administrative units as states, census tracts, and then households. Because of the successive stages in cluster sampling, this approach is often called **multistage sampling**.

For a given number of cases, cluster sampling tends to be less accurate than simple or stratified random sampling. Despite this disadvantage, cluster sampling is more economical and practical than other types of probability sampling, particularly when the population is large and widely dispersed.

Example of cluster or multistage sampling:
Salsberry and Reagan (2007) performed secondary analysis of data from the National Longitudinal Survey of Youth's Child-Mother dataset to examine the relationship between maternal prenatal smoking and weight and their children's subsequent weight in adolescence. The original nationally representative sample of women, first interviewed in 1979, was selected using a multistage design in which administrative units, then households, then people were sampled.

Systematic Sampling

Systematic sampling involves the selection of every kth case from a list, such as every 10th person on a patient list. Systematic sampling designs can be applied in such a way that an essentially random sample is drawn. First, the size of the population is divided by the size of the desired sample to obtain the sampling interval width. The **sampling interval** is the standard distance between the selected elements. For instance, if we wanted a sample of 50 from a population of 5,000, our sampling interval would be 100 (5,000/50 = 100). In other words, every 100th case on the sampling frame would be sampled. Next, the first case would be selected randomly (e.g., by using a table of random numbers). If the random number chosen were 73, the people corresponding to numbers 73, 173, 273, and so forth would be included in the sample. Systematic sampling conducted in this manner is essentially identical to simple random sampling and often is preferable because the same results are obtained in a more convenient manner.

Example of a systematic sample:
Gillespie and colleagues (2007) studied resilience in operating room (OR) nurses. The researchers sent a survey to 1,430 nurses—every other member of the professional association for OR nurses in Australia.

Evaluation of Probability Sampling

Probability sampling is the only viable method of obtaining representative samples. If all the elements in the population have an equal probability of being selected, then the resulting sample is likely to do a good job of representing the population. A further advantage is that probability sampling allows researchers to estimate the magnitude of sampling error. **Sampling error** refers to differences between population values (e.g., the average age of the population) and sample values (e.g., the average age of the sample).

The great drawbacks of probability sampling are its inconvenience and complexity. It is usually beyond the scope of most researchers to sample using a probability design, unless the population is narrowly defined—and if it *is* narrowly defined, probability sampling may seem like "overkill." Probability sampling is the preferred and most respected method of obtaining sample elements, but it is often impractical.

> **TIP**
>
> The quality of the sampling plan is of particular importance in survey research, because the purpose of surveys is to obtain descriptive information about the prevalence or average values for a population. All national surveys, such as the National Health Interview Survey in the United States, use probability samples (usually cluster samples). Probability samples are rarely used in experimental and quasi-experimental studies.

Sample Size in Quantitative Studies

Sample size—the number of subjects in a sample—is a major issue in conducting and evaluating quantitative research. No simple equation can determine how large a sample is needed, but quantitative researchers often strive for the largest sample possible. The larger the sample, the more representative it is likely to be. Every time researchers calculate a percentage or an average based on sample data, the purpose is to estimate a population value. The larger the sample, the smaller the sampling error.

Let us illustrate this with an example of estimating monthly aspirin consumption in a nursing home (Table 12.3). The population is 15 nursing home residents whose aspirin consumption averages 16 per month. Two simple random samples with sample sizes of 2, 3, 5, and 10 were drawn from the population of 15 residents. Each sample average on the right represents an estimate of the population average, which we know is 16. (Under ordinary circumstances, the population value would be unknown, and we would draw only one sample.) With a sample size of 2, our estimate might have been wrong by as many as 8 aspirins (sample 1B). As the sample size increases, the average gets closer to the population value, and differences in the estimates between samples A and B get smaller. As the sample size increases, the probability of getting a deviant sample diminishes because large samples provide the opportunity to counterbalance atypical values.

Researchers can estimate how large their samples should be to adequately test their research hypotheses through **power analysis** (Cohen, 1988). A simple example can illustrate basic principles of power analysis. Suppose a researcher were testing a new intervention to help people quit smoking; smokers would be randomly assigned to either an experimental or a control group. The question is, "How many subjects should be used in this study?" When using power analysis, researchers estimate how large the group difference will be (e.g., the difference in the average

TABLE 12.3	COMPARISON OF POPULATION AND SAMPLE VALUES AND AVERAGES: NURSING HOME ASPIRIN CONSUMPTION EXAMPLE		
NUMBER IN GROUP	GROUP	VALUES (INDIVIDUAL NUMBER OF ASPIRINS CONSUMED)	AVERAGE
15	Population	2, 4, 6, 8, 10, 12, 14, 16, 18, 20, 22, 24 26, 28, 30	16.0
2	Sample 1A	6, 14	10.0
2	Sample 1B	20, 28	24.0
3	Sample 2A	16, 18, 8	14.0
3	Sample 2B	20, 14, 26	20.0
5	Sample 3A	26, 14, 18, 2, 28	17.6
5	Sample 3B	30, 2, 26, 10, 4	14.4
10	Sample 4A	22, 16, 24, 20, 28, 14, 28, 20, 4	15.8
10	Sample 4B	12, 18, 8, 10, 16, 6, 28, 14, 30, 22	16.4

number of cigarettes smoked in the week after the intervention). This estimate might be based on previous research or on a pilot test. When expected differences are large, it does not take a large sample to ensure that the differences will be revealed in a statistical analysis; but when small differences are predicted, large samples are needed. For new areas of research, group differences are likely to be small. In our example, if a small group difference in postintervention smoking were expected, the sample size needed to test the effectiveness of the new program, assuming standard statistical criteria, would be about 800 smokers (400 per group). If medium differences were expected, the total sample size would still need to be several hundred smokers.

Statistical conclusion validity is threatened when samples are too small, and researchers run the risk of gathering data that will not support their hypotheses—even when those hypotheses are correct. Large samples are no assurance of accuracy, however. With nonprobability sampling, even a large sample can harbor extensive bias. The famous example illustrating this point is the 1936 U.S. presidential poll conducted by the magazine *Literary Digest,* which predicted that Alfred M. Landon would defeat Franklin D. Roosevelt by a landslide. A sample of about 2.5 million people participated in this poll, but biases arose because the sample was drawn from telephone directories and automobile registrations during a Depression year when only the well-to-do (who favored Landon) had a car or telephone.

A large sample cannot correct for a faulty sampling design; nevertheless, a large nonprobability sample is preferable to a small one. When critiquing quantitative studies, you must assess both the sample size and the sample selection method to judge how representative the sample likely was.

> **TIP**
>
> The sampling plan is often one of the weakest aspects of quantitative studies. Most nursing studies use samples of convenience, and many are based on samples that are too small to provide an adequate test of the research hypotheses. Power analysis is not used by many nurse researchers, and research reports typically offer no justification for the size of the study sample. Small samples run a high risk of leading researchers to erroneously reject their research hypotheses. Therefore, you should be especially prepared to critique the sampling plan of studies that fail to support research hypotheses.

SAMPLING IN QUALITATIVE RESEARCH

Qualitative studies almost always use small, nonrandom samples. This does not mean that qualitative researchers are unconcerned with the quality of their samples, but rather that they use different considerations in selecting study participants.

The Logic of Qualitative Sampling

Quantitative research is concerned with measuring attributes and relationships in a population, and therefore a representative sample is desirable so that the findings can be generalized to the population. The aim of most qualitative studies is to discover *meaning* and to uncover multiple realities, and so generalizability is not a guiding consideration.

Qualitative researchers ask such sampling questions as: "Who would be an information-rich data source for my study?" "To whom should I talk, or what should I observe, to maximize my understanding of the phenomenon?" A critical first step in qualitative sampling is selecting settings with high potential for information richness.

As the study progresses, new sampling questions emerge, such as the following: "Whom can I talk to or observe who would (1) confirm my understandings; (2) challenge or modify my understandings; or (3) enrich my understandings?" Thus, as with the overall design in qualitative studies, sampling design is an emergent one that capitalizes on early information to guide subsequent direction.

> **TIP**
>
> As with quantitative researchers, qualitative researchers often identify eligibility criteria for their studies. Although they do not articulate an explicit population to whom results are intended to be generalized, qualitative researchers do establish the kinds of people who are eligible to participate in their research.

Types of Qualitative Sampling

Qualitative researchers usually eschew probability samples. A random sample is not the best method of selecting people who will make good informants, that is, people who are knowledgeable, articulate, reflective, and willing to talk at length with researchers. Various nonprobability sampling designs have been used by qualitative researchers.

Convenience and Snowball Sampling

Qualitative researchers often begin with a convenience sample, which is sometimes referred to as a *volunteer sample*. Volunteer samples are especially likely to be used when researchers need to have potential participants come forward and identify themselves. For example, if we wanted to study the experiences of people with frequent nightmares, we might have difficulty readily identifying potential participants. In such a situation, we might recruit sample members by placing a notice on a bulletin board, in a newspaper, or on the Internet, requesting people with nightmares to contact us. In this situation, we would be less interested in obtaining a representative sample of people with nightmares, than in obtaining a diverse group representing various experiences with nightmares.

Sampling by convenience is often efficient, but it is not usually a preferred sampling approach, even in qualitative studies. The key aim in qualitative studies is to extract the greatest possible information from the small number of informants in the sample, and a convenience sample may not provide the most information-rich sources. However, convenience sample may be an economical way to begin the sampling process.

Example of a convenience sample:

Woodman and Radzyminski (2007) explored the experiences of women following breast reduction surgery. A convenience sample of nine women was recruited during their follow-up visits.

Qualitative researchers also use snowball sampling, asking early informants to make referrals for other study participants. This method is sometimes referred to as *nominated sampling* because it relies on the nominations of others already in the sample. A weakness of this approach is that the eventual sample might be restricted to a rather small network of acquaintances. Moreover, the quality of the referrals may be affected by whether the referring sample member trusted the researcher and truly wanted to cooperate.

Example of a snowball sample:

Yu (2007) explored the influence of the Chinese culture on attitudes toward sexual behavior among British-born Chinese teenagers. Snowball sampling was used to identify 20 teenagers and their Chinese-born parents.

Purposive Sampling

Qualitative sampling may begin with volunteer informants and may be supplemented with new participants through snowballing, but many qualitative studies eventually evolve to a purposive (or *purposeful*) sampling strategy—to a strategy in which researchers deliberately choose the cases or types of cases that will best contribute to the information needs of the study. That is, regardless of how initial participants are selected, qualitative researchers often strive to select sample members purposefully based on the information needs emerging from the early findings. Who to sample next depends on who has been sampled already.

Within purposive sampling, several strategies have been identified (Patton, 2002), only some of which are mentioned here. Note that researchers themselves do not necessarily refer to their sampling plans with Patton's labels; his classification shows the kind of diverse strategies qualitative researchers have adopted to meet the conceptual needs of their research:

➤ **Maximum variation sampling** involves deliberately selecting cases with a wide range of variation on dimensions of interest.

➤ *Extreme (deviant) case sampling* provides opportunities for learning from the most unusual and extreme informants (e.g., outstanding successes and notable failures).

➤ *Typical case sampling* involves the selection of participants who illustrate or highlight what is typical or average.

➤ *Criterion sampling* involves studying cases who meet a predetermined criterion of importance.

Maximum variation sampling is often the sampling mode of choice in qualitative research because it is useful in documenting the scope of a phenomenon and in identifying important patterns that cut across variations. Other strategies can also be used advantageously, however, depending on the nature of the research question.

Example of maximum variation sampling:
Spilsbury and colleagues (2007) performed an in-depth study of patients' perceptions of the effect of pressure ulcers on their quality of life. The sample of 23 patients was deliberately selected to be varied in terms of gender, age, type of ward, reasons for hospital admission, and anatomical site of the pressure ulcer.

> **TIP**
> A qualitative research report will not necessary use such terms as "maximum variation sampling," but may describe the researcher's efforts to select a diverse sample of participants.

A strategy of sampling confirming and disconfirming cases is another purposive strategy that is often used toward the end of data collection in qualitative studies. As researchers note trends and patterns in the data, emerging conceptualizations may need to be checked. **Confirming cases** are additional cases that fit researchers' conceptualizations and strengthen credibility. **Disconfirming cases** are new cases that do not fit and serve to challenge researchers' interpretations. These "negative" cases may offer new insights about how the original conceptualization needs to be revised or expanded.

> **TIP**
>
> Some qualitative researchers appear to call their sample *purposive* simply because they "purposely" selected people who experienced the phenomenon of interest. However, exposure to the phenomenon is an eligibility criterion—the population of interest is composed of people with that exposure. If the researcher then recruits *any* person with the desired experience, the sample is selected by convenience, not purposively. Purposive sampling implies an intent to carefully choose *particular* exemplars or *types* of people who can best enhance the researcher's understanding of the phenomenon.

Theoretical Sampling

Theoretical sampling is a method of sampling that is most often used in grounded theory studies. Theoretical sampling involves decisions about what data to collect next and where to find those data to develop an emerging theory optimally. The basic question in theoretical sampling is: "What groups or subgroups should the researcher turn to next?" (Glaser, 1978). Groups are chosen as they are needed for their relevance in furthering the emerging conceptualization. These groups are not chosen before the research begins but only as they are needed for their theoretical relevance in developing further emerging categories.

Theoretical sampling is not the same as purposeful sampling. The objective of theoretical sampling is to discover categories and their properties and to offer new insights about interrelationships that occur in the substantive theory.

Example of a theoretical sampling:
Crigger and Meek (2007) used theoretical sampling in their grounded theory study of the process that occurs after nurses perceive that they have made a mistake in their clinical practice. After interviewing and analyzing data from their first three respondents, the researchers realized the theoretical importance of nurses' decision to stay in hospital practice. They specifically sought to include in their sample nurses who no longer practiced in hospital settings.

Sample Size in Qualitative Research

There are no rules for sample size in qualitative research—sample size is usually determined based on informational needs. Hence, a guiding principle in sampling is **data saturation**—that is, sampling to the point at which no new information is obtained and redundancy is achieved. Morse (2000) has noted that the number of participants needed to reach saturation depends on a number of factors. For example, the broader the scope of the research question, the more participants will likely be needed. Data quality can also affect sample size. If participants are good informants who are able to reflect on their experiences and communicate effectively, saturation can be achieved with a relatively small sample. Also, if longitudinal data are collected, fewer participants may be needed, because each will provide a greater amount of information. Type of sampling strategy may also be relevant. For example, a larger sample is likely to be needed with maximum variation sampling than with typical case sampling. Sample size also depends on the type of qualitative inquiry, as discussed next.

Sampling in the Three Main Qualitative Traditions

There are similarities among the various qualitative traditions with regard to sampling: samples are usually small, probability sampling is not used, and final sampling decisions usually take place in the field during data collection. However, there are some differences as well.

Sampling in Ethnography

Ethnographers may begin by initially adopting a "big net" approach—that is, mingling with and having conversations with as many members of the culture under study as possible. Although they may converse with many people (usually 25 to 50), ethnographers often rely heavily on a smaller number of **key informants**, who are highly knowledgeable about the culture and who develop special, ongoing relationships with the researcher. These key informants are often the researcher's main link to the "inside."

Key informants are chosen purposively, guided by the ethnographer's informed judgments, although sampling may become more theoretical as the study progresses. Developing a pool of potential key informants often depends on ethnographers' ability to construct a relevant framework. For example, an ethnographer might decide to seek out different types of key informants based on their *roles* (e.g., health care practitioners, advocates). Once a pool of potential key informants is developed, key considerations for final selection are their level of knowledge about the culture and how willing they are to collaborate with the ethnographer in revealing and interpreting the culture.

Sampling in ethnography typically involves more than selecting informants. To understand a culture, ethnographers have to decide not only *whom* to sample, but *what* to sample as well. For example, ethnographers make decisions about observing *events* and *activities*, about examining *records* and *artifacts*, and about exploring *places* that provide clues about the culture. Key informants can play an important role in helping ethnographers decide what to sample.

Example of an ethnographic sample:

Sobralske (2006) conducted an ethnographic study exploring health care seeking beliefs and behaviors of Mexican American men living in Washington state. The researchers participated in activities within the Mexican American community, and then recruited participants through community organizations, religious groups, schools, and personal contacts. The sample consisted of eight key informants who varied in terms of acculturation, occupation, educational levels, and interests. The sample also included 28 secondary research participants, who were men and women with insight into health care seeking beliefs and actions of Mexican American men. The secondary participants helped to validate the findings from the key informants.

Sampling in Phenomenological Studies

Phenomenologists tend to rely on very small samples of participants—typically 10 or fewer. There is one guiding principle in selecting the sample for a phenomenological study: all participants must have experienced the phenomenon and must be able to articulate what it is like to have lived that experience. Although phenomenological researchers seek participants who have had the targeted experiences, they also want to explore diversity of individual experiences. Thus, they may specifically look for people with demographic or other differences who have shared a common experience.

Example of a sample in a phenomenological study:
Sigurgeirsdottir and Halldorsdottir (2008) studied the existential struggle, needs, and experiences of patients in rehabilitation. Their purposive sample of 12 patients spanning an age range from 26 to 85 years and included men and women and patients with chronic and acute problems.

Interpretive phenomenologists may, in addition to sampling people, sample artistic or literary sources. Experiential descriptions of the phenomenon may be selected from a wide array of literature, such as poetry, novels, biographies, autobiographies, diaries, and journals. These sources can help increase phenomenologists' insights into the phenomena under study. Art—including paintings, sculpture, film, photographs, and music—is viewed as another source of lived experience. Each artistic medium is viewed as having its own specific language or way of expressing the experience of the phenomenon.

Sampling in Grounded Theory Studies

Grounded theory research is typically done with samples of about 20 to 40 people, using theoretical sampling. The goal in a grounded theory study is to select informants who can best contribute to the evolving theory. Sampling, data collection, data analysis, and theory construction occur concurrently, and so study participants are selected serially and contingently (i.e., contingent on the emerging conceptualization). Sampling might evolve as follows:

1. The researcher begins with a general notion of where and with whom to start. The first few cases may be solicited purposively, by convenience, or through snowballing.

2. In the early part of the study, a strategy such as maximum variation sampling might be used to gain insights into the range and complexity of the phenomenon under study.

3. The sample is adjusted in an ongoing fashion. Emerging conceptualizations help to inform the sampling process.

4. Sampling continues until saturation is achieved.

5. Final sampling often includes a search for confirming and disconfirming cases to test, refine, and strengthen the theory.

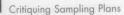

Example of sampling in a grounded theory study:
Montgomery and colleagues (2006) performed a grounded theory study of mothering while receiving treatment for serious mental illness. The sample consisted of 21 mothers receiving professional mental health treatment. After the first eight interviews were completed, the researchers used theoretical sampling to capture the range of mothering experiences—for example, they specifically sought to interview women who did not live with their children.

CRITIQUING SAMPLING PLANS

In coming to conclusions about the quality of evidence that a study yields, the sampling plan—particularly for a quantitative study—merits special scrutiny. If the sample is seriously biased or too small, the findings may be misleading or just plain wrong.

In critiquing a description of a sampling plan, you should consider two issues. The first is whether the researcher has adequately described the sampling strategy. Ideally, research reports should include a description of the following:

➤ The type of sampling approach used (e.g., convenience, snowball, purposive, simple random)

➤ The population under study and the eligibility criteria for sample selection in quantitative studies; the nature of the setting and study group in qualitative ones (qualitative studies may also articulate eligibility criteria);

➤ The number of participants in the study and a rationale for the sample size

➤ A description of the main characteristics of participants (e.g., age, gender, medical condition, and so forth)

➤ In quantitative studies, the number and characteristics of potential subjects who declined to participate in the study.

If the description of the sample is inadequate, you may not be in a position to deal with the second and principal issue, which is whether the researcher made good sampling decisions. And, if the description is incomplete, it will be difficult to draw conclusions about whether the evidence can be applied in your clinical practice.

Critiquing Quantitative Sampling Plans

The sampling plan in a quantitative study should be scrutinized with respect to its effects on the various types of study validity. If a sample is small, statistical conclusion validity will likely be undermined. If the eligibility criteria are tightly constrained, this could benefit internal validity—but probably to the detriment of external validity.

As noted earlier, a key criterion for assessing the adequacy of a sampling plan in quantitative research is whether the sample is representative of the population.

You will never know for sure, of course, but if the sampling strategy is weak or if the sample size is small, there is reason to suspect some bias. When researchers have adopted a sampling plan in which the risk for bias is high, they should take steps to estimate the direction and degree of this bias so that readers can draw some informed conclusions.

Even with a rigorous sampling plan, the sample may contain some bias if not all people invited to participate in a study agree to do so. If certain segments of the population refuse to participate, then a biased sample can result, even when probability sampling is used. The research report ideally should provide information about **response rates** (i.e., the number of people participating in a study relative to the number of people sampled), and about possible **nonresponse bias**—differences between participants and those who declined to participate (also sometimes referred to as *response bias*). In a longitudinal study, attrition bias should be reported.

In developing the sampling plan, quantitative researchers make decisions about the specification of the population as well as the selection of the sample. If the target population is defined broadly, researchers may have missed opportunities to control confounding variables, and the gap between the accessible and the target population may be too great. Your job as reviewer is to come to conclusions about the reasonableness of generalizing the findings from the researcher's sample to the accessible population and from the accessible population to a broader target population. If the sampling plan is seriously flawed, it may be risky to generalize the findings at all without replicating the study with another sample.

Box 12.1 presents some guiding questions for critiquing the sampling plan of a quantitative research report. ✖

BOX 12.1 GUIDELINES FOR CRITIQUING QUANTITATIVE SAMPLING DESIGNS

1. Is the population under study identified and described? Are eligibility criteria specified? Are the sample selection procedures clearly delineated?
2. What type of sampling plan was used? Would an alternative sampling plan have been preferable? Was the sampling plan one that could be expected to yield a representative sample?
3. How were subjects recruited into the sample? Does the method suggest potential biases?
4. Did some factor other than the sampling plan (e.g., a low response rate) affect the representativeness of the sample?
5. Are possible sample biases or weaknesses identified?
6. Are key characteristics of the sample described (e.g., mean age, percent female)?
7. Is the sample size sufficiently large to support statistical conclusion validity? Was the sample size justified on the basis of a power analysis or other rationale?
8. Does the sample support inferences about external validity? To whom can the study results reasonably be generalized?

Critiquing Qualitative Sampling Plans

In a qualitative study, the sampling plan can be evaluated in terms of its adequacy and appropriateness (Morse, 1991). *Adequacy* refers to the sufficiency and quality of the data the sample yielded. An adequate sample provides data without any "thin" spots. When researchers have truly obtained saturation, informational adequacy has been achieved, and the resulting description or theory is richly textured and complete.

Appropriateness concerns the methods used to select a sample. An appropriate sample is one resulting from the identification and use of study participants who can best supply information according to the conceptual requirements of the study. Researchers must use a strategy that will yield the fullest possible understanding of the phenomenon of interest. A sampling approach that excludes negative cases or that fails to include participants with unusual experiences may not meet the information needs of the study.

Another important issue to consider concerns the potential for transferability of the findings. The degree of transferability of study findings is a direct function of the similarity between the sample of the original study and the people at another site to which the findings might be applied. *Fittingness* is the degree of congruence between these two groups. Thus, in critiquing a report, you should see whether the researcher provided an adequately thick description of the sample and the context in which the study was carried out so that someone interested in transferring the findings could make an informed decision.

Further guidance in critiquing qualitative sampling decisions is presented in Box 12.2.

BOX 12.2 GUIDELINES FOR CRITIQUING QUALITATIVE SAMPLING DESIGNS

1. Is the setting or context adequately described? Is the setting appropriate for the research question?

2. Are the sample selection procedures clearly delineated? What type of sampling strategy was used?

3. Were the eligibility criteria for the study specified? How were participants recruited into the study? Did the recruitment strategy yield information-rich participants?

4. Given the information needs of the study—and, if applicable, its qualitative tradition— was the sampling approach appropriate? Are dimensions of the phenomenon under study adequately represented?

5. Is the sample size adequate and appropriate for the qualitative tradition of the study? Did the researcher indicate that saturation had been achieved? Do the findings suggest a richly textured and comprehensive set of data without any apparent "holes" or thin areas?

6. Are key characteristics of the sample described (e.g., age, gender)? Is a rich description of participants and context provided, allowing for an assessment of the transferability of the findings?

In the following sections, we describe the sampling plans of two nursing studies, followed by some questions to guide critical thinking.

EXAMPLE 1 ■ Sampling In a Quantitative Study

Study

Quality of life of older adults in Canada and Brazil (Paskulin and Molzahn, 2007).

Purpose

This study examined factors contributing to quality of life (QOL) of older adults in Canada and Brazil. The specific research questions were: "Are there differences in QOL of older adults in selected regions of Brazil and Canada?" "Do such factors as health satisfaction, meaning in life, opportunities for leisure, satisfaction with personal relationships, and adequacy of financial resources contribute to perceptions of QOL in both countries?"

Design

The researchers collected data via a cross-sectional survey. The Canadian survey was completed through mailed questionnaires, whereas the Brazilian survey involved in-home interviews. Participants in both countries completed the short form of the World Health Organization QOL scale (WHOQOL-BREF), an instrument specifically designed to measure quality of life across cultures.

Sampling Plan

Efforts were made to collect data from random samples of older people (age 60 or older) in relatively affluent coastal regions of both countries. Somewhat different strategies were required, however, because the lack of appropriate databases in Brazil made a mail survey there impossible. In Canada, letters inviting participation were mailed to a stratified random sample of older adults listed in the Ministry of Health Services Client Registry in British Columbia. The registry includes names and personal information about all people receiving health care services in the province. Invitations were mailed to 420 people, of whom 251 responded positively and were mailed a questionnaire. In the end, completed questionnaires were returned by 202 people, for a response rate of 48.1%. In Brazil, data were collected through a door-to-door household survey of older adults in the Northwest Health Region of Porto Alegre. To enhance the representativeness of the sample, 100 of 700 streets were randomly selected. After randomly selecting a side and section of each of the 100 streets, three elders from each sampled street segment were sought. A total of 379 elders were invited to participate; 76 refused, 15 were unable to respond to questions in the interview, and 288 completed the survey. The response rate in Brazil was thus 68.4%. The researchers had hoped to achieve a total sample of 300 participants in each country. Although their final sample fell short of this goal, they did a power analysis suggesting that a sample of about 500 people would be adequate for their analysis. The mean age in both countries was about 72, but in other respects the samples differed. For example, there were more men in the Canadian sample (47% versus 33%), more Canadians than Brazilians were married or partnered (66% versus 47%), and the Canadian respondents were better educated.

Key Findings

■ Ratings on overall QOL were higher in the Canadian sample, as were scores on subscales measuring physical, psychological, and environmental aspects of QOL.

■ Health satisfaction was the strongest contributor to QOL in both countries.

CRITICAL THINKING SUGGESTIONS*:

*See the Student Resource CD-ROM for a discussion of these questions.

1. Answer the relevant questions from Box 12.1 regarding this study.
2. Also, consider the following targeted questions, which may further sharpen your critical thinking skills and assist you in understanding this study:
   a. The report did not specifically note what the stratifying variables were for the Canadian sample selection. What might you recommend, assuming that basic demographic information was available?
   b. The report did not mention whether the stratified random sampling of Canadians was proportionate or disproportionate. What would you recommend?
   c. Why do you think the response rate was higher in Brazil than in Canada?
   d. Identify some of the major potential sources of bias in the final samples of Canadians and Brazilians.
   e. How might demographic differences in the two countries have affected the QOL results?
3. If the results of this study are valid and reliable, what might be some of the uses to which the findings could be put in clinical practice?

EXAMPLE 2 ■ Sampling in a Qualitative Study

Study

Relational patterns of couples living with chronic pelvic pain from endometriosis (Butt and Chesla, 2007).

Research Purpose

This study investigated responses in couples' relationships in living with chronic pelvic pain from the women's diagnosed endometriosis.

Method

Butt and Chesla conducted their inquiry within the tradition of interpretive phenomenology. A sample of women and their partners were interviewed in depth to explore the participants' illness understanding, symptom experience, and relational responses to the disease. Each partner was interviewed separately, and then joint interviews were conducted about 4 weeks later. Interviews lasted up to 2 hours each.

Sampling Plan

The sample was composed of 13 women in a partnered or married relationship who had experienced pelvic pain from endometriosis for at least 6 months, and their partners. To be included, the women had to speak English, be at least 18 years of age, and had to have lived with their partners for at least a year. Recruitment was specifically designed to enlist participants from diverse treatment sites, socioeconomic groups, and ethnicities. Participants were recruited from public and private treatment providers and clinics, and in informational and support groups for endometriosis. Interested parties responded to informational flyers via telephone, and arrangements were made to discuss the details of the study and to obtain consent. All 13 women and their partners participated in individual and joint interviews. Recruitment stopped after extensive data had been gathered in the 39 interviews and when the researchers found "repetitive patterns and themes" in their data. The sample included women, aged 23 to 48, who had lived with their partners between 1 and 23 years. Two had children. About 60% of the women were European Americans, and 92% were employed for pay. Nearly half the sample had annual household incomes in excess of $100,000.

Key Findings

- The results suggested that living with chronic pelvic pain from endometriosis was a physically and emotionally difficult and painful experience for the couples.
- Five different patterns of relationships were observed: (1) together but alone; (2) battling endometriosis together; (3) conjoined through disability; (4) totalized by caregiving; and (5) engaged in mutual care.

CRITICAL THINKING SUGGESTIONS:

1. Answer the relevant questions from Box 12.2 regarding this study.
2. Also, consider the following targeted questions, which may further sharpen your critical thinking skills and assist you in understanding this study:
    a. Do you think it was a strength or weakness of the sampling plan to use different treatment sites to recruit participants? Why?
    b. According to the eligibility criteria, would same-sex partners have been eligible for this study?
    c. Comment on the variation the researchers achieved in type of study participants.
3. If the results of this study are valid and trustworthy, what might be some of the uses to which the findings could be put in clinical practice?

EXAMPLE 3 ■ Sampling in the Quantitative Study in Appendix A

1. Read the method section from Howell and colleagues' (2007) study ("Anxiety, anger, and blood pressure in children") in Appendix A of this book, and then answer the relevant questions in Box 12.1.
2. Also, consider the following targeted questions, which may further sharpen your critical thinking skills and assist you in assessing aspects of the study's merit:
    a. What type of sampling plan might have improved the representativeness of the sample in this study?
    b. Identify some of the major potential sources of bias in the sample.

EXAMPLE 4 ■ Sampling in the Qualitative Study in Appendix B

1. Read the method section from Beck's (2006) study ("The anniversary of birth trauma") in Appendix B of this book, and then answer the relevant questions in Box 12.2.
2. Also, consider the following targeted questions, which may further sharpen your critical thinking skills and assist you in assessing aspects of the study's merit:
    a. Comment on the characteristics of the participants, given the purpose of the study.
    b. Comment on Beck's statements (in the section labeled "Procedure") regarding response rates.
    c. Do you think that Beck should have limited her sample to women from one country only? Provide a rationale for your answer.

CHAPTER REVIEW

Key new terms introduced in the chapter, together with a summary of major points, are presented in this section. In addition, Chapter 12 of the accompanying *Study Guide for Essentials of Nursing Research,* 7th edition offers various exercises and study suggestions for reinforcing concepts presented in this chapter. For additional review, see the Student Self-Study Review Questions section of the Student Resource CD-ROM provided with this book.

Key New Terms

Accessible population	Population	Sampling error
Cluster sampling	Power analysis	Simple random sampling
Consecutive sampling	Probability sampling	Snowball sampling
Convenience sampling	Purposive (purposeful)	Strata
Data saturation	sampling	Stratified random
Eligibility criteria	Quota sampling	sampling
Maximum variation	Response rate	Systematic sampling
sampling	Sample size	Target population
Nonprobability sampling	Sampling	Theoretical sampling
Nonresponse bias	Sampling bias	

Summary Points

➤ **Sampling** is the process of selecting a portion of the **population**, which is an entire aggregate of cases. An **element** is the basic unit of a population about which information is collected—usually humans in nursing research.

➤ **Eligibility criteria** (including both **inclusion criteria** and **exclusion criteria**) are used to define population characteristics.

➤ Researchers usually sample from an **accessible population**, but should identify the **target population** to which they would like to generalize their results.

➤ A key consideration in assessing a sample in a quantitative study is its **representativeness**—the extent to which the sample is similar to the population and avoids bias. **Sampling bias** refers to the systematic overrepresentation or underrepresentation of some segment of the population.

➤ The principal types of **nonprobability sampling** (wherein elements are selected by nonrandom methods) are convenience, quota, consecutive, and purposive sampling. Nonprobability sampling designs are convenient and economical; a major disadvantage is their potential for bias.

➤ **Convenience sampling** uses the most readily available or most convenient group of people for the sample. **Snowball sampling** is a type of convenience sampling in which referrals for potential participants are made by those already in the sample.

➤ **Quota sampling** divides the population into homogeneous **strata** (subpopulations) to ensure representation of the subgroups in the sample; within each stratum, subjects are sampled by convenience.

➤ **Consecutive sampling** involves taking *all* of the people from an accessible population who meet the eligibility criteria over a specific time interval, or for a specified sample size.

➤ In **purposive** (or *judgmental*) **sampling**, participants are hand-picked to be included in the sample based on the researcher's knowledge about the population.

➤ **Probability sampling** designs, which involve the random selection of elements from the population, yield more representative samples than nonprobability designs and permit estimates of the magnitude of **sampling error**.

➤ **Simple random sampling** involves the random selection of elements from a **sampling frame** that enumerates all the elements; **stratified random sampling** divides the population into homogeneous subgroups from which elements are selected at random.

➤ **Cluster sampling** (or **multistage sampling**) involves the successive selection of random samples from larger to smaller units.

➤ **Systematic sampling** is the selection of every *k*th case from a list. By dividing the population size by the desired sample size, the researcher establishes the **sampling interval**, which is the standard distance between the selected elements.

➤ In quantitative studies, researchers should use a **power analysis** to estimate **sample size** needs. Large samples are preferable to small ones because larger samples enhance statistical conclusion validity and tend to be more representative, but even large sample do not *guarantee* representativeness.

➤ Qualitative researchers use the conceptual demands of the study to select articulate and reflective informants with certain types of experience in an emergent way, capitalizing on early learning to guide subsequent sampling decisions.

➤ Qualitative researchers most often use **purposive sampling** to guide them in selecting data sources that maximize information richness. Various purposive sampling strategies have been used by qualitative researchers.

➤ One purposive strategy is **maximum variation sampling**, which entails purposely selecting cases with a wide range of variation. Another important strategy is **sampling confirming and disconfirming cases** (i.e., selecting cases that enrich and challenge the researchers' conceptualizations).

➤ Other types of purposive sampling include *extreme case sampling* (selecting the most unusual or extreme cases); *typical case sampling* (selecting cases that illustrate what is typical); and *criterion sampling* (studying cases that meet a predetermined criterion of importance).

➤ Samples in qualitative studies are typically small and based on information needs. A guiding principle is **data saturation**, which involves sampling to the point at which no new information is obtained and redundancy is achieved.

➤ Ethnographers make numerous sampling decisions, including not only *who* to sample but *what* to sample (e.g., activities, events, documents, artifacts); decision-making is often aided by their *key informants* who serve as guides and interpreters of the culture.

➤ Phenomenologists typically work with a small sample of people (often 10 or fewer) who meet the criterion of having lived the experience under study.

➤ Grounded theory researchers typically use **theoretical sampling** in which sampling decisions are guided in an ongoing fashion by the emerging theory. Samples of about 20 to 40 people are typical in grounded theory studies.

➤ Criteria for evaluating qualitative sampling are informational adequacy and appropriateness.

STUDIES CITED IN CHAPTER 12

Butt, F. S., & Chesla, C. (2007). Relational patterns of couples living with chronic pelvic pain from endometriosis. *Qualitative Health Research, 17,* 571–585.

Crigger, N., & Meek, V. (2007). Toward a theory of self-reconciliation following mistakes in nursing practice. *Journal of Nursing Scholarship, 39,* 177–183.

Ekwall, A., & Hallberg, I. (2007). The association between caregiving satisfaction, difficulties and coping among older family caregivers. *Journal of Clinical Nursing, 16,* 832–844.

Fraser, C., & Polito, S. (2007). A comparative study of self-efficacy in men and women with multiple sclerosis. *Journal of Neuroscience Nursing, 39,* 102–106.

Gillespie, B., Chaboyer, W., Wallis, M., & Grimbeek, P. (2007). Resilience in the operating room: Developing a testing of a resilience model. *Journal of Advanced Nursing, 59,* 427–438.

Lindgren, T., Fukouka, Y., Rankin, S., Cooper, B., Carroll, D., & Munn, Y. (2008). Cluster analysis of elderly cardiac patients' prehospital symptomatology. *Nursing Research, 57,* 14–23.

Montgomery, P., Tompkins, C., Forchuk, C., & French, S. (2006). Keeping close: Mothering with serious mental illness. *Journal of Advanced Nursing, 54,* 20–28.

Nachreiner, N., Hansen, H., Okano, A., Gerberich, S., Ryan, A., McGovern, P. et al. (2007). Difference in work-related violence by nurse license type. *Journal of Professional Nursing, 23,* 290–300.

O'Meara, D., Mireles-Cabodevila, E., Frame, E., Hummell, A., Hammel, J. Dweik, R. et al. (2008). Evaluation of delivery of enteral nutrition in critically ill patients receiving mechanical ventilation. *American Journal of Critical Care, 17,* 53–61.

Paskulin, L., & Molzahn, A. (2007). Quality of life of older adults in Canada and Brazil. *Western Journal of Nursing Research, 29,* 10–26.

Pieper, B., Templin, T., & Ebright, J. (2006). Chronic venous insufficiency in HIV-positive persons with and without a history of injection drug use. *Advances in Skin & Wound Care, 19,* 37–42.

Salsberry, P., & Reagan, P. (2007). Taking the long view: The prenatal environment and early adolescent overweight. *Research in Nursing & Health, 30,* 297–307.

Sigurgeirsdottir, J., & Halldorsdottir, S. (2008). Existential struggle and self-reported needs of patients in rehabilitation. *Journal of Advanced Nursing, 61,* 384–392.

Sobralske, M.C. (2006). Health care seeking among Mexican American men. *Journal of Transcultural Nursing, 17,* 129–138.

Spilsbury, K., Nelson, A., Cullum, N., Iglesias, C., Nixon, J., & Mason, S. (2007). Pressure ulcers and their treatment and effect on quality of life. *Journal of Advanced Nursing, 57,* 494–504.

Van den Heede, K., Clarke, S., Sermeus, W., Vleugels, A., & Aiken, L. (2007). International experts' perspectives on the state of the nurse staffing and patient outcomes literature. *Journal of Nursing Scholarship, 39,* 290–297.

Woodman, R., & Radzyminski, S. (2007). Women's perception of life following breast reduction. *Plastic Surgical Nursing, 27,* 85–92.

Yu, J. (2007). British-born Chinese teenagers: The influence of Chinese ethnicity on their attitudes toward sexual behavior. *Nursing & Health Sciences, 9,* 69–75.

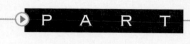

Data Collection

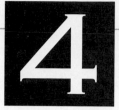

CHAPTER

13   Data Collection Methods

STUDENT OBJECTIVES

On completing this chapter, you will be able to:

➤ Evaluate a researcher's decision to use existing data or to collect new data

➤ Discuss the dimensions along which data collection approaches vary

➤ Identify phenomena that lend themselves to self-reports, observation, and physiologic measurement

➤ Distinguish between and evaluate structured and unstructured self-reports; open-ended and closed-ended questions; and interviews and questionnaires

➤ Distinguish between and evaluate structured and unstructured observations and describe various methods of collecting, sampling, and recording observational data

➤ Describe the major features and advantages of biophysiologic measures

➤ Critique a researcher's decisions regarding the data collection plan (degree of structure, general method, mode of administration) and its implementation

➤ Define new terms in the chapter

The phenomena in which researchers are interested must be translated into data that can be analyzed. Without high-quality data collection methods, the accuracy of the evidence is subject to challenge. This chapter discusses the challenging task of collecting data for research purposes.

OVERVIEW OF DATA COLLECTION AND DATA SOURCES

Alternative data collection methods vary along several dimensions that we discuss in this introductory section.

Existing Data Versus Original Data

Most researchers collect original data generated specifically for the study, but sometimes they can take advantage of existing data. Secondary analyses, for example, rely on data that have been gathered by others. Historical researchers and meta-analysts also rely on available data.

Existing **records** are an important data source for nurse researchers. A wealth of data gathered for other than research purposes can be fruitfully exploited to answer research questions. Hospital records, patient charts, care plan statements, and the like all constitute rich data sources to which nurse researchers may have access.

The most salient advantage of records is that they are economical; the collection of original data is often time-consuming and costly. On the other hand, when researchers are not responsible for collecting data, they may be unaware of the records' biases. If the available records are not the entire set of all possible such records, researchers must question how representative existing records are. Another problem confronting researchers in the United States is the increasing difficulty of gaining access to institutional records because of privacy rules (Health Insurance Portability and Accountability Act [HIPAA]).

> **TIP**
>
> The difference between using records and doing secondary analyses is that researchers doing a secondary analysis typically have a ready-to-analyze data set, whereas researchers using records have to assemble the data set, and considerable coding and data manipulation usually are necessary.

Example of a study using records:
Heavey and colleagues (2008) used data from 4,237 charts of economically disadvantaged young women attending a family planning clinic to explore demographic factors (e.g., age, race) and economic ones (e.g., health insurance) associated with differences in contraceptive choices.

Major Types of Data Collection Methods

If existing data are unsuitable for a research question, researchers must collect new data. In developing their data collection plan, researchers make many important decisions, including one about the basic type of data to gather. Three types have been used most frequently by nurse researchers: self-reports, observations, and bio-physiologic measures. **Self-reports** are participants' responses to questions posed by the researcher, as in an interview. Direct **observation** of people's behaviors, characteristics, and circumstances is an alternative to self-reports for certain research questions. Nurses also use **biophysiologic measures** to assess important clinical variables. Self-reports are the most common data collection approach in both qualitative and quantitative nursing studies.

In quantitative studies, researchers decide upfront how to operationalize their variables and gather their data. Their data collection plans are almost always "cast in stone" before a single piece of data is collected.

Qualitative researchers typically go into the field knowing the most likely sources of data, but they do not rule out other possible data sources that might come to light as data collection progresses. Table 13.1 compares data collection features in the three main qualitative traditions. Ethnographers almost always triangulate data from various sources, with observation and interviews being the most important methods. Ethnographers also gather or examine products of the culture under study, such as documents, records, artifacts, photographs, and so on. Phenomenologists and grounded theory researchers rely primarily on in-depth interviews with individual participants, although observation also plays a role in some grounded theory studies.

TABLE 13.1 ⊙	**COMPARISON OF DATA COLLECTION IN THREE QUALITATIVE TRADITIONS**		
ISSUE	ETHNOGRAPHY	PHENOMENOLOGY	GROUNDED THEORY
Types of data	Primarily observation and interviews, plus artifacts, documents, photographs, genealogies, maps, social network diagrams	Primarily in-depth interviews, sometimes diaries, other written materials	Primarily individual interviews, sometimes group interviews, observation, participant diaries, documents
Unit of data collection	Cultural system	Individuals	Individuals
Data collection points	Mainly longitudinal	Mainly cross-sectional	Cross-sectional or longitudinal
Length of time for data collection	Typically long, many months or years	Typically moderate	Typically moderate
Salient field issues	Gaining entrée, determining a role, learning how to participate, reactivity, encouraging candor, loss of objectivity, premature exit, reflexivity	Bracketing one's views, building rapport, encouraging candor, listening while preparing what to ask next, keeping "on track," handling emotionality	Building rapport, encouraging candor, listening while preparing what to ask next, keeping "on track," handling emotionality

Key Dimensions of Data Collection Methods

Regardless of type of data collected in a study, data collection methods vary along four dimensions: structure, quantifiability, researcher obtrusiveness, and objectivity.

➤ *Structure.* In structured data collection, the same information is gathered from all participants in a comparable, prespecified way. Sometimes, however, it is more appropriate to allow participants to reveal relevant information in a naturalistic way.

➤ *Quantifiability.* Data that will be analyzed statistically must be quantifiable. Structured data collection approaches tend to yield data that are more easily quantified.

➤ *Obtrusiveness.* Data collection methods differ in the degree to which researchers are obtrusive in their efforts and participants are aware of their status as study participants.

➤ *Objectivity.* Quantitative researchers generally strive for methods that are as objective as possible. In qualitative research, however, the subjective judgment of the investigator is considered a valuable tool.

The research question often dictates where on these four dimensions the data collection method will lie. For example, questions that are best suited for a phenomenological study tend to use methods that are low on structure, quantifiability, and objectivity, whereas research questions appropriate for a survey tend to require methods that are high on all four dimensions. However, researchers often have latitude in designing appropriate data collection plans.

> **TIP**
>
> Most data that are analyzed quantitatively actually begin as qualitative data. If a researcher asked respondents if they have been severely depressed, moderately depressed, somewhat depressed, or not at all depressed in the past week, they answer in words, not numbers. The words are transformed, through a coding process, into quantitative categories.

SELF-REPORTS

A lot of information can be gathered by questioning people. If, for example, we wanted to learn about patients' diets or exercise habits, we would likely gather data by asking them relevant questions. The unique ability of humans to communicate verbally on a sophisticated level makes direct questioning a particularly important part of nurse researchers' data collection repertoire.

Qualitative Self-Report Techniques

Qualitative researchers use flexible methods of gathering self-report data. They do not have a set of questions that must be asked in a specific order and worded in a given way. Instead, they start with general questions and allow respondents to tell their stories in a naturalistic fashion. In other words, qualitative self-reports, usually obtained through interviews, tend to be conversational. Unstructured interviews, which are used by researchers in all qualitative research traditions, encourage respondents to define the important dimensions of a phenomenon and to elaborate on what is relevant to them, rather than being guided by investigators' *a priori* notions of relevance.

Types of Qualitative Self-Reports

There are several approaches to collecting qualitative self-report data. Completely **unstructured interviews** are used when researchers have no preconceived view of the content or flow of information to be gathered. Their aim is to elucidate respondents' perceptions of the world without imposing their own views. Researchers begin by asking a broad **grand tour question** such as, "What happened when you first learned that you had AIDS?" Subsequent questions are guided by initial responses. Ethnographic and phenomenological studies often use unstructured interviews.

Semi-structured (or *focused*) **interviews** are used when researchers have a list of topics or broad questions that must be addressed in an interview. Interviewers use a written **topic guide** (or *interview guide*) to ensure that all question areas are covered. The interviewer's function is to encourage participants to talk freely about all the topics on the guide.

Example of a semi-structured interview:
Brown and colleagues (2008) explored the perceived impact of childhood leukemia on the career development and expectations of young adult survivors via semi-structured interviews with 11 young men and women. Examples of questions they asked are: "How, if at all, has your cancer diagnosis affected your educational plans?" and "Tell me about your future" (p. 21)

Focus group interviews are interviews with groups of about 5 to 10 people whose opinions and experiences are solicited simultaneously. The interviewer (or *moderator*) guides the discussion according to a topic guide. The advantages of a group format are that it is efficient and can generate a lot of dialogue—although not everyone is comfortable sharing their views or experiences in front of a group. Focus groups have been used by researchers in many qualitative traditions, and can play a particularly important role in feminist, critical theory, and participatory action research.

Example of focus group interviews:
Sivan and colleagues (2008) conducted a focus group study to learn about how parents from different racial or ethnic and income groups view children's behavior problems and two instruments used to assess them. Fifteen focus groups (separate ones for mothers and fathers from three racial or ethnic backgrounds) were conducted at an urban medical center. An example of a question from the interview guide is: "If you saw a child aged 2 to 4 years old in your neighborhood and you said to yourself, 'Wow, that kid's got problems!' what behavior would you be seeing?" (p. 23).

Life histories are narrative self-disclosures about individual life experiences. With this approach, researchers ask respondents to describe, often in chronologic sequence, their experiences regarding a specified theme, either orally or in writing. Some researchers have used this approach to obtain a total life health history.

Personal **diaries** have long been used as a source of data in historical research. It is also possible to generate new data for a study by asking participants to maintain a diary or journal over a specified period. Diaries can be useful in providing an intimate description of a person's everyday life. The diaries may be completely unstructured; for example, individuals who have undergone organ transplantation could be asked simply to spend 10 to 15 minutes a day jotting down their thoughts. Frequently, however, subjects are requested to make entries into a diary regarding some specific aspect of their experience, sometimes in a semi-structured format.

Example of diaries:

Bray (2007) explored the inpatient experiences of adolescents, aged 13 to 16, during their hospitalization for a planned surgery. The youth were asked to keep unstructured diaries of their experiences during their hospital stay, and they were also interviewed 2 weeks after discharge. The diaries provided data and also served to aid discussion in the interviews.

The **critical incidents technique** is a method of gathering information about people's behaviors in specific circumstances. The technique focuses on a factual *incident*—an observable and integral episode of human behavior; *critical* means that the incident must have had a discernible impact on some outcome. The technique differs from other self-report approaches in that it focuses on something specific about which respondents can be expected to testify as expert witnesses. Generally, data on 100 or more critical incidents are collected, but this typically involves interviews with a much smaller number of people, because each participant can often describe multiple incidents.

Example of a critical incident study:

Sharoff (2008) used the critical incident technique in a study of holistic nurses' use of complementary and alternative modalities in the care of their clients. Participants were instructed: "Please think of an important event in your practice where you utilized a modality. Please reflect on how this experience affected you in your practice as a holistic nurse. Please briefly describe this incident" (p. 19).

The **think aloud method** has been used to collect data about cognitive processes, such as thinking, problem-solving, and decision-making. This method involves having people use audio-recording devices to talk about decisions as they are being made or while problems are being solved, over an extended period (e.g., throughout a shift). The method produces an inventory of decisions and underlying processes as they occur in a naturalistic context.

Gathering Qualitative Self-Report Data

Researchers gather narrative self-report data to develop a construction of a phenomenon that is consistent with that of participants. This goal requires researchers to take steps to overcome communication barriers and to enhance the flow of meaning. For example, researchers should strive to learn about special jargon and idioms of the group under study before collecting data.

Although qualitative interviews are conversational in nature, this does not mean that researchers enter into them casually. The conversations are purposeful ones that require advance preparation. For example, the wording of questions should make sense to respondents and reflect their world view. In addition to being good questioners, researchers must be good listeners. Only by attending carefully to what respondents are saying can in depth interviewers develop appropriate follow-up questions.

Unstructured interviews are typically long, sometimes lasting several hours. The issue of how best to record such abundant information is a difficult one. Some researchers take notes during the interview, filling in the details after the interview is completed—but this method is risky in terms of data accuracy. Most prefer tape recording the interviews for later transcription. Although some respondents are self-conscious when their conversation is recorded, they typically forget about the presence of recording equipment after a few minutes.

Quantitative Self-Report Techniques

Structured approaches to collecting self-report data are appropriate when researchers know in advance exactly what they need to know and can frame appropriate questions to obtain the needed information. Structured self-report data are usually collected by means of a formal, written document—an **instrument**. The instrument is known as an **interview schedule** when the questions are asked orally in a face-to-face or telephone format and as a **questionnaire** when respondents complete the instrument themselves.

Question Form

In a totally structured instrument, respondents are asked to respond to the same questions in the same order. **Closed-ended questions** (or *fixed-alternative questions*) are ones in which the **response alternatives** are prespecified by the researcher. The alternatives may range from a simple yes or no to complex expressions of opinion. The purpose of such questions is to ensure comparability of responses and to facilitate analysis.

Many structured instruments, however, also include some **open-ended questions**, which allow participants to respond to questions in their own words. When open-ended questions are included in questionnaires, respondents must write out their responses. In interviews, the interviewer writes down responses verbatim or uses a tape-recorder for later transcription. Some examples of open-ended and closed-ended questions are presented in Box 13.1.

Closed-ended questions are more difficult to construct than open-ended ones but easier to analyze. Closed-ended questions are also more efficient: people can complete more closed-ended questions than open-ended ones in a given amount of

BOX 13.1 EXAMPLES OF QUESTION TYPES

Open-ended Questions
- What led to your decision to stop smoking?
- Please describe your experiences on the day you were discharged from the hospital.

Dichotomous question

Have you been hospitalized as an inpatient at any time in the past 5 years?
- ❏ 1. Yes
- ❏ 2. No

Multiple-choice question

How important is it to you to avoid a pregnancy at this time?
- ❏ 1. Extremely important
- ❏ 2. Very important
- ❏ 3. Somewhat important
- ❏ 4. Not important

Cafeteria question

People have different opinions about the use of estrogen replacement therapy for women at menopause. Which of the following statements best represents your point of view?
- ❏ 1. Estrogen replacement is dangerous and should be banned.
- ❏ 2. Estrogen replacement has undesirable side effects that suggest the need for caution in its use.
- ❏ 3. I am undecided about my views on estrogen replacement.
- ❏ 4. Estrogen replacement has many beneficial effects that merit its use.
- ❏ 5. Estrogen replacement is a wonder treatment that should be administered routinely to most menopausal women.

Rank-order question

People value different things in life. Below is a list of things that many people value. Please indicate their order of importance to you by placing a "1" beside the most important, "2" beside the second-most important, and so on.
- _____ Career achievement/work
- _____ Family relationships
- _____ Friendships, social interactions
- _____ Health
- _____ Money, material wealth
- _____ Religion

Forced-choice question

Which statement most closely represents your point of view?
- ❏ 1. What happens to me is my own doing.
- ❏ 2. Sometimes I feel I don't have enough control over my life.

Rating question

On a scale from 0 to 10, where 0 means "extremely dissatisfied" and 10 means "extremely satisfied," how satisfied were you with the nursing care you received during your hospital stay?

Extremely dissatisfied   Extremely satisfied

0 1 2 3 4 5 6 7 8 9 10

time. In questionnaires, respondents may be unwilling to compose lengthy written responses to open-ended questions. The major drawback of closed-ended questions is that researchers might overlook some potentially important responses. Closed-ended questions also can be superficial. Open-ended questions allow for richer information if the respondents are verbally expressive and cooperative. Finally, some respondents object to choosing from alternatives that do not reflect their opinions precisely.

Instrument Construction

In drafting (or borrowing) questions for a structured instrument, researchers must carefully monitor the wording of each question for clarity, sensitivity to respondents' psychological state, absence of bias, and (in questionnaires) reading level. Questions must be sequenced in a psychologically meaningful order that encourages cooperation and candor.

Draft instruments are usually critically reviewed by peers or colleagues and then pretested with a small sample of respondents. A *pretest* is a trial run to determine whether the instrument is useful in generating desired information. The development and pretesting of self-report instruments can take many months to complete.

Interviews Versus Questionnaires

Researchers using structured self-reports must decide whether to use interviews or questionnaires, and the decision can affect the findings and the quality of the evidence. Questionnaires, relative to interviews, have the following advantages:

➤ Questionnaires are less costly and require less time and effort to administer; this is a particular advantage if the sample is geographically dispersed. Internet questionnaires are especially economical and are likely to be an increasingly important means of distributing questionnaires.

➤ Questionnaires offer the possibility of anonymity or greater perceived privacy, which may be crucial in obtaining information about unconventional behavior or embarrassing traits.

➤ The absence of an interviewer avoids biases reflecting respondents' reaction to the interviewer rather than to the questions themselves.

Example of mailed questionnaires:
Kennedy-Malone and colleagues (2008) surveyed a random sample of gerontologic nurse practitioners (GNPs) to identify their prescribing patterns and other practice characteristics. Questionnaires were mailed to 1,000 GNPs.

The strengths of interviews outweigh those of questionnaires:

➤ Response rates tend to be high in face-to-face interviews. Respondents are less likely to refuse to talk to an interviewer than to ignore a questionnaire, especially a mailed questionnaire. Low response rates can lead to bias because respondents are rarely a random subset of the original sample. In the mailed questionnaire study of GNPs described earlier (Kennedy-Malone, 2008), the response rate was 47%.

➤ Many people simply cannot fill out a questionnaire; examples include young children, the blind, and the very elderly. Interviews are feasible with most people.

➤ Questions are less likely to be misinterpreted by respondents because interviewers can determine whether questions have been understood.

➤ Interviewers can produce additional information through observation of respondents' living situation, degree of cooperativeness, and so on—all of which can be useful in interpreting responses.

Most advantages of face-to-face interviews also apply to telephone interviews. Complicated or detailed instruments are not well suited to telephone interviewing, but for relatively brief instruments, telephone interviews combine relatively low costs with high response rates.

Example of personal interviews:
Coe and colleagues (2007) studied predictors of Pap test use among women living on Hopi reservations in Arizona. Data were gathered through face-to-face interviews with 559 women. Over 91% of the women who were contacted agreed to be interviewed.

TIP
Even in interview situations, participants are sometimes asked some of their questions in a questionnaire format. Questions that are deeply personal (e.g., about sexuality) or that may require some reflection (e.g., about loneliness) are sometimes easier to answer privately on a form than to express aloud to an interviewer.

Scales and Other Forms of Structured Self-Reports

Several special types of structured self-report are used by nurse researchers. These include composite social-psychological scales, vignettes, and Q sorts.

Scales

Social-psychological scales are often incorporated into questionnaires or interview schedules. A **scale** is a device that assigns a numeric score to people along a continuum, like a scale for measuring weight. Social-psychological scales quantitatively discriminate among people with different attitudes, perceptions, and psychological traits.

The most common scaling technique is the **Likert scale**, which consists of several declarative statements (**items**) that express a viewpoint on a topic. Respondents are asked to indicate how much they agree or disagree with the statement.

Table 13.2 presents an illustrative six-item Likert scale for measuring attitudes toward condom use. In this example, agreement with positively worded statements is assigned a higher score. The first statement is positively worded; agreement

TABLE 13.2	EXAMPLE OF A LIKERT SCALE TO MEASURE ATTITUDES TOWARD CONDOMS							
		RESPONSES†					**SCORE**	
DIRECTION OF SCORING*	**ITEM**	SA	A	?	D	SD	**PERSON 1** (✓)	**PERSON 2** (✕)
+	1. Using a condom shows you care about your partner.		✓			✕	4	1
−	2. My partner would be angry if I talked about using condoms.				✕	✓	5	3
−	3. I wouldn't enjoy sex as much if my partner and I used condoms.				✕	✓	4	2
+	4. Condoms are a good protection against AIDS and other sexually transmitted diseases.			✓	✕		3	2
+	5. My partner would respect me if I insisted on using condoms.	✓				✕	5	1
−	6. I would be too embarrassed to ask my partner about using a condom.				✕	✓	5	2
	Total score						26	11

* Researchers would not indicate the direction of scoring on a Likert scale administered to participants. The scoring direction is indicated in this table for illustrative purposes only.
† SA, strongly agree; A, agree; ?, uncertain; D, disagree; SD, strongly disagree

indicates a favorable attitude toward condom use. Because there are five response alternatives, a score of 5 would be given to someone strongly agreeing, 4 to someone agreeing, and so forth. The responses of two hypothetical respondents are shown by a check or an X, and their item scores are shown in the right-hand columns. Person 1, who agreed with the first statement, has a score of 4, whereas person 2, who strongly disagreed, has a score of 1. The second statement is negatively worded, and so scoring is reversed—a 1 is assigned for strongly agree, and so forth. This reversal is necessary so that a high score consistently reflects positive attitudes toward condom use.

A person's total score is determined by summing item scores (these scales are sometimes called **summated rating scales)**. In our example, person 1 has a much more positive attitude toward condoms (total score = 26) than person 2 (total score = 11). Summing item scores makes it possible to make fine discriminations among people with different opinions. A single Likert item allows people to be put into only five categories. A six-item scale, such as the one in Table 13.2, permits finer gradation—from a minimum possible score of 6 (6 × 1) to a maximum possible score of 30 (6 × 5).

Example of a Likert scale:

Gomez and colleagues (2007) administered the Death Anxiety Scale, a 20-item Likert scale, to a sample of over 700 men and women. Examples of items on this scale include "I get upset when I am in a cemetery" and "I frequently think of my own death."

Another technique for measuring attitudes is the **semantic differential** (SD). With the SD, respondents are asked to rate concepts (e.g., dieting, exercise) on a series of *bipolar adjectives,* such as good/bad, effective/ineffective, important/unimportant. Respondents place a check at the appropriate point on a seven-point scale that extends from one extreme of the dimension to the other. SDs are flexible and easy to construct, and the concept being rated can be virtually anything— a person, concept, controversial issue, and so on. The scoring procedure for SD responses is similar to that for Likert scales. Scores from 1 to 7 are assigned to each bipolar scale response, with higher scores generally associated with the positively worded adjective. Responses are then summed across the bipolar scales to yield a total score.

Example of a semantic differential:

Fitzgerald and colleagues (2008) developed and tested the Diabetes Semantic Differential Scales, which involves having patients and providers rate 18 diabetes care concepts on 9 sets of bipolar adjectives. For example, one stimulus is "Help with diabetes from family" and adjective pairs include tense/relaxed, unsafe/safe, and weak/strong.

Another type of psychosocial measure is the **visual analog scale** (VAS), which can be used to measure subjective experiences, such as pain, fatigue, and dyspnea. The VAS is a straight line, the end anchors of which are labeled as the extreme limits of the sensation or feeling being measured (Figure 13.1). Participants mark a point on the line corresponding to the amount of sensation experienced. Traditionally, a VAS line is 100 mm in length, which makes it easy to derive a score from 0 to 100 by simply measuring the distance from one end of the scale to the mark on the line.

Example of a visual analog scale:

Litherland and Schiotz (2007) conducted a randomized controlled trial (RCT) to test patient discomfort with two alternative single use catheters among 196 women undergoing urethral catheterization of the urinary bladder. Patient discomfort was measured using a VAS.

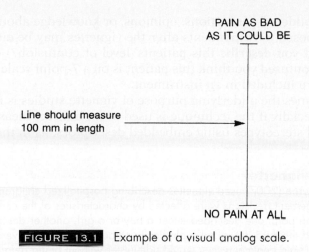

PAIN AS BAD
AS IT COULD BE

Line should measure
100 mm in length

NO PAIN AT ALL

FIGURE 13.1   Example of a visual analog scale.

Scales such as those we have described permit researchers to efficiently quantify subtle gradations in the strength or intensity of individual characteristics. Scales can be administered either verbally or in writing and thus can be used with most people. Scales are susceptible to several common problems, however, many of which are referred to as **response set biases**. The most important biases include the following:

➤ *Social desirability response set bias*—a tendency to misrepresent attitudes or traits by giving answers that are consistent with prevailing social views

➤ *Extreme response set bias*—a tendency to consistently express extreme attitudes or feelings (e.g., strongly agree), leading to distortions because extreme responses may be unrelated to the trait being measured

➤ *Acquiescence response set bias*—a tendency to agree with statements regardless of their content by some people (*yea-sayers*). The opposite tendency for other people (*nay-sayers*) to disagree with statements independently of the question content is less common.

These biases can be reduced through such strategies as *counterbalancing* positively and negatively worded statements, developing sensitively worded questions, creating a permissive, nonjudgmental atmosphere, and guaranteeing the confidentiality of responses.

TIP

Most quantitative studies that collect self-report data involve one or more social-psychological scales. Typically, the scales are ones that were developed previously by other researchers.

Vignettes

Another self report approach involves the use of **vignettes**, which are brief descriptions of events or situations to which respondents are asked to react. The descriptions, which can either be fictitious or based on fact, are structured to elicit information about respondents' perceptions, opinions, or knowledge about a phenomenon. The questions posed to respondents after the vignettes may be either open-ended (e.g., How would you describe this patients' level of confusion?) or closed-ended (e.g., Rate how confused you think this patient is on a 7-point scale). Usually three to five vignettes are included in an instrument.

Sometimes the underlying purpose of vignette studies is not revealed to participants, especially if the technique is used as an indirect measure of attitudes, prejudices, and stereotypes using embedded descriptors, as in the following example.

Example of a vignette:

Griffin, Polit, and Byrne (2007) used vignettes describing hospitalized children to determine if pediatric nurses' pain management decisions were affected by characteristics of the children. The three vignettes described children in pain: one described either a boy or a girl, another described a white or African American child, and the third described a physically attractive or unattractive child. Nurses answered questions about the pain treatments they would administer without being aware that the children's characteristics had been experimentally manipulated.

Vignettes are an economic means of eliciting information about how people might behave in situations that would be difficult to observe in daily life. The principal problem with vignettes concerns the validity of responses. If respondents describe how they would react in a situation portrayed in the vignette, how accurate is that description of their actual behavior?

Q Sorts

In a **Q sort**, participants are presented with a set of cards on which words or statements are written. Participants are asked to sort the cards along a specified bipolar dimension, such as agree or disagree. Typically, there are between 50 and 100 cards to be sorted into 9 or 11 piles, with the number of cards to be placed in each pile predetermined by the researcher. The sorting instructions and objects to be sorted in a Q sort can vary. For example, patients could be asked to rate nursing behaviors on a most-to-least helpful continuum, or trauma patients could be asked to rate aspects of their treatment on a most-to-least distressing continuum.

Q sorts are versatile and can be applied to a wide variety of problems. Requiring people to place a predetermined number of cards in each pile eliminates many response biases that can occur in Likert Scales. On the other hand, it is difficult and time-consuming to administer Q sorts to a large sample of people. Some critics argue that the forced distribution of cards according to researchers' specifications is artificial and excludes information about how participants would ordinarily distribute their responses.

Example of a Q sort:

Herron-Marx and co-researchers (2007) used a Q sort to explore women's experiences of enduring postnatal perineal and pelvic floor morbidity. Statements for the 36 cards to be sorted into 9 piles on an agree or disagree continuum were developed from an earlier in-depth study with a sample of postpartum women. An example of a statement in the card sort is: "My perineum sometimes feels dry."

Evaluation of Self-Report Methods

Self-report techniques—the most common method of data collection in nursing studies—are strong with respect to their directness. If researchers want to know how people feel or what they believe, the most direct approach is to ask them. Moreover, self-reports frequently yield information that would be difficult, or impossible, to gather by other means. Behaviors can be directly *observed*, but only if people are willing to engage in them publicly. Furthermore, observers can only observe behaviors occurring at the time of the study; self-report instruments can gather retrospective data about activities and events occurring in the past or about behaviors in which participants plan to engage in the future.

Despite these advantages, self-report methods have some weaknesses. The most serious issue concerns the validity and accuracy of self-reports: How can we be sure that respondents feel or act the way they say they do? How can we trust the information that respondents provide, particularly if the questions ask them to admit to potentially undesirable traits? Investigators often have no choice but to assume that most respondents have been frank. Yet, we all have a tendency to present ourselves in the best light, and this may conflict with the truth. When reading research reports, you should be alert to potential biases in self-reported data, particularly with respect to behaviors or feelings that society judges to be controversial or wrong.

You should also be aware of the merits of unstructured and structured self-reports. In general, unstructured (qualitative) interviews are of greatest utility when a new area of research is being explored. A qualitative approach allows researchers to examine what the basic issues are, how sensitive or controversial the topic is, and how individuals conceptualize and talk about a phenomenon.

Qualitative self-reports are extremely time-consuming and demanding, however, and they are not appropriate for capturing the measurable aspects of a phenomenon, such as incidence (e.g., the percentage of women who experience postpartum depression [PPD]), frequency (how often symptoms of PPD are experienced); duration (e.g., average time period during which PPD is present), or magnitude (e.g., degree of severity of PPD). Structured self-reports are also appropriate when researchers want to test hypotheses concerning relationships.

OBSERVATION

For some research questions, direct observation of people's behavior is an alternative to self-reports, especially in clinical settings. Observational methods can be used to gather such information as the conditions of individuals (e.g., the sleep–wake state of patients); verbal communication (e.g., exchange of information at change-of-shift report); nonverbal communication (e.g., body language); activities (e.g., geriatric patients' self-grooming activities); and environmental conditions (e.g., noise levels in nursing homes).

In observational studies, researchers have flexibility with regard to several important dimensions:

➤ *Focus of the observation*. The focus can be on broadly defined events (e.g., patient mood swings), or on small, highly specific behaviors (e.g., gestures, facial expressions).

➤ *Concealment.* Researchers do not always tell people they are being observed, because awareness of being observed may cause people to behave atypically, thereby jeopardizing the validity of the observations. The problem of behavioral distortions owing to the known presence of an observer is called **reactivity**.

➤ *Duration.* Some observations can be made in a short period of time, but others, particularly those in ethnographic studies, may require months or years in the field.

➤ *Method of recording observations.* Observations can be made through the human senses and then recorded by paper-and-pencil methods, but they can also be done with sophisticated equipment (e.g., video equipment, audio recording equipment, computers).

As with self-report techniques, an important dimension for observational methods is degree of structure—that is, whether the observational data are amenable to qualitative or quantitative analysis.

Qualitative Observational Methods

Qualitative researchers collect observational data with a minimum of structure and researcher-imposed constraints. Skillful, unstructured observation permits researchers to see the world as the study participants see it, to develop a rich understanding of the phenomena of interest, and to grasp the subtleties of cultural variation.

Naturalistic observations often are made in field settings through **participant observation**. A participant observer participates in the functioning of the group under study and strives to observe and record information within the contexts and experiences that are relevant to participants. By assuming a participating role, observers may have insights that would have eluded more passive or concealed observers. Not all qualitative observational studies use *participant* observation; some unstructured observations involve watching and recording unfolding behaviors without the observers' participation in activities. Most qualitative observations, however, do involve some participation, particularly in ethnographic and grounded theory research.

TIP

Some research reports state that participant observation was used, even though the description of methods suggests that observation but not participation was involved. Some researchers appear to use the term "participant observation" inappropriately to refer to all unstructured observations conducted in the field.

The Observer–Participant Role in Participant Observation

In participant observation, the role that observers play in the group under study is important because their social position determines what they are likely to see. The extent of the observers' actual participation in a group is best thought of as a continuum. At one extreme is complete immersion in the setting, with researchers assuming full participant status; at the other extreme is complete separation, with researchers as onlookers. Researchers may, in some cases, assume a fixed position on this continuum throughout the study, but often researchers' role as participants evolves over the course of the field work. Leininger and McFarland (2006) describe a participant observer's role as evolving through a four-phase sequence:

1. Primarily observation and active listening
2. Primarily observation with limited participation
3. Primarily participation with continued observation
4. Primary reflection and reconfirmation of findings with informants

In the initial phase, researchers observe and listen to those under study, allowing observers and participants to get more comfortable in interacting. In phase 2, observation is enhanced by a modest degree of participation in the social group. In phase 3, researchers strive to become more active participants, learning by the experience of doing rather than just watching and listening. In phase 4, researchers reflect on the total process of what transpired.

Observers must overcome at least two major hurdles in assuming a satisfactory role vis-à-vis participants. The first is to gain entrée into the social group under investigation; the second is to establish rapport and develop trust within that group. Without gaining entrée, the study cannot proceed; but without the trust of the group, the researcher will typically be restricted to "front stage" knowledge—that is, information distorted by the group's protective facades. The goal of participant observers is to "get back stage"—to learn about the true realities of the group's experiences and behaviors. On the other hand, being a fully participating member does not *necessarily* offer the best perspective for studying a phenomenon—just as being an actor in a play does not offer the most advantageous view of the performance.

Example of participant–observer roles:

Tutton and colleagues (2008) undertook an ethnographic study of professional nursing culture on a trauma unit, from the perspective of both nurses and patients. Participant observation was one of the methods used, over 16 periods of observation. The researchers "took the role of observer as participant. This involved sitting quietly in one corner of the room, but participating in conversations when invited and undertaking minor tasks such as moving foot stools and getting drinks" (p. 147).

Gathering Participant Observation Data

Participant observers typically place few restrictions on the nature of the data collected, but they often do have a broad plan for the types of information to be gathered. Among the aspects of an observed activity likely to be considered relevant are the following:

1. *The physical setting—"where" questions.* Where is the activity happening? What are the main features of the setting? What is the context within which behavior unfolds?

2. *The participants—"who" questions.* Who is present? What are their characteristics and roles? Who is given access to the setting?

3. *Activities—"what" questions.* What is going on? What are participants doing? What methods do they use to communicate, and how frequently do they do so?

4. *Frequency and duration—"when" questions.* When did the activity begin and end? Is the activity a recurring one and, if so, how regularly does it recur?

5. *Process—"how" questions.* How is the activity organized? How does the event unfold?

6. *Outcomes—"why" questions.* Why is the activity happening, or why is it happening in this manner? What did not happen (especially if it ought to have happened) and why?

The next decision is to identify a way to sample observations and to select observational locations. Researchers generally use a combination of positioning approaches. *Single positioning* means staying in a single location for a period to observe transactions in that location. *Multiple positioning* involves moving around the site to observe behaviors from different locations. *Mobile positioning* involves following a person throughout a given activity or period.

Because participant observers cannot be in more than one place at a time, observation is usually supplemented with information from unstructured interviews. For example, informants may be asked to describe what went on in a meeting the observer was unable to attend, or to describe an event that occurred before the observer entered the field. In such cases, the informant functions as the observer's observer.

Recording Observations

The most common forms of record keeping for participant observation are logs and field notes, but photographs and videotapes may also be used. A **log** (or *field diary*) is a daily record of events and conversations. **Field notes** are broader and more interpretive. Field notes represent the observer's efforts to record information and to synthesize and understand the data.

Field notes can be categorized according to their purpose. *Descriptive notes* (or *observational notes*) are objective descriptions of events and conversations, and the contexts within which they occurred. The term **thick description** is often used to characterize the goal of participation observers' descriptive notes.

Reflective notes document researchers' personal experiences, reflections, and progress in the field, and can serve a number of different purposes. *Theoretic notes* document interpretive efforts to attach meaning to observations. *Methodologic notes* are reminders about how subsequent observations should be made. *Personal notes* are comments about the researcher's own feelings during the research process. Box 13.2 presents examples of various types of field notes from Beck's (2002) study of mothering twins and triplets.

The success of any participant observation study depends on the quality of the logs and field notes. It is clearly essential to record observations as quickly as possible, but participant observers cannot usually record information by openly carrying a clipboard or a tape-recorder because this would undermine their role as ordinary participants. Observers must develop skills in making detailed mental notes that can later be written or tape-recorded.

BOX 13.2 EXAMPLE OF FIELD NOTES FOR UNSTRUCTURED OBSERVATIONS (FROM A GROUNDED THEORY STUDY)

Observational Notes: O.L. attended the mothers of multiples support group again this month but she looked worn out today. She wasn't as bubbly as she had been at the March meeting. She explained why she wasn't doing as well this month. She and her husband had just found out that their house has lead-based paint in it. Both twins do have increased lead levels. She and her husband are in the process of buying a new home.

Theoretical Notes: So far all the mothers have stressed the need for routine in order to survive the first year of caring for twins. Mothers, however, have varying definitions of routine. I.R. had the firmest routine with her twins. B.L. is more flexible with her routine, i.e., the twins are always fed at the same time but aren't put down for naps or bed at night at the same time. Whenever one of the twins wants to go to sleep is fine with her. B.L. does have a daily routine in regards to housework. For example, when the twins are down in the morning for a nap, she makes their bottles up for the day (14 bottles total).

Methodologic Notes: The first sign-up sheet I passed around at the Mothers of Multiples Support Group for women to sign up to participate in interviews for my grounded theory study only consisted of two columns: one for the mother's name and one for her telephone number. I need to revise this sign-up sheet to include extra columns for the age of the multiples, the town where the mother lives, and older siblings and their ages. My plan is to start interviewing mothers with multiples around 1 year of age so that the moms can reflect back over the process of mothering their infants for the first 12 months of their lives.

Right now I have no idea of the ages of the infants of the mothers who signed up to be interviewed. I will need to call the nurse in charge of this support group to find out the ages.

Personal Notes: Today was an especially challenging interview. The mom had picked the early afternoon for me to come to her home to interview her because that is the time her 2-year-old son would be napping. When I arrived at her house her 2-year-old ran up to me and said hi. The mom explained that he had taken an earlier nap that day and that he would be up during the interview. So in the living room with us during our interview were her two twin daughters (3 months old) swinging in the swings and her 2-year-old son. One of the twins was quite cranky for the first half hour of the interview. During the interview the 2-year-old sat on my lap and looked at the two books I had brought as a little present. If I didn't keep him occupied with the books, he would keep trying to reach for the microphone of the tape recorder.

From Beck, C. T. (2002). Releasing the pause button: Mothering twins during the first year of life. *Qualitative Health Research, 12,* 593–608.

Quantitative Observational Methods

Structured observation involves the use of formal instruments and protocols that dictate what to observe, how long to observe it, and how to record the data. Unlike participant observation, structured observation is not intended to capture a broad slice of ordinary life, but rather to document specific behaviors, actions, and events. The creativity of structured observation lies not in the observation itself but rather in the formulation of a system for accurately categorizing, recording, and encoding the observations. Because structured techniques depend on plans developed before the actual observation, they are not appropriate when researchers have limited knowledge about the phenomena under investigation.

TIP

Researchers often use structured observations in situations in which study participants cannot be asked questions—or cannot be expected to provide reliable answers. Many structured observational instruments are designed to capture the behaviors of infants and children, or older people whose communication skills are impaired.

Categories and Checklists

The most common approach to making structured observations is to use a category system for classifying observed phenomena. A **category system** represents a method of recording in a systematic fashion the behaviors and events of interest that transpire within a setting.

Some category systems are constructed so that *all* observed behaviors within a specified domain (e.g., body positions and movements) can be classified into one and only one category. A contrasting technique is to develop a system in which only particular types of behavior (which may or may not be manifested) are categorized. For example, if we were studying autistic children's aggressive behavior, we might develop such categories as "strikes another child" or "throws objects around the room." In this category system, many behaviors—all that are nonaggressive—would not be classified, and some children may exhibit *no* aggressive actions. Nonexhaustive systems are adequate for many purposes, but one risk is that resulting data might be difficult to interpret. When a large number of behaviors are not categorized, the investigator may have difficulty placing categorized behavior into perspective.

Example of nonexhaustive categories:
Liaw and colleagues (2006) studied changes in patterns of infants' distress at different phases of a routine tub bath in the neonatal intensive care unit (NICU). The researchers developed a system to categorize behavioral signs of distress (jerks, tremors, grimaces, arching). Behaviors unrelated to distress were not categorized.

One of the most important requirements of a category system is the careful and explicit operational definition of the behaviors and characteristics to be observed. Each category must be carefully explained, giving observers clear-cut criteria for assessing the occurrence of the phenomenon. Even with detailed definitions of categories, observers often are faced with making numerous on-the-spot inferences. Virtually all category systems require observer inference, to greater or lesser degree.

Example of moderately high observer inference:
Uitterhoeve and colleagues (2008) videotaped oncology nurses interacting with actors playing the role of patients. The videotaped encounters were coded for nurses' responses to patients' cues. Nurses' responses were coded according to both function and form. Function, for example, involved coding whether the patient's cue was *explored*, *acknowledged* but not explored, or elicited a *distancing* response.

Category systems are the basis for constructing a **checklist**, which is the instrument observers use to record observed phenomena. The checklist is usually formatted with the list of behaviors or events from the category system on the left and space for tallying the frequency or duration of occurrence of behaviors on the right. The task of the observer using an exhaustive category system (such as the one in the previous example) is to place *all* observed behaviors in one category for each integral unit of behavior (e.g., a sentence in a conversation, a time interval). With nonexhaustive category systems, categories of behaviors that may or may not be manifested by participants are listed. The observer's tasks are to watch for instances of these behaviors and to record their occurrence.

Rating Scales

Another approach to structured observations is to use a **rating scale**, which is a tool that requires observers to rate some phenomena in terms of points along a descriptive continuum. The observer may be required to make ratings of behavior at intervals throughout the observation or to summarize an entire event or transaction after the observation is completed.

Rating scales can be used as an extension of checklists, in which the observer records not only the occurrence of some behavior but also some qualitative aspect of it, such as its magnitude or intensity. When rating scales are coupled with a category scheme in this fashion, considerably more information about the phenomena under investigation can be obtained. The disadvantage of this approach is that it places an immense burden on observers.

Example of observational ratings:
The NEECHAM Confusion Scale, an observational measure for recording the presence and severity of acute confusion, has subscales that involve behavioral ratings. For example, one rating in the Processing subscale concerns alertness or responsiveness; ratings are from 0 (responsiveness depressed) to 4 (full attentiveness). The NEECHAM has been used for both clinical and research purposes. For example, Bond and colleagues (2006) used NEECHAM scores as their measure of delirium with 76 hospitalized patients with cancer. Observers used the scale at admission, during hospitalization, and at discharge.

Observational Sampling

Researchers must decide when to apply their structured observational systems. Observational sampling methods provide a mechanism for obtaining representative examples of the behaviors being observed. One system is **time sampling**, which involves the selection of time periods during which observations will occur. Time frames may be selected systematically (e.g., every 30 seconds at 2-minute intervals) or at random.

With **event sampling,** researchers select integral behaviors or events to observe. Event sampling requires researchers to either have knowledge about the occurrence of events or be in a position to wait for their occurrence. Examples of integral events that may be suitable for event sampling include shift changes of nurses in a hospital and cardiac arrests in the emergency room. This sampling approach is preferable to time sampling when the events of interest are infrequent and may be missed if time sampling is used. When behaviors and events are relatively frequent, however, time sampling enhances the representativeness of the observed behaviors.

Example of event sampling:
Cakmak and Kuguoglu (2007) used structured observations to compare the breastfeeding patterns of mothers who had had a vaginal birth with those who had delivered by cesarean section. Observations were made for the first three breastfeeding sessions of 200 mothers of healthy neonates.

Evaluation of Observational Methods

Certain research questions are better suited to observation than to self-reports, such as when people cannot adequately describe their own behaviors. This may be the case when people are unaware of their own behavior (e.g., stress-induced behavior), when behaviors are emotionally laden (e.g., grieving behavior), or when people are not capable of reporting their actions (e.g., young children or the mentally ill). Observational methods have an intrinsic appeal for directly capturing behaviors and events. Moreover, nurses are often in a position to watch people's behaviors and may, by training, be especially sensitive observers.

Several of the shortcomings of observational methods have already been mentioned. These include possible ethical problems and reactivity of the observed when the observer is conspicuous. One of the most pervasive problems, however, is the vulnerability of observations to bias. A number of factors interfere with objective observations, including the following:

➤ Emotions, prejudices, and values of the observer may lead to faulty inference.

➤ Personal views may color what is seen in the direction of what observers want to see.

➤ Anticipation of what is to be observed may affect what is perceived.

➤ Hasty decisions may result in erroneous classifications or ratings.

Observational biases probably cannot be eliminated, but they can be minimized through careful observer training.

Both unstructured and structured observational methods have advantages and disadvantages. Qualitative observational methods have the potential of yielding rich insights into human behaviors and social situations. Skillful participant observers can "get inside" a situation and thoroughly scrutinize its complexities. On the other hand, observer bias may pose a threat; once researchers begin to participate in a group's activities, the possibility of emotional involvement becomes a salient issue. Participant observers may develop a myopic view on issues of importance to the group. Another issue is that qualitative observational methods are more dependent on the observational and interpersonal skills of the observer.

Qualitative observational methods are especially profitable for in-depth research in which the investigator wishes to establish an adequate conceptualization of the important issues in a social setting or to develop hypotheses. Structured observation is better suited to formal hypothesis testing regarding measurable aspects of human behaviors.

BIOPHYSIOLOGIC MEASURES

Clinical nursing studies involve biophysiologic instruments, both for creating independent variables (e.g., an intervention using biofeedback equipment) and for measuring dependent variables. For the most part, our discussion focuses on the use of biophysiologic measures as dependent (outcome) variables.

Nursing studies in which biophysiologic measures have been used include a wide variety of purposes. Examples include studies of basic biophysiologic processes, explorations of the ways in which nursing actions and interventions affect physiologic outcomes, product assessments, studies to evaluate the measurement of biophysiologic information gathered by nurses, and studies of the correlates of physiologic functioning in patients with health problems.

Types of Biophysiologic Measures

Biophysiologic measures include both *in vivo* and *in vitro* measures. *In vivo* measures are those performed directly within or on living organisms, such as blood pressure, body temperature, and vital capacity measurement. *In vivo* instruments are available to measure all bodily functions, and technologic advances continue to improve the ability to measure biophysiologic phenomena more accurately, and conveniently.

Example of a study with in vivo measures:
Li and colleagues (2008) studied hypertension control and predictors of medication adherence in older Chinese immigrants living in the United States. A key outcome measure was blood pressure (BP) control, defined as the average BP (averaged over two readings) of less than 140/90 mm Hg.

With *in vitro* measures, data are gathered from participants by extracting biophysiologic material from them and subjecting it to analysis by specialized laboratory technicians. *In vitro* measures include chemical measures (e.g., the measurement of hormone, sugar, or potassium levels); microbiologic measures (e.g., bacterial counts and identification); and cytologic or histologic measures (e.g., tissue biopsies).

Example of a study with *in vitro* measures:
Ward and colleagues (2008) examined children's nocturnal sleep and nap behaviors in relation to salivary cortisol levels sampled midmorning and afternoon after naps in child care centers. Problem napping and disruptive behaviors were associated with higher afternoon cortisol levels.

Evaluation of Biophysiologic Measures

Biophysiologic measures offer a number of advantages to nurse researchers, including the following:

➤ Biophysiologic measures are relatively accurate and precise, especially compared with psychological measures, such as self-report measures of anxiety, pain, and so forth.

➤ Biophysiologic measures are objective. Two nurses reading from the same spirometer output are likely to record identical tidal volume measurements, and two spirometers are likely to produce the same readouts. Patients cannot easily distort measurements of biophysiologic functioning.

➤ Biophysiologic instrumentation provides valid measures of targeted variables; thermometers can be relied on to measure temperature and not blood volume, and so forth. For nonbiophysiologic measures, there are typically concerns about whether an instrument is really measuring the target concept.

Biophysiologic measures are plentiful, tend to be accurate and valid, and are extremely useful in clinical nursing studies. However, care must be exercised in using them with regard to practical, ethical, medical, and technical considerations.

IMPLEMENTING A DATA COLLECTION PLAN

In addition to selecting methods for collecting data, researchers must develop and implement a plan for gathering and recording the data. This involves decisions that could affect the quality of the data being collected.

One important decision concerns who will collect the data. Researchers often hire assistants to collect data rather than doing it themselves. This is especially likely to be the case in large-scale quantitative studies. In other studies, nurses or other health care staff are asked to assist in the collection of data. From your perspective as a consumer, the critical issue is whether the people collecting data are able to produce valid and accurate data. In any research endeavor, adequate training and monitoring of data collectors is essential—and this may even include self-training and trial runs. Also, blinding of data collectors (withholding information about study hypotheses or group assignments) is a good strategy in most quantitative studies.

Another issue concerns the circumstances under which data are gathered. For example, it may be critical to ensure privacy. In most cases, it is important for researchers to create a nonjudgmental atmosphere in which participants are encouraged to be candid or behave naturally. Again, you as a consumer must ask whether there is anything about the way in which the data are collected that could create bias or otherwise affect data quality. In evaluating the data collection plan of a study, then, you should critically appraise not only the actual methods chosen but also the procedures used to collect and record the data.

CRITIQUING DATA COLLECTION METHODS

The goal of a data collection plan is to produce data that are of exceptional quality. Every decision researchers make about the data collection methods and procedures is likely to affect data quality—and hence the quality of the overall study. These decisions should be critiqued in drawing conclusions about the study's capacity to answer the research questions or test study hypotheses.

It may, however, be difficult to perform a thorough critique of data collection methods in studies reported in journals because researchers' descriptions are seldom detailed owing to space constraints in journals. Thus, one aspect of a critique is likely to involve an appraisal of how much information the research report provided about the data collection methods used. Although space constraints in journals make it impossible for researchers to elaborate their methods fully, researchers do have a responsibility to communicate basic information about their approach so that readers can better assess the quality of evidence that the study yields.

Degree of structure is especially important in your assessment of a data collection plan. Researchers' decisions about structure are based on considerations

---

BOX 13.3 GUIDELINES FOR CRITIQUING DATA COLLECTION PLANS

1. Given the research question and the characteristics of participants, did the researchers use the best method of capturing study phenomena (i.e., self-reports, observation, biophysiologic measures)? Was triangulation of methods used appropriately (i.e., Were multiple methods sensibly used)?

2. Did the researchers make good data collection decisions with regard to structure, quantification, researcher obtrusiveness, and objectivity?

3. If self-report methods were used, did the researchers make good decisions about the specific methods used to solicit information (e.g., in-person interviews, focus group interviews, mailed questionnaires, Internet questionnaires, and so on)? For structured self-reports, was there an appropriate mix of questions and composite scales?

4. Were efforts made to enhance data quality in collecting the self-report data (e.g., Were efforts made to reduce or to evaluate response biases? Was the reading level of the instruments appropriate, for self-administered questionnaires)?

5. If observational methods were used, did the report adequately describe what the observations entailed? What did the researcher actually observe, in what types of setting did the observations occur, and how often and over how long a period were observations made? Were risks of observational bias addressed? How much inference was required of the observers, and was this appropriate?

6. Were biophysiologic measures used in the study, and was this appropriate? Did the researcher appear to have the skills necessary for proper interpretation of biophysiologic measures?

7. How were data recorded? What efforts were made to ensure high accuracy in recording information? For example, were interviews tape-recorded and transcribed?

8. Did the report provide adequate information about data collection procedures? Were data collectors judiciously chosen and properly trained? Where and under what circumstances were data gathered? Were data gathered in a manner that promoted high-quality responses (e.g., in terms of privacy, efforts to put respondents at ease)?

that you can often evaluate. For example, in a questionnaire situation, respondents who are not articulate may have difficulty answering questions that force them to compose lengthy answers. Other considerations include the amount of time available (structured instruments are more efficient); the expected sample size (qualitative interviews and observations are difficult to analyze with large samples); the status of existing information on the topic (in a new area of inquiry, an unstructured approach may be preferred); and, most important, the nature of the research question.

Another important issue is the *mix* of data collection approaches. Triangulation of methods is often extremely desirable, especially in qualitative research. Thus, an important issue to consider in evaluating unstructured data collection is whether the types and amount of data collected are sufficiently rich to support an in-depth, holistic understanding of the phenomena under study.

Finally, it is important to evaluate the actual procedures used to collect and record the data. This means considering who collected the data, how they were trained, whether formal instruments were adequately pretested, in what types of setting data collection occurred, and whether efforts were made to reduce biases. Guidelines for critiquing the data collection methods of a nursing study are presented in Box 13.3.

RESEARCH EXAMPLES AND CRITICAL THINKING ACTIVITIES

In this section, we provide details about the data collection plan for a quantitative and a qualitative study, followed by some questions to guide critical thinking.

EXAMPLE 1 ■ Data Collection in a Quantitative Study

Study

An intervention for multiethnic obese parents and overweight children (Berry et al., 2007).

Purpose

This study assessed the effects of the addition of coping skills training for obese multiethnic parents who, along with their overweight children aged 7 to 17, were enrolled in a weight management program. The outcomes of interest included health behavior outcomes of the parents and clinical weight-related outcomes for both parents and children.

Design

A total of 80 parent–child dyads were randomly assigned to an experimental or control group. Parents and children in both groups received a nutrition and exercise program, and 12 weeks of exercise classes. Parents in the experimental group received an additional 6 weeks of coping skills training taught by an advanced practice nurse.

Data Collection Plan

Data were collected at baseline, and at 3 months and 6 months post-baseline. Two trained research assistants, blinded to study group, collected parent and child outcome data on height and weight (for calculating body mass index [BMI]), body fat percentage (BFP), and pedometer steps. BFP was obtained using the Tanita Body Fat Analyzer Scale, which uses leg-to-leg bioimpedance analysis (a low-level electrical signal that is passed through the body using foot electrodes). Pedometer steps were measured using an Accusplit Eagle 170 Deluxe Activity Pedometer that counts steps, walking distance in miles, and number of calories burned. Parents' health behavior outcomes were assessed through three self-report scales. The Family Assessment Device (FAD) is a 60-item measure encompassing six family functioning dimensions (e.g., problem-solving, communication, behavior control). The Eating Self-Efficacy Scale (ESES) is a 25-item scale that asks participants to rate their difficulty controlling eating from 1 (*no difficulty*) to 7 (*difficulty*). The third scale was the Health-Promoting Lifestyle Profile II (HPLP II), a 48-item four-point Likert scale that measures the frequency of health-promoting behaviors in six subscales (e.g., exercise, nutrition, stress management). Study participants also completed a demographic questionnaire at baseline that asked questions about parents' ethnicity, religion, socioeconomic status, and about children's age, birth order, and health problems.

Key Findings

- At 6 months post-baseline, parents in the experimental group had significantly lower BMI and BFP, and higher numbers of pedometer steps, than parents in the control group.
- Experimental group parents also had significantly greater improvements in several health behavior measures, such as stress management and behavior control.
- Differences in children's outcomes were not statistically significant, but there was a trend toward decreased BMI and BFP in the experimental group.

CRITICAL THINKING SUGGESTIONS*:

*See the Student Resource CD-ROM for a discussion of these questions.

1. Answer the relevant questions in Box 13.3 in terms of this study.
2. Also, consider the following targeted questions, which may further sharpen your critical thinking skills and assist you in assessing aspects of the study's merit:
   a. Comment on factors that could have biased the data in this study.
   b. Comment on the researchers' overall data collection plan in terms of the timing of the data collection.
3. If the results of this study are valid and reliable, what might be some of the uses to which the findings could be put in clinical practice?

EXAMPLE 2 ■ Data Collection in a Qualitative Study

Study

Black non-Hispanic mothers' perceptions about the promotion of infant-feeding methods by nurses and physicians (Cricco-Lizza, 2006); Exemplar: The milk of human kindness: WIC influence on the infant-feeding decisions of Black non-Hispanic women (Cricco-Lizza, 2007).

Purpose

The overall purpose of this study was to explore the context of Black women's infant feeding decisions within an urban Women, Infants, and Children (WIC) clinic.

Design

Cricco-Lizza undertook an ethnographic study that involved 18 months of field work in a New York metropolitan area WIC clinic.

Data Collection Plan

The main forms of data collection for this study were unstructured self-reports (interviews and informal conversations) and participant observation. With regard to the observational data, Cricco-Lizza observed the WIC clinic operations, focusing in particular on the interactions of 130 Black mothers with their babies, significant others, other WIC mothers, and WIC staff. Observations occurred in the waiting room and in group nutrition education classes. Observation sessions—63 in total—were each about 2 hours long and took place two to three times per week at varying times and days. While observing the mothers in the clinic waiting room, the researcher also initiated informal discussions with some of them about their infant-feeding beliefs and motherhood experiences. Data obtained through observation were recorded as field notes. After completing an observation session, the researcher immediately constructed an outline of salient events that was later expanded to included specific, detailed information about behaviors, conversations, and the setting. Field notes were typed up shortly after each session. From the group of 130 women who were observed, Cricco-Lizza purposively selected 11 key informants who were willing to be interviewed several times. In-depth interviews (which were tape recorded and then transcribed) were conducted during pregnancy, during the early postpartum period, and again 1 month later. The interviews, which followed a formal protocol, captured a range of information about the childbirth experience and infant-feeding beliefs and practices. Six women used formula feeding and five women breastfed their infants. Formal interviews were supplemented by informal interviews and telephone conversations with the key informants. Informal meetings occurred in the women's homes, hospitals, malls, and the WIC clinic. A total of 147 telephone conversations occurred, and the calls provided rich information about important events that happened unexpectedly in the women's lives. Notes from the conversations were recorded immediately. The researcher had between 11 and 32 "data points" (formal and informal interviews) for each key informant. Throughout data collection, the researcher made no recommendations about infant-feeding methods. All data were collected by the researcher herself, and she personally verified the accuracy of each transcribed interview, line by line. Thousands of pages of transcribed interviews and field notes were amassed during the study.

Findings

- The WIC clinic environment set a positive tone for the delivery of service, and the mothers saw the clinic as an important source of support.
- WIC influenced the women's infant-feeding decisions. Despite the fact that WIC provided free formula that facilitated bottle-feeding, personalized breastfeeding promotion by trusted WIC staff resulted in breastfeeding decisions by many women.
- However, informants reported limited breastfeeding education and support from nurses and physicians during the childbearing period.

CRITICAL THINKING SUGGESTIONS:

1. Answer the relevant questions in Box 13.3 in terms of this study.
2. Also, consider the following targeted questions, which may further sharpen your critical thinking skills and assist you in assessing aspects of the study's merit:
   a. How likely is it that the researcher's presence at the WIC clinic affected the women's behaviors? Comment on Cricco-Lizza's role as a participant observer.
   b. Comment on the researcher's observational sampling plan.
   c. Comment on factors that could have biased the data in this study.
   d. Comment on the researcher's overall data collection plan in terms of the amount of information gathered and the timing of the data collection.

3. If the results of this study are trustworthy, what might be some of the uses to which the findings could be put in clinical practice?

EXAMPLE 3 ■ Data Collection in the Quantitative Study in Appendix A

1. Read the method section from Howell and colleagues' (2007) study ("Anxiety, anger, and blood pressure in children") in Appendix A of this book, and then answer the relevant questions in Box 13.3.
2. Also, consider the following targeted questions, which may further sharpen your critical thinking skills and assist you in assessing aspects of the study's merit:
   a. Could any of the variables in this study have been measured by observation? Should they have been?
   b. Comment on factors that could have biased the data in this study.
   c. Comment on the fact that the researchers took a single blood pressure measurement from each child.

EXAMPLE 4 ■ Data Collection in the Qualitative Study in Appendix B

1. Read the method section from Beck's (2006) study ("The anniversary of birth trauma") in Appendix B of this book, and then answer the relevant questions in Box 13.3.
2. Also, consider the following targeted questions, which may further sharpen your critical thinking skills and assist you in assessing aspects of the study's merit:
   a. Could any of the variables in this study have been measured by observation? Should they have been?
   b. Did Beck's study involve a "grand tour" question?

CHAPTER REVIEW
....

Key new terms introduced in the chapter, together with a summary of major points, are presented in this section. In addition, Chapter 13 of the accompanying *Study Guide for Essentials of Nursing Research,* 7th edition offers various exercises and study suggestions for reinforcing concepts presented in this chapter. For additional review, see the Student Self-Study Review Questions section of the Student Resource CD-ROM provided with this book. ●

Key New Terms
....

Category system	Focus group interview	Likert Scale
Checklist	Grand tour question	Log
Closed-ended question	Instrument	Observational methods
Critical incidents technique	Interview schedule	Open-ended question
Field notes	Item	Q sort
	Life history	Rating scale

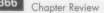

Reactivity
Response alternatives
Response set bias
Scale
Self-report

Semantic differential
Semi-structured
    interview
Summated rating scale
Think aloud technique

Topic guide
Unstructured
    interview
Vignette
Visual analog scale

Summary Points

- Some researchers use existing data in their studies—for example, those doing historical research, secondary analyses, or analyses of available **records**.

- Data collection methods vary on four dimensions: structure, quantifiability, researcher obtrusiveness, and objectivity.

- The three principal data collection methods for nurse researchers are self-reports, observations, and biophysiologic measures.

- Self-reports, which involve directly questioning study participants, are the most widely used method of collecting data for nursing studies.

- In qualitative studies, self-reports include completely **unstructured interviews**, which are conversational discussions on the topic of interest; **semi-structured** (or *focused*) **interviews**, using a broad **topic guide**; **focus group interviews**, which involve discussions with small groups; **life histories**, which encourage respondents to narrate their life experiences regarding some theme; **diaries**, in which respondents are asked to maintain daily records about some aspects of their lives; the **critical incidents technique**, which involve probes about the circumstances surrounding an incident that is critical to an outcome of interest; and the **think aloud method**, which involves having people talk about decisions as they are making them.

- Structured self-reports for quantitative studies involve a formal **instrument**—a **questionnaire** or **interview schedule**—that may contain **open-ended questions** (which permit respondents to respond in their own words) and **closed-ended questions** (which offer respondents **response alternatives** from which to choose).

- Questionnaires are less costly than interviews, offer the possibility of anonymity, and run no risk of interviewer bias; however, interviews yield higher response rates, are suitable for a wider variety of people, and provide richer data than questionnaires.

- Social-psychological **scales** are self-report tools for quantitatively measuring the intensity of such characteristics as personality traits, attitudes, needs, and perceptions.

- **Likert scales** (or **summated rating scales**) present respondents with a series of **items** worded favorably or unfavorably toward a phenomenon; responses indicating level of agreement or disagreement with each statement are scored and summed into a composite score.

➤ The **semantic differential (SD)** technique consists of a series of scales with bipolar adjectives (e.g., good/bad) along which respondents rate their reactions toward phenomena.

➤ A **visual analog scale (VAS)** is used to measure subjective experiences (e.g., pain, fatigue) along a 100 mm line designating a bipolar continuum.

➤ Scales are versatile and powerful but are susceptible to **response set biases**— the tendency of some people to respond to items in characteristic ways, independently of item content.

➤ **Vignettes** are brief descriptions of some event, person, or situation to which respondents are asked to react.

➤ With a **Q sort**, respondents sort a set of statements on cards into piles according to specified criteria.

➤ **Observational methods**, which include both structured and unstructured procedures, are techniques for acquiring data through the direct observation of phenomena.

➤ One type of unstructured observation is **participant observation**, in which the researcher gains entrée into a social group and participates to varying degrees in its functioning while making in-depth observations of activities and events. **Logs** of daily events and **field notes** of the observer's experiences and interpretations constitute the major data collection instruments.

➤ Structured observations for quantitative studies dictate what the observer should observe; they often involve **checklists**—tools based on **category systems** for recording the appearance, frequency, or duration of prespecified behaviors or events. Observers may also use **rating scales** to rate phenomena along a dimension of interest (e.g., energetic or lethargic).

➤ Structured observations often use a sampling plan (e.g., **time sampling** or **event sampling**) for selecting the behaviors, events, and conditions to be observed.

➤ Observational techniques are a versatile and important alternative to self-reports, but observational biases can pose a threat to the validity and accuracy of observational data.

➤ Data may also be derived from **biophysiologic measures**, which can be classified as either *in vivo* measurements (those performed within or on living organisms) or *in vitro* measurements (those performed outside the organism's body, such as blood tests). Biophysiologic measures have the advantage of being objective, accurate, and precise.

➤ In developing a data collection plan, the researcher must decide who will collect the data, how the data collectors will be trained, and what the circumstances for data collection will be.

STUDIES CITED IN CHAPTER 13

Beck, C. T. (2002). Releasing the pause button: Mothering twins during the first year of life. *Qualitative Health Research, 12*, 593–608.

Berry, S., Savoye, M., Melkus, G., & Grey, M. (2007). An intervention for multiethnic obese patients and overweight children. *Applied Nursing Research, 20,* 63–71.

Bond, S., Neelon, V., & Belyea, M. (2006). Delirium in hospitalized older patients with cancer. *Oncology Nursing Forum, 33,* 1075–1083.

Bray, L. (2007). Experiences of young people admitted for planned surgery. *Paediatric Nursing, 19,* 14–18.

Brown, C., Pikler, V., Lavish, L., Keune, K., & Hutto, C. (2008). Surviving childhood leukemia: Career, family, and future expectations. *Qualitative Health Research, 18,* 19–30.

Cakmak, H., & Kuguoglu, S. (2007). Comparison of the breastfeeding patterns of mothers who delivered their babies per vagina and via cesarean section. *International Journal of Nursing Studies, 44,* 1128–1137.

Coe, K., Martin, L., Nuvayestewa, L., Attakai, A., Papenfuss, M., DeZapien, J., et al. (2007). Predictors of Pap test use among women living on the Hopi reservation. *Health Care for Women International, 28,* 764–781.

Cricco-Lizza, R. (2006). Black non-Hispanic mothers' perceptions about the promotion of infant-feeding methods by nurses and physicians. *Journal of Obstetric, Gynecologic, & Neonatal Nursing, 35,* 173–180.

Cricco-Lizza, R. (2007). Exemplar: The milk of human kindness: WIC influence on the infant-feeding decisions of Black non-Hispanic women. In P. L. Munhall (Ed.). *Nursing research: A qualitative perspective* (4th ed.). Sudbury, MA: Jones & Bartlett, pp. 331–348.

Fitzgerald, J., Stansfield, R., Tang, T., Oh, M., Frohna, A., Armbruster, B., et al. (2008). Patient and provider perceptions of diabetes: Measuring and evaluating differences. *Patient Education and Counseling, 70,* 118–125.

Gomez, J., Hidalgo, M., & Tomas-Sabado, J. (2007). Using polytomous item response models to assess death anxiety. *Nursing Research, 56,* 89–96.

Griffin, R., Polit, D., & Byrne, M. (2007). Stereotyping and nurses' recommendations for treating pain in hospitalized children. *Research in Nursing & Health, 30,* 655–666.

Heavey, E., Moysich, K., Hyland, A., Druschel, C., & Sill, M. (2008). Differences in contraceptive choice among female adolescents at a state-funded family planning clinic. *Journal of Midwifery & Women's Health, 53,* 45–52.

Herron-Marx, S., Williams, A., & Hicks, C. (2007). A Q methodology study of women's experience of enduring postnatal perineal and pelvic floor morbidity. *Midwifery, 23,* 322–334.

Kennedy-Malone, L., Fleming, M., & Penny, J. (2008). Prescribing patterns of gerontological nurse practitioners in the United States. *Journal of the American Academy of Nurse Practitioners, 20,* 28–34.

Li, W.W., Wallhagen, M., & Froelicher, E. (2008). Hypertension control, predictors of medication adherence and gender differences in older Chinese immigrants. *Journal of Advanced Nursing, 61,* 326–335.

Liaw, J., Yang, L. Yuh, Y., & Yin, T. (2006). Effects of tub bathing procedures on preterm infants' behavior. *Journal of Nursing Research, 14,* 297–305.

Litherland, A., & Schiotz, H. (2007). Patient-perceived discomfort with two coated urinary catheters. *British Journal of Nursing, 16,* 284–287.

Sharoff, L. (2008). Exploring nurses' perceived benefits of utilizing holistic modalities for self and clients. *Holistic Nursing Practice, 22,* 15–24.

Sivan, A., Ridge, A., Gross, D., Richardson, R., & Cowell, J. (2008). Analysis of two measures of child behavior problems by African American, Latino, and non-Hispanic Caucasian parents of young children. *Journal of Pediatric Nursing, 23,* 20–27.

Tutton, E., Seers, K., & Langstaff, D. (2008). Professional nursing culture on a trauma unit: Experiences of patients and staff. *Journal of Advanced Nursing, 61,* 145–153.

Uitterhoeve, R., de Leeuw, J., Bensing, J., Heaven, C., Borm, G., deMulder, P., et al. (2008). Cue-responding behaviours of oncology nurses in video-simulated interviews. *Journal of Advanced Nursing, 61,* 71–80.

Ward, T., Gay, C., Alkon, A., Anders, T., & Lee, K. (2008). Nocturnal sleep and daytime nap behaviors in relation to salivary cortisol levels and temperament in preschool-age children attending child care. *Biological Research for Nursing, 9,* 244–253.

14 Measurement and Data Quality

STUDENT OBJECTIVES

On completing this chapter, you will be able to:

➤ Describe the major characteristics of measurement and identify major sources of measurement error

➤ Describe aspects of reliability and validity, and specify how each aspect can be assessed

➤ Interpret the meaning of reliability and validity

➤ Describe the function and meaning of sensitivity, specificity, and likelihood ratios

➤ Evaluate the overall quality of a measuring tool used in a study

➤ Define new terms in the chapter

An ideal data collection procedure is one that captures a construct in a way that is accurate, truthful, and sensitive. Few data collection procedures match this ideal perfectly. In this chapter, we discuss criteria for evaluating the quality of data obtained with structured instruments.

MEASUREMENT

Quantitative studies derive data through the measurement of variables, and so we begin by briefly discussing the concept of measurement.

What Is Measurement?

Measurement involves rules for assigning numbers to *qualities* of objects to designate the *quantity* of the attribute. Attributes do not inherently have numeric values; humans invent rules to measure attributes. Many quantitative researchers concur with a statement by early American psychologist L. L. Thurstone: "Whatever exists, exists in some amount and can be measured." Attributes are not constant; they vary from day to day, from situation to situation, or from one person to another. This variability is capable of a numeric expression that signifies *how much* of an attribute is present.

Measurement requires numbers to be assigned to objects according to *rules*. Rules for measuring temperature, weight, and other physical attributes are familiar to us. Rules for measuring many variables for nursing studies, however, have to be created. Whether data are collected by observation, self-report, or some other method, researchers must specify the criteria according to which numbers are to be assigned.

Advantages of Measurement

A major strength of measurement is that it removes guesswork and ambiguity in gathering and communicating information. Consider how handicapped health care professionals would be in the absence of measures of body temperature, blood pressure, and so on. Without such measures, subjective evaluations of clinical outcomes would have to be used. Because measurement is based on explicit rules, resulting information tends to be objective, that is, it can be independently verified. Two people measuring the weight of a person using the same scale would likely get identical results. Not all measures are completely objective, but most incorporate mechanisms for minimizing subjectivity.

Measurement also makes it possible to obtain reasonably precise information. Instead of describing Nathan as "tall," we can depict him as being 6 feet 3 inches tall. If necessary, we could achieve even greater precision. Such precision allows researchers to make fine distinctions among people with different degrees of an attribute.

Finally, measurement is a language of communication. Numbers are less vague than words and can thus communicate information more clearly. If a researcher reported that the average oral temperature of a sample of patients was "somewhat high," different readers might develop different conceptions about the sample's physiologic state. If the researcher reported an average temperature of 99.6°F, however, there is no ambiguity.

Levels of Measurement

In this chapter, we discuss the overall concept of measurement and describe how measurements can be evaluated. In the next chapter we consider what researchers *do* with their measurements in their statistical analyses. The statistical operations available to researchers depend on a variable's **level of measurement**. There are four major classes, or levels, of measurement.

Nominal measurement, the lowest level, involves using numbers simply to categorize attributes. Examples of variables that are nominally measured include gender and blood type. The numbers used in nominal measurement do not have quantitative meaning. If we coded males as 1 and females as 2, the numbers would not have quantitative implications—the number 2 does not mean "more than" 1. Nominal measurement provides information only about categorical equivalence and nonequivalence and so the numbers cannot be treated mathematically. It is nonsensical, for example, to compute the average gender of the sample by adding the numeric values of the codes and dividing by the number of participants.

Ordinal measurement ranks objects based on their relative standing on an attribute. If a researcher orders people from heaviest to lightest, this is ordinal measurement. As another example, consider this ordinal coding scheme for measuring ability to perform activities of daily living: 1 = completely dependent; 2 = needs another person's assistance; 3 = needs mechanical assistance; and 4 = completely independent. The numbers signify incremental ability to perform activities of daily living independently. Ordinal measurement does not, however, tell us how much greater one level is than another. For example, we do not know if being completely independent is twice as good as needing mechanical assistance. As with nominal measures, the mathematic operations permissible with ordinal-level data are restricted.

Interval measurement occurs when researchers can specify the ranking of objects on an attribute *and* the distance between those objects. Most educational and psychological tests yield interval-level measures. For example, the Stanford-Binet Intelligence Scale—a standardized intelligence (IQ) test used in many countries—is an interval measure. A score of 140 on the Stanford-Binet is higher than a score of 120, which, in turn, is higher than 100. Moreover, the difference between 140 and 120 is presumed to be equivalent to the difference between 120 and 100. Interval scales expand analytic possibilities: interval-level data can be averaged meaningfully, for example. Many sophisticated statistical procedures require interval measurements.

Ratio measurement is the highest level. Ratio scales, unlike interval scales, have a rational, meaningful zero and therefore provide information about the absolute magnitude of the attribute. The Fahrenheit scale for measuring temperature (interval measurement) has an arbitrary zero point. Zero on the thermometer does not signify the absence of heat; it would not be appropriate to say that 60°F is twice as hot as 30°F. Many physical measures, however, are ratio measures with a real zero. A person's weight, for example, is a ratio measure. It is acceptable to say that someone who weighs 200 pounds is twice as heavy as someone who weighs 100 pounds. Statistical procedures suitable for interval data are also appropriate for ratio-level data.

Example of different measurement levels:
Lyon and co-researchers (2008) examined whether there were different patterns and levels of cytokines (signaling molecules that mediate and regulate immunity) between women with breast cancer and women with a negative breast biopsy. In the context of this study, the women's breast cancer status was a dichotomous nominal-level variable. Stage of cancer (I through IV) for the women with cancer was an ordinal variable. The women's age and cytokine levels (e.g., interleukin-6) were ratio variables. There were no interval-level variables in this study.

Researchers usually strive to use the highest levels of measurement possible—especially for their dependent variables—because higher levels yield more information and are amenable to more powerful analyses than lower levels.

HOW-TO-TELL TIP

How can you tell the measurement level of a variable? A variable is *nominal* if the values could be interchanged (e.g., 1 = male, 2 = female OR 1 = female, 2 = male—the codes are arbitrary). A variable is usually *ordinal* if there is a quantitative ordering of values AND if there are only a small number of values (e.g., very important, important, not too important, unimportant). A variable is usually considered *interval* if it is measured with a composite scale or psychological test. A variable is *ratio-level* if it makes sense to say that one value is twice that of another (e.g., 100 mg is twice as much as 50 mg).

Errors of Measurement

Researchers work with fallible measures. Both the procedures involved in taking measurements and the objects being measured are susceptible to influences that can alter the resulting data. Scores from even the best measuring instruments have a certain degree of error. We can think of every piece of quantitative data as consisting of two parts: a true component and an error component. This can be written as an equation, as follows:

$$\text{Obtained score} = \text{True score} \pm \text{Error}$$

The **obtained** (or *observed*) **score** could be, for example, a patient's heart rate or score on an anxiety scale. The **true score** is the true value that would be obtained if it were possible to have an infallible measure. The true score is hypothetical—it can never be known because measures are *not* infallible. The final term in the equation is the **error of measurement**. The difference between true and obtained scores is the result of distorting factors. Some errors are random or variable, whereas others are systematic, representing a source of *bias*. The most common factors contributing to measurement error are the following:

➤ *Situational contaminants*. Scores can be affected by the conditions under which they are produced. For example, environmental factors (e.g., temperature, lighting, time of day) can be sources of measurement error.

➤ *Response-set biases*. Relatively enduring characteristics of respondents can interfere with accurate measurements (see Chapter 13).

➤ *Transitory personal factors*. Temporary states, such as fatigue, hunger, or mood, can influence people's motivation or ability to cooperate, act naturally, or do their best.

➤ *Administration variations*. Alterations in the methods of collecting data from one person to the next can affect obtained scores. For example, if some physiologic measures are taken before a feeding and others are taken after a feeding, then measurement errors can potentially occur.

➤ *Item sampling*. Errors can be introduced as a result of the sampling of items used to measure an attribute. For example, a student's score on a 100-item test of research methods will be influenced somewhat by *which* 100 questions are included.

This list is not exhaustive, but it illustrates that data are susceptible to measurement error from a variety of sources.

RELIABILITY

The reliability of a quantitative measure is a major criterion for assessing its quality. **Reliability** is the consistency with which an instrument measures the attribute. If a scale weighed a person at 120 pounds one minute and 150 pounds the next, we would consider it unreliable. The less variation an instrument produces in repeated measurements, the higher its reliability.

Reliability also concerns a measure's accuracy. An instrument is reliable to the extent that its measures reflect true scores—that is, to the extent that measurement errors are absent from obtained scores. A reliable instrument maximizes the true score component and minimizes the error component of an obtained score.

Three aspects of reliability are of interest to quantitative researchers: stability, internal consistency, and equivalence.

Stability

The *stability* of an instrument is the extent to which similar results are obtained on two separate occasions. The reliability estimate focuses on the instrument's susceptibility to extraneous influences over time, such as participant fatigue. Assessments of stability are made through **test–retest reliability** procedures. Researchers administer the same measure to a sample twice and then compare the scores.

TABLE 14.1	FICTITIOUS DATA FOR TEST–RETEST RELIABILITY OF SELF-ESTEEM SCALE	
SUBJECT NUMBER	TIME 1	TIME 2
1	55	57
2	49	46
3	78	74
4	37	35
5	44	46
6	50	56
7	58	55
8	62	66
9	48	50
10	67	63
		$r = .95$

Suppose, for example, we were interested in the stability of a self-report scale that measured self-esteem. Because self-esteem is a fairly stable attribute that does not change much from one day to another, we would expect a reliable measure of it to yield consistent scores on two different days. As a check on the instrument's stability, we administer the scale 2 weeks apart to a sample of 10 people. Fictitious data for this example are presented in Table 14.1.

The scores on the two tests are not identical but, on the whole, differences are not large. Researchers compute a **reliability coefficient**, a numeric index that quantifies an instrument's reliability, to objectively determine how small the differences are. Reliability coefficients (designated as r) range from .00 to 1.00.* The higher the value, the more reliable (stable) is the measuring instrument. In the example shown in Table 14.1, the reliability coefficient is .95, which is quite high.

> **TIP**
> Reliability coefficients higher than .70 are often considered satisfactory, but coefficients greater than .80 are far preferable.

---

*Computation procedures for reliability coefficients are not presented in this textbook, but formulas can be found in Polit (1996) or Waltz et al. (2005). Although reliability coefficients can technically be less than .00 (i.e., a negative value), they are almost invariably a number between .00 and 1.00.

Test–retest reliability is relatively easy to compute, but a major problem with this approach is that many traits do change over time, independently of the instrument's stability. Attitudes, mood, knowledge, and so forth can be modified by experiences between two measurements. Thus, stability indexes are most appropriate for relatively enduring characteristics, such as temperament. Even with such traits, test–retest reliability tends to decline as the interval between the two administrations increases.

Example of test–retest reliability:
Welch and colleagues (2006) developed the Beliefs about Dietary Compliance Scale to measure perceived benefits and barriers to limiting dietary sodium. The 1-week test–retest reliability was .68 for the "Benefits" subscale and .86 for the "Barriers" subscale.

Internal Consistency

Scales and tests that involve summing item scores are almost always evaluated for their internal consistency. Ideally, scales are composed of items that all measure the one unitary attribute and nothing else. On a scale to measure nurses' empathy, it would be inappropriate to include an item that measures diagnostic competence. An instrument may be said to be **internally consistent** to the extent that its items measure the same trait.

Internal consistency reliability is the most widely used reliability approach among nurse researchers. This approach is the best means of assessing an especially important source of measurement error in psychosocial instruments, the sampling of items. Internal consistency is usually evaluated by calculating **coefficient alpha** (or **Cronbach's alpha**). The normal range of values for coefficient alpha is between .00 and +1.00. The higher the reliability coefficient, the more accurate (internally consistent) the measure.

Example of internal consistency reliability:
Frasure (2008) conducted a systematic review of instruments designed to measure nurses' attitudes toward research utilization. Frasure concluded that one of the strongest scales was the Research Utilization in Nursing Survey. This scale has five subscales, with alphas ranging from .77 to .91.

Equivalence

Equivalence, in the context of reliability assessment, primarily concerns the degree to which two or more independent observers or coders agree about the scoring on an instrument. With a high level of agreement, the assumption is that measurement errors have been minimized.

The degree of error can be assessed through **interrater** (or *interobserver*) **reliability** procedures, which involve having two or more trained observers or coders

make simultaneous, independent observations. An index of equivalence or agreement is then calculated with these data to evaluate the strength of the relationship between the ratings. When two independent observers score some phenomenon congruently, the scores are likely to be accurate and reliable.

Example of interrater reliability:
Polit and Beck (2008) examined whether there was evidence of gender bias in published nursing studies. They independently coded 47 variables for a sample of studies; their degree of agreement ranged from 88% to 100%.

Interpretation of Reliability Coefficients

Reliability coefficients are important indicators of an instrument's quality. Unreliable measures reduce statistical power and hence affect statistical conclusion validity. If data fail to support a hypothesis, one possibility is that the instruments were unreliable—not necessarily that the expected relationships do not exist. Knowledge about an instrument's reliability thus is critical in interpreting research results, especially if research hypotheses are not supported.

Various things affect an instrument's reliability. For example, reliability is related to sample heterogeneity. The more homogeneous the sample (i.e., the more similar the scores), the lower the reliability coefficient will be. Instruments are designed to measure differences among those being measured, and if sample members are similar to one another, it is more difficult for the instrument to discriminate reliably among those with varying degrees of the attribute. A depression scale will be less reliable with a homeless group than with a general sample. Also, longer scales (those with more items) tend to be more reliable than shorter ones.

Finally, reliability estimates vary according to the procedure used to obtain them. Estimates of reliability computed by different procedures are not identical, and so it is important to consider which aspect of reliability is most important for the attribute being measured.

Example of different reliability estimates:
Rossen and Gruber (2007) developed a scale to measure older adults' self-efficacy in relocating to independent living communities. Their 32-item scale had a test–retest reliability of .70 over a 2-week period. Cronbach's alpha for the total scale was .97.

> **TIP**
> Many psychosocial scales contain two or more **subscales**, each of which tap distinct, but related, concepts (e.g., a measure of independent functioning might include subscales for motor activities, communication, and socializing). The reliability of the subscales is typically assessed and, if subscale scores are summed for an overall score, the scale's overall reliability would also be assessed.

VALIDITY

The second important criterion for evaluating a quantitative instrument is its validity. **Validity** is the degree to which an instrument measures what it is supposed to measure. When researchers develop an instrument to measure hopelessness, how can they be sure that resulting scores validly reflect this construct and not something else, such as depression?

Reliability and validity are not totally independent qualities of an instrument. *A measuring device that is unreliable cannot possibly be valid*. An instrument cannot validly measure an attribute if it is erratic and inaccurate. An instrument can, however, be reliable without being valid. Suppose we wanted to assess patients' anxiety by measuring the circumference of their wrists. We could obtain highly accurate and precise measurements of wrist circumferences, but such measures would not be valid indicators of anxiety. Thus, the high reliability of an instrument provides no evidence of its validity; low reliability of a measure *is* evidence of low validity.

TIP

Many methodologic studies are designed to determine the quality of instruments used by clinicians or researchers. In these **psychometric assessments**, information about the instrument's reliability and validity is carefully documented.

As with reliability, validity has a number of aspects. One aspect is known as face validity. **Face validity** refers to whether the instrument looks as though it is measuring the appropriate construct, especially to people who will be completing the instrument.

Example of face validity:
Johnson and colleagues (2008) developed an instrument to measure cognitive appraisal of health among survivors of stroke. One part of the development process involved assessing the face validity of the items on the scale. Stroke survivors were asked a series of open-ended questions regarding their health appraisal after completing the scale, and then the themes that emerged were compared with the content of scale items to assess the congruence of key constructs.

Although it is good for an instrument to have face validity, three other aspects of validity are of greater importance in assessments of an instrument: content validity, criterion-related validity, and construct validity.

Content Validity

Content validity concerns the degree to which an instrument has an appropriate sample of items for the construct being measured and adequately covers the construct domain. Content validity is crucial for tests of knowledge, where the content validity question is: "How representative are the questions on this test of the universe of questions on this topic?"

Content validity is also relevant in measures of complex psychosocial traits. Researchers designing a new instrument should begin with a thorough conceptualization of the construct so the instrument can capture the full content domain. Such a conceptualization might come from rich first-hand knowledge, an exhaustive literature review, or findings from a qualitative inquiry.

An instrument's content validity is necessarily based on judgment. No totally objective methods exist for ensuring the adequate content coverage of an instrument, but it is increasingly common to use a panel of substantive experts to evaluate the content validity of new instruments. Researchers typically calculate a **content validity index** (CVI) that indicates the extent of expert agreement. We have suggested a CVI value of .90 as the standard for establishing excellence in a scale's content validity (Polit & Beck, 2006).

Example of using a content validity index:
Bu and Wu (2008) developed a scale to measure nurses' attitudes toward patient advocacy. The content validity of their 84-item scale was rated by seven experts (a bioethicist, patient advocacy researchers, measurement experts). The scale's CVI was calculated to be .85.

Criterion-Related Validity

In **criterion-related validity** assessments, researchers seek to establish a relationship between scores on an instrument and some external criterion. The instrument, whatever abstract attribute it is measuring, is said to be valid if its scores correspond strongly with scores on the criterion.

After a criterion is established, validity can be estimated easily. A **validity coefficient** is computed by using a mathematic formula that correlates scores on the instrument with scores on the criterion variable. The magnitude of the coefficient is an estimate of the instrument's validity. These coefficients (r) range between .00 and 1.00, with higher values indicating greater criterion-related validity. Coefficients of .70 or higher are desirable.

Sometimes a distinction is made between two types of criterion-related validity. **Predictive validity** refers to an instrument's ability to differentiate between people's performances or behaviors on a future criterion. When a school of nursing correlates students' incoming high school grades with their subsequent grade-point averages, the predictive validity of high school grades for nursing school performance is being evaluated. **Concurrent validity** refers to an instrument's ability to distinguish among people who differ in their present status on some criterion. For example, a psychological test to differentiate between patients in a mental institution who could and could not be released could be correlated with current behavioral ratings of health care personnel. The difference between predictive and concurrent validity, then, is the difference in the timing of obtaining measurements on a criterion.

Validation via the criterion-related approach is most often used in applied or practically oriented research. Criterion-related validity is helpful in assisting decision makers by giving them some assurance that their decisions will be effective, fair, and, in short, valid.

Example of predictive validity:
Perraud and co-researchers (2006) developed a scale—the Depression Coping Self-Efficacy Scale—to measure depressed individuals' confidence in their ability to follow treatment recommendations. Scale scores at discharge from a psychiatric hospital were found to be predictive of rehospitalization 6 to 8 weeks later.

Construct Validity

As discussed in Chapter 9, **construct validity** is a key criterion for assessing the quality of a study, and construct validity has most often been linked to measurement issues. The key construct validity questions with regard to measurement are: "What is this instrument really measuring?" and "Does it validly measure the abstract concept of interest?" The more abstract the concept, the more difficult it is to establish construct validity, however; at the same time, the more abstract the concept, the less suitable it is to rely on criterion-related validity. What objective criterion is there for such concepts as empathy, role conflict, or separation anxiety?

Construct validation is essentially a hypothesis-testing endeavor, typically linked to a theoretical perspective about the construct. In validating a measure of death anxiety, we would be less concerned with its relationship to a criterion than with its correspondence to a cogent conceptualization of death anxiety.

Construct validation can be approached in several ways, but it always involves logical analysis and testing relationships predicted on the basis of firmly grounded conceptualizations. Constructs are explicated in terms of other abstract concepts; researchers make predictions about the manner in which the target construct will function in relation to other constructs.

One approach to construct validation is the **known-groups technique**. In this procedure, groups that are expected to differ on the target attribute are administered the instrument, and group scores are compared. For instance, in validating a measure of fear of the labor experience, the scores of primiparas and multiparas could be contrasted. Women who had never given birth would likely experience more anxiety than women who had already had children; one might question the validity of the instrument if such differences did not emerge.

Another method involves examining relationships based on theoretical predictions. Researchers might reason as follows: According to theory, construct X is related to construct Y; scales A and B are measures of constructs X and Y, respectively; scores on the two scales are related to each other, as predicted by the theory; therefore, it is inferred that A and B are valid measures of X and Y. This logical analysis is fallible, but it does offer supporting evidence.

Another approach to construct validation employs a statistical procedure known as **factor analysis**, which is a method for identifying clusters of related items on a scale. The procedure is used to identify and group together different measures of some underlying attribute and to distinguish them from measures of different attributes.

In summary, construct validation employs both logical and empirical procedures. As with content validity, construct validity requires a judgment pertaining to what the instrument is measuring. Construct validity and criterion-related validity share an empirical component, but, in the latter case, there is a pragmatic, objective criterion with which to compare a measure rather than a second measure of an abstract theoretical construct.

Example of construct validation:
Weiss and co-researchers (2006) adapted the Perceived Readiness for Discharge after Birth Scale (PRDBS). They examined the construct validity of the scale using the known-groups approach, comparing several groups of mothers hypothesized to differ in their perceived readiness for discharge—for example, breastfeeding versus bottle-feeding mothers, primiparas versus multiparas, and those with and without clinical variances during postpartum hospitalization. Factor analysis was also used to further assess construct validity.

Interpretation of Validity

As with reliability, validity is not an all-or-nothing characteristic of an instrument. An instrument does not possess or lack validity; it is a question of degree. An instrument's validity is not proved, established, or verified but rather is supported to a greater or lesser extent by evidence.

Strictly speaking, researchers do not validate an instrument but rather an application of it. A measure of anxiety may be valid for presurgical patients on the day of an operation but may not be valid for nursing students on the day of a test. Of course, some instruments may be valid for a wide range of uses with different types of samples, but each use requires new supporting evidence. The more evidence that can be gathered that an instrument is measuring what it is supposed to be measuring, the more confidence people will have in its validity.

TIP
In quantitative studies involving self-report or observational instruments, the research report usually provides validity and reliability information from an earlier study—often a study conducted by the person who developed the instrument. If the sample characteristics in the original study and the new study are similar, the citation provides valuable information about data quality in the new study. Ideally, researchers should also compute new reliability coefficients for the actual research sample.

SENSITIVITY AND SPECIFICITY

Reliability and validity are the two most important criteria for evaluating quantitative instruments, but researchers sometimes need to consider other qualities. In particular, for screening and diagnostic instruments—be they self-report, observational, or biophysiologic—sensitivity and specificity need to be evaluated.

Sensitivity is the ability of a measure to identify a "case" correctly, that is, to screen in or diagnosis a condition correctly. A measure's sensitivity is its rate of yielding "true positives." **Specificity** is the measure's ability to identify noncases correctly, that is, to screen *out* those without the condition. Specificity is an instrument's rate of yielding "true negatives." To determine an instrument's sensitivity and specificity, researchers need a reliable and valid criterion of "caseness" against which scores on the instrument can be assessed.

> **TIP**
>
> There is, unfortunately, a tradeoff between the sensitivity and specificity of an instrument. When sensitivity is increased to include more true-positive cases the number of false-negative cases increases. Therefore, a critical task is to develop the appropriate *cut-off point* (i.e., the score value used to distinguish cases and noncases). Instrument developers use sophisticated procedures to make such a determination.

To illustrate, suppose we wanted to evaluate whether adolescents' self-reports about their smoking were accurate, and we asked 100 teenagers aged 13 to 15 about whether they had smoked a cigarette in the previous 24 hours. The "gold standard" for nicotine consumption is cotinine levels in a body fluid, and so let us assume that we did a urinary cotinine assay. Some fictitious data are shown in Table 14.2.

Sensitivity, in this example, is calculated as the proportion of teenagers who said they smoked *and* who had high concentrations of cotinine, divided by all real

TABLE 14.2 **FICTITIOUS DATA TO ILLUSTRATE SENSITIVITY, SPECIFICITY, AND LIKELIHOOD RATIOS**

SELF-REPORTED SMOKING	URINARY COTININE LEVEL		
	Positive (Cotinine >200 ng/mL)	Negative (Cotinine ≤ 200 ng/mL)	TOTAL
Yes, smoked	A (true positive) 20	B (false positive) 10	A + B 30
No, did not smoke	C (false negative) 20	D (true negative) 50	C + D 70
Total	A + C ("real" positives) 40	B + D ("real" negatives) 60	A + B + C + D 100

Sensitivity = A/(A + C)   = .50
Specificity = D/(B + D)   = .83
Likelihood ratio—positive (LR+) = sensitivity/(1 − specificity)   = 2.99
Likelihood ratio—negative (LR−) = (1 − sensitivity)/specificity   = .60

smokers as indicated by the urine test. Put another way, it is the true–positive findings divided by all *real*–positive findings. In this case, there was considerable under-reporting of smoking and so the sensitivity of the self-report was only .50. Specificity is the proportion of teenagers who accurately reported they did not smoke, or the true–negative findings, divided by all *real*–negative findings. In our example, specificity is .83. There was considerably less over-reporting of smoking ("faking bad") than under-reporting ("faking good"). (Sensitivity and specificity are sometimes reported as percentages rather than proportions, simply by multiplying the proportions by 100.)

> **TIP**
>
> It is difficult to establish standards of acceptability for sensitivity and specificity. Both should be as high as possible, but the establishment of cut-off points may need to take into account the financial and emotional costs of having tests with false–positive versus false–negative results.

In the medical community, reporting **likelihood ratios** has come into favor because it summarizes the relationship between specificity and sensitivity in a single number. The likelihood ratio addresses the question, "How much more likely are we to find that an indicator is positive among those *with* the outcome of concern compared with those for whom the indicator is negative?" For a positive test result, then, the likelihood ratio (LR+) is the ratio of true–positive results to false–positive results. The formula for LR+ is sensitivity, divided by 1 minus specificity. For the data in Table 14.2, LR+ is 2.99: we are about three times as likely to find that a self-report of smoking really *is* for a true smoker than it is for a non-smoker. For a negative test result, the likelihood ratio (LR−) is the ratio of false–negative results to true–negative results. For the data in Table 14.2, the LR− is .60. In this example, we are about half as likely to find that a self-report of non-smoking is false than we are to find that it reflects a true nonsmoker. When a test is high on both sensitivity and specificity (which is not especially true in our example), the LR+ value is high and the LR− value is low.

Example of likelihood ratios:
Holland and co-researchers (2006) developed and validated a screening instrument to determine early in a hospital stay the adult patients who would need specialized discharge planning services. In the sample of nearly 1,000 patients used to develop the instrument, the sensitivity was 79% and the specificity was 76%. The LR+ was 3.29 and the LR− was 0.27.

CRITIQUING DATA QUALITY IN QUANTITATIVE STUDIES

If data are seriously flawed, the study cannot contribute useful evidence. Therefore, in drawing conclusions about a study and its evidence, it is important to consider whether researchers have taken appropriate steps to collect data that accurately reflect reality. Research consumers have the right—indeed, the obligation—to ask:

"Can I trust the data?" "Do the data accurately and validly reflect the construct under study?"

Information about data quality should be provided in every quantitative research report, because it is not possible to come to conclusions about the quality of evidence of the study without such information. Reliability estimates are usually reported because they are easy to communicate. Ideally—especially for composite scales—the report should provide reliability coefficients based on data from the study itself, not just from previous research. Interrater or interobserver reliability is especially crucial for coming to conclusions about data quality in observational studies. The values of the reliability coefficients should, of course, be sufficiently high to support confidence in the findings. It is especially important to scrutinize reliability information in studies with nonsignificant findings because the unreliability of measures can undermine statistical conclusion validity.

Validity is more difficult to document in a report than reliability. At a minimum, researchers should defend their choice of existing measures based on validity information from the developers, and they should cite the relevant publication. If a study used a screening or diagnostic measure, information should also be provided about its sensitivity and specificity.

Box 14.1 provides some guidelines for critiquing aspects of data quality of quantitative measures. The guidelines are available in the Toolkit on the accompanying *Student Resource CD-ROM* for your use and adaptation. ✖

BOX 14.1 GUIDELINES FOR CRITIQUING DATA QUALITY IN QUANTITATIVE STUDIES

1. Is there congruence between the research variables as conceptualized (i.e., as discussed in the introduction of the report) and as operationalized (i.e., as described in the method section)?

2. If operational definitions (or scoring procedures) are specified, do they clearly indicate the rules of measurement? Do the rules seem sensible? Were data collected in such a way that measurement errors were minimized?

3. Does the report offer evidence of the reliability of measures? Does the evidence come from the research sample itself, or is it based on other studies? If the latter, is it reasonable to conclude that data quality would be similar for the research sample as for the reliability sample (e.g., are sample characteristics similar)?

4. If reliability is reported, which estimation method was used? Was this method appropriate? Should an alternative or additional method of reliability appraisal have been used? Is the reliability sufficiently high?

5. Does the report offer evidence of the validity of the measures? Does the evidence come from the research sample itself, or is it based on other studies? If the latter, is it reasonable to believe that data quality would be similar for the research sample as for the validity sample (e.g., are the sample characteristics similar)?

6. If validity information is reported, which validity approach was used? Was this method appropriate? Does the validity of the instrument appear to be adequate?

7. If there is no reliability or validity information, what conclusion can you reach about the quality of the data in the study?

8. If a diagnostic or screening tool was used, is information provided about its sensitivity and specificity, and were these qualities adequate?

9. Were the research hypotheses supported? If not, might data quality play a role in the failure to confirm the hypotheses?

▶ RESEARCH EXAMPLES AND CRITICAL THINKING ACTIVITIES

In this section, we provide details about the development and testing of an instrument, followed by some questions to guide critical thinking.

EXAMPLE 1 ■ Instrument Development and Psychometric Assessment

Studies

Postpartum Depression Screening Scale: Development and psychometric testing (Beck & Gable, 2000); Further validation of the Postpartum Depression Screening Scale (Beck & Gable, 2001a).

Background

Beck studied postpartum depression (PPD) in a series of qualitative studies, using both a phenomenological approach (1992, 1996) and a grounded theory approach (1993). Based on her in-depth understanding of PPD, she began to develop a scale that could be used to screen for PPD, the Postpartum Depression Screening Scale (PDSS). Working with Gable, an expert psychometrician, Beck developed, refined, and validated the scale, and had it translated into Spanish (Beck & Gable, 2000, 2001a, 2001b, 2001c, 2003, 2005).

Scale Development

The PDSS is a Likert scale designed to tap seven dimensions, such as sleeping or eating disturbances and mental confusion. A 56-item pilot form of the PDSS was initially developed with 8 items per dimension. Beck's program of research on PPD and her knowledge of the literature were used for specifying the domain and for drafting items to operationalize the construct.

Content Validity

Content validity was enhanced by using direct quotes from the qualitative studies as items on the scale (e.g., "I felt like I was losing my mind"). The pilot form was subjected to two content validation procedures, and feedback from these procedures led to some revisions.

Construct Validity

The PDSS was administered to a sample of 525 new mothers in 6 states (Beck & Gable, 2000). The PDSS was finalized as a 35-item scale with 7 subscales, each with 5 items. This version of the PDSS was subjected to factor analyses, which involved a validation of Beck's hypotheses about how individual items mapped onto underlying constructs. In a subsequent study, Beck and Gable (2001a) administered the PDSS and other depression scales to 150 new mothers and tested hypotheses about how scores on the PDSS would correlate with scores on other scales, and these analyses suggested good construct validity.

Criterion-Related Validity

In the second study, Beck and Gable correlated scores on the PDSS with an expert clinician's diagnosis of PPD for each woman. The validity coefficient was .70.

Internal Consistency Reliability

In both studies, Beck and Gable evaluated the internal consistency reliability of the PDSS and its subscales. Subscale reliability was high, ranging from .83 to .94 in the first study and from .80 to .91 in the second study.

Sensitivity and Specificity

In the second validation study, Beck and Gable examined the sensitivity and specificity of the PDSS at different cut-off points, using the expert clinician's diagnosis to establish true–positive findings and true–negative findings for PPD. In the validation study, 46 of the 150 mothers had a diagnosis of major or minor depression. To illustrate the tradeoffs the researchers made, a cut-off score of 95 on the PDSS yielded a sensitivity of .41, meaning that only 41% of the women actually diagnosed with PPD would be identified. Yet a score of 95 had a specificity of 1.00, meaning that all cases *without* an actual PPD diagnosis would be accurately screened out. At the other extreme, a cut-off score of 45 had a 1.00 sensitivity but only .28 specificity (i.e., 72% false–positive), an unacceptable rate of overdiagnosis. Based on their results, Beck and Gable recommended a cut-off score of 60, which would accurately screen in 91% of PPD cases, and would mistakenly screen in 28% who do not have PPD. Beck and Gable determined that using this cut-off point would have correctly classified 85% of their sample.

Spanish Translation

Beck (Beck & Gable, 2003, 2005) collaborated with translation experts to develop a Spanish version of the PDSS. The English and Spanish versions were administered to a bilingual sample of 34 people, in random order. Scores on the two versions were highly congruent. The alpha reliability coefficient was .95 for the total Spanish scale, and ranged from .76 to .90 for the subscales. The cut-off point for the Spanish version was also determined to be 60.

CRITICAL THINKING SUGGESTIONS*:

*See the Student Resource CD-ROM for a discussion of these questions.

1. Answer questions 3 to 6 and 8 from Box 14.1 regarding this study.
2. Also, consider the following targeted questions, which may further sharpen your critical thinking skills and assist you in understanding this study:
   a. What is the level of measurement of scores on the PDSS?
   b. Was the criterion-related validity effort an example of concurrent or predictive validity?
   c. The researchers determined that there should be seven subscales to the PDSS. Why do you think this might be the case?
   d. Each item on the PDSS is scored on a 5-point scale from 1 to 5. What is the range of possible scores on the scale, and what is the range of possible scores on each subscale?
   e. Comment on the researchers credentials for undertaking this study together, and on the appropriateness of their overall effort.
3. What might be some of the uses to which the scale could be put in clinical practice?

EXAMPLE 2 ■ Measurement and Data Quality in the Study in Appendix A

1. Read the "Instruments" subsection from Howell and colleagues' (2007) study ("Anxiety, anger, and blood pressure in children") in Appendix A of this book, and then answer the relevant questions in Box 14.1.
2. Also, consider the following targeted questions, which may further sharpen your critical thinking skills and assist you in assessing aspects of the study's merit:
   a. What could the researchers have done to assess the quality of height and weight measurements? Should they have done this?
   b. What are some potential sources of measurement error in the measurement of trait anger, trait anxiety, and anger expression in this study?
   c. What is the level of measurement of the key variables in this study?

CHAPTER REVIEW

Key new terms introduced in the chapter, together with a summary of major points, are presented in this section. In addition, Chapter 14 of the accompanying *Study Guide for Essentials of Nursing Research*, 7th edition offers various exercises and study suggestions for reinforcing concepts presented in this chapter. For additional review, see the Student Self-Study Review Questions section of the Student Resource CD-ROM provided with this book.

Key New Terms

Coefficient alpha
Construct validity
Content validity
Content validity index (CVI)
Criterion-related validity
Cronbach's alpha
Error of measurement
Face validity
Factor analysis

Internal consistency
Interval measurement
Interobserver reliability
Level of measurement
Likelihood ratio
Known-groups technique
Measurement
Nominal measurement
Ordinal measurement

Psychometric assessment
Ratio measurement
Reliability
Reliability coefficient
Sensitivity
Specificity
Test–retest reliability
Validity
Validity coefficient

Summary Points

➤ **Measurement** involves the assignment of numbers to objects to represent the amount of an attribute, using a specified set of rules.

➤ There are four **levels of measurement**: (1) **nominal measurement**—the classification of attributes into mutually exclusive categories; (2) **ordinal measurement**—the ranking of objects based on their relative standing on an attribute; (3**) interval measurement**—indicating not only the rank of objects but the distance between them; and (4) **ratio measurement**—distinguished from interval measurement by having a rational zero point.

➤ **Obtained scores** from an instrument consist of a **true score** component (the value that would be obtained for a hypothetical perfect measure of the attribute) and an error component, or **error of measurement**, that represents measurement inaccuracies.

➤ Few quantitative measuring instruments are infallible. Sources of measurement error include situational contaminants, response-set biases, and transitory personal factors, such as fatigue.

➤ **Reliability**, a primary criterion for assessing a quantitative instrument, is the degree of consistency or accuracy with which an instrument measures an attribute. The higher the reliability of an instrument, the lower the amount of error in obtained scores.

➤ Different methods are used to assess an instrument's reliability and to compute a **reliability coefficient**. Reliability coefficients typically range from .00 to 1.00, and should be at least .70 (but preferably greater than .80) to be considered satisfactory.

➤ The **stability** aspect of reliability, which concerns the extent to which an instrument yields the same results on repeated administrations, is evaluated by **test–retest procedures.**

➤ **Internal consistency** reliability, which refers to the extent to which all the instrument's items are measuring the same attribute, is usually assessed with **Cronbach's alpha**.

➤ When the reliability assessment focuses on **equivalence** between observers in rating or coding behaviors, estimates of **interrater** (or **interobserver**) **reliability** are obtained.

➤ **Validity** is the degree to which an instrument measures what it is supposed to be measuring.

➤ **Face validity** refers to whether the instrument appears, on the face of it, to be measuring the appropriate construct.

➤ **Content validity** is concerned with the sampling adequacy of the content being measured. Expert ratings on the relevance of items can be used to compute a **content validity index** (**CVI**).

➤ **Criterion-related validity** (which includes both **predictive validity** and **concurrent validity**) focuses on the correlation between the instrument and an outside criterion.

➤ **Construct validity**, an instrument's adequacy in measuring the focal construct, is a hypothesis-testing endeavor. One construct validation method, the **known-groups technique**, contrasts scores of groups hypothesized to differ on the attribute; another is **factor analysis**, a statistical procedure for identifying unitary clusters of items.

➤ Sensitivity and specificity are important criteria for screening and for diagnostic instruments. **Sensitivity** is the instrument's ability to identify a case correctly (i.e., its rate of yielding true–positive results). **Specificity** is the instrument's ability to identify noncases correctly (i.e., its rate of yielding true–negative results). Other related indexes, **likelihood ratios**, are frequently used in medical research.

➤ A **psychometric assessment** of a new instrument is usually undertaken to gather evidence about validity, reliability, and other assessment criteria.

STUDIES CITED IN CHAPTER 14

Beck, C. T. (1992). The lived experience of postpartum depression: A phenomenological study. *Nursing Research, 41*, 166–170.

Beck, C. T. (1993). Teetering on the edge: A substantive theory of postpartum depression. *Nursing Research, 42*, 42–48.

Beck, C. T. (1996). Postpartum depressed mothers interacting with their children. *Nursing Research, 45*, 98–104.

Beck, C. T., & Gable, R. K. (2000). Postpartum Depression Screening Scale: Development and psychometric testing. *Nursing Research, 49,* 272-282.

Beck, C. T., & Gable, R. K. (2001a). Further validation of the Postpartum Depression Screening Scale. *Nursing Research, 50,* 155–164.

Beck, C. T., & Gable, R. K. (2003). Postpartum Depression Screening Scale: Spanish version. *Nursing Research, 52,* 296–306.

Beck, C. T., & Gable, R. K. (2005). Screening performance of the Postpartum Depression Screening Scale—Spanish version. *Journal of Transcultural Nursing, 16*(4), 331–338.

Bu, X., & Wu, Y. (2008). Development and psychometric evaluation of the instrument: Attitude Toward Patient Advocacy. *Research in Nursing & Health, 31,* 63–75.

Frasure, J. (2008). Analysis of instruments measuring nurses' attitudes toward research utilization: A systematic review. *Journal of Advanced Nursing, 61,* 5–18.

Holland, D., Harris, M., Leibson, C., Pankrantz, V., & Krichbaum, K. (2006). Development and validation of a screen for specialized discharge planning services. *Nursing Research, 55,* 62–71.

Johnson, E., Bakas, T., & Lyon, B. (2008). Cognitive Appraisal of Health Scale. *Clinical Nurse Specialist, 22,* 12–18.

Lyon, D., McCain, N., Walter, J., & Schubert, C. (2008). Cytokine comparisons between women with breast cancer and women with a negative breast biopsy. *Nursing Research, 57,* 51–58.

Perraud, S., Fogg, L., Kopytko, E., & Gross, D. (2006). Predictive validity of the Depression Coping Self-Efficacy Scale (DCSES). *Research in Nursing & Health, 29,* 147–160.

Polit, D., & Beck, C. (2008). Is there gender bias in nursing research? *Research in Nursing & Health 31,* 417–427.

Rossen, E., & Gruber, K. (2007). Development and psychometric testing of the relocation self-efficacy scale. *Nursing Research, 56,* 244–251.

Weiss, M., Ryan, P., & Lokken, L. (2006). Validity and reliability of the Perceived Readiness for Discharge After Birth Scale. *Journal of Obstetric, Gynecologic, & Neonatal Nursing, 35,* 34–45.

Welch, J., Bennett, S., Delp, R., & Agarwal, R. (2006). Benefits of and barriers to dietary sodium adherence. *Western Journal of Nursing Research, 28,* 162–180.

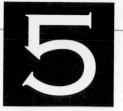

PART 5

Data Analysis and Interpretation

15 Statistical Analysis of Quantitative Data

STUDENT OBJECTIVES

On completing this chapter, you will be able to:

➤ Describe the characteristics of frequency distributions, and identify and interpret various descriptive statistics

➤ Describe the logic and purpose of parameter estimation, and interpret confidence intervals

➤ Describe the logic and purpose of tests of statistical significance, describe hypothesis testing procedures, and interpret *p* values

➤ Specify the appropriate applications for *t*-tests, analysis of variance, chi-squared tests, and correlation coefficients and interpret the meaning of the calculated statistics

➤ Describe the applications and principles of multiple regression and analysis of covariance

➤ Understand the results of simple statistical procedures described in a research report

➤ Define new terms in the chapter

The data collected in a study do not by themselves answer research questions or test research hypotheses. Data need to be systematically analyzed so that trends and patterns can be detected. This chapter describes procedures for analyzing quantitative data, and Chapter 17 discusses the analysis of qualitative data.

DESCRIPTIVE STATISTICS

Without statistics, quantitative data would be a chaotic mass of numbers. Statistical procedures enable researchers to organize, interpret, and communicate numeric information. Statistics are either descriptive or inferential. **Descriptive statistics** are used to synthesize and describe data. Averages and percentages are examples of descriptive statistics. When such indexes are calculated on data from a population, they are called **parameters**. A descriptive index from a sample is a **statistic.** Most scientific questions are about parameters; researchers calculate statistics to estimate them and use **inferential statistics** to make inferences about the population.

A set of data can be described in terms of three characteristics: the shape of the distribution of values, central tendency, and variability. Central tendency and variability are dealt with in subsequent sections.

Frequency Distributions

Data that are not analyzed or organized are overwhelming. It is not even possible to discern general trends in the data without some structure. Consider the 60 numbers in Table 15.1. Let us assume that these numbers are the scores of 60 preoperative patients on a six-item measure of anxiety—scores that are on an interval scale. Visual inspection of the numbers in this table provides little insight on patients' anxiety.

Frequency distributions are a method of imposing order on numeric data. A **frequency distribution** is a systematic arrangement of numeric values from the lowest to the highest, together with a count (or percentage) of the number of times each

TABLE 15.1	PATIENTS' ANXIETY SCORES								
22	27	25	19	24	25	23	29	24	20
26	16	20	26	17	22	24	18	26	28
15	24	23	22	21	24	20	25	18	27
24	23	16	25	30	29	27	21	23	24
26	18	30	21	17	25	22	24	29	28
20	25	26	24	23	19	27	28	25	26

TABLE 15.2	FREQUENCY DISTRIBUTION OF PATIENTS' ANXIETY SCORES	
SCORE (X)	FREQUENCY (f)	PERCENTAGE (%)
15	1	1.7
16	2	3.3
17	2	3.3
18	3	5.0
19	2	3.3
20	4	6.7
21	3	5.0
22	4	6.7
23	5	8.3
24	9	15.0
25	7	11.7
26	6	10.0
27	4	6.7
28	3	5.0
29	3	5.0
30	2	3.3
	N = 60	100.0%

value was obtained. The 60 anxiety scores are presented as a frequency distribution in Table 15.2. This arrangement makes it convenient to see the highest and lowest scores, the most common score, where the scores clustered, and how many patients were in the sample (total sample size is typically designated as **N** in research reports). None of this was easily discernible before the data were organized.

Some researchers display frequency data graphically in a *frequency polygon* (Fig. 15.1). In such graphs, scores typically are on the horizontal line, with the lowest value on the left, and frequency counts or percentages are on the vertical line. Data distributions can be described by their shapes. **Symmetric distribution** occurs if, when folded over, the two halves of a frequency polygon would be superimposed (Fig. 15.2). In an asymmetric or **skewed distribution**, the peak is off center, and one tail is longer than the other. When the longer tail is pointed toward

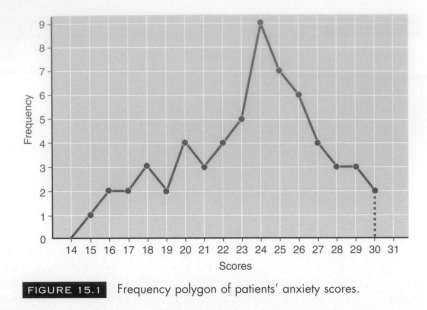

Frequency polygon of patients' anxiety scores.

the right, the distribution has a **positive skew**, as in the first graph of Figure 15.3. Personal income is an example of a positively skewed attribute. Most people have moderate incomes, with only a few people with high incomes at the right end of the distribution. If the longer tail points to the left, the distribution has a **negative skew**, as in the second graph in Figure 15.3. Age at death is an example of a negatively skewed attribute. Here, most people are at the far right end of the distribution, with relatively few people dying at an early age.

Another aspect of a distribution's shape concerns how many peaks or high points it has. A *unimodal distribution* has one peak (graph A, Figure 15.2), whereas a *multimodal distribution* has two or more peaks—that is, two or more values of high frequency. A multimodal distribution with two peaks is a *bimodal distribution*, illustrated in graph B of Figure 15.2.

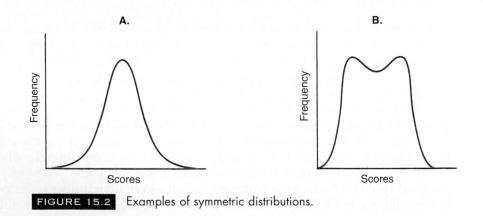

Examples of symmetric distributions.

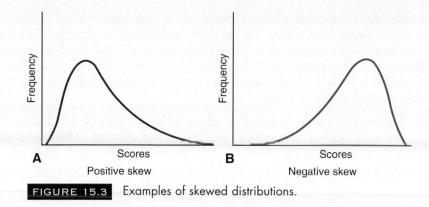

FIGURE 15.3   Examples of skewed distributions.

A distribution of particular interest is the **normal distribution** (sometimes called *a bell-shaped curve*). A normal distribution is symmetric, unimodal, and not very peaked, as illustrated in graph A of Figure 15.2. Many human attributes (e.g., height, intelligence) approximate a normal distribution.

Central Tendency

Frequency distributions are a good way to organize data and clarify patterns, but often a pattern is less useful than an overall summary. Researchers usually ask such questions as, "What is the average oxygen consumption of myocardial infarction patients during bathing?" or "What is the average weight loss of patients with cancer?" Such questions seek a single number that best represents a distribution of values. Because an index of typicalness is more likely to come from the center of a distribution than from an extreme, such indexes are called measures of **central tendency**. Lay people use the term *average* to refer to central tendency, but researchers avoid this term because there are three indexes of central tendency: the mode, the median, and the mean.

➤ **Mode:** The mode is the number that occurs most frequently in a distribution. In the following distribution, the mode is 53:

50 51 51 52 53 53 53 53 54 55 56

The value of 53 occurred four times, a higher frequency than for other numbers. The mode of the patients' anxiety scores in Table 15.2 was 24. The mode, in other words, identifies the most "popular" value. The mode is used most often to describe typical or high-frequency values for nominal measures.

➤ **Median:** The median is the point in a distribution that divides scores in half. Consider the following set of values:

2 2 3 3 4 5 6 7 8 9

The value that divides the cases in half is midway between 4 and 5, and thus 4.5 is the median. For the patient anxiety scores, the median is 24, the same as the mode. An important characteristic of the median is that it does not take into account individual values and is thus insensitive to extremes. In the above set of numbers, if the value of 9 were changed to 99, the median would remain 4.5. Because of this property, the median is the preferred index of central tendency to describe a highly skewed distribution. In research reports, the median may be abbreviated as *Md* or *Mdn*.

➤ **Mean:** The mean is equal to the sum of all values divided by the number of participants—what people refer to as the average. The mean of the patients' anxiety scores is 23.4 (1405 ÷ 60). As another example, here are the weights of eight people:

$$85 \ 109 \ 120 \ 135 \ 158 \ 177 \ 181 \ 195$$

In this example, the mean is 145. Unlike the median, the mean is affected by the value of every score. If we were to exchange the 195-lb person for one weighing 275 lb, the mean weight would increase from 145 to 155 lb. A substitution of this kind would leave the median unchanged. In research reports, the mean is often symbolized as M or $\bar{X}$ (e.g., $\bar{X} = 145$).

For interval-level or ratio-level measurements, the mean, rather than the median or mode, is usually the statistic reported. Of the three indexes, the mean is the most stable: if repeated samples were drawn from a population, the means would fluctuate less than the modes or medians. Because of its stability, the mean usually is the best estimate of a population central tendency. When a distribution is highly skewed, however, the mean does not characterize the center of the distribution; in such situations, the median is preferred. For example, the median is a better central tendency measure of family income than the mean because income is positively skewed.

Variability

Two distributions with identical means could differ markedly with respect to shape (e.g., how skewed they are) and how spread out the data are (i.e., how different people are from one another on an attribute). This section describes the **variability** of distributions.

Consider the two distributions in Figure 15.4, which represent hypothetical scores for students from two schools on an IQ test. Both distributions have a mean of 100, but the patterns are different. School A has a wide range of scores, with some below 70 and some above 130. In school B, by contrast, there are few low or high scores. School A is more **heterogeneous** (i.e., more variable) than school B, and school B is more **homogeneous** than school A. Researchers compute an index of variability to express the extent to which scores in a distribution differ from one another. The most common indexes are the range and standard deviation.

➤ **Range:** The range is the highest score minus the lowest score in a distribution. In the example of the patients' anxiety scores, the range is 15 (30 − 15). In the distributions in Figure 15.4, the range for school A is about 80 (140 − 60), whereas the range for school B is about 50 (125 − 75). The chief virtue of the

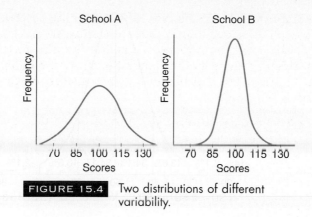

FIGURE 15.4 Two distributions of different variability.

range is its ease of computation. Because it is based on only two scores, however, the range is unstable: from sample to sample from the same population, the range tends to fluctuate considerably. Moreover, the range ignores score variations between the two extremes. In school B of Figure 15.4, if a single student obtained a score of 60 and another obtained a score of 140, the range of both schools would then be 80, despite large differences in heterogeneity. For these reasons, the range is used largely as a gross descriptive index.

➤ **Standard deviation:** The most widely used variability index is the standard deviation. Like the mean, the standard deviation is calculated based on every value in a distribution.[*] The standard deviation summarizes the *average* amount of deviation of values from the mean. In the anxiety scale example, the standard deviation is 3.725.[**] In research reports, the standard deviation is often abbreviated as *s* or *SD*.

TIP

Occasionally, the standard deviation is simply shown in relation to the mean without a formal label. For example, the patients' anxiety scores might be shown as $M = 23.4$ (3.7) or $M = 23.4 \pm 3.7$, where 23.4 is the mean and 3.7 is the standard deviation.

A standard deviation is more difficult to interpret than the range. For the SD of the anxiety scores, you might ask, 3.725 *what*? What does the number mean? We can answer these questions from several angles. First, the SD is an index of how variable scores in a distribution are and so if (for example) male and female nursing students had means of 23 on the anxiety scale, but their SDs were 7 and 3,

---

[*] Formulas for computing the standard deviation, as well as other statistics discussed in this chapter, are not shown in this textbook. The emphasis here is on helping you to understand statistical applications. References at the end of the book can be consulted for computation formulas (e.g., Polit, 1996).

[**] Research reports occasionally refer to an index of variability known as the **variance**. The variance is simply the value of the standard deviation squared. In the example of the patients' anxiety scores, the variance is 3.725^2, or 13.88.

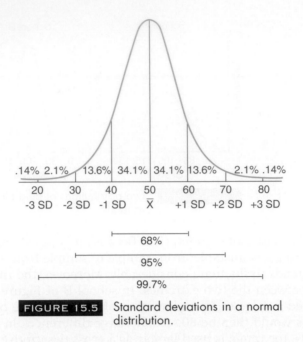

.14% 2.1% 13.6% 34.1% 34.1% 13.6% 2.1% .14%

20	30	40	50	60	70	80
-3 SD	-2 SD	-1 SD	$\overline{X}$	+1 SD	+2 SD	+3 SD

68%

95%

99.7%

FIGURE 15.5 Standard deviations in a normal distribution.

respectively, we would immediately know that the females were more homogeneous (i.e., their scores were more similar to one another).

The standard deviation represents the *average* of deviations from the mean. The mean tells us the single best point for summarizing an entire distribution, and a standard deviation tells us how much, on average, the scores deviate from that mean. In the anxiety scale example, they deviated by an average of just under 4 points. A standard deviation might thus be interpreted as an indication of our degree of error when we use a mean to describe an entire sample.

In normal and near-normal distributions, there are roughly three standard deviations above and below the mean. Suppose we had a normal distribution with a mean of 50 and an SD of 10 (Fig. 15.5). In such a distribution, a fixed percentage of cases fall within certain distances from the mean. Of all cases, 68% fall within 1 SD above and below the mean. Thus, in this example, nearly 7 of 10 scores are between 40 and 60. In a normal distribution, 95% of the scores fall within 2 SDs from the mean. Only a handful of cases—about 2% at each extreme—lie more than 2 SDs from the mean. Using this figure, we can see that a person with a score of 70 achieved a higher score than about 98% of the sample.

TIP

Descriptive statistics (percentages, means, standard deviations, and so on) are used for various purposes, but are most often used to summarize sample characteristics, describe key research variables, and document methodologic features (e.g., response rates). They are seldom used to answer research questions—inferential statistics are usually used for this purpose.

TABLE 15.3	EXAMPLE OF DESCRIPTIVE STATISTICS: SELECTED PSYCHOSOCIAL RISKS AND RESOURCES FOR LOW-INCOME WOMEN		
	N	RANGE OF ACTUAL SCORES	MEAN (SD)
Stress (Prenatal Psychosocial Profile, PPP)	130	11–54	18.3 (5.7)
Depression (Beck Depression Inventory)	128	2–59	13.6 (9.9)
Spirituality (Spiritual Perspective Scale)	130	14–60	48.0 (9.2)
Total social support (PPP scale)	129	13–132	98.8 (30.5)

Adapted from Jesse, D. E., Graham, M., & Swanson, M. (2006). Psychosocial and spiritual factors associated with smoking and substance use during pregnancy in African American and white low-income women. *Journal of Obstetric, Gynecologic, & Neonatal Nursing, 35*(1), 68–77.

Example of descriptive statistics:

Table 15.3 presents descriptive statistics based on data from a Jesse and colleagues' (2006) study of factors related to smoking and substance use during pregnancy among low-income women. The table shows, for four psychosocial risk or resource factors, the actual range of scores, mean scores, and SDs. We can see from this table that the scores were heterogeneous, and that most distributions were skewed. For example, the mean on the spirituality scale (48.0) was much higher than the midpoint between the lowest and highest value (37.0), indicating a negative skew.

Bivariate Descriptive Statistics

So far, our discussion has focused on *univariate* (one-variable) *descriptive statistics*. The mean, mode, and standard deviation describe one variable at a time. *Bivariate* (two-variable) *descriptive statistics* describe relationships between two variables.

Contingency Tables

A **contingency table** (or **crosstab**) is a two-dimensional frequency distribution in which the frequencies of two variables are *crosstabulated*. Suppose we had data on patients' sex and whether they were nonsmokers, light smokers (<1 pack of cigarettes a day), or heavy smokers (≥1 pack a day). The question is whether there is a tendency for men to smoke more heavily than women, or vice versa (i.e., whether there is a *relationship* between smoking and sex). Fictitious data on these two variables are shown in a contingency table in Table 15.4. Six **cells** are created by placing one variable (sex) along one dimension and the other variable (smoking status) along the other dimension. After subjects' data are allocated to the appropriate cells, percentages are computed. The crosstab allows us to see at a glance that, in this sample, women were more likely than men to be nonsmokers (45.4% versus 27.3%) and less likely to be heavy smokers (18.2% versus 36.4%). Contingency tables usually are used with nominal data or ordinal data that have few ranks. In the present example, sex is nominal, and smoking status, as defined, is ordinal.

TABLE 15.4 ▶ **CONTINGENCY TABLE FOR SEX AND SMOKING STATUS RELATIONSHIP**

| | SEX | | | | | |
| | WOMEN | | MEN | | TOTAL | |
SMOKING STATUS	n	%	n	%	n	%
Nonsmoker	10	45.4	6	27.3	16	36.4
Light smoker	8	36.4	8	36.4	16	36.4
Heavy smoker	4	18.2	8	36.4	12	27.3
TOTAL	22	100.0	22	100.0	44	100.0

Correlation

Relationships between two variables are usually described through **correlation** procedures. The correlation question is: To what extent are two variables related to each other? For example, to what degree are anxiety test scores and blood pressure measures related? This question can be answered quantitatively by calculating a **correlation coefficient**, which describes the *intensity* and *direction* of a relationship.

Two variables that are related are height and weight: tall people tend to weigh more than short people. The relationship between height and weight would be a *perfect relationship* if the tallest person in a population was the heaviest, the second tallest person was the second heaviest, and so on. The correlation coefficient summarizes how "perfect" a relationship is. The possible values for a correlation coefficient range from −1.00 through .00 to +1.00. If height and weight were perfectly correlated, the correlation coefficient expressing this would be 1.00 (the actual correlation coefficient is in the vicinity of .50 to .60 for a general population). Height and weight have a **positive relationship** because greater height tends to be associated with greater weight.

When two variables are unrelated, the correlation coefficient is zero. One might anticipate that women's shoe size is unrelated to their intelligence. Women with large feet are as likely to perform well on IQ tests as those with small feet. The correlation coefficient summarizing such a relationship would presumably be in the vicinity of .00.

Correlation coefficients between .00 and −1.00 express a **negative** (*inverse*) **relationship**. When two variables are inversely related, increments in one variable are associated with decrements in the second. For example, there is a negative correlation between depression and self-esteem. This means that, on average, people with *high* self-esteem tend to be *low* on depression. If the relationship were perfect (i.e., if the person with the highest self-esteem score had the lowest depression score and so on), then the correlation coefficient would be −1.00. In actuality, the relationship between depression and self-esteem is moderate—usually in the vicinity of −.40 or −.50. Note that the higher the *absolute value* of the coefficient (i.e., the value disregarding the sign), the stronger the relationship. A correlation of −.80, for instance, is much stronger than a correlation of +.20.

The most commonly used **correlation** index is the **product–moment correlation coefficient** (also referred to as **Pearson's** *r*), which is computed with interval or ratio measures. It is difficult to offer guidelines on what should be interpreted as strong or weak relationships, because it depends on the variables. If we were to measure patients' body temperature both orally and rectally, a correlation (*r*) of .70 between the two measurements would be low. For most psychosocial variables (e.g., stress and severity of illness), however, an *r* of .70 would be rather high. Perfect correlations (+1.00 and −1.00) are extremely rare.

TIP

Validity coefficients, such as those described in Chapter 14, are usually calculated using Pearson's correlation coefficients.

In research reports, correlation coefficients are often reported in tables displaying a two-dimensional **correlation matrix**, in which variables are displayed in both rows and columns. To read a correlation matrix, one finds the row for one variable and reads across until the row intersects with the column for another variable, as described in the following example.

Example of a correlation matrix:
Lee and colleagues (2007) conducted a study to examine interrelationships among mothers' characteristics, paternal support, and mothers' interactions with their medically fragile infants. Table 15.5, adapted from their report, presents a correlation matrix for some key study variables.

This table lists, on the left, four variables: mothers' positive involvement with their infant (variable 1), mother's education (2), mothers' depressive symptoms (3), and fathers' support (4). The numbers in the top row, from 1 to 4, correspond to the four variables: 1 is maternal positive involvement, and so on. The correlation matrix shows, in column 1, the correlation coefficient between maternal involvement and all variables. At the intersection of row 1, column 1, we find 1.00, which simply indicates that maternal involvement scores are perfectly correlated with themselves. The next entry in the first column is the value of *r* between maternal involvement and maternal education. The value of .28 (which can be read as +.28) indicates a modest, positive relationship between these two variables: women with more education had a slight tendency to demonstrate more positive involvement with their infants. The next entry in column 1 shows a negative correlation between maternal involvement and maternal depression (−.38), indicating a tendency for higher depression to be associated with less positive involvement.

Describing Risk

The evidence-based practice (EBP) movement has made clinical decision-making based on research findings an important issue. There are a number of descriptive statistical indexes that can be used to interpret findings and facilitate such decision-making. Many of these indexes involve calculating changes in risk—for example, a change in risk after exposure to a potentially beneficial intervention. The indexes

TABLE 15.5	EXAMPLE OF A CORRELATION MATRIX: STUDY OF MEDICALLY FRAGILE INFANTS AT 6 MONTHS ($N = 59$)			
VARIABLE	1	2	3	4
1. Mother's positive involvement with infant	1.00			
2. Mother's education	.28	1.00		
3. Mother's depressive symptoms	−.38	−.22	1.00	
4. Father's social support/helpfulness	.20	.17	−.38	1.00

Adapted from Table 3 of Lee et al. (2007).

described in this section are often not reported in nursing research articles, but they are routinely described in books on EBP.

In this section, we focus on describing dichotomous outcomes (e.g., had a fall/did not have a fall) in relation to exposure or nonexposure to a beneficial treatment or protective factor. This situation results in a 2×2 contingency table with four cells. The four cells in the contingency table in Table 15.6 are labeled so that various indexes can be explained. *Cell a* is the number with an undesirable outcome

TABLE 15.6	INDEXES OF RISK AND ASSOCIATION IN A 2×2 CONTINGENCY TABLE		
EXPOSURE TO AN INTERVENTION OR PROTECTIVE FACTOR	OUTCOME		TOTAL
	YES (Undesirable Outcome)	NO (Desirable Outcome)	
Yes (Exposed)	a	b	a + b
No (Not Exposed)	c	d	c + d
TOTAL	a + c	b + d	a + b + c + d

Absolute Risk, exposed group (AR_E)	$= a/(a + b)$		
Absolute Risk, non-exposed group (AR_{NE})	$= c/(c + d)$		
Absolute Risk Reduction (ARR)	$= (c/(c + d)) - (a/(a + b))$	Or	$AR_{NE} - AR_E$
Odds Ratio (OR)	$= \dfrac{ad}{bc}$	Or	$\dfrac{a/b}{c/d}$

(e.g., death) in an intervention/protected group; *cell b* is the number with a desirable outcome (e.g., survival) in an intervention/protected group; and *cells c* and *d* are the two outcome possibilities for a nontreated or unprotected group. We can now explain the meaning and calculation of some indexes that are of interest to clinicians. The Toolkit on the accompanying CD-ROM includes additional indexes. ⊗

TIP

Note that the computations shown in Table 15.6 specifically reflect *risk* indexes that assume that exposure to an intervention or protective factor will be beneficial, and that information for the *undesirable* outcome (risk) will be in cells a and c. If good outcomes rather than risks are put in cells a and c, the formulas would have to be modified. As a general rule, to use the formulas shown in Table 15.6, the cell in the lower left corner (cell c) should be hypothesized to reflect the highest number of undesirable outcomes.

Absolute Risk

Absolute risk can be computed for both those exposed to an intervention or protective factor, and for those not exposed. **Absolute risk** is simply the proportion of people who experienced an undesirable outcome in each group. To illustrate, suppose 200 smokers were randomly assigned to a smoking cessation intervention or to a control group (Table 15.7). Smoking status 3 months after the intervention is the outcome variable. In this example, the absolute risk of continued smoking is .50

TABLE 15.7	HYPOTHETICAL DATA FOR SMOKING CESSATION INTERVENTION EXAMPLE		
EXPOSURE TO INTERVENTION	OUTCOME		TOTAL
	CONTINUED SMOKING	STOPPED SMOKING	
Yes (experimental group)	50	50	100
No (control group)	80	20	100
TOTAL	130	70	200

Absolute risk, exposed group (AR_E) $= 50/100 = .50$

Absolute risk, non-exposed group (AR_{NE}) $= 80/100 = .80$

Absolute risk reduction (ARR) $= .80 - .50 = .30$

Odds ratio (OR) $= \dfrac{(50/50)}{(80/20)} = .25$

in the intervention group and .80 in the control group. In the absence of the intervention, 20% of those in the experimental group would presumably have stopped smoking anyway, but the intervention boosted the rate to 50%.

Absolute Risk Reduction

The **absolute risk reduction (ARR)** index represents a comparison of the two risks. It is computed by subtracting the absolute risk for the exposed group from the absolute risk for the unexposed group. This index indicates the estimated proportion of people who would be spared from the undesirable outcome through exposure to an intervention or protective factor. In our example, the value of ARR is .30: 30% of the control group subjects presumably would have stopped smoking if they had received the intervention, over and above the 20% who stopped without the intervention.

TIP

An index known as the **risk ratio** (RR) or *relative risk* is another risk index. The RR is the estimated proportion of the original risk of an adverse outcome (in our example, continued smoking) that persists when people are exposed to the intervention. Computations and an expanded discussion of relative risk are available on the Toolkit of the accompanying CD-ROM.

Odds Ratio

The odds ratio (OR) is the most widely-reported risk index, even though it is less intuitively meaningful than other risk indexes. The **odds**, in this context, is the proportion of subjects *with* the adverse outcome relative to those *without* it. In our example, the odds of continued smoking for the experimental group is 50 (the number who continued smoking) divided by 50 (the number who stopped), or 1. The odds for the control group is 80 divided by 20, or 4. The **odds ratio** is the ratio of these two odds, or .25 in our example. The estimated odds of continuing to smoke are one-fourth as high for those in the intervention group as among those in the control group. Turned around, we could say that the estimated odds of continued smoking is four times higher among smokers who do not get the intervention as among those who do. Odds ratios can also be computed when the independent variable is not dichotomous. For instance, we could estimate the OR for having a low birthweight infant among mothers in three different age groups (20 or younger, 21 to 30, and 31 and older), using one of the groups as a reference. In the following example, the control group was the reference group for three intervention groups.

Example of odds ratios:
Champion and colleagues (2007) conducted a randomized clinical trial (RCT) to test methods of increasing mammography adherence among women who had not had a mammography in the previous 15 months. Women were randomized to one of four groups: usual care, tailored telephone counseling, tailored print, and tailored print *and* telephone counseling. Compared with usual care, all intervention groups increased mammography adherence, with ORs ranging from 1.60 to 1.91.

INTRODUCTION TO INFERENTIAL STATISTICS

Descriptive statistics are useful for summarizing data, but researchers usually do more than simply describe. **Inferential statistics**, which are based on the *laws of probability*, provide a means for drawing conclusions about a population, given data from a sample.

Sampling Distributions

When using a sample to estimate population characteristics, it is important to obtain a sample that is representative, and random sampling is the best means of securing such samples. Inferential statistics are based on the assumption of random sampling from populations—although this assumption is widely violated.

Even with random sampling, however, sample characteristics are seldom identical to those of the population. Suppose we had a population of 30,000 nursing school applicants whose mean score on a standardized entrance examination was 500 with a standard deviation of 100. Now suppose we do not know these parameters, but must estimate them based on scores from a random sample of 25 students. Should we expect a mean of exactly 500 and a standard deviation of 100 for the sample? It would be improbable to obtain identical values. Our sample mean might be, for example, 505. If we drew a completely new random sample of 25 students and computed the mean, we might obtain a value of 497. Sample statistics fluctuate and are unequal to the population parameter because of sampling error. Researchers need a way to determine whether sample statistics are good estimates of population parameters.

To understand the logic of inferential statistics, we must perform a mental exercise. Consider drawing a sample of 25 students from the population of applicants, calculating a mean score, replacing the students, and drawing a new sample. If we drew 5,000 samples, we would have 5,000 means (data points) that we could use to construct a frequency polygon (Figure 15.6). This distribution is called a **sampling distribution of the mean**. A sampling distribution is theoretical, because in practice no one *actually* draws consecutive samples from a population and plots their means. Statisticians have shown that (1) sampling distributions of means are normally distributed and (2) the mean of a sampling distribution equals the population mean. In our example, the mean of the sampling distribution is 500, the same as the population mean.

Remember that when scores are normally distributed, 68% of the cases fall between +1 SD and −1 SD from the mean. Thus, for a sampling distribution of means, the probability is 68 out of 100 that any randomly drawn sample mean lies between +1 SD and −1 SD of the population mean. The problem is to determine the standard deviation of the sampling distribution—which is called the **standard error of the mean** (or SEM). The word *error* signifies that the sample means contain some error as estimates of the population mean. The smaller the standard error (i.e., the less variable the sample means), the more accurate are the means as estimates of the population value.

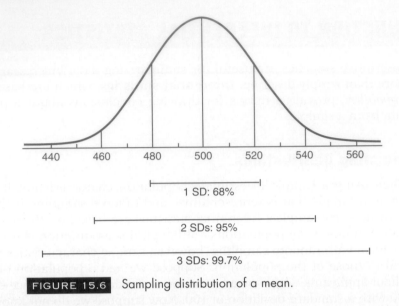

FIGURE 15.6 Sampling distribution of a mean.

Because no one actually constructs a sampling distribution, how can its standard deviation be computed? Fortunately, there is a formula for estimating the SEM from data from a single sample, using two pieces of information: the standard deviation for the sample and sample size. In the present example, the SEM is 20 (Figure 15.6), which represents an estimate of how much sampling error there would be from one sample mean to another in an infinite number of samples of 25 students.

We can now estimate the probability of drawing a sample with a certain mean. With a sample size of 25 and a population mean of 500, the chances are about 95 out of 100 that a sample mean would fall between the values of 460 and 540—2 SDs above and below the mean. Only 5 times out of 100 would the mean of a randomly selected sample of 25 applicants be greater than 540 or less than 460. In other words, only 5 times out of 100 would we be likely to draw a sample whose mean deviates from the population mean by more than 40 points.

Because the SEM is partly a function of sample size, we need only increase sample size to increase the accuracy of our estimate. Suppose that instead of using a sample of 25 applicants to estimate the population mean, we used a sample of 100. With this many students, the standard error of the mean would be 10, not 20—and the probability would be about 95 in 100 that a sample mean would be between 480 and 520. The chances of drawing a sample with a mean very different from that of the population are reduced as sample size increases because large numbers promote the likelihood that extreme cases will cancel each other out.

You may be wondering why you need to learn about these abstract statistical notions. Consider, though, that what we are talking about concerns how likely it is that a researcher's results are accurate. As an intelligent consumer, you need to evaluate critically how believable research evidence is so that you can decide whether to incorporate it into your nursing practice. The concepts underlying the standard error are important in such an evaluation and are related to issues we stressed in Chapter 12 on sampling. First, the more homogeneous the population is on the critical attribute (i.e., the smaller the standard deviation), the more likely it is that results calculated from a sample will be accurate. Second, the larger the sample size, the greater is the likelihood of accuracy. The concepts discussed in this section are the basis for drawing conclusions about statistical evidence.

Estimation of Parameters

Statistical inference consists of two techniques: estimation of parameters and hypothesis testing. Parameter estimations are infrequently presented in nursing research reports, but that situation is changing. The emphasis on EBP has heightened interest among practitioners in learning not only whether a hypothesis was supported (via traditional hypothesis tests) but also the estimated value of a population parameter and the level of accuracy of the estimate (via parameter estimation). Most medical research journals *require* that estimation information be reported because it is more useful to clinicians, reflecting the view that this approach offers information about both clinical and statistical significance. In this section we present some general concepts relating to parameter estimation and offer some examples based on one-variable descriptive statistics.

Point Estimation

Parameter estimation is used to estimate a parameter—for example, a mean, a proportion, or a mean difference between two groups (e.g., experimental and control subjects). Estimation can take two forms: point estimation or interval estimation. *Point estimation* involves calculating a single statistic to estimate the population parameter. To continue with the earlier example, if we calculated the mean entrance examination score for a sample of 25 applicants and found that it was 510, then this would be the point estimate of the population mean.

Confidence Intervals

Point estimates convey no information about margin of error and so inferences about the accuracy of the parameter estimate cannot objectively be made. *Interval estimation* of a parameter is useful because it indicates a range of values within which the parameter has a specified probability of lying. With interval estimation, researchers construct a **confidence interval** (**CI**) around the estimate; the upper and lower limits are called **confidence limits**. Constructing a confidence interval around a sample mean establishes a range of values for the population value and the probability of being right—the estimate is made with a certain degree of confidence. By convention, researchers usually use either a 95% or a 99% confidence interval.

TIP

Confidence intervals address one of the key EBP questions for appraising evidence presented in Box 2.1: How *precise* is the estimate of effects?

Calculating confidence limits around a mean involves the SEM. As shown in Figure 15.6, 95% of the scores in a normal distribution lie within about 2 SDs (more precisely, 1.96 SDs) from the mean. In our example, if the point estimate for mean test scores is 510 and the SD is 100, the SEM for a sample of 25 would be 20. We can build a 95% confidence interval with this formula: CI 95% = $(\bar{X} \pm 1.96 \times SEM)$. That is, the confidence is 95% that the population mean lies between the values equal to 1.96 times the SEM, above and below the sample mean. In the example at hand, we would obtain the following:

$$CI\ 95\% = (510 \pm (1.96 \times 20.0))$$

$$CI\ 95\% = (510 \pm (39.2))$$

$$CI\ 95\% = (470.8\ to\ 549.2)$$

The final statement may be read as follows: the confidence is 95% that the population mean is between 470.8 and 549.2.

Confidence intervals reflect how much risk researchers are willing to take of being wrong. With a 95% CI, researchers accept the probability that they will be wrong five times out of 100. A 99% CI sets the risk at only 1% by allowing a wider range of possible values. The formula is:CI 99% = $(\bar{X} \pm 2.58 \times SEM)$. The 2.58 reflects the fact that 99% of all cases in a normal distribution lie within ±2.58 SD units from the mean.

In our example, the 99% CI would be 458.4 to 561.6. In random samples with 25 subjects, 99 out of 100 CIs so constructed would contain the population mean. The price of having a lower risk of being wrong is reduced specificity. With a 95% interval, the range of the CI was only about 80 points; with a 99% interval, the range is more than 100 points.

The acceptable risk of error depends on the nature of the problem, but for most studies, a 95% confidence interval is sufficient. Confidence intervals may be—and often are—constructed around indexes of risk, such as the OR.

Example of confidence intervals:
Carruth and colleagues (2006) examined the proportion of farm women failing to obtain cervical cancer screening in three southern states. They presented failure rates (failure to obtain a pap smear within the past 3 years) for women in different age, race, and education groups in the three states, along with 95% CI values. For example, for all women in Louisiana, the failure rate was 27.9 (24.5, 31.3), whereas in Texas the rate was 19.6 (15.6, 22.6).

Hypothesis Testing

Statistical **hypothesis testing** provides objective criteria for deciding whether research hypotheses should be accepted as true or rejected as false. Suppose we hypothesized that maternity patients exposed to a film on breastfeeding would breastfeed longer than mothers who did not see the film. We find that the mean number of days of breastfeeding is 131.5 for 25 experimental subjects and 125.1 for 25 control subjects. Should we conclude that the hypothesis has been supported? True, group differences are in the predicted direction, but perhaps in another sample the group means would be nearly identical. Two explanations for the observed outcome are possible: (1) the film is truly effective in encouraging breastfeeding or (2) the difference in this sample was due to chance factors (e.g., differences in the characteristics of the two groups even before the film was shown, reflecting a selection bias).

The first explanation is the researcher's *research hypothesis*, and the second is the *null hypothesis*. The null hypothesis, it may be recalled, states that there is no relationship between the independent and dependent variables. Statistical hypothesis testing is basically a process of disproof or rejection. It cannot be demonstrated directly that the research hypothesis is correct. But it is possible to show, using theoretical sampling distributions, that the null hypothesis has a high probability of being incorrect, and such evidence lends support to the research hypothesis. Hypothesis testing helps researchers to make objective decisions about study results—that is, to decide whether results are likely to reflect chance differences or hypothesized effects.

The rejection of the null hypothesis, then, is what researchers seek to accomplish through **statistical tests**. Although null hypotheses are accepted or rejected on the basis of sample data, the hypothesis is made about population values. The real interest in testing hypotheses, as in all statistical inference, is to use a sample to make inferences about a population.

Type I and Type II Errors

Researchers decide whether to accept or reject the null hypothesis by determining how probable it is that observed group differences are due to chance. Because information about the population is not available, it cannot be asserted flatly that the null hypothesis is or is not true. Researchers must be content to say that hypotheses are either *probably* true or *probably* false. Statistical inferences are based on incomplete information; hence, there is always a risk of making an error.

Researchers can make two types of error: rejecting a true null hypothesis or accepting a false null hypothesis. Figure 15.7 summarizes the possible outcomes of researchers' decisions. Researchers make a **Type I error** by rejecting the null

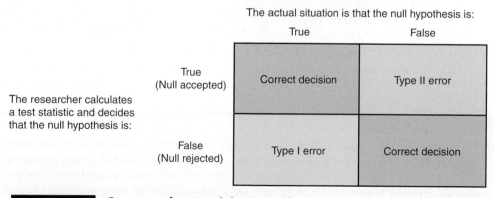

FIGURE 15.7 Outcomes of statistical decision-making.

hypothesis that is, in fact, true. For instance, if we concluded that the film was effective in promoting breastfeeding when, in fact, group differences were due to sampling error, we would have made a Type I error—a false–positive conclusion. Conversely, we might conclude that observed differences in breastfeeding were caused by random sampling fluctuations when the film actually did have an effect. Acceptance of a false null hypothesis is called a **Type II error**—a false–negative conclusion.

Level of Significance

Researchers do not know when they have made an error in statistical decision-making. The validity of a null hypothesis could be known only by collecting data from the population, in which case there would be no need for statistical inference.

Researchers control the degree of *risk* for a Type I error by selecting a **level of significance**, which indicates the probability of making a Type I error. The two most frequently used levels of significance (referred to as **alpha** or α) are .05 and .01. With a .05 significance level, we accept the risk that of 100 samples from a population, a true null hypothesis would be wrongly rejected 5 times. In 95 of 100 cases, however, a true null hypothesis would be correctly accepted. With a .01 significance level, the risk of making a Type I error is lower: In only 1 sample out of 100 would we wrongly reject the null hypothesis. By convention, the minimal acceptable alpha level for scientific research is .05.

> **TIP**
>
> Levels of significance are analogous to the CI values described earlier—an alpha of .05 is analogous to the 95% CI, and an alpha of .01 is analogous to the 99% CI.

Naturally, researchers would like to reduce the risk of committing both types of error. Unfortunately, lowering the risk of a Type I error increases the risk of a Type II error. The stricter the criterion for rejecting a null hypothesis, the greater the probability of accepting a false null hypothesis. However, researchers can reduce the risk of a Type II error simply by increasing their sample size.

The probability of committing a Type II error, referred to as **beta** (β), can be estimated through *power analysis,* the same procedure we mentioned in Chapter 12 in connection with sample size. *Power* refers to the ability of a statistical test to detect true relationships, and is the complement of beta (that is, power equals $1 - \beta$). The standard criterion for an acceptable risk for a Type II error is .20, and thus researchers ideally use a sample size that gives them a minimum power of .80.

> **TIP**
>
> Many nursing studies have small samples and thus have insufficient power to achieve statistical conclusion validity. Quantitative researchers should do a power analysis before starting their study, but many do not. If a research report indicates that a research hypothesis was not supported by the data, consider whether a Type II error might have occurred as a result of inadequate sample size.

Tests of Statistical Significance

In hypothesis testing, researchers use study data to compute a **test statistic**. For every test statistic, there is a theoretical sampling distribution, analogous to the sampling distribution of means. Hypothesis testing uses theoretical distributions to establish *probable* and *improbable* values for the test statistics, which are used to accept or reject the null hypothesis.

An example from our study of gender bias in nursing research (Polit & Beck, 2008) will illustrate the process. We tested the hypothesis that females are overrepresented as participants in nursing studies—that is, that the average percentage of females across published studies in four leading journals was greater than 50%. We found, using a consecutive sample of 259 studies from 4 nursing research journals over a 2-year period, that the mean percentage of females was 75.3. Using statistical procedures, we could test the hypothesis that the mean of 75.3 is not merely a chance fluctuation from the population mean of 50.0.

In hypothesis testing, researchers assume that the null hypothesis is true and then gather evidence to disprove it. Assuming a mean percentage of 50.0 for the entire population of recently published nursing studies, a theoretical sampling distribution can be constructed. For simplicity, let us say that the standard error of the mean in this example is 2.0 (in our study, the SEM was actually less than 2.0). This is shown in Figure 15.8. Based on normal distribution characteristics, we can determine probable and improbable values of sample means from the population of nursing studies. If, as is assumed according to the null hypothesis, the population mean is 50.0, 95% of all sample means would fall between 46.0 and 54.0 (i.e., within about 2 SDs above and below the mean of 50.0). The obtained sample mean of 75.3 lies in the region considered *improbable* if the null hypothesis were correct—in fact, any value greater than 54.0% female would be improbable if the true population mean were 50.0 when the criterion of improbability is an alpha level of .05. The *improbable* range beyond 2 SDs corresponds to only 5% (100% – 95%) of the

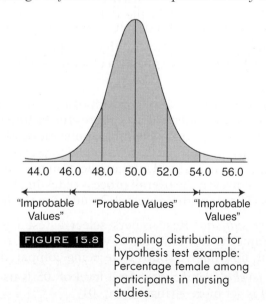

44.0   46.0   48.0   50.0   52.0   54.0   56.0

"Improbable   "Probable Values"   "Improbable
Values"   Values"

FIGURE 15.8 Sampling distribution for hypothesis test example: Percentage female among participants in nursing studies.

sampling distribution. In our study, the probability of obtaining a value of 75.3% female by chance alone was actually less than 1 in 10,000. We thus rejected the null hypothesis that the mean percentage of females in nursing studies was 50.0. We would not be justified in saying that we had *proved* the research hypothesis because the possibility of having made a Type I error remains—but the possibility is, in this case, remote.

Researchers reporting the results of hypothesis tests state whether their findings are **statistically significant**. The word *significant* should not be read as important or meaningful. In statistics, the term *significant* means that obtained results are not likely to have been the result of chance, at some specified level of probability. A **nonsignificant result** means that any observed difference or relationship could have been the result of a chance fluctuation.

> **TIP**
> It may help to keep in mind that inferential statistics are just a tool to help us evaluate whether study results are likely to be *real* and replicable, or simply spurious.

Parametric and Nonparametric Tests

Most tests that we discuss in this chapter—and also most tests used by researchers—are **parametric tests**. Parametric tests have three attributes, they (1) focus on population parameters; (2) involve certain assumptions about variables being analyzed, such as the assumption that they are normally distributed in the population; and (3) require measurements on at least an interval scale.

Nonparametric tests, by contrast, do not estimate parameters and involve less restrictive assumptions about the shape of the distribution of the critical variables. Nonparametric tests are most often used when the data have been measured on a nominal or ordinal scale or when the data distribution is markedly skewed—or when the sample size is too small to be confident about the shape of the distribution Parametric tests are more powerful than nonparametric tests and are generally preferred when variables are measured on at least the interval scale and the sample size is not small.

Overview of Hypothesis Testing Procedures

In the next section, a few statistical procedures for testing research hypotheses are discussed. The emphasis is on explaining applications of statistical tests and on interpreting their meaning rather than on explaining computations.

Each statistical test has a particular application and can be used only with certain kinds of data; however, the overall process of testing hypotheses is basically the same for all tests. The steps that researchers take are the following:

1. *Selecting a test statistic*. Researchers select a test based on such factors as whether a parametric test is justified, which levels of measurement were used, and, if relevant, how many groups were being compared.

2. *Specifying the level of significance*. An α level of .05 is usually chosen, but sometimes the level is set more stringently at .01.

3. *Computing a test statistic.* Researchers then calculate a test statistic based on the collected data.

4. *Determining degrees of freedom.* The term **degrees of freedom (df)** is used throughout hypothesis testing to refer to the number of observations free to vary about a parameter. The concept is too complex for full elaboration here, but computing degrees of freedom is easy.

5. *Comparing the test statistic to a tabled value.* Theoretical distributions have been developed for all test statistics, and values for these distributions are available in tables for specified degrees of freedom and level of significance. The *tabled* value enables researchers to determine whether the *computed* value is beyond what is probable if the null hypothesis is true. If the absolute value of the computed statistic is larger than the tabled value, the results are statistically significant; if the computed value is smaller, the results are nonsignificant.

When a computer is used for the analysis, as is almost always the case, researchers follow only the first step and then give commands to the computer. The computer calculates the test statistic, degrees of freedom, and the *actual* probability that the relationship being tested is owing to chance. For example, the computer may print that the probability (p) of an experimental group doing better on a measure of postoperative recovery than the control group on the basis of chance alone is .025. This means that fewer than 3 of 100 times (or only 25 of 1,000 times) would a group difference of the size observed occur by chance. This computed probability can then be compared with the desired level of significance. In the present example, if the significance level were .05, the results would be significant because .025 is more stringent than .05. Any computed probability greater than .05 (e.g., .15) indicates a nonsignificant relationship (sometimes abbreviated *NS*)—that is, one that could have occurred on the basis of chance in more than 5 of 100 samples.

BIVARIATE STATISTICAL TESTS

Researchers use a variety of statistical tests to make inferences about the validity of their hypotheses. The most frequently used bivariate tests are briefly described and illustrated.

t-Tests

A common research situation is the comparison of two groups of people on a dependent variable. The procedure used to test the statistical significance of a difference between the means of two groups is the parametric test called the *t*-**test**.

Suppose we wanted to test the effect of early discharge of maternity patients on perceived maternal competence. We administer a scale of perceived maternal competence at discharge to 20 primiparas who had a vaginal delivery: 10 who remained in the hospital 25 to 48 hours (regular discharge group) and 10 who were discharged 24 hours or less after delivery (early discharge group). Data for this example are presented in Table 15.8. The mean scores for these two groups are 25.0 and 19.0,

TABLE 15.8 ▶	FICTITIOUS DATA FOR *t*-TEST EXAMPLE: SCORES ON A PERCEIVED MATERNAL COMPETENCE SCALE	
REGULAR-DISCHARGE MOTHERS		**EARLY-DISCHARGE MOTHERS**
30		23
27		17
25		22
20		18
24		20
32		26
17		16
18		13
28		21
29		14
Mean = 19.0		Mean = 25.0
	$t = 2.86$, $df = 18$, $p = .011$	

respectively. Are these differences *real* (i.e., would they be found in the population of early-discharge and later-discharge mothers?), or do group differences reflect chance fluctuations? The 20 scores for this sample vary from one mother to another. Some variability reflects individual differences in perceived maternal competence. Some variability might be caused by measurement error (e.g., the scale's low reliability), some could result from participants' moods on a particular day, and so forth. The research question is: Can a significant portion of the variability be attributed to the independent variable—time of discharge from the hospital? The *t*-test allows us to make inferences about this question objectively.

The formula for calculating the *t* statistic uses group means, variability, and sample size. The computed value of *t* for the data in Table 15.8 is 2.86. Degrees of freedom in this example are equal to the total sample size minus 2 ($df = 20 - 2 = 18$). For an α level of .05, the tabled value of *t* with 18 degrees of freedom is 2.10. *This value establishes an upper limit to what is probable if the null hypothesis is true.* Thus, the calculated *t* of 2.86, which is larger than the tabled value of *t*, is improbable (i.e., statistically significant). We can now say that the primiparas discharged early had significantly lower perceived maternal competence than those who were not discharged early. The group difference in perceived maternal competence is sufficiently large that it is unlikely to reflect merely chance fluctuations. In fewer than 5 of 100 samples would a difference in means this great be found by chance alone. In fact, the actual p value is .011: only in about 1 of 100 samples would this large of a difference be found by chance.

The situation we just described calls for an *independent groups t-test*: mothers in the two groups were different people, independent of each other. There are situations for which this type of t-test is not appropriate. For example, if means for a single group of people measured before and after an intervention were being compared, researchers would compute a *paired t-test* (also called a *dependent groups t-test*), using a different formula.

Example of t-tests:
Jukkala & Henly (2007) developed scales to measure nurses' knowledge of, experience in, and comfort with neonatal resuscitation. They compared scores on these three scales for different subgroups of nurses, for example, urban versus rural nurses. The two groups did not differ in terms of mean scores on the knowledge scale ($t = -0.91$, $df = 68$, $p > .05$), but urban nurses had significantly higher scores than rural nurses on the experience scale ($t = 4.75$, $p < .001$) and the comfort scale ($t = 2.59$, $p = .012$).

As an alternative to t-tests, confidence intervals can be constructed around the difference between two means. The results provide information about both statistical significance (i.e., whether the null hypothesis should be rejected) and precision of the estimated difference. In the example in Table 15.8, we can construct CIs around the mean difference value in maternal competence scores of 6.0 ($25.0 - 19.0$). For a 95% CI, the confidence limits in our example are 1.6 and 10.4: we can be 95% confident that the true difference between population means for early- and regular-discharge mothers lies somewhere between these values.

With CI information, we learn the range within which the mean difference probably lies and we can also see that the mean difference is significant at the .05 level *because the range does not include 0.* Given that there is a 95% probability that the mean difference is not lower than 1.6, this means that there is less than a 5% probability that there is no difference at all—thus, the null hypothesis can be rejected.

Analysis of Variance

Analysis of variance (ANOVA) is used to test mean group differences of three or more groups. ANOVA decomposes the variability of a dependent variable into two components: variability attributable to the independent variable (e.g., group status) and variability due to all other sources (e.g., individual differences, measurement error). Variation *between* groups is contrasted with variation *within* groups to yield an **F ratio** statistic.

Suppose we were comparing the effectiveness of different interventions to help people stop smoking. One group of smokers receives intensive nurse counseling (group A); a second group is treated by a nicotine patch (group B); and a third control group receives no special treatment (group C). The dependent variable is 1-day

TABLE 15.9	FICTITIOUS DATA FOR ONE-WAY ANOVA EXAMPLE: NUMBER OF CIGARETTES SMOKED IN 1 DAY, POST-TREATMENT				
GROUP A NURSE COUNSELING		GROUP B NICOTINE PATCH		GROUP C UNTREATED CONTROLS	
28	19	0	27	33	35
0	24	31	0	54	0
17	0	26	3	19	43
20	21	30	24	40	39
35	2	24	27	41	36
Mean$_A$ = 16.6		Mean$_B$ = 19.2		Mean$_C$ = 34.0	
$F = 4.98$, $df = 2, 27$, $p = .01$					

cigarette consumption measured 1 month after the intervention. Thirty smokers who wish to quit smoking are randomly assigned to one of the three conditions. The null hypothesis is that the population means for posttreatment cigarette smoking is the same for all three groups, and the research hypothesis is inequality of means. Table 15.9 presents fictitious data for each subject. The mean numbers of post-treatment cigarettes consumed are 16.6, 19.2, and 34.0 for groups A, B, and C, respectively. These means are different, but are they significantly different—or do differences reflect random fluctuations?

An ANOVA applied to these data yields an F ratio of 4.98. For $\alpha = .05$ and $df = 2$ and 27 (2 df between groups and 27 df within groups), the tabled F value is 3.35. Because our obtained F value of 4.98 exceeds 3.35, we reject the null hypothesis that the population means are equal. The *actual* probability, as calculated by a computer, is .014. Group differences in posttreatment cigarette smoking are beyond chance expectations. In only 14 of 1,000 samples would differences this great be obtained by chance alone.

The data support the hypothesis that different treatments were associated with different cigarette smoking, but we cannot tell from these results whether treatment A was significantly more effective than treatment B. Statistical analyses known as **multiple comparison procedures** (or **post hoc tests**) are needed. Their function is to isolate the differences between group means that are responsible for rejecting the overall ANOVA null hypothesis. Note that it is *not* appropriate to use a series of *t*-tests (group A versus B, A versus C, and B versus C) because this increases the risk of a Type I error.

ANOVA also can be used to test the effect of two (or more) independent variables on a dependent variable, such as when a factorial experimental design has been used. Suppose we wanted to determine whether the two smoking cessation interventions (nurse counseling and nicotine patch) were equally effective for men and women. We randomly assign males and females, separately, to the two modes of treatment conditions, without a control condition. Suppose the analysis revealed the following about two *main effects*: On average, people in the nurse counseling group smoked less than those in the nicotine patch group (19.0 versus 25.0), and, overall, females smoked less than males (21.0 versus 23.0). In addition, there is an *interaction effect*: Female smoking was especially low in the counseling condition (mean = 16.0), whereas male smoking was especially high in that condition (mean = 30.0). By performing a *two-way ANOVA* on these data, it would be possible to test the statistical significance of these differences.

A type of ANOVA known as **repeated measures ANOVA (RM-ANOVA)** is often used when the means being compared are means at different points in time (e.g., mean blood pressure at 2, 4, and 6 hours after surgery). This is analogous to a paired *t*-test, extended to three or more points of data collection, because the same people are being measured multiple times. When two or more groups are measured several times, a repeated measures ANOVA provides information about a main effect for time (Do the measures change significantly over time, irrespective of group?); a main effect for groups (Do the group means differ significantly, irrespective of time?); and an interaction effect (Do the groups differ more at certain times?).

Example of an RM-ANOVA:
Fife and co-researchers (2008) tested an intervention, for people living with HIV and their partners, to facilitate adaptive coping. Data on coping and other outcomes were gathered at baseline, immediately after the intervention, and 3 months later. RM-ANOVA was used to assess the effect of the intervention, with treatment group as the between-group factor, and time as the repeated measure factor. There were several significant interaction effects, indicating that those in the treatment group changed significantly more over time than those in the control group. For example, the increases in the number of coping strategies from time 1 to time 2 was significantly different for the two groups ($F = 9.2$, $p = .004$).

Chi-Squared Test

The **chi-squared** (χ^2) **test** is used to test hypotheses about the proportion of cases in different categories, as in a contingency table. For example, suppose we were studying the effect of nursing instruction on patients' compliance with a self-medication regimen. Nurses implement a new instructional strategy based on Orem's Self-Care Model with 100 randomly assigned experimental patients, whereas 100 control group patients get usual instruction. The research hypothesis is that a higher proportion of people in the treatment than in the control condition will be compliant. Some fictitious data for this example are presented in Table 15.10, which shows that 60% of those in the experimental group were compliant, compared with 40% in the control group. But is this 20 percentage point difference statistically significant (i.e., likely to be "real"?).

The chi-squared statistic is computed by summing differences between the *observed frequencies* in each cell (such as those in Table 15.10) and the *expected frequencies*—the frequencies that would be expected if there were *no* relationship between the two variables. In this example, the value of the χ^2 statistic is 8.00,

TABLE 15.10	OBSERVED FREQUENCIES FOR CHI-SQUARE EXAMPLE		
	GROUP		
PATIENT COMPLIANCE	EXPERIMENTAL	CONTROL	TOTAL
Compliant	60	40	100
Noncompliant	40	60	100
TOTAL	100	100	200

$\chi^2 = 8.00$, $df = 1$, $p = .005$

which we can compare with the value from a theoretical chi-squared distribution. With $df = 1$ in this example, the tabled value from a theoretical chi-squared distribution that must be exceeded to establish significance at the .05 level is 3.84. The obtained value of 8.00 is substantially larger than would be expected by chance (the actual $p = .005$). We can conclude that a significantly larger proportion of experimental patients than control patients were compliant.

Example of chi-squared test:
Zaybak and Khorshid (2008) used a crossover design to examine the effect of different durations of subcutaneous heparin injections (30 seconds versus 10 seconds) on bruising. Bruising occurred in 64% of the 30-second injections compared with 42% of the 10-second injections. The difference was statistically significant, $\chi^2 = 4.8$, $p = .02$.

As with means, it is possible to construct confidence intervals around the difference between two proportions. In our example, the group difference in proportion compliant was .20. The 95% CI in this example is .06 to .34. We can be 95% confident that the true population difference in compliance rates between those exposed to the intervention and those not exposed is between 6% and 34%. This interval does not include 0%, so we can be 95% confident that group differences are "real" in the population.

Correlation Coefficients

Pearson's r is both descriptive and inferential. As a descriptive statistic, r summarizes the magnitude and direction of a relationship between two variables. As an inferential statistic, r tests hypotheses about population correlations; the null hypothesis is that there is no relationship between two variables (i.e., that the population $r = .00$).

Suppose we were studying the relationship between patients' self-reported level of stress (higher scores imply more stress) and the pH level of their saliva. With a sample of 50 patients, we find that $r = -.29$. This value indicates a tendency for people with high stress scores to have lower pH levels than those with low stress scores. But we need to ask whether this finding can be generalized to the population. Does the coefficient of $-.29$ reflect a random fluctuation, observed only in this particular sample, or is the relationship significant? Degrees of freedom for correlation coefficients equal N minus 2, which is 48 in this example. The tabled value for r with $df = 48$ and $\alpha = .05$ is .2803. Because the absolute value of the calculated r is .29, the null hypothesis can be rejected. There is a modest but significant relationship between patients' self-reported level of stress and the acidity of their saliva.

Confidence intervals can be constructed around Pearson's rs. In our example, the 95% CI around the r of .29 for stress levels and saliva pH, with a sample of 50 subjects, is .01 to .53. Because the lower confidence limit is greater than .00, we can see that the correlation in this example was statistically significant at the .05 level—but note that the range of possible values for the population r is very large because of the small sample size.

Example of Pearson's r:
Litwinczuk and Groh (2007) examined the relationship between spirituality, purpose in life, and well-being in HIV-positive persons. They found that spirituality was significantly correlated with purpose in life ($r = .295$, $df = 44$, $p = .049$), but not with well-being ($r = .261$, $df = 44$, $p = .084$) in their sample of 46 HIV positive men and women.

Effect Size Indexes

To enhance statistical conclusion validity, researchers can estimate the sample size they need in a study by conducting an upfront *power analysis*, and thereby minimize the risk of a Type II error. Power analysis concepts are also useful in after-the-fact descriptions of results. As with the risk indexes described earlier, **effect size indexes** provide readers and clinicians with estimates about the magnitude of effects within the research sample—an important issue in EBP (see Box 2.1). Effect size information can be crucial because, with large samples, even miniscule effects can be statistically significant at dramatic levels. *P* values tell you whether results are likely to be *real*, but effect sizes can suggest whether they are important. Effect size estimates play an important role in meta-analyses, as we discuss in Chapter 19.

It is beyond this scope of this book to explain effect sizes in detail, but we can offer an illustration. One frequently used effect size indicator is called d, an index that summarizes the magnitude of differences in means in a two-group situation, such as the means of an experimental and control group on outcomes like blood pressure or anxiety scores. The d statistic could thus be calculated to estimate effect size in conjunction with t-tests. A d of zero indicates no effect—the means of the two groups being compared are the same. Although theoretically the value of d can be greater than 1, in practice, d values are typically more modest. By convention, a d of .20 or less is considered *small*, a d of .50 is considered *moderate*, and a d of .80 or greater is considered large.

Different effect size indexes, and different associated conventions, are associated with different situations. The key point is that they encapsulate information about how powerful the effect of an independent variable is on a dependent variable.

Example of calculated effect size:
Bennett and colleagues (2008) tested the effectiveness of a telephone motivational interviewing intervention to increase physical activity and improve self-efficacy for exercise in rural adults using an experimental design. The researchers presented *d* values to indicate the magnitude of the intervention's effects. For example, the effect of the intervention on self-efficacy for exercise was statistically significant and fairly substantial, $d = .62$.

Guide to Bivariate Statistical Tests

The selection of a statistical test depends on several factors, such as the number of groups and the levels of measurement of the research variables. To aid you in evaluating the appropriateness of statistical tests used by nurse researchers, a chart summarizing key features of the major bivariate tests is presented in Table 15.11. This table includes only the tests mentioned in this chapter, which are the most frequently used statistical tests in nursing research. An expanded version of this table that includes a few tests not mentioned in this chapter is available in the toolkit. ✖

MULTIVARIATE STATISTICAL ANALYSIS

Many nurse researchers now use complex **multivariate statistics** to analyze their data. We use the term *multivariate* to refer to analyses dealing with at least three—but usually more—variables simultaneously. The evolution to more sophisticated methods of analysis has resulted in increased rigor in nursing studies, but one unfortunate side effect is that it has become more challenging for novice consumers to understand research reports.

Given the introductory nature of this text and the fact that many of you are not proficient with even simple statistical tests, it is not possible to describe in detail the complex analytic procedures that now appear in nursing journals. However, we present some basic information that might assist you in reading reports in which two commonly used multivariate statistics are used: multiple regression and analysis of covariance (ANCOVA).

TABLE 15.11 ◗ GUIDE TO MAJOR BIVARIATE STATISTICAL TESTS				
			MEASUREMENT LEVEL	
NAME	TEST STATISTIC	PURPOSE	INDEPENDENT VARIABLE	DEPENDENT VARIABLE
t-test for independent groups	t	To test the difference between the means of two independent groups (e.g., experimental vs. control, men vs. women)	Nominal	Interval, Ratio
t-test for paired groups	t	To test the difference between the means of a paired group (e.g., pretest vs. posttest for same people)	Nominal	Interval, Ratio
Analysis of variance (ANOVA)	F	To test the difference among means of 3+ independent groups, or means for 2+ independent variables (as in a factorial experiment)	Nominal	Interval, Ratio
Repeated measures ANOVA	F	To test the difference among means of 3+ related groups (e.g., over time)	Nominal	Interval, Ratio
Pearson's correlation coefficient	r	To test the existence of a relationship between two variables	Interval, Ratio	Interval, Ratio
Chi-squared test	χ^2	To test the difference in proportions in 2+ independent groups	Nominal (or ordinal, few categories)	Nominal (or ordinal, few categories)

Multiple Regression

Correlations enable researchers to make predictions. For example, if the correlation between secondary school grades and nursing school grades were .60, nursing school administrators could make predictions—albeit imperfect predictions—about applicants' future academic performance. Researchers often strive to improve their ability to predict a dependent variable by including more than one independent variable in the analysis.

As an example, we might predict that infant birthweight is related to amount of maternal prenatal care. We could collect data on birthweight and number of prenatal visits and then compute a correlation coefficient to determine whether a significant relationship between the two variables exists (i.e., whether prenatal care would help predict infant birthweight). Birthweight is affected by many other factors, however, such as gestational period and mothers' smoking behavior. Many researchers, therefore, perform a **multiple regression analysis** that allows them to explain or predict a dependent variable with multiple independent variables. In multiple regression, the dependent variables are interval- or ratio-level variables. Independent variables (also called **predictor variables** in multiple regression) are either interval- or ratio-level variables or dichotomous nominal-level variables, such as male or female.

When several independent variables are used to predict a dependent variable, the resulting statistic is the **multiple correlation coefficient,** symbolized as R. Unlike the bivariate correlation coefficient r, R does not have negative values. R varies from .00 to 1.00, showing the *strength* of the relationship between several independent variables and a dependent variable, but not *direction*.

There are several ways of evaluating R. One is to determine whether R is statistically significant—that is, whether the overall relationship between the independent variables and the dependent variable is likely to be real, or the result of chance sampling fluctuations. This is done through the computation of an F statistic that can be compared with tabled F values.

A second way of evaluating R is to determine whether the addition of new independent variables adds further predictive power. For example, we might find that the R between infant birthweight on the one hand and maternal weight and prenatal care on the other is .30. By adding a third independent variable—let us say maternal smoking behavior—R might increase to .36. Is the increase from .30 to .36 statistically significant? In other words, does knowing whether the mother smoked during her pregnancy *really* improve our understanding of birthweight variation, or does the larger R value simply reflect factors peculiar to this sample? Multiple regression provides a way of answering this question.

The magnitude of the R statistic is also informative. Researchers would like to predict a dependent variable perfectly. In our example, if it were possible to identify all the factors that lead to differences in infants' weight, we could collect relevant data and get an R of 1.00. The value of R in nursing studies is usually much smaller—seldom higher than .70. An interesting feature of R is that, when squared, it can be interpreted as the proportion of the variability in the dependent variable explained by the predictors. In predicting birthweight, if we achieved an R of .60 ($R^2 = .36$), we could say that the independent variables accounted for just over one-third (36%) of the variation in birthweights. Two-thirds of the variability, however, was caused by factors not identified or measured. Researchers usually report multiple correlation results in terms of R^2 rather than R.

Example of multiple regression analysis:

Wall (2007), in her study of community-dwelling people with chronic obstructive pulmonary disease (COPD), studied the relationship between several physiologic and psychosocial variables on the one hand and functional performance on the other. Using multiple regression, she found, for example, that the person's age and severity of pulmonary disease were significant predictors of functional performance. Overall, the R^2 between predictor variables and functional performance was .46.

TABLE 15.12 ⏵	EXAMPLE OF MULTIPLE REGRESSION ANALYSIS: FUNCTIONAL PERFORMANCE SCORES AMONG COMMUNITY-DWELLING PEOPLE WITH COPD, REGRESSED ON DEMOGRAPHIC, PHYSIOLOGIC, AND PSYCHOSOCIAL PREDICTORS ($N = 119$)				
PREDICTOR VARIABLE*	b	SE	BETA (β)	P
Age	−.023	.005	−.322	<.001
Sex (males = 0, females = 1)	−.233	.091	−.189	.012
Comorbidity scores	−.173	.172	−.073	.319
$FEV_{1\% \ predicted}$	.009	.003	.242	.001
Depression scores	−.575	.086	−.707	<.001
Anxiety scores	.057	.059	.088	.335
Happiness level	.070	.089	.071	.428
Life satisfaction level	.012	.060	.017	.847
Perceived social support	−.001	.028	−.002	.979
Mastery scores	−.011	.015	−.067	.462

$F = 11.06$; $df = 9, 108$; $p < .001$; $R^2 = .51$; adjusted $R^2 = .46$.

* Except for the variable *sex*, higher values correspond to "more" of the variable; the value of the constant in this regression model is not shown in this table.
Adapted from Table 2 of Wall (2007).

Some additional findings from this study are summarized in Table 15.12. Multiple regressions yield information about whether each independent variable is related significantly to the dependent variable. In Table 15.12, the first column shows that the analysis used 10 variables to predict the functional performance scores for 119 people with COPD. The next column shows the values for *b*, which are the *regression coefficients* associated with each predictor. These coefficients, computed from raw study data, could be used to actually predict functional performance in a new sample of patients—but they are not values you need to be concerned with in interpreting a regression table. The next column shows the standard error (SE) of the regression coefficients. When the regression coefficient (*b*) is divided by the SE, the result is a value for the *t* statistic, which can be used to determine the significance of individual predictors. In our table, the *t* values are not shown (although they were included in Wall's table). Nevertheless, we can compute them from information in the table; for example, the value of *t* for the predictor *age* would be −4.60 (that is, −.023 ÷ .005 = −4.60). This is highly significant, as shown in the last column: the probability (*p*) is less than 1 in 1,000 that the relationship between patient's age and functional performance is spurious. The table indicates that, as age increases, functional performance *decreases*, as indicated by the minus sign on the coefficient. Three other predictor variables were significantly related to functional performance: the less severe the disease as measured by $FEV_{1\%predicted}$, and the lower the level of depression, the higher the functional performance. Sex was also significant. This variable was coded with a 1 for female patients and 0 for male patients. Because the sign on the coefficient is negative, it means that men were significantly more likely than women to have higher functional performance scores. Other predictors in the analysis (e.g., comorbidity scores) were not significantly related to functional performance, once other factors were taken into consideration.

Multiple regression analysis indicates whether an independent variable is significantly related to the dependent variable *even when* the other predictor variables are controlled—a concept we explain more fully in the next section. In this example, sex was a significant predictor of functional performance, even when age, depression, and the other seven variables were controlled. Thus, multiple regression, like analysis of covariance (discussed next), is a means of statistically controlling confounding variables.

The fourth column of Table 15.12 shows the value of the *beta* (β) *coefficients* for each predictor. Although it is beyond the scope of this textbook to explain beta coefficients in detail, suffice it to say that, unlike the *b* regression coefficients, betas are all in the same measurement units and their absolute values are sometimes used to compare the relative importance of predictors. In this particular sample, and with these particular predictors, the variable *depression* was the best predictor of functional performance ($\beta = -.707$), and the variable *age* was the second best predictor ($\beta = -.322$).

At the bottom of the table, we see that the value of F of 11.06 for the overall regression equation, with 9 and 108 *df*, was highly significant, $p < .001$. The value of R^2 is .51, but after adjustments are made for sample size and number of predictors, the value is reduced to .46. Thus, 46% of the variance in average functional performance scores among persons with COPD in this sample is explained by the combined effect of the 10 predictors. The remaining 54% of variation is explained by other factors that were not measured in this study.

Analysis of Covariance

Analysis of covariance (ANCOVA), which combines features of ANOVA and multiple regression, is used to control confounding variables statistically—that is to "equalize' groups being compared. This approach can be especially valuable in certain situations, as when a nonequivalent control group design is used. The initial equivalence of the experimental and comparison groups in these studies is uncertain and so researchers must consider whether group differences in outcomes reflect preexisting group differences. When control through randomization is lacking, ANCOVA offers the possibility of *post hoc* statistical control.

Because the idea of statistical control may mystify you, we will explain the underlying principle with a simple illustration. Suppose we were interested in testing the effectiveness of a special exercise program on physical fitness, using employees of two companies as subjects. Employees of one company receive the exercise intervention, and those of the second company do not. The employees' score on a physical fitness test is the dependent variable. The research question is: "Can some of the group difference in performance on the physical fitness test be attributed to participation in the special program?" Physical fitness is also related to other, extraneous characteristics of the study participants (e.g., their age)—characteristics that might differ between the two groups of employees.

Figure 15.9 illustrates how ANCOVA works. The large circles represent total variability (i.e., the total extent of individual differences) in physical fitness scores for all study participants. A certain amount of variability is the result of age: Younger people tend to perform better on the test than older ones. This relationship is represented by the overlapping small circle on the left in part A of the figure. Another part of the variability can be explained by participation in the exercise program, represented here by the overlapping small circle on the right. In part A, the fact that the two small circles (age and program participation) *themselves* overlap indicates that there is a relationship between these two variables. In other words, people in the intervention group are, on average, either older or younger than those in the comparison group. Because this age difference could distort the results of the study, age should be controlled.

ANCOVA can do this by statistically removing the effect of the confounding variable (age) on physical fitness. This is designated in part A of Figure 15.9 by the darkened area of the large circle. Part B illustrates that the analysis would examine the effect of program participation on fitness scores *after* removing the effect of age (called a *covariate*). With the variability associated with age removed, we get a more precise estimate of the intervention's effect on physical fitness. Note that there is still a lot of individual variability (the bottom half of the large circle) that is not explained. This means that analytic precision could be further enhanced by controlling additional confounding variables (e.g., weight, diet, smoking). ANCOVA can control multiple confounding variables.

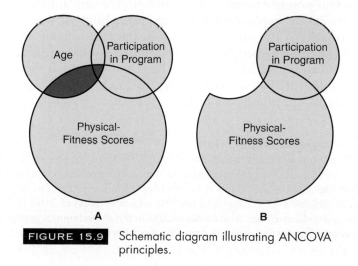

FIGURE 15.9 Schematic diagram illustrating ANCOVA principles.

Analysis of covariance tests the significance of differences between group means after adjusting scores on the dependent variable to eliminate the effect of the covariates. This adjustment uses multiple regression procedures. ANCOVA produces F statistics—one to test the significance of the covariates and another to test the significance of group differences—that can be compared with tabled values of F to determine whether to accept or reject the null hypothesis.

ANCOVA, like multiple regression analysis, is an extremely powerful and useful analytic technique for controlling confounding influences on dependent measures. ANCOVA can be used with true experimental designs, because randomization does not guarantee that groups are totally equivalent. Baseline measures of the dependent variables make particularly good covariates.

Example of ANCOVA:
Liu and co-researchers (2008) compared men and women, and patients in different age groups, with regard to health-related quality of life (QOL) following kidney transplantation. ANCOVA was used to compare mean group scores on a health-related scale, using amount of time after transplant as the covariate.

Other Multivariate Techniques

Other multivariate techniques increasingly are being used in nursing studies. We mention a few techniques briefly to acquaint you with terms you might encounter in the research literature.

Logistic Regression

Logistic regression analyzes the relationships between multiple independent variables and a nominal-level dependent variable (e.g., compliant versus noncompliant). It is similar to multiple regression, although it employs a different statistical estimation procedure that many prefer for nominal-level dependent variables. Logistic regression transforms the probability of an event occurring (e.g., that a woman will practice breast self-examination or not) into its *odds* (i.e., into the ratio of one event's probability relative to the probability of a second event). After further transformations, the analysis examines the relationship of the independent variables to the transformed dependent variable. For each predictor, the logistic regression yields an odds ratio, which is the factor by which the odds change for a unit change in the predictors. Logistic regression yields odds ratios for each predictor and CI information around the ORs.

Example of logistic regression:
Nyamathi and colleagues (2008) tested the efficacy of a nurse case-managed intervention on adherence to latent tuberculosis infection treatment among homeless adults, using multiple logistic regression. The intervention was found to be effective for many subgroups of participants. For example, the adjusted OR (adjusted for background and site characteristics) of 2.60 (95% CI = 1.69, 4.02) for African Americans indicated that African Americans in the experimental group were more than twice as likely as those in the control group to complete the tuberculosis treatment.

Factor Analysis

Factor analysis, as noted in Chapter 14, is widely used by researchers seeking to develop, refine, or validate complex instruments. The major purpose of factor analysis is to reduce a large set of variables into a smaller, more manageable set. Factor analysis disentangles complex interrelationships among variables and identifies which variables "go together" as unified concepts or factors. For example, suppose we developed 50 Likert statements to measure men's attitudes toward a vasectomy. It would not be appropriate to combine all 50 items to form a scale score because there are various dimensions, or themes, to men's attitudes toward vasectomy. One dimension may relate to the issue of masculinity and virility, another may concern the loss of ability to reproduce, and so on. These various dimensions should serve as the basis for constructing subscales, and factor analysis offers an objective, empirical method for doing so.

Example of factor analysis:
Lynn and colleagues (2007) developed the Patient's Assessment of Quality Scale—Acute Care Version as a measure of nursing care quality. They administered the original 90 items to 1,470 patients, and responses were factor analyzed. The analysis revealed five underlying factors: Individuation, Nurse Characteristics, Caring, Environment, and Responsiveness.

Multivariate Analysis of Variance

Multivariance analysis of variance (MANOVA) is the extension of ANOVA to more than one dependent variable. This procedure is used to test the significance of differences between the means of two or more groups on two or more dependent variables, considered simultaneously. For instance, if we wanted to compare the effect of two alternative methods of exercise on both blood pressure and heart rate, then a MANOVA would be appropriate. Covariates can also be included, in which case the analysis would be called a **multivariate analysis of covariance (MANCOVA)**.

Causal Modeling

Causal modeling involves the development and statistical testing of a hypothesized explanation of the causes of a phenomenon, usually with nonexperimental data. **Path analysis**, which is based on multiple regression, is a widely used approach to causal modeling. Alternative methods of testing causal models are also being used by nurse researchers, the most important of which is **structural equations modeling (SEM)**. Both SEM and path analysis are highly complex statistical techniques whose utility relies on a sound underlying causal theory.

Guide to Multivariate Statistical Analyses

In selecting a multivariate analysis, researchers attend to such issues as the number of independent variables, the number of dependent variables, the measurement level of all variables, and the desirability of controlling confounding variables. Table 15.13 is an aid to help you evaluate the appropriateness of multivariate statistics used in research reports. This chart includes the major multivariate analyses used by nurse researchers.

TABLE 15.13	GUIDE TO SELECTED MULTIVARIATE ANALYSES						
		MEASUREMENT LEVEL OF VARIABLES*			NUMBER OF VARIABLES*		
TEST NAME	PUPROSE	IV	DV	COVAR	IVs	DVs	COVAR
Multiple regression	To test the relationship between 2+ IVs and 1 DV; to predict a DV from 2+ IVs	N, I, R	I, R	—	2+	1	—
Analysis of covariance (ANCOVA)	To test the difference between the means of 2+ groups, while controlling for 1+ covariate	N	I, R	N, I, R	1+	1	1+
Logistic regression	To test the relationship between 2+ IVs and 1 DV; to predict the probability of an event; to estimate relative risk	N, I, R	N	—	2+	1	—
Factor analysis	To determine the dimensionality or structure of a set of variables						
Multivariate analysis of variance (MANOVA)	To test the difference between the means of 2+ groups for 2+ DVs simultaneously	N	I, R	—	1+	2+	—
Multivariate analysis of covariance (MANCOVA)	To test the difference between the means of 2+ groups for 2+ DVs simultaneously, while controlling for 1+ covariate	N	I, R	N, I, R	1+	2+	1+

*Variables: IV, independent variable; DV, dependent variable; Covar., covariate.

†Measurement levels: N, nominal; I, interval; R, ratio.

READING AND UNDERSTANDING STATISTICAL INFORMATION

Statistical findings are communicated in the results section of research reports and are reported in the text as well as in tables (or, less frequently, figures). This section provides some assistance in reading and interpreting statistical information.

Tips on Reading Text with Statistical Information

There are usually several types of information reported in the results section. First, there are descriptive statistics, which typically provide an overview of participants' characteristics. Information about the subjects' background enables readers to draw conclusions about the groups to which the findings might be generalized. Second, some researchers provide statistical information for evaluating the extent of any biases. For example, researchers sometimes compare the characteristics of people who did and did not agree to participate in the study (e.g., using t-tests). Or, in a quasi-experimental design, evidence of the preintervention comparability of the experimental and comparison groups helps readers to evaluate the study's internal validity. Inferential statistics relating to the research questions or hypotheses are then presented. Supplementary analyses are sometimes presented to help unravel the meaning of the results.

The text of research reports usually provides certain information about the statistical tests, including (1) which test was used, (2) the value of the calculated statistic, (3) degrees of freedom, and (4) level of statistical significance. Examples of how the results of various statistical tests would likely be reported in the text are shown below.

1. t-test: $\quad\quad\quad\quad t = 1.68; df = 160; p = .09$

2. Chi-squared: $\quad\quad \chi^2 = 16.65; df = 2; p < .001$

3. Pearson's r: $\quad\quad r = .36; df = 100; p < .01$

4. ANOVA: $\quad\quad\quad F = 0.18; df = 1, 69, NS$

Note that the significance level is sometimes reported as the *actual* computed probability that the null hypothesis is correct, as in example 1—which is the preferred approach. In this case, the observed group differences could be found by chance in 9 of 100 samples; thus, this result is not statistically significant because the differences have an unacceptably high chance of being spurious. The probability level is sometimes reported simply as falling below or above the researchers' significance criterion, as in examples 2 and 3. In both cases, the results are statistically significant because the probability of obtaining such results by chance alone is less than 1 in 100. Note that you need to be careful to read the symbol that follows the p value (the probability value) correctly: The symbol $<$ means less than—that is, the results are statistically significant; the symbol $>$ means greater than—that is, the results are not statistically significant. When results do not achieve statistical significance at the desired level, researchers may simply indicate that the results were not significant (NS), as in example 4.

Statistical information usually is noted parenthetically in a sentence describing the findings, as in the following example: The patients in the experimental group had a significantly lower rate of infection than those in the control group ($\chi^2 = 5.41, df = 1, p = .02$). In reading research reports, it is not important to absorb numeric information for actual test statistics. For example, the actual value of χ^2 has no inherent interest. What is important is to grasp whether the statistical tests indicate that the research hypotheses were accepted as probably true (as demonstrated by significant results) or rejected as probably false (as demonstrated by nonsignificant results).

Tips on Reading Statistical Tables

The use of tables allows researchers to condense a lot of statistical information into a compact space and also prevents redundancy. Consider, for example, putting information from a correlation matrix (see Table 15.5) into the text: "The correlation between mother's positive involvement and mother's education was .28; the correlation between mothers' positive involvement and mothers' depression was −.38 . . ."

Unfortunately, although tables are efficient, they may be daunting, partly because of the absence of standardization. There is no universally accepted method of presenting *t*-test information, for example, and so each table may present a new deciphering challenge. Another problem is that some researchers try to include an enormous amount of information in their tables; we deliberately used tables of relative simplicity as examples in this chapter.

We know of no magic solution for helping you to comprehend statistical tables, but we have a few suggestions. First, read the text and the tables simultaneously because the text may help to unravel what the table is trying to communicate. Second, before trying to understand the numbers in a table, try to glean as much information as possible from the accompanying words. Table titles and footnotes often communicate critical pieces of information. The table headings should be carefully reviewed because these indicate what the variables in the analysis are (often listed in the far left-hand column of the table as row labels, as in Table 15.3 and Table 15.12) and what statistical information is included (often specified in the top row as the column headings, as in these same two tables). Third, you may find it helpful to consult the glossary of symbols found on the last page of the Glossary to determine the meaning of a statistical symbol included in a report table. Note that not all symbols were described in this chapter; therefore, it may be necessary to refer to a statistics textbook, such as that of Polit (1996) or Munro and colleagues (2004), for further information. We recommend that you devote some extra time to making sure you have grasped what the tables are conveying and that, for each table, you write out a sentence or two that summarizes some of the tabular information in "plain English."

TIP

In tables, probability levels associated with the significance tests are sometimes presented directly (e.g., $p < .05$), as in Table 15.12. Here, the significance of each test is indicated in the last column, headed "*p*." However, researchers often indicate significance levels in tables through asterisks placed next to the value of the test statistic. By convention, one asterisk usually signifies $p < .05$, two asterisks signify $p < .01$, and three asterisks signify $p < .001$ (there is usually a key at the bottom of the table that indicates what the asterisks mean). Thus, a table might show: $t = 3.00$, $p < .01$ *or* $t = 3.00^{**}$. The absence of an asterisk would signify a nonsignificant result.

CRITIQUING QUANTITATIVE ANALYSES

For novice research consumers, it is often difficult to critique statistical analyses. We hope this chapter has helped to demystify what statistics are all about, but we also recognize the limited scope of this presentation. Although it would be unreasonable to expect you now to be adept at evaluating statistical analyses, there are certain things you should routinely look for in reviewing research reports. Some specific guidelines are presented in Box 15.1. ✪

One aspect of the critique should focus on which analyses were reported in the article. Researchers generally perform many more analyses than can be presented in a short journal article. You should determine whether the reported statistical

---

BOX 15.1 GUIDELINES FOR CRITIQUING STATISTICAL ANALYSES

1. Did the descriptive statistics in the report sufficiently describe the major key variables and background characteristics of the sample? Were the correct descriptive statistics used—for example, was a mean presented when percentages would have been more informative?

2. Were statistical analyses used advantageously to strengthen conclusions about the study's internal validity (e.g., to test for selection bias or attrition bias)?

3. In general, does the report provide a rationale for the use of the chosen statistical strategies? Does the report contain sufficient information for you to judge whether appropriate statistics were used?

4. Does the report include any inferential statistics? If inferential statistics were not used, should they have been?

5. Was information provided about both hypothesis testing and parameter estimation (i.e., confidence intervals)? Were effect sizes (or risk indexes) reported? Overall, did the statistics reported provide readers and potential users of the study results with sufficient information about the evidence the study yielded?

6. Were any multivariate procedures used? If not, should they have been used—for example, would the internal validity of the study be strengthened by statistically controlling confounding variables?

7. Were the selected statistical tests appropriate, given the level of measurement of the variables and the nature of the hypotheses?

8. Were the results of any statistical tests significant? What do the tests tell you about the plausibility of the research hypotheses? Were effects sizeable? What do the effects suggest about the clinical importance of the findings?

9. Were the results of any statistical tests nonsignificant? Is it plausible that these reflect Type II errors? What factors might have undermined the study's statistical conclusion validity?

10. Was there an appropriate amount of statistical information? Were findings clearly and logically organized? Were tables or figures used judiciously to summarize large amounts of statistical information? Are the tables clearly presented, with good titles and carefully labeled column headings? Is the information presented in the text and the tables redundant?

TABLE 15.14	EFFECTS OF MUSIC THERAPY ON PHYSIOLOGIC AND PSYCHOLOGICAL OUTCOMES[a]			
OUTCOME	INTERVENTION GROUP MEAN (N = 36)	CONTROL GROUP MEAN (N = 49)	F or t	p
State Anxiety Scores			F = 14.34*	.0004
Day 1 AM	12.8	17.6		
Day 1 PM	14.5	17.1		
Day 2 AM	13.5	17.6		
Pain Ratings			F = 7.33*	.009
Day 1 AM	2.2	3.2		
Day 1 PM	2	3.2		
Day 2 AM	2.1	3.2		
Heart Rate			F**	.76
Day 1 AM	82	81		
Day 1 PM	81	81		
Day 2 AM	81	83		
Diastolic BP			F**	.11
Day 1 AM	56	62		
Day 1 PM	56	59		
Day 2 AM	57	61		
Parenteral morphine equivalents, Days 1–3 (mg)	69	61	t**	.34

* The F values are for experimental-control group comparisons within an RM-ANOVA; the Fs for main effects over time, and interaction effects, were not reported.
** The actual values of these statistics were not reported.
[a] Based on Sendelbach et al. (2006).

information adequately describes the sample and reports the results of statistical tests for all hypotheses. Another presentational issue concerns the researcher's judicious use of tables to summarize statistical information.

A thorough critique also addresses whether researchers used the appropriate statistics. Tables 15.12 and 15.14 provide summaries of the most frequently used statistical tests—although we do not expect that you will readily be able to determine the appropriateness of the tests used in a study without further statistical instruction. The major issues to consider are the number of independent and dependent variables, the levels of measurement of the research variables, and the number of groups (if any) being compared.

If researchers did not use a multivariate technique, you should consider whether the bivariate analysis adequately tests the relationship between the independent and dependent variables. For example, if a *t*-test or ANOVA was used, could the internal validity of the study have been enhanced through the statistical control of confounding variables, using ANCOVA? The answer will almost always be "yes."

Finally, you can be alert to possible exaggerations or subjectivity in the reported results. Researchers should never claim that the data proved, verified, confirmed, or demonstrated that the hypotheses were correct or incorrect. Hypotheses should be described as being *supported* or *not supported, accepted* or *rejected*.

The main task for beginning consumers in reading a results section of a research report is to understand the meaning of the statistical tests. What do the quantitative results indicate about the researcher's hypothesis? How believable are the findings? The answer to such questions form the basis for interpreting the research results, a topic discussed in Chapter 16.

RESEARCH EXAMPLES AND CRITICAL THINKING ACTIVITIES

In this section we provide details about analytic portion of a study, followed by some questions to guide critical thinking.

EXAMPLE 1 ■ Descriptive and Bivariate Inferential Statistics

Study

Effects of music therapy on physiological and psychological outcomes for patients undergoing cardiac surgery (Sendelbach et al., 2006).

Statement of Purpose

The purpose of this study was to compare the effects of a relaxing music intervention, versus a quiet and uninterrupted rest period, on pain intensity, anxiety, physiologic indicators, and opioid consumption among patients who had had cardiac surgery.

Methods

Patients undergoing coronary artery bypass (CAB), valve replacement surgery, or both in one of three midwestern hospitals were recruited to participate in the study. A total of 86 patients were randomly assigned to a music/relaxation intervention group or to a control group. Patients in the intervention group were told to assume a comfortable position and were read a script that encouraged relaxation. Then they listened to a tape of relaxing music by headphones for 20 minutes. The intervention occurred each morning and afternoon on three postoperative days (POD). Those in the control group were advised to rest in bed in a comfortable position for 20 minutes. For both groups, measures for pain intensity, anxiety, heart rate, and blood pressure were obtained immediately before and after each intervention period. Medication usage was obtained from patients' charts.

Descriptive Statistics

The researchers presented descriptive statistics (means and percentages) to describe the characteristics of sample members before the intervention. For example, the mean age of the participants was 63.3 (SD = 13.5). As described by the authors, "the typical subject was 63 years old, male (69.8%), had CAB surgery (69.8%), and had seldom used music therapy (81.2%)" (p. 196).

Analysis of Bias

The researchers tested the preintervention comparability of the two groups to assess the risk of selection bias. The groups were similar for most of the characteristics examined. For example, the mean age of the experimental and control group subjects was 62.3 and 64.7 years, respectively, and the t-test for this analysis was nonsignificant ($p = .43$). However, there was a nearly significant difference with regard to type of procedure: those in the control group were more likely to have a joint CAB–valve procedure (19.6%) than those in the intervention group (4.0%); the chi-squared test yielded a $p = .051$.

Hypothesis Tests

The researchers used RM-ANOVA to compare group differences in pain, anxiety, blood pressure, and heart rate over time. Because of a high rate of missing data, the RM-ANOVA was done for only three time periods: the morning and afternoon of POD 1, and the morning of POD 2. Selected results are summarized in Table 15.14. The analysis indicated that those in the experimental had significantly lower state anxiety scores than those in the control group throughout the three time periods ($F = 14.34$, $df = 1, 83$, $p = .0004$). For example, in the morning of the first postoperative day, the average anxiety score was 13.5 in the intervention group, compared with 17.6 in the control group. In only 4 of 10,000 samples would the group differences in anxiety scores have occurred by chance alone. The intervention group also had significantly lower pain ratings at all three time periods ($p = .009$). Group differences for heart rate and blood pressure were not significantly different. Differences in opioid consumption, measured in milligrams of parenteral morphine equivalents, were also not significantly different according to the t-tests. The researchers concluded that patients recovering from cardiac surgery may benefit from music therapy.

CRITICAL THINKING SUGGESTIONS*:

*See the Student Resource CD-ROM for a discussion of these questions.

1. Answer the relevant questions from Box 15.1 regarding this study.
2. Also, consider the following targeted questions, which may further sharpen your critical thinking skills and assist you in understanding this study:
   a. Were the two groups (experimentals versus controls) comparable in terms of the proportion male and female? (The p value for the chi-squared test for differences in proportions was .065).
   b. The group difference in opioid use was not statistically significant. State the findings for this outcome in words, including information about the means and p value.
   c. In the actual report for this study, there are two figures showing experimental-control group differences over time in pain and anxiety. Create a comparable figure charting differences in diastolic blood pressure.
3. What might be some of the uses to which the findings could be put in clinical practice?

EXAMPLE 2 ■ Statistical Analysis in the Study in Appendix A

1. Read the "Results" section of Howell and colleagues' (2007) study ("Anxiety, anger, and blood pressure in children") in Appendix A of this book, and then answer the relevant questions in Box 15.1.

2. Also, consider the following targeted questions, which may further sharpen your critical thinking skills and assist you in assessing aspects of the study's merit:
   a. In reporting information about scale scores for boys and girls (Table 1), the researchers stated that "Boys had higher mean anger scores but lower mean anxiety scores than girls." Did the researchers test whether the sex differences were statistically significant? What test was used or would have been used?
   b. Looking at Table 1, write one or two sentences about the results for diastolic blood pressure, making sure to mention SD values.
   c. In Table 2, do the results indicate a significant relationship between scores on any of the anger scales with any blood pressure measurements? If yes, which ones and what are the levels of significance? Which variable was most highly correlated with systolic blood pressure (SBP) and diastolic blood pressure (DBP)?
   d. Several multiple regression analyses were performed to predict blood pressure values, including separate analyses for the boys and girls. Were height and weight (two of the predictor variables) better able to predict SBP and DBP values for the boys or for the girls in this study? (Note: we have presented a table with multiple regression analysis results from this study on the accompanying CD-ROM). 💿

CHAPTER REVIEW

Key new terms introduced in the chapter, together with a summary of major points, are presented in this section. In addition, Chapter 15 of the *Study Guide for Essentials of Nursing Research,* 7th edition offers various exercises and study suggestions for reinforcing concepts presented in this chapter. For additional review, see the Student Self-Study Review Questions section of the Student Resource CD-ROM provided with this book. 💿

Key New Terms

Alpha (α)
Analysis of covariance (ANCOVA)
Analysis of variance (ANOVA)
Beta (β)
Central tendency
Chi-squared test
Confidence interval (CI)
Correlation
Correlation coefficient
Correlation matrix
Crosstab
Degrees of freedom
Descriptive statistics

Effect size
F ratio
Factor analysis
Frequency distribution
Hypothesis testing
Inferential statistics
Level of significance
Logistic regression
Mean
Median
Mode
Multiple regression analysis
Multivariate statistics
N

Negative relationship
Negative skew
Nonparametric test
Nonsignificant result (NS)
Odds ratio (OR)
p value
Parametric test
Pearson's r
Positive relationship
Positive skew
Predictor variables
r
R^2
Range

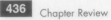

Sampling distribution of
   the mean
Skewed distribution
Standard deviation

Statistical test
Statistically significant
Symmetric distribution
Test statistic

t-test
Type I error
Type II error
Variability

Summary Points

- **Descriptive statistics** enable researchers to summarize and describe quantitative data.

- In **frequency distributions**, numeric values are ordered from lowest to highest, together with a count of the number (or percentage) of times each value was obtained.

- Data for a variable can be completely described in terms of the shape of the distribution, central tendency, and variability.

- The shape of a distribution can be **symmetric** or **skewed**, with one tail longer than the other; it can also be unimodal with one peak (i.e., one value of high frequency), or multimodal with more than one peak. A **normal distribution** (bell-shaped curve) is symmetric, unimodal, and not too peaked.

- Measures of **central tendency** represent the average or typical value of a set of scores. The **mode** is the value that occurs most frequently in the distribution; the **median** is the point above which and below which 50% of the cases fall; and the **mean** is the arithmetic average of all scores. The mean is usually the preferred measure of central tendency because of its stability.

- Measures of **variability**—how spread out the data are—include the **range** and **standard deviation (SD)**. The range is the distance between the highest and lowest scores. The SD indicates how much, on average, scores deviate from the mean.

- A **contingency table** is a two-dimensional frequency distribution in which the frequencies of two nominal- or ordinal-level variables are **cross-tabulated**.

- **Correlation coefficients** describe the direction and magnitude of a relationship between two variables, and range from −1.00 (perfect *negative correlation*) through .00 to +1.00 (perfect *positive correlation*). The most frequently used correlation coefficient is **Pearson's *r***, used with interval- or ratio-level variables.

- Statistical indexes that describe the magnitude of exposure to risk factors or interventions provide useful information for making clinical decisions. The most commonly reported risk index is the **odds ratio (OR)**. which is the ratio of the odds for an exposed versus unexposed group, with the *odds* reflecting the proportion of people with the adverse outcome relative to those without it.

- **Inferential statistics**, which are based on laws of probability, allow researchers to make inferences about a population based on data from a sample; they offer a framework for deciding whether the sampling error that results from sampling fluctuation is too high to provide reliable population estimates.

➤ The **sampling distribution of the mean** is a theoretical distribution of the means of an infinite number of same-sized samples drawn from a population. Sampling distributions are the basis for inferential statistics.

➤ The **standard error of the mean (SEM)**—the standard deviation of this theoretical distribution—indicates the degree of average error of a sample mean; the smaller the standard error, the more accurate are the estimates of the population value.

➤ Statistical inference consists of two major types of approaches: estimating parameters and testing hypotheses. **Parameter estimation** is used to estimate a population parameter.

➤ Point estimation provides a single value of a population estimate (e.g., a mean or an odds ratio). Interval estimation provides the upper and lower limits of a range of values—the **confidence interval (CI)**—between which the population value is expected to fall, at a specified probability level. Most often, the 95% CI is reported, which indicates that there is a 95% probability that the true population value lies between the upper and lower confidence limit.

➤ **Hypothesis testing** through statistical tests enables researchers to make objective decisions about relationships between variables.

➤ The *null hypothesis* states that no relationship exists between the variables and that any observed relationship is due to chance fluctuations; rejection of the null hypothesis lends support to the research hypothesis. In testing hypotheses, researchers compute a **test statistic** and then determine whether the statistic falls at or beyond a critical region on the relevant theoretical distribution. The value of the test statistic indicates whether the null hypothesis is "improbable."

➤ A **Type I** error occurs if a null hypothesis is incorrectly rejected (false–positive findings). A **Type II error** occurs when a null hypothesis that should be rejected is accepted (false–negative findings).

➤ Researchers control the risk of making a Type I error by establishing a **level of significance** (or **alpha** level), which is the probability that such an error will occur. The .05 level (the conventional standard) means that in only 5 of 100 samples would the null hypothesis be rejected when it should have been accepted.

➤ The probability of committing a Type II error is **beta** (β). Power, the ability of a statistical test to detect true relationships, is the complement of beta (i.e., power equals $1 - \beta$). The standard criterion for an acceptable level of power is .80.

➤ Results from hypothesis tests are either significant or nonsignificant; **statistically significant** means that the obtained results are not likely to be caused by chance fluctuations at a given probability level (*p* **value**).

➤ **Parametric tests** involve the estimation of at least one parameter, assumptions of normally distributed variables, and the use of interval or ratio data; **nonparametric tests** are used when the normality of the distribution cannot be assumed.

➤ Two common statistical tests are the *t*-test and **analysis of variance (ANOVA)**, both of which can be used to test the significance of the difference between group means; ANOVA is used when there are three or more groups (one-way

ANOVA) or when there is more than one independent variable (e.g., two-way ANOVA). **Repeated measured ANOVA** (RM-ANOVA) is used when data are collected over multiple time periods.

➤ The **chi-squared test** is used to test hypotheses about differences in proportions.

➤ Pearson's *r* can be used to test whether a correlation is significantly different from zero.

➤ *Power analysis* can be used at the outset of a study to estimate how large a sample is required to avoid a Type II error. Power analysis concepts are also used after the fact to calculate an **effect size** (e.g., the *d* index), which summarizes the strength of the effect of an independent variable (e.g., an intervention) on the dependent variable.

➤ Confidence intervals can be constructed around almost any computed statistic, including differences between means, differences between proportions, and correlation coefficients. CI information is valuable to clinical decision-makers, who need to know more than whether differences are probably real.

➤ **Multivariate statistics** are increasingly being used in nursing research to untangle complex relationships among three or more variables.

➤ **Multiple regression analysis** is a method for understanding the effect of two or more **predictor** (independent) **variables** on a continuous dependent variable. The multiple correlation coefficient (**R**), can be squared to estimate the proportion of variability in the dependent variable accounted for by the predictors.

➤ **Analysis of covariance** (**ANCOVA**) permits researchers to control confounding variables (called *covariates*) before determining whether group differences are statistically significant.

➤ Other multivariate procedures used by nurse researchers include **logistic regression**, **factor analysis**, **multivariate analysis of variance (MANOVA)**, as well as causal modeling procedures, such as path analysis and structural equations modeling.

STUDIES CITED IN CHAPTER 15

Bennett, J., Young, H., Nail, L., Winter-Stone, K., & Hanson, G. (2008). A telephone only motivational intervention to increase physical activity in rural adults. *Nursing Research, 57*, 24–32.

Carruth, A., Browning, S., Reed, D., Skarke, L., & Sealey, L. (2006). The impact of farm lifestyle and health characteristics. *Nursing Research, 55*, 121–127.

Champion, V., Skinner, C., Hui, S., Monahan, P., Juliar, B., Daggy, J. et al. (2007). The effect of telephone versus print tailoring for mammography adherence. *Patient Education and Counseling, 65*, 416–423.

Fife, B., Scott, L., Fineberg, N., & Zwicki, B. (2008). Promoting adaptive coping by persons with HIV disease: Evaluation of a patient/partner intervention model. *Journal of the Association of Nurses in AIDS Care, 19*, 75–84.

Jesse, D.E., Graham, M., & Swanson, M. (2006). Psychosocial and spiritual factors associated with smoking and substance use during pregnancy in African American and white low-income women. *Journal of Obstetric, Gynecologic, & Neonatal Nursing, 35*, 68–77.

Jukkala, A., & Henly, S. (2007). Readiness for neonatal resuscitation: Measuring knowledge, experience, and comfort level. *Applied Nursing Research, 20*, 78–85.

Lee, T., Holditch-Davis, D., & Miles, M. (2007). The influence of maternal and child characteristics and paternal support on interactions of mothers and their medically fragile infants. *Research in Nursing & Health, 30,* 17–30.

Litwinczuk, K., & Groh, C. (2007). The relationship between spirituality, purpose in life, and well-being in HIV-positive persons. *Journal of the Association of Nurses in AIDS Care, 18,* 13–22.

Liu, H., Feurer, I., Dwyer, K., Speroff, T., Shaffer, D., & Pinson, C. W. (2008). The effects of gender and age on health-related quality of life following kidney transplantation. *Journal of Clinical Nursing, 17,* 82–89.

Lynn, M., McMillen, B., & Sidani, S. (2007). Understanding and measuring patients' assessment of the quality of nursing care. *Nursing Research, 56,* 159–166.

Nyamathi, A., Nahid, P., Berg, J., Burrage, J., Christiani, A., Aqtash, S. et al. (2008). Efficacy of nurse case-managed intervention for latent tuberculosis among homeless subsamples. *Nursing Research, 57,* 33–39.

Polit, D., & Beck, C. (2008). Is there gender bias in nursing research? *Research in Nursing & Health, 31,* 417–427.

Sendelbach, S., Halm, M., Doran, K., Miller, E., & Gaillard, P. (2006). Effects of music therapy on physiological and psychological outcomes for patients undergoing cardiac surgery. *Journal of Cardiovascular Nursing, 21*(3), 194–200.

Wall, M. P. (2007). Predictors of functional performance in community-dwelling people with COPD. *Journal of Nursing Scholarship, 39,* 222–228.

Zaybak, A., & Khorshid, L. (2008). A study on the effect of the duration of subcutaneous heparin injection on bruising and pain. *Journal of Clinical Nursing, 17,* 378–385.

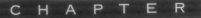

CHAPTER

16 Rigor and Interpretation in Quantitative Research

STUDENT OBJECTIVES

On completing this chapter, you will be able to:

➣ Describe the dimensions of an interpretation of quantitative research results

➣ Describe the mindset conducive to a critical interpretation of research results

➣ Identify approaches to an assessment of the credibility of quantitative results, and undertake such an assessment

➣ Critique researchers' interpretation of their results in the discussion section of a report

➣ Define new terms in the chapter

For quantitative nursing studies, this chapter brings us back full circle. Early in this book, we provided some guidance on the challenges of designing and doing rigorous research (Chapter 4). We described the development of research questions (Chapter 6) and devoted subsequent chapters to the methods researchers use to address them. In this chapter, we consider researchers' answers to research questions, and what to make of them—returning to some issues discussed in Chapter 2 on evidence-based nursing practice, and to the guidelines for critiquing studies in Chapter 4.

INTERPRETATION OF QUANTITATIVE RESULTS

The analysis of quantitative data provides the study **results**, which are summarized in the *results* section of a research article. Researchers present their *interpretations* of the results in the *discussion* section of their reports. Discussion sections are important in helping readers make sense of study findings, but should not be considered a substitute for your own efforts at interpretation because it is difficult for researchers to be totally objective in their interpretations. Moreover, discussion sections are brief because of journal page constraints.

This chapter offers some guidance to help you in interpreting quantitative results and in critiquing discussion sections of research articles. Another aim of this chapter is to encourage you to think critically about all aspects of a quantitative study. At this point, you have gained some understanding and appreciation of the theoretical, methodologic, and analytic components of a study, and are better positioned to apply the critiquing guidelines we provided in Table 4.1 than you were earlier. A research critique provides the foundation for an informed interpretation of the results. Statistical results need to be thoroughly understood, and then evaluated within the context of the aims of the project, its theoretical basis, the existing body of related research evidence, and the strengths and limitations of the research methods.

Aspects of Interpretation

It is not an easy or straightforward task to interpret quantitative research results. Interpreting the results of a study involves attending to six different but overlapping considerations, which intersect with the "Questions for Appraising the Evidence" presented in Box 2.1:

➤ The credibility and accuracy of the results
➤ The precision of the estimate of effects
➤ The magnitude of effects and importance of the results
➤ The meaning of the results, especially with regard to causality
➤ The generalizability of the results
➤ The implications of the results for nursing practice, theory development, or further research

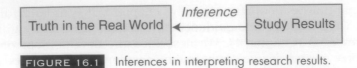

FIGURE 16.1   Inferences in interpreting research results.

Before discussing these considerations, we want to remind you about the role of inference in research thinking and interpretation.

Inference and Interpretation

As noted in Chapter 4, an *inference* is the act of drawing conclusions based on limited information, using logical reasoning processes. Interpreting research findings involves making a series of inferences. In research, virtually everything is a "stand-in" for something else. A sample is a stand-in for a population, a scale for a concept yields scores that are stand-ins for an attribute being measured, and so on.

Figure 16.1 shows that research findings are meant to reflect "truth in the real world"—the findings themselves are intended to be "stand-ins" for the true state of affairs. Inferences about the real world are valid, however, to the extent that the researchers have made rigorous methodologic decisions in selecting proxies and controlling sources of bias. We use versions of Figure 16.1 several times in this chapter to illustrate the kinds of questions interpreters could ask in drawing conclusions about whether study findings really do reflect "truth in the real world."

The Interpretive Mindset

Evidence-based practice (EBP) involves integrating current best evidence from rigorous research into clinical decision-making. EBP encourages clinicians to think critically about a course of action, and to challenge the status quo, when such a challenge is warranted based on a careful assessment of "best evidence." Thinking critically, and demanding evidence, are also part of research interpreters' job. Just as clinicians must ask, "What *evidence* is there that this intervention or strategy will yield positive results?" so must interpreters ask, "What *evidence* is there that the results are real and true?"

Figure 16.2 presents a simplified schema illustrating this process, in this case for a situation involving an evidence-based clinical intervention. This figure illustrates evidence integration with the results of only two studies on the effectiveness of an intervention, but in reality there typically would be multiple pieces of evidence. (Integration of evidence is discussed in Chapter 19). The important point of this figure is that evidence for *clinical decisions* involves making inferences about study results, which in turn are based on inferences from the evidence on *methodologic decisions*.

To be a good interpreter of research results, one must begin with a skeptical attitude and a null hypothesis. *The "null hypothesis" in interpretation is that the results are wrong and the evidence is flawed.* The "research hypothesis" is that the evidence can be trusted and used in practice because the results reflect the truth.

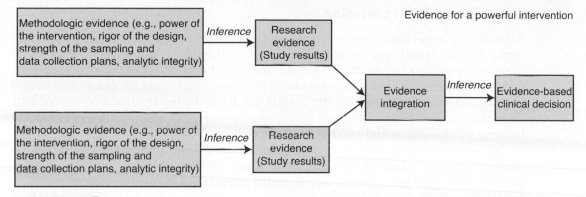

Evidence for a powerful intervention

FIGURE 16.2 Schema for evidence-based pathway for clinical decisions about a nursing intervention.

Interpreters decide whether the null hypothesis or the research hypothesis has more merit by critically examining the methodologic evidence. The greater the evidence that the researcher's design and methods were sound, the less plausible is the null hypothesis that the results are not right.

TIP

In critically interpreting study results, it is not inappropriate to adopt the attitude reflected in the Missourian slogan "Show me!" You should expect researchers to "show you" that their design is strong, their measurements are reliable and valid, their sample is adequately large and representative, and that their analysis is sufficiently powerful.

CREDIBILITY OF QUANTITATIVE RESULTS

One of the most important interpretive tasks is to assess whether the results are *right*. This corresponds to the first question we posed in Chapter 2 (Box 2.1) within an EBP context: "What is the quality of the evidence (i.e., how rigorous and reliable is it?")." If the results are judged not to be credible, the remaining interpretive issues (the meaning, magnitude, precision, or generalizability, and implications of results) are not likely to be relevant.

A credibility assessment requires a careful analysis of the study's methodologic and conceptual limitations and strengths. To come to a conclusion about whether the results closely approximate "truth in the real world," each aspect of the study—its research design, intervention design, sampling plan, measurement and data collection plan, and analytic approach—all must be subjected to critical scrutiny.

There are various ways to approach the issue of credibility, including the use of the critiquing guidelines we have offered throughout this book, and the global critiquing protocol presented in Table 4.1. We share some additional perspectives in this chapter.

Proxies and Interpretation

Researchers begin with ideas and constructs, and then devise ways to operationalize them. The constructs are linked to the actual methodologic outcomes in a series of approximations, each of which is subject to critical evaluation because at each step there is a potential for inadequate correspondence and outright error. The better the proxies, the more credible the results are likely to be. In this section, we will illustrate successive proxies using sampling concepts, to highlight the potential for inferential challenges and validity problems.

When researchers formulate their research questions or hypotheses, the population of interest is typically abstract. Actual specifications for the target population are not delineated until later, when eligibility criteria are defined. For example, suppose we wanted to test the effectiveness of an intervention to increase physical activity levels in low-income women. Figure 16.3 shows the series of steps between the abstract population construct (low-income women) and the actual women who participate and provide study data. Using data from the actual sample on the far right, the researcher would like to make inferences about the effectiveness of the intervention for a broader group, but each proxy along the way represents a potential problem for achieving the desired inference. In interpreting a study, readers must consider how *plausible* it is that the actual sample reflects the recruited sample, the accessible population, the target population, and then the population construct.

Table 16.1 presents a description of a hypothetical scenario in which the researchers moved from a target population of low-income women, to an actual sample of 161 women who participated in the study. The table shows some questions that a person trying to make inferences about the study results might ask. Answers to these questions would affect the interpretation of whether the intervention *really* is effective with low-income women—or only with extremely motivated, cooperative welfare recipients from two neighborhoods of Los Angeles who recently got approved for public assistance.

As Figure 16.3 suggests, researchers make a series of methodologic decisions that affect the inferences that can be made, and these decisions must be carefully scrutinized in interpreting whether the results are credible. However, participant behavior and external circumstances also affect the results and need to be considered in the interpretation. In our example in Table 16.1, 300 women were recruited for the study, but only 161 provided usable data for the analyses. The final sample

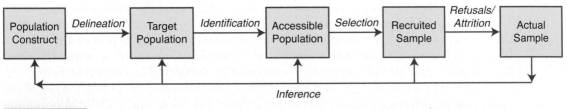

FIGURE 16.3 Inferences about populations: from analysis sample to the population.

TABLE 16.1 ⏵ SUCCESSIVE SERIES OF PROXIES IN SAMPLING		
ELEMENT	DESCRIPTION	POSSIBLE INFERENTIAL CHALLENGES
Population construct	Low-income women	
Target population	All women who receive public assistance (cash welfare) in California	⇝ Why only welfare recipients—why not the working poor? ⇝ Why California?
Accessible population	All women who receive public assistance in Los Angeles and who speak English or Spanish	⇝ Why Los Angeles? ⇝ What about non-English/ non-Spanish speakers?
Recruited sample	A consecutive sample of 300 female welfare recipients (English or Spanish speaking) who applied for benefits in January, 2009 at two randomly selected welfare offices in Los Angeles	⇝ Why only new applicants—what about women with long-term receipt? ⇝ Why only two offices? Are these representative? ⇝ Is January a typical month?
Actual sample	161 women from the recruited sample who fully participated in the study	⇝ Who refused to participate (or was too ill, and so on) and why? ⇝ Who dropped out of the study, and why?

of 161 almost surely would differ in important ways from the 139 who were not in the study, and these differences affect inferences about the worth of the study evidence.

Fortunately, researchers are increasingly being required to document participant flow in their studies—especially in intervention studies. Guidelines called the Consolidated Standards of Reporting Trials or **CONSORT guidelines** have been adopted by major medical and nursing journals to help readers track study participants. CONSORT flow charts, when available, should be carefully scrutinized in interpreting study results. Regrettably, providing such information has not become routine in reports of nonexperimental studies.

Example of a CONSORT flow chart:

Bennett and colleagues (2008) tested the effectiveness of a telephone-only motivational intervention designed to increase physical activity in rural adults. Figure 16.4 shows the progression of study participants through the study, from 138 originally assessed for eligibility to 72 who provided final data for analysis. As this figure clearly shows, a total of 52 people who were originally assessed were not actually enrolled in the study, for a variety of reasons, such as refusals and failure to meet eligibility criteria. Some of those enrolled did not actually participate in the study ($N = 5$ in the two groups), others were lost in follow-up ($N = 5$), and others were excluded because they did not complete the final survey ($N = 14$).

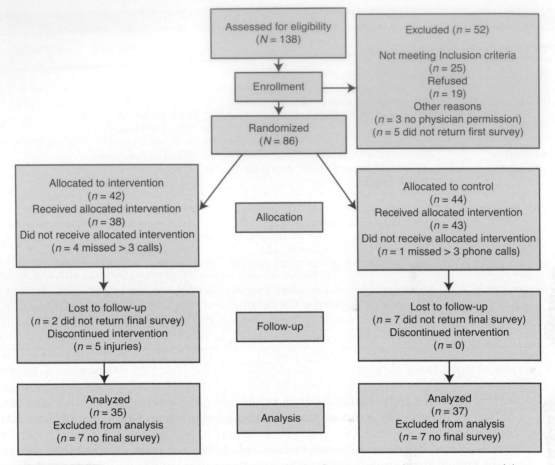

FIGURE 16.4 Example of a Consolidated Standards of Reporting Trials (CONSORT) guidelines flow chart: Flow of participants in a telephone-only motivational interview intervention study to increase physical activity. (Bennett et al., 2008, p. 27.)

We illustrated how successive proxies in a study, from the abstract to the concrete, can affect inferences with regard to sampling, but we might well have chosen other types of methodologic decisions. To reinforce our concept, Figure 16.5 shows another example relating to inferences about an intervention. As with our previous illustration, the researcher would move from an abstraction on the left (here, a "theory" about why an intervention might have certain beneficial outcomes), through the design of protocols that purport to operationalize the theory, to the actual implementation and use of the intervention on the right. The researcher wants the right side of the figure to be a good proxy for the left side—and the interpreter's job is to assess the plausibility that the researcher was successful in the transformation.

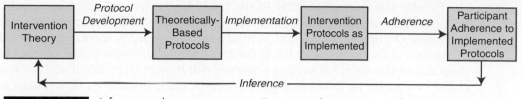

FIGURE 16.5 Inferences about interventions: From actual operations to the theory.

Credibility and Validity

Inference and validity are inextricably linked. As the research methodology experts Shadish and colleagues (2002) have stated, "We use the term *validity* to refer to the approximate truth of an inference" (p. 34). To be careful interpreters, readers must search for evidence within the study that the desired inferences are, in fact, valid. Part of this process involves giving consideration to alternative and potentially competing hypotheses about the credibility and meaning of the results.

In Chapter 9 we discussed four key types of validity that play a central role in assessing the credibility of study results: statistical conclusion validity, internal validity, external validity, and construct validity. Let us use our sampling example (Figure 16.2 and Table 16.1) to demonstrate the relevance of methodologic decisions to all four types of validity—and hence to inferences about study results.

First, let us consider construct validity—a term that has relevance not only for the measurement of research constructs but also for many aspects of a study. In our example, the population construct was *low-income women*, which led to population eligibility criteria stipulating public assistance recipients in California. There are, however, many other alternative operationalizations of the population construct (e.g., California women living in families below the official poverty level). Construct validity, it may be recalled, involves inferences from the particulars of the study to higher-order constructs. So it is fair to ask, "Do the specified eligibility criteria adequately capture the population construct, low-income women?"

Statistical conclusion validity—the extent to which correct inferences can be made about the existence of "real" relationships between key variables—is also affected by sampling decisions. To be safe, researchers should do a power analysis at the outset to estimate how large a sample is needed. In our example, let us say we assumed (based on previous research) that the effect size for the exercise intervention would be small-to-moderate, with $d = .40$. For a power of .80, with risk of a Type I error set at .05, we would need a sample of about 200 participants. The actual sample of 161 yields a nearly 30% risk of a Type II error (i.e., falsely concluding that the intervention was not successful).

External validity—the generalizability of the results—is clearly affected by sampling decisions and outcomes. To whom would it be safe to generalize the results in this example—to the population construct of low-income women? to all welfare recipients in California? to all new welfare recipients in Los Angeles who speak English or Spanish? Inferences about the extent to which the study results correspond to "truth in the real world" must take sampling decisions and sampling problems (e.g., recruitment difficulties) into account.

Finally, the internal validity of the study (the extent to which a causal connection between variables can be inferred) is also affected by sample composition. In particular (in this example), differential attrition would be a concern. Were those in the intervention group more likely (or less likely) than those in the control group to drop out of the study? If so, any observed differences in physical activity outcomes could be caused by individual differences in the groups (e.g., differences in motivation), rather than by the intervention itself.

Methodologic decisions and the careful implementation of those decisions— whether they be about sampling, intervention design, measurement, research design, or analysis—inevitably affect the rigor of a study. And all of them can affect the four types of validity, and hence the interpretation of the results.

Credibility and Bias

Part of a researcher's job in designing and conducting a study is to translate abstract constructs into plausible and meaningful proxies. Another major job concerns efforts to eliminate, reduce, or control biases—or, as a last resort, to detect and understand them. As a reader of research reports, your job is to be on the hunt for biases, and to factor them into your assessment of the credibility of the results.

Biases are factors that create distortions and that undermine researchers' efforts to capture and reveal "truth in the real world." Biases are pervasive. It is not so much a question of whether there *are* biases in a study, so much as what types of bias are present, and how extensive, sizeable, and systematic the biases are. We have discussed many types of bias in this book—some reflect design inadequacies (e.g., selection bias), others reflect recruitment or sampling problems (e.g., nonresponse bias), others are related to measurement (e.g., social desirability). To our knowledge, there is no comprehensive listing of biases that might arise in the context of a study, but we have devised a list of some of the biases and errors mentioned in this book (Table 16.2). This table does not represent an effort to create an all-inclusive list, but rather is meant to serve as a reminder of some of the problems to consider in interpreting study results.

TIP

The Toolkit on the accompanying CD-ROM includes a longer list of biases, including many that were not described in this book. We have provided definitions and notes for all biases listed. It is important to recognize that different disciplines and different writers may use different names for the same or similar biases. The actual names are not important—what is important is to understand how different forces can distort the results and affect inferences. ⊗

Credibility and Corroboration

Earlier we noted that research interpreters should seek evidence to disconfirm the "null hypothesis" that the research results of a study are wrong. Some evidence to discredit the null hypothesis comes from the plausibility that proxies were good

TABLE 16.2	SELECTED LIST OF MAJOR POTENTIAL BIASES OR ERRORS IN QUANTITATIVE STUDIES IN FOUR RESEARCH DOMAINS		
RESEARCH DESIGN	**SAMPLING**	**MEASUREMENT**	**ANALYSIS**
Expectation bias	Sampling error	Social desirability bias	Type I error
Hawthorne effect	Volunteer bias	Acquiescence bias	Type II error
Contamination of treatments	Nonresponse bias	Nay-sayers bias	
Carryover effects		Extreme response set bias	
Noncompliance bias		Recall or memory bias	
Selection bias		Reactivity	
Attrition bias		Observer biases	
History bias			

stand-ins for abstractions or idealized methods. Other evidence involves ruling out validity threats and biases. Yet another strategy is to seek corroboration for the results.

Corroboration can come from both internal and external sources, and the concept of *replication* is an important one in both cases. Interpretations are aided by considering prior research on the topic, for example. Interpreters can examine whether the study results replicate (are congruent with) those of other studies. Discrepancies in study results may help to support the "null hypothesis" of erroneous results, whereas consistency across studies discredits it.

Researchers can pursue opportunities for replication themselves. For example, in multisite studies, if the results are similar across sites, this suggests that something "real" is occurring with some regularity. Triangulation can be another form of replication and sometimes can help to corroborate results in quantitative studies. For example, if there are multiple measures of an important outcome, and the results are similar across the different measures, then there can perhaps be greater confidence that the results are "real" and do not reflect some peculiarity of an instrument or data collection procedure. If the results are different, this could provide support for the null hypothesis that the results are wrong—but it could reflect a problem with one of the measures. When mixed results occur, interpreters must dig deeper to try to uncover the reason.

Finally, we are strong advocates of mixed methods studies, a special type of triangulation. When findings from the analysis of qualitative data are consistent with the results of statistical analyses, internal corroboration can be especially powerful and persuasive.

OTHER ASPECTS OF INTERPRETATION

If a critical assessment of how the study was designed and conducted leads you to accept that the results are probably "real," you have gone a long way in interpreting the study findings. Other interpretive tasks depend on a conclusion that the accuracy of the results is at least plausible.

Precision of the Results

The results of statistical hypothesis test indicate whether an observed relationship or group difference is probably real and likely to be replicable with another sample. A p value in hypothesis testing is a measure of how strong the evidence is that the study's null hypothesis is false—it is not an estimate of any quantity that is of direct relevance to practicing nurses. Thus, a p value offers information that is important, but incomplete.

Confidence intervals, by contrast, communicate information about how precise (or imprecise) the study results are. Dr. David Sackett, a founding father of the EBP movement, had this to say about confidence intervals: "P values on their own are . . . not informative . . . By contrast, CIs indicate the strength of evidence about quantities of direct interest, such as treatment benefit. They are thus of particular relevance to practitioners of evidence-based medicine" (2000, p. 232). It seems likely that nurse researchers will increasingly report CI information in the years ahead because of the value of this information for interpreting study results and assessing their potential utility for nursing practice.

Magnitude of Effects and Importance

In quantitative studies, results that support the researcher's hypotheses are described as *significant*. A careful analysis of study results involves an evaluation of whether, in addition to being statistically significant, the effects are large and clinically important.

Attaining statistical significance does not necessarily mean that the results are meaningful to nurses and clients. Statistical significance indicates that the results are unlikely to be due to chance—not that they are necessarily important. With large samples, even modest relationships are statistically significant. For instance, with a sample of 500, a correlation coefficient of .10 is significant at the .05 level, but a relationship this weak may have little practical value. When assessing the importance of the findings, interpreters of research results must pay attention to actual numeric values and also, if available, to effect sizes. We expect that, like CIs, effect size information will increasingly be included in nursing reports to address the important EBP question (Box 2.1): "What *is* the evidence—what is the magnitude of effects?"

The absence of statistically significant results, conversely, does not always mean that the results are unimportant—although because nonsignificant results could reflect a Type II error, the case is more complex. Suppose we compared two alternative procedures for making a clinical assessment (e.g., body temperature). Suppose further that we retained the null hypothesis, that is, found no statistically significant differences between the two methods. If an effect size analysis suggested a very small effect size for the differences *despite a large sample size*, we might be justified in concluding that the two procedures yield equally accurate assessments. If one of these procedures is more efficient or less painful than the other, nonsignificant findings could indeed be clinically important. Nevertheless, corroboration in replication studies would be needed before firm conclusions could be reached.

Example of contrasting statistical and clinical significance:
Jezewski and Feng (2007) surveyed 579 emergency room nurses in four states about their knowledge of (and confidence with) advance directives. The found that several nurse characteristics (e.g., education, whether they had a direct care role) were significantly related to their knowledge and confidence. By inspecting the actual values of the regression coefficients, however, they concluded that "the clinical significance of these relationships is questionable" (p. 138).

The Meaning of Quantitative Results

In quantitative studies, statistical results are in the form of test statistic values, *p* levels, effect sizes, and confidence intervals, to which researchers and consumers must attach meaning (if they have concluded that these results are credible). Many questions about the meaning of statistical results reflect a desire to interpret causal connections.

Interpreting what results mean is not typically a challenge in descriptive studies. For example, suppose we found that, among patients undergoing electroconvulsive therapy (ECT), the percentage who experience an ECT-induced headache is 59.4% (95% CI = 56.3, 63.1). This result is directly meaningful and interpretable. But if we found that headache prevalence is significantly lower in a cryotherapy intervention group than among patients given acetaminophen, we would need to interpret what the results mean. In particular, we need to interpret whether it is plausible that cryotherapy *caused* the reduced prevalence of headaches. Clearly, internal validity is a key issue in interpreting the meaning of results with a potential for causal inference—even if the results have previously been deemed to be "real" (i.e., statistically significant).

In this section, we discuss the interpretation of various research outcomes within a hypothesis testing context. The emphasis is on the issue of causal interpretations. In thinking about interpretations of causality, we encourage you to review the criteria for causal relationships discussed in Chapter 9.

> **TIP**
>
> We point out once again that even if researchers have not formally stated hypotheses in the introduction of a report, they nevertheless had an underlying hypothesis if they used inferential statistical tests, because that is what such tests are designed to do—test hypotheses.

Interpreting Hypothesized Results

Interpreting the meaning of statistical results is often easiest when hypotheses are supported. Such interpretations have been partly accomplished beforehand because, in developing hypotheses, researchers have already brought together prior findings, a theoretical framework, and logical reasoning. This groundwork forms the context within which more specific interpretations are made. Nevertheless, a few caveats should be kept in mind.

First, it is important to be conservative in drawing conclusions from the results and to avoid the temptation of going beyond the data to explain what results mean. An example might help to explain what we mean by "going beyond" the data. Suppose we hypothesized that pregnant women's anxiety level about labor and delivery is correlated with the number of children they have already borne. The data reveal that a significant negative relationship between anxiety levels and parity ($r = -.40$) exists. We interpret this to mean that increased experience with childbirth results in decreased anxiety. Is this conclusion supported by the data? The conclusion appears to be logical, but in fact, there is nothing in the data that leads directly to this interpretation. An important, indeed critical, research precept is *correlation does not prove causation*. The finding that two variables are related offers no evidence suggesting which of the two variables—if either—caused the other. In our example, perhaps causality runs in the opposite direction, that is, that a woman's anxiety level influences how many children she bears. Or perhaps a third variable not examined in the study, such as the woman's relationship with her husband, causes or influences both anxiety and number of children. As discussed in Chapter 9, inferring causality is especially difficult in studies that have not used an experimental design.

Alternative explanations for the findings should always be considered and, if possible, researchers themselves should test rival hypotheses directly. If competing interpretations can be ruled out, so much the better, but every angle should be examined to see if one's own explanation has been given adequate competition. Remember that threats to internal validity reflect competing explanations for what the results might mean and need thorough consideration.

Empirical evidence supporting research hypotheses never constitutes *proof* of their veracity. Hypothesis testing is probabilistic. There is always a possibility that observed relationships resulted from chance—that is, that there has been a Type I error. Researchers must be tentative about their results and about interpretations of them. Thus, even when the results are in line with expectations, researchers should draw conclusions with restraint and should give due consideration to limitations identified in assessing the accuracy of the results.

Example of corroboration of a hypothesis:

Coleman (2007) used the Health Belief Model to guide his cross-sectional study of factors related to high-risk sexual behaviors in African American men infected with HIV. Consistent with the model, Coleman found (among other things) that self-efficacy about condom use was significantly related to condom use, and stated that self-efficacy and other factors "were observed to be key determinants of condom use during sexual activity" (p. 113).

This study is a good example of the challenges of interpreting findings in correlational studies. The researchers' interpretation was that self-efficacy was a factor that *determined* ("caused") whether a man infected with HIV would use a condom. This is a conclusion supported by earlier research, and consistent with a well-respected theory of health behavior. Yet there is nothing in the data that would rule out the possibility that a person's use of condoms *determined* self-efficacy, or that some other factor caused both condom use and higher self-efficacy. Coleman's interpretation is certainly plausible, and even likely to be correct, but his cross-sectional design makes it difficult to totally rule out other explanations. A major threat to the internal validity of the inference in this study is temporal ambiguity.

Interpreting Nonsignificant Results

Nonsignificant results pose interpretative problems because statistical tests are geared toward disconfirmation of the null hypothesis. Failure to reject a null hypothesis can occur for many reasons, and the real reason is usually difficult to discern. The null hypothesis *could* actually be true, for example. The nonsignificant result, in this case, accurately reflects the absence of a relationship among research variables. On the other hand, the null hypothesis could be false, in which case a Type II error has been committed.

Retention of a false null hypothesis can result from a variety of methodologic problems, such as poor internal validity, an anomalous sample, a weak statistical procedure, or unreliable measures. In particular, failure to reject null hypotheses is often a consequence of insufficient power, usually reflecting too small a sample size.

In any event, a retained null hypothesis should not be considered as proof of the *absence* of relationships among variables. *Nonsignificant results provide no evidence of the truth or the falsity of the hypothesis.* Interpreting the meaning of nonsignificant results can, however, be aided by considering such factors as sample size and effect size estimates.

Example of nonsignificant results:

Griffin, Polit, and Byrne (2007) hypothesized that stereotypes about children (based on children's gender, race, and physical attractiveness) would influence pediatric nurses' perceptions of children's pain and their pain treatment recommendations. None of the hypotheses was supported (i.e., there was no evidence of stereotyping). The conclusion that stereotyping was, in fact, essentially absent was bolstered by the fact that the randomly selected sample was rather large—334 nurses—and nurses were blinded to the manipulation (child characteristics). Effect sizes were extremely low and offered additional support for the conclusion that stereotyping was absent.

Because statistical procedures are designed to provide support for rejecting null hypotheses, these procedures are not well-suited for testing *actual* research hypotheses about the absence of relationships between variables or about equivalence between groups. Yet sometimes this is exactly what researchers want to do—and this is especially true in clinical situations in which the goal is to determine if one practice is just as effective as another. When the actual research hypothesis is null (i.e., a prediction of no group difference or no relationship), stringent additional strategies must be used to provide supporting evidence. In particular, it is imperative to compute effect sizes and confidence intervals as a means of illustrating that the risk of a Type II error was small. There may also be clinical standards that can be used to corroborate that nonsignificant—but predicted—results can be accepted as consistent with the research hypothesis.

Example of support for a hypothesized nonsignificant result:

Medves and O'Brien (2004) conducted a clinical trial to test the hypothesis that thermal stability would be comparable for infants bathed for the first time by a parent or by a nurse. As predicted, differences in temperature change between newborns bathed by nurses or parents were not statistically significant. The researchers provided additional support for concluding that heat loss was not associated with who bathed the newborn by indicating that a power analysis had been used to determine sample size needs and that parents for the two groups of infants were comparable demographically. Also, although the prebath temperatures of the infants in the two groups were significantly different, the researchers used initial temperature as a covariate to control these differences. Finally, they made an *a priori* determination that a change in temperature of 1°C would be clinically significant; at four points in time after the bath, the group differences in temperature were never this large; thus, the small differences were judged clinically insignificant.

Interpreting Unhypothesized Significant Results

Unhypothesized significant results can occur in two situations. The first involves exploring relationships that were not considered during the design of the study. For example, in examining correlations among variables in a data set, a researcher might notice that two variables that were not central to the research questions were nevertheless significantly correlated—and interesting. To interpret this finding, it would be wise to consult the literature to determine if other investigators had observed similar relationships.

Example of a serendipitous significant finding:

Quinn (2005) studied delay in seeking care for symptoms of acute myocardial infarction (MI). She noted that "the relationship of type of MI experienced with time to seek care was a serendipitous finding when correlations were performed examining the relationship of all clinical variables with time to seek care" (p. 289). She explored this unexpected finding in further analyses.

The second situation is more perplexing, and it does not happen often: obtaining results *opposite* to those hypothesized. For instance, a researcher might hypothesize that individualized teaching about AIDS risks is more effective than group instruction, but the results might indicate that the group method was significantly better. Some researchers view such situations as awkward or embarrassing, but research should not be undertaken primarily to corroborate researchers' predictions, but rather to arrive at truth and enhance understanding. There is no such thing as a study whose results "came out wrong" if they reflect the truth.

When significant findings are opposite to what was hypothesized, it is less likely that the methods are flawed than that the reasoning or theory is problematic. The interpretation of such findings should involve comparisons with other research, a consideration of alternate theories, and a critical scrutiny of the research methods.

Example of unhypothesized significant results:
Willem and colleagues (2007) studied Belgian nurses' job satisfaction and factors that might affect it. One hypothesis was that the more formalization there was in a hospital, the less satisfied nurses would be with task requirements, organizational policies, and interaction among colleagues. However, formalization was found to be significantly associated with *higher* satisfaction on these dimensions.

Interpreting Mixed Results

Interpretation is often complicated by *mixed results*: some hypotheses are supported by the data, but others are not. Or a hypothesis may be accepted with one measure of the dependent variable, but rejected with a different measure. When only some results run counter to a theoretical position or conceptual scheme, the research methods are the first aspect of the study deserving critical scrutiny. Differences in the validity and reliability of the various measures may account for such discrepancies, for example. On the other hand, mixed results may suggest that a theory needs to be qualified, or that certain constructs within the theory need to be reconceptualized. Mixed results sometimes present opportunities for making conceptual advances because efforts to make sense of disparate pieces of evidence may lead to a breakthrough.

Example of mixed results:
Pearson (2007) hypothesized that a low value on the ankle-brachial index (ABI) (<.90 mm Hg) would be associated with the presence of cardiac disease, carotid disease, claudication, and diabetes in women. Using data from a sample of 810 women, she found that a low ABI value was significantly related to moderate to severe carotid artery stenosis, but was not significantly associated with cardiac disease, diabetes, or claudication. The large sample minimized the risk that the failure to support some hypotheses resulted from a Type II error.

In summary, interpreting the meaning of research results is a demanding task, but it offers the possibility of unique intellectual rewards. In essence, interpreters must play the role of scientific detectives, trying to make pieces of the puzzle fit together so that a coherent picture emerges.

Generalizability of the Results

Researchers are rarely interested in discovering relationships among variables for a specific group of people at a specific point in time. If a new nursing intervention is found to be successful, others will want to adopt it. Therefore, an important interpretive question is whether the intervention will "work" or whether the relationships will "hold" in other settings, with other people. Part of the interpretive process involves asking the question, "To what groups, environments, and conditions can the results of the study reasonably be applied?"

In interpreting the study with regard to the generalizability of the results, it is useful to consider our earlier discussion about proxies. For which higher-order constructs, which populations, which settings, or which versions of an intervention were the study operations good "stand-ins"?

Implications of the Results

Once you have reached conclusions about the credibility, precision, importance, meaning, and generalizability of the results, you are ready to draw inferences about their implications. You might consider the implications of the findings with respect to future research (What should other researchers working in this area do—what is the right "next step," or what methods would yield more credible results?) or theory development (What are the implications for nursing theory?). However, you are most likely to consider the implications for nursing practice (How, if at all, should the results be used by other nurses in their practice?).

Clearly, all of the dimensions of interpretation that we have discussed are critical in evidence-based nursing practice. With regard to generalizability, it may not be enough to ask a broad question about to whom the results could apply—you need to ask, Are these results relevant to *my* particular clinical situation? Of course, if you have reached the conclusion that the results have limited credibility or importance, they may be of little utility to your practice.

CRITIQUING INTERPRETATIONS

In the discussion section of research reports related to nursing, researchers offer their interpretation of the findings and discuss what the findings might imply for nursing. When critiquing a study, your own interpretation and inferences can be contrasted against those of the researchers.

As a reviewer, you should be wary if the discussion section fails to point out any limitations. Researchers are in the best position to detect and assess the impact of sampling deficiencies, practical constraints, data quality problems, and so on, and it is a professional responsibility to alert readers to these difficulties. Moreover, when researchers acknowledge methodologic shortcomings, readers know that these limitations were considered in interpreting the results. Of course, researchers are unlikely to note all relevant shortcomings of their own work. Thus, the inclusion of comments about study limitations in the discussion section, although important, does not relieve you of the responsibility of identifying limitations on your own. Your task as a reviewer is to develop your own interpretation and assessment of limitations, to challenge conclusions that do not appear to be warranted by the results, and to indicate how the study's evidence could have been enhanced.

You should also carefully scrutinize any interpretations of causality, particularly in nonexperimental studies. Sometimes even the titles of reports suggest a potentially inappropriate inference of a causal connection. If the title of a nonexperimental study includes terms such as "the effect of . . .," or "the impact of . . .," this may signal the need for critical scrutiny of the researcher's inferences.

BOX 16.1 GUIDELINES FOR CRITIQUING INTERPRETATIONS/DISCUSSIONS IN QUANTITATIVE RESEARCH REPORTS

Interpretation of the Findings

1. Did the researchers discuss the limitations of the study and their possible effects on the credibility of the results? In discussing limitations, were all key threats to the study's validity and biases covered? Did the interpretations take limitations into account?

2. What types of evidence were offered in support of the interpretation, and was that evidence persuasive? If results were "mixed," were possible explanations offered? Were results interpreted in light of findings from other studies?

3. Did the researchers make any unjustifiable causal inferences? Were alternative explanations for the findings considered? Were the rationales for rejecting these alternatives convincing?

4. Did the interpretation take into account the precision of the results and the magnitude of effects? Did the researchers distinguish between practical and statistical significance?

5. Did the researchers draw any unwarranted conclusions about the generalizability of the results?

Implications of the Findings and Recommendations

6. Did the researchers discuss the study's implications for clinical practice, nursing theory, or future nursing research? Did they make specific recommendations?

7. If yes, are the stated implications appropriate, given the study's limitations and the magnitude of the effects—as well as evidence from other studies? Are there important implications that the report neglected to include?

In addition to comparing your interpretation with that of the researchers, your critique should also draw conclusions about the stated implications of the study. Some researchers make grandiose claims or offer unfounded recommendations on the basis of modest results. Some guidelines for evaluating researchers' interpretation are offered in Box 16.1. ⊗

RESEARCH EXAMPLES AND CRITICAL THINKING ACTIVITIES

In this section we provide details about the interpretive portion of a study, followed by some questions to guide critical thinking.

EXAMPLE 1 ■ Interpretation in a Quantitative Study

Study

Relaxation and music reduce pain following intestinal surgery (Good et al., 2005).

Statement of Purpose

The purpose of the study was to test the efficacy of three alternative interventions for pain relief following intestinal (INT) surgery: relaxation, chosen music, and both combined. Gate control theory of pain provided the theoretical context for the study.

Method

A sample of 217 patients from 4 hospitals who had undergone INT surgery were randomly assigned to 1 of 4 conditions: a chosen music intervention, a jaw relaxation intervention, combined intervention, or a standard care control group. Fifty of the patients were lost to follow-up, leaving a final analysis sample of 167 patients. The primary outcome variables were patients' pain sensation and pain distress, both measured on a 100-mm visual analog scale. Pain measurements were taken at multiple points, including preoperatively, before, during and after ambulation for 2 days postsurgery, and before and after a rest period for 2 days after surgery. Additional measures included pulse and respiratory rates and self-reported sleep quality. Patients in the treatment groups were also asked questions about their reactions to the treatment.

Analyses

The researchers analyzed potential selection biases by comparing the patients in the four groups on pretest pain measures. Although the groups were not significantly different, the baseline measures were used as covariates in the principal analyses to improve precision of estimated effects. Patients who completed the study were compared with those who dropped out on major demographic variables, and no significant differences were found. With baseline pain statistically controlled, the researchers found lower pain scores in the three treatment groups, taken together, than in the control group on both days at the preparatory to and postrest phases, but not at postambulation. Differences in pain among the three treatment groups, however, were nonsignificant. There were no group differences on other outcome measures, such as respiratory or pulse rate or sleep quality.

The researchers did additional exploratory analyses, which they noted should be interpreted cautiously. They undertook subgroup analyses that explored whether the treatments had different effects for patients with different baseline pain levels. They found that, on day 2, the treatment effect was significant at postambulation for both those categorized as being in high and in low pain before surgery. The researchers' analysis of impressionistic data also reinforced their conclusion that the effects of relaxation therapy or music were beneficial. For example, 96% of those in the three treatment groups reported that the treatment was helpful for pain, and 62% reported that it helped them feel more in control of their pain.

The researchers also presented information about clinical significance. For example, they computed effect sizes, and found most to be in the small-to-moderate range. Effect sizes were larger for those who were initially in greater pain. Clinical effects were also estimated by calculating the percentage decrease in pain sensation and distress between treatment and control group members. Differences were about 16% to 40% lower among those in intervention groups than among controls who used pain medication alone.

Discussion

Here are a few excerpts from the Discussion section of this report:

"In these INT surgery patients, relaxation, music, and the combination reduced pain at rest and at several ambulatory points on postoperative days 1 and 2. Subgroup analyses of those with high and low pain on day 2 showed further effects at post-ambulation and post-recovery, which suggests that the initial lack of effect may be related to the large variance in pain scores. Thus the interventions provided many patients with clinically significant relief, which was supported by exit reports of helpfulness . . ." (p. 248).

"The positive effects at rest are generally consistent with those of other studies of abdominal, orthopaedic, and GYN [gynecologic] surgical patients who were not studied during ambulation . . . Evidence at most data points supported the Good and Moore (1996) theoretical proposition that nonpharmacological modalities (relaxation, music, or their combination), in addition to analgesics, are helpful for satisfactory pain relief . . ." (p. 249).

"It is recommended that researchers try longer listening times during the first 2 days to see if a larger dose improves pain, physiological measures, opioid uptake, side effects, sleep, recovery, and complications . . . " (p. 249).

"The results can be generalized to populations of INT surgery patients that are similar to this one: middle-aged Caucasian males and females undergoing specific surgeries in urban and suburban hospitals in the U.S...With similar effects, it is recommended that nurses give patients choices among these interventions, encourage sequential use, and suggest using the music to relax or distract from pain." (p. 249).

CRITICAL THINKING SUGGESTIONS*:

*See the Student Resource CD-ROM for a discussion of these questions. 👤

1. Answer the relevant questions from Box 16.1 regarding this study. (We encourage you to read the report in its entirety, especially the discussion section, to answer these questions).
2. Also, consider the following targeted questions, which may further sharpen your critical thinking skills and assist you in understanding this study:
   a. Comment on the statistical conclusion validity of this study.
   b. The researchers originally hypothesized that patients who received the combination of music and relaxation treatments would have less pain than patients who receive single treatments. Comment on what the results suggest about this hypothesis.
3. What might be some of the uses to which the findings could be put in clinical practice?

📺 EXAMPLE 2 ■ Discussion Section in the Study in Appendix A

1. Read the "Discussion" section of Howell and colleagues' (2007) study ("Anxiety, anger, and blood pressure in children") in Appendix A of this book, and then answer the relevant questions in Box 16.1.
2. Also, consider the following targeted questions, which may further sharpen your critical thinking skills and assist you in assessing aspects of the study's merit:
   a. Were there any statistically significant correlations that were unanticipated or unhypothesized in this study? Did the researchers discuss them? If yes, do you agree with their interpretation?
   b. Comment on the researchers' recommendations about gender-specific research in the discussion section.

📺 EXAMPLE 3 ■ Quantitative Study in Appendix C

Read McGillion and colleagues' (2008) study ("Randomized controlled trial of a psychoeducation program for the self-management of chronic cardiac pain") in Appendix C (on the accompanying Student Resource CD-ROM) and then address the following suggested activities or questions.

1. Before reading our critique, which accompanies the full report on the CD-ROM, either write your own critique or prepare a list of what you think are the major strengths and weaknesses of the study. Pay particular attention to validity threats and various types of bias. Then contrast your critique or list with ours. Remember that you (or your instructor) do not necessarily have to agree with all of the points made in our critique, and that you may identify strengths and weaknesses that we overlooked. You may find the broad critiquing guidelines in Table 4-1 helpful.

2. Write a short summary of how credible, important, and generalizable you find the study results to be. Your summary should conclude with your interpretation of what the results mean, and what their implications are for nursing practice. Contrast your summary with the discussion section in the report itself.

3. In selecting studies to include with this textbook, we avoided choosing poor-quality studies. Studies with numerous flaws would have been easier to critique, but we did not wish to embarrass any nurse researchers. In the questions below, we offer some "pretend" scenarios in which the researchers for the study in Appendix C made different methodologic decisions than the ones they in fact did make. Write a paragraph or two critiquing these "pretend" decisions, pointing out how these alternatives would have affected the rigor of the study and the inferences that could be made.

   a. Pretend that the researchers had been unable to randomize subjects to treatments. The design, in other words, would be a nonequivalent control group quasi-experiment, with different conditions for patients in different pre-existing groups.

   b. Pretend that 130 participants were randomized (this is what actually did happen), but that only 80 participants remained in the study 3 months after random assignment.

   c. Pretend that the HRQL and the SAQ were psychometrically weaker—for example, that they had reliabilities less than .70.

CHAPTER REVIEW

Key new terms introduced in the chapter, together with a summary of major points, are presented in this section. In addition, Chapter 16 of the *Study Guide for Essentials of Nursing Research*, 7th edition offers various exercises and study suggestions for reinforcing concepts presented in this chapter. For additional review, see the Student Self-Study Review Questions section of the Student Resource CD-ROM provided with this book.

Key New Terms

CONSORT guidelines   Results

Summary Points

➤ The interpretation of quantitative research **results** (the outcomes of the statistical analyses) typically involves consideration of (1) the credibility of the results; (2) precision of estimates of effects; (3) magnitude of effects; (4) underlying meaning of the results; (5) generalizability of results; and (6) implications for future research, theory development, and nursing practice.

❧ Inference is central to interpretation. The particulars of the study—especially the methodologic decisions made by researchers—affect the inferences that can be made about the correspondence between study results and "truth in the real world."

❧ A cautious and even skeptical outlook is appropriate in drawing conclusions about the credibility and meaning of study results.

❧ An assessment of a study's credibility can involve various approaches, one of which involves an evaluation of the degree of congruence between abstract constructs or idealized methods on the one hand, and the proxies actually used on the other.

❧ Credibility assessments can also involve a careful assessment of study rigor through an analysis of validity threats and various biases that could undermine the accuracy of the results.

❧ Corroboration (replication) of results, through either internal or external sources, is another approach in a credibility assessment.

❧ Researchers can facilitate interpretations by carefully documenting methodologic decisions and the outcomes of those decisions (e.g., by using the **CONSORT guidelines** to document participant flow).

❧ In their discussions of study results, researchers should themselves always point out known study limitations, but readers should draw their own conclusions about the rigor of the study and about the plausibility of alternative explanations for the results.

STUDIES CITED IN CHAPTER 16

Bennett, J., Young, H., Nail, L., Winter-Stone, K., & Hanson, G. (2008). A telephone only motivational intervention to increase physical activity in rural adults. *Nursing Research, 57,* 24–32.

Coleman, C. (2007). Health beliefs and high-risk sexual behaviors among HIV infected African American men. *Applied Nursing Research, 20,* 110–115.

Good, M., Anderson, G., Ahn, S., Cong, X., & Stanton-Hicks, M. (2005). Relaxation and music reduce pain following intestinal surgery. *Research in Nursing & Health, 28,* 240–251.

Griffin, R., Polit, D., & Byrnes, M. (2007). Stereotyping and nurses' treatment of children's pain. *Research in Nursing & Health, 30,* 655–666.

Jezewski, M., & Feng, J. (2007). Emergency nurses' knowledge, attitudes, and experiential survey on advance directives. *Applied Nursing Research, 20,* 132–139.

Medves, J. M., & O'Brien, B. (2004). The effect of bather and location of first bath on maintaining thermal stability in newborns. *Journal of Obstetric, Gynecologic, & Neonatal Nursing, 33,* 175–182.

Pearson, T. L. (2007). Correlation of ankle-brachial index values with carotid disease, coronary disease, and cardiovascular risk factors in women. *Journal of Cardiovascular Nursing, 22,* 436–439.

Quinn, J. (2005). Delay in seeking care for symptoms of acute myocardial infarction: Applying a theoretical model. *Research in Nursing & Health, 28,* 283–294.

Willem, A., Buelens, M., & DeJongue, I. (2007). Impact of organizational structure on nurses' job satisfaction. *International Journal of Nursing Studies, 44,* 1011–1020.

17 Analysis of Qualitative Data

STUDENT OBJECTIVES

On completing this chapter, you will be able to:

➤ Describe prototypical qualitative analysis styles and understand the intellectual processes involved in qualitative analysis

➤ Describe activities that qualitative researchers perform to manage and organize their data

➤ Discuss the procedures used to analyze qualitative data, including both general procedures and those used in ethnographic, phenomenological, and grounded theory research

➤ Assess the adequacy of researchers' descriptions of their analytic procedures and evaluate the suitability of those procedures

➤ Define new terms in the chapter

Qualitative data are derived from narrative materials, such as verbatim transcripts from in-depth interviews, participant observers' field notes, or personal diaries. This chapter describes methods for analyzing such qualitative data.

INTRODUCTION TO QUALITATIVE ANALYSIS

Qualitative analysis is a labor-intensive activity that requires creativity, conceptual sensitivity, and sheer hard work. In this section, we discuss some general considerations relating to qualitative analysis.

Qualitative Analysis Challenges

The purpose of data analysis, regardless of the type of data or underlying research tradition, is to organize, provide structure to, and elicit meaning from the data. Qualitative data analysis is a particularly challenging enterprise, for three major reasons. First, there are no universal rules for analyzing qualitative data. The absence of standard analytic procedures makes it difficult to explain how to do such analyses, and how to present findings in a way that their validity is apparent. Some of the procedures that we describe in the next chapter are important tools for enhancing the trustworthiness of the analysis.

The second challenge of qualitative analysis is the enormous amount of work required. Qualitative analysts must organize and make sense of pages and pages of narrative materials. In a multimethod study by one of us (Polit), the qualitative data consisted of transcribed interviews with over 100 low-income women discussing life stressors and health problems. The transcriptions ranged from 30 to 50 pages, resulting in more than 3,000 pages that had to be read and reread, organized, integrated, and interpreted.

A third challenge is that doing qualitative analysis well requires powerful inductive skills (inducing universals from particulars) and creativity. A good qualitative analyst must have the skill to discern patterns and to weave them together into a unified whole in an insightful way.

The final challenge comes in reducing data for reporting purposes. Quantitative results can often be summarized in a few tables. Qualitative researchers, by contrast, must balance the need to be concise with the need to maintain the richness and evidentiary value of their data.

TIP

Qualitative analyses are more difficult to *do* than quantitative ones, but qualitative findings are usually easier to understand than quantitative ones because the stories are often told in everyday language. Qualitative analyses are often harder to appraise than quantitative analyses, however, because readers cannot know first-hand if researchers adequately captured thematic patterns in the data.

Analysis Styles

Crabtree and Miller (1999) observed that there are nearly as many qualitative analysis strategies as there are qualitative researchers, but they identified three major styles, ranging from one that is more standardized to one that is more intuitive. The three prototypical styles are:

➤ *Template analysis style*. In this style, researchers develop a **template** to which the narrative data are applied. Researchers begin with a rudimentary template or coding guide before collecting data, but revise it as more data are gathered. The analysis of the data, sorted according to the template, is interpretive, not statistical. This style is most likely to be adopted by researchers whose research tradition is ethnography, ethology, discourse analysis, and ethnoscience.

➤ *Editing analysis style*. Researchers using an editing style act as interpreters who read through the data in search of meaningful segments and units. Once they identify segments, they develop a **category scheme** and corresponding codes that can be used to sort and organize the data. The researchers then search for patterns and structures that connect the categories. Researchers whose research traditions are grounded theory, phenomenology, and ethnomethodology use procedures that fall within the editing analysis style.

➤ *Immersion/crystallization style*. This style involves the analyst's total immersion in (and reflection of) the text materials, resulting in an intuitive crystallization of the data. This highly interpretive, subjective style is sometimes encountered in hermeneutic or critical inquiries.

Researchers seldom use terms such as *template analysis style* or *editing style* in their reports (although there are exceptions). These terms are primarily *post hoc* characterizations of styles adopted by qualitative researchers.

The Qualitative Analysis Process

The analysis of qualitative data is an active and interactive process. Qualitative researchers typically scrutinize their data carefully and deliberately, often reading the data over and over in a search for meaning and deeper understanding. Insights and theories cannot emerge until researchers become completely familiar with their data. Morse and Field (1995) noted that qualitative analysis is a "process of fitting data together, of making the invisible obvious, of linking and attributing consequences to antecedents. It is a process of conjecture and verification, of correction and modification, of suggestion and defense" (p. 126).

QUALITATIVE DATA MANAGEMENT AND ORGANIZATION

Qualitative analysis is supported and facilitated by several tasks that help to organize and manage the mass of narrative data, as described next.

Transcribing Qualitative Data

Audiotaped interviews and field notes are major data sources in qualitative studies. Verbatim transcription of the tapes is a critical step in preparing for data analysis, and researchers must ensure that transcriptions are accurate and validly reflect the totality of the interview experience.

Transcription errors are almost inevitable, which means that researchers need to check the accuracy of transcribed data. When checking for transcription accuracy, researchers should listen to the taped interview. Researchers should begin data analysis with the best-possible quality data, which requires careful training of transcribers, ongoing feedback, and continuous efforts to verify accuracy.

Developing a Category Scheme

Qualitative researchers begin their analysis by organizing their data (i.e., by developing a method to classify and index their data). Researchers must be able to gain access to parts of the data, without having repeatedly to reread the data set in its entirety. This phase of data analysis is essentially reductionist—data must be converted to smaller, more manageable units that can be retrieved and reviewed.

The most widely used procedure is to develop a category scheme and then to code data according to the categories. A preliminary category system (a template) is sometimes drafted before data collection, but more typically qualitative analysts develop categories based on a scrutiny of actual data. There are no easy guidelines for this task. Developing a high-quality category scheme involves a careful reading of the data, with an eye to identifying underlying concepts and clusters of concepts. The nature of the categories may vary in level of detail or specificity, as well as in level of abstraction.

Researchers whose aims are primarily descriptive tend to use categories that are fairly concrete. For example, the category scheme may focus on differentiating various types of actions or events, or different phases in a chronologic unfolding of an experience. In developing a category scheme, related concepts are often grouped together to facilitate the coding process.

Example of a descriptive category scheme:

Perry and colleagues (2008) did a descriptive qualitative study about factors influencing women's participation in a 12-week walking program, the Heart-to-Heart program. Data were gathered from field notes and focus group sessions with women who participated in the program. Data were analyzed inductively and coded into two broad descriptive categories, barriers and motivators to adopting a walking program. Subcategories were specific barriers or motivators. For example, the three main "barrier" categories were (1) balancing family and self; (2) chronic illness; and (3) illness or injury breaking the routine.

Studies designed to develop a theory are more likely to involve abstract, conceptual categories. In creating conceptual categories, researchers must break the data into segments, closely examine them, and compare them with other segments for similarities and dissimilarities to determine what the meaning of those phenomena are. (This is part of the process is referred to as *constant comparison* by grounded theory researchers.) The researcher asks questions, such as the following about discrete events, incidents, or statements:

➤ What is this?

➤ What is going on?

➤ What does it stand for?

➤ What else is like this?

➤ What is this distinct from?

Important concepts that emerge from close examination of the data are then given a label that forms the basis for a category scheme. These names are necessarily abstractions, but the labels are usually sufficiently graphic that the nature of the material to which they refer is clear—and often provocative.

Example of a conceptual category scheme:
Box 17.1 shows the category scheme developed by Beck (2006) to code data from her Internet interviews on the anniversary of birth trauma (the full study is in Appendix B). The coding scheme included four major thematic categories with subcodes. For example, an excerpt that described a mother's feelings of dread and anxiety during the days leading up to the anniversary of her traumatic birth would be coded 1A, the category for "plagued with an array of distressing thoughts and emotions." (Note that Beck's original coding scheme, shown in Box 17.1, was further developed and made more parsimonious during the analysis stage. For example, codes 2D, 2E, and 2F, were collapsed into a larger category called "Various ways to make it through the day." Table 2 in the full report [Appendix B] shows several significant statements that exemplify this broader category).

TIP

A good category scheme is crucial to the analysis of qualitative data. Without a high-quality category scheme, researchers cannot retrieve their narrative information. Unfortunately, research reports rarely present the category scheme for readers to critique, but they may provide information about its development. This, in turn, may help you evaluate its adequacy (e.g., researchers may say that the scheme was reviewed by peers or developed and independently verified by two or more researchers).

Coding Qualitative Data

Once a category scheme has been developed, the data are read in their entirety and coded for correspondence to the categories—a task that is seldom straightforward. Researchers may have difficulty deciding the most appropriate code, or may not fully comprehend the underlying meaning of some aspect of the data. It may take several readings of the material to grasp its nuances.

Also, researchers often discover in going through the data that the initial category scheme was incomplete. It is common for categories to emerge that were not initially identified. When this happens, it is risky to assume that the category was absent in materials that have already been coded. A concept might not be identified

---

BOX 17.1   BECK'S (2006) CODING SCHEME FOR THE ANNIVERSARY OF BIRTH TRAUMA

Theme 1. The Prologue: An Agonizing Time
A. Plagued with an array of distressing thoughts and emotions
B. Physically taking a toll
C. Clocks, calendars, and seasons playing key roles
D. Ruminating about the day their babies had been born

Theme 2: The Actual Day: A Celebration of a Birthday or Torment of an Anniversary
A. Concept of time taking center stage
B. Not knowing how to celebrate her child's birthday
C. Tormented by powerful emotions
D. Scheduled birthday party on a different day
E. Consumed with technical details of the birthday party
F. Need to physically get away on the birthday

Theme 3: The Epilogue: A Fragile State
A. Surviving the actual anniversary took a heavy toll
B. Needed time to recuperate
C. Crippling emotions lingered
D. Sense of relief

Theme 4: Subsequent Anniversaries: For Better or Worse

A. Each birthday slightly easier to cope with
B. No improvement noted
C. Worrying about future birthdays
D. Each anniversary is a lottery; a time bomb.

---

as salient until it has emerged three or four times. In such a case, it would be necessary to reread all previously coded material to have a truly complete grasp of that category.

Another issue is that narrative materials usually are not linear. For example, paragraphs from transcribed interviews may contain elements relating to three or four different categories, embedded in a complex fashion.

Example of a multitopic segment:
An example of a multitopic segment of an interview from Beck's (2006) anniversary of birth trauma study is shown in Figure 17.1. The codes in the margin represent codes from the category scheme presented in Box 17.1.

Manual Methods of Organizing Qualitative Data

Various procedures have been used to organize and manage qualitative data. Before the advent of computer programs for qualitative data management, the most usual procedure was the development of **conceptual files**. This approach involves creating a physical file for each category, and then cutting out and inserting into the file all of the materials relating to that category. Researchers can then retrieve all of the content on a particular topic by reviewing the applicable file folder.

"I have experienced one anniversary of the trauma of Anna's birth. During the summer I remember looking at the calendar, fearing her birthday would take place on the same day of her birth (Wednesday). Hearing the word "October" or seeing the word in writing gave me chills.	1C
Prior to the anniversary I grew very sentimental about our hospital experience and would delve into piles of photos, hospital memorabilia and reading birth stories. Instead of feeling validated or better, it seemed to kick the grief into high gear. I felt very alone. My closet contained all the hospital stuff and when I was sad or alone I would go there, ironically, to feel even more alone. I didn't feel anyone would ever understand.	1A
Time was definitely a traumatic concept during the anniversary. There is sooo much emphasis on time in the birthing process, so this seemed to carry and surface on and	1C
around her birthday. I found myself linking the time of day to what happened that evening, driving to the hospital, number of dilation to the minute and when my water was broken. I	1D
would see commercials for a television show and feel scared, knowing it played during the time of my laboring. Even today, a clock reading 8:47 will turn my stomach upside down."	1C,1A

FIGURE 17.1 Coded excerpt from Beck's (2006) study.

The creation of such conceptual files is clearly a cumbersome and labor-intensive task. This is particularly true when segments of the narrative materials have multiple codes, such as the excerpt shown in Figure 17.1. In this situation, there would need to be three copies of the second paragraph—one for each file corresponding to the three codes that were used (1A, 1C, 1D). Researchers must also be sensitive to the need to provide sufficient context that the cut-up material can be understood. Thus, it is often necessary to include material preceding or following the directly relevant materials.

Computer Programs for Managing Qualitative Data

Computer assisted qualitative data analysis software (CAQDAS) can help to remove some of the work of cutting and pasting pages of narrative material. Dozens of CAQDAS have been developed. These programs permit the entire data file to be entered onto the computer, each portion of an interview or observational record coded, and then portions of the text corresponding to specified codes retrieved and printed (or shown on a screen) for analysis. The software can also be used to examine relationships between codes. Software cannot, however, *do* the coding, and it cannot tell the researcher how to analyze the data. Researchers must continue their role as analysts and critical thinkers.

Computer programs offer many advantages for managing qualitative data, but some people prefer manual methods because they allow researchers to get closer to the data. Others have raised objections to having a process that is basically cognitive turned into an activity that is mechanical and technical. Despite concerns, many researchers have switched to computerized data management. Proponents insist that it frees up their time and permits them to pay greater attention to more important conceptual issues.

Example of using computers to manage qualitative data:
Feely and colleagues (2007) studied people's perceptions of living with depression. They used a popular software called NVivo to manage their data, which had been collected in focus group and personal interviews with people diagnosed with depression.

ANALYTIC PROCEDURES

Data *management* in qualitative research is reductionist in nature: It involves converting large masses of data into smaller, more manageable segments. By contrast, qualitative data *analysis* is constructionist: It is an inductive process that involves putting segments together into meaningful conceptual patterns. Although there are various approaches to qualitative data analysis, some elements are common to several of them. We provide some general guidelines, followed by a description of procedures used by ethnographers, phenomenologists, and grounded theory researchers.

It should be noted that qualitative researchers who conduct studies that are not based in a specific research tradition sometimes say that a **content analysis** was performed. Qualitative content analysis is the analysis of the content of narrative data to identify prominent themes and patterns among the themes—primarily using either a template or editing analysis style.

Example of a content analysis:
Zanchetta and colleagues (2007) undertook a content analysis of semistructured interviews with 15 older men with prostate cancer to understand the information strategies they used to understand and deal with the disease.

A General Analytic Overview

The analysis of qualitative materials begins with a search for broad categories or themes. In their review of how the term *theme* is used among qualitative researchers, DeSantis and Ugarriza (2000) offered this definition: "A **theme** is an abstract entity that brings meaning and identity to a current experience and its variant manifestations. As such, a theme captures and unifies the nature or basis of the experience into a meaningful whole" (p. 362).

Themes emerge from the data. They often develop within categories of data (i.e., within categories of the coding scheme used for indexing materials), but may also cut across them. For example, in Beck's anniversary of birth trauma (2006) study (see Box 17.1) one theme that emerged was mothers' fragile state after the actual day of the anniversary was over, which included 3B (needing time to recuperate) and 3D (sense of relief).

The search for themes involves not only discovering commonalities across participants, but also seeking natural variation. Themes are never universal. Researchers must attend not only to what themes arise but also to how they are patterned. Does the theme apply only to certain types of people or in certain communities? In certain contexts? At certain periods? What are the conditions that precede the observed phenomenon, and what are the apparent consequences of it? In other words, the qualitative analyst must be sensitive to *relationships* within the data.

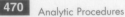

> **TIP**
>
> Qualitative researchers often use major themes as the subheadings in the results section of their reports. For example, in their analysis of diaries that nurses wrote to help critically ill patients understand their intensive care unit (ICU) experience, Roulin and colleagues (2007) identified four main themes that were used to organize their results section: "Sharing the story," "Sharing the presence," "Sharing feelings," and "Sharing through support."

Researchers' search for themes, regularities, and patterns in the data can sometimes be facilitated by charting devices that enable them to summarize the evolution of behaviors, events, and processes. For example, for qualitative studies that focus on dynamic experiences—such as decision-making—it is often useful to develop flow charts or time-lines that highlight time sequences, major decision points and events, and factors affecting the decisions.

The identification of key themes and categories is seldom a tidy, linear process—iteration is almost always necessary. That is, researchers derive themes from the narrative materials, go back to the materials with the themes in mind to see if the materials really do fit, and then refine the themes as necessary. Sometimes apparent insights early in the process have to be abandoned.

Example of abandoning an early conceptualization:
Strang and colleagues' (2006) studied the experiences of family caregivers of people with dementia. They wrote: "We coded data categories in stages with each stage representing a higher level of conceptual complexity . . . the interplay within the caregiver dyad reminded us of *dancing*. As the analysis progressed, the dance metaphor failed to fully represent the increasingly complex nature of the interactions between caregiver and the family member with dementia. We abandoned it completely" (p. 32).

Some qualitative researchers use metaphors as an analytic strategy, as the preceding example suggests. A **metaphor** is a symbolic comparison, using figurative language to evoke a visual analogy. Metaphors can be a powerfully creative and expressive tool for qualitative analysts, although they can run the risk of "supplanting creative insight with hackneyed cliché masquerading as profundity" (Thorne & Darbyshire, 2005, p. 1111).

Example of a metaphor:
Bakitas (2007) conducted a study of the symptom experience of chemotherapy-induced peripheral neuropathy (CIPN) in patients undergoing chemotherapy. She used the metaphor of *background noise* as an overarching metaphor that captured the essence of CIPN symptom experiences. The CIPN was usually kept in the "background" and was overshadowed by other symptom or treatment effects. Support for the noise metaphor came from participants' own comparison of CIPN to sound.

A further step involves validation. In this phase, the concern is whether the themes inferred accurately represent the perspectives of the study participants. Several validation procedures can be used, which we will discuss in Chapter 18. If more than one researcher is working on the study, sessions in which the themes are reviewed and specific cases discussed can be highly productive. Such investigator triangulation cannot ensure thematic validity, but it can minimize idiosyncratic biases.

In validating and refining themes, some researchers introduce **quasi-statistics**— a tabulation of the frequency with which certain themes or insights are supported by the data. The frequencies cannot be interpreted in the same way as frequencies generated in survey studies because of imprecision in the enumeration of the themes, but, as Becker (1970) pointed out,

> Quasi-statistics may allow the investigator to dispose of certain troublesome null hypotheses. A simple frequency count of the number of times a given phenomenon appears may make untenable the null hypothesis that the phenomenon is infrequent. A comparison of the number of such instances with the number of negative cases— instances in which some alternative phenomenon that would not be predicted by his theory appears—may make possible a stronger conclusion, especially if the theory was developed early enough in the observational period to allow a systematic search for negative cases (p. 81).

Example of tabulating data:
Barnes and Aguilar (2007) studied recently arrived Cuban refugees' perceptions of community-level support in Texas. Twenty Cuban adult refugees were interviewed about their experiences. One question area involved the refugees' perceptions about what type of support was most needed during the first 5 years of resettlement. One-quarter thought practical support (housing, food) was needed first, another quarter thought emotional support was needed first, and "fully half of respondents thought both forms of support were needed simultaneously" (p. 232).

> **TIP**
> Although relative few qualitative researchers make formal efforts to quantify features of their data, be alert to quantitative implications when you read a qualitative report. Qualitative researchers routinely use words such as "some," "most," or "many" in characterizing the experiences and actions of study participants, which implies some level of quantification.

In the final analysis stage, researchers strive to weave the thematic pieces together into an integrated whole. The various themes need to be interrelated to provide an overall structure (e.g., a theory or integrated description) to the data. The integration task is a difficult one, because it demands creativity and intellectual rigor if it is to be successful.

Ethnographic Analysis

Analysis begins from the moment ethnographers set foot in the field. Ethnographers are continually looking for *patterns* in the behavior and thoughts of the participants, comparing one pattern against another, and analyzing many patterns simultaneously. As they analyze patterns of everyday life, ethnographers acquire a deeper understanding of the culture being studied. Maps, flowcharts, and organizational charts are also useful tools that help to crystallize and illustrate the data being collected. Matrices (two-dimensional displays) can also help to highlight a comparison graphically, to cross-reference categories, and to discover emerging patterns.

Spradley's (1979) research sequence is often used for data analysis in an ethnographic study. His method is based on the premise that language is the primary means that relates meaning in a culture. The task of ethnographers is to describe cultural symbols and to identify their coding rules. His sequence of 12 steps, which includes both data collection and data analysis, is as follows:

1. Locating an informant
2. Interviewing an informant
3. Making an ethnographic record
4. Asking descriptive questions
5. Analyzing ethnographic interviews
6. Making a domain analysis
7. Asking structural questions
8. Making a taxonomic analysis
9. Asking contrast questions
10. Making a componential analysis
11. Discovering cultural themes
12. Writing the ethnography

Thus, in Spradley's method there are four levels of data analysis, the first of which is *domain analysis*. **Domains**, which are units of cultural knowledge, are broad categories that encompass smaller categories. During this first level of data analysis, ethnographers identify relational patterns among terms in the domains that are used by members of the culture. The ethnographer focuses on the cultural meaning of terms and symbols (objects and events) used in a culture, and their interrelationships.

In *taxonomic analysis*, the second level of data analysis, ethnographers decide how many domains the data analysis will encompass. Will only one or two domains be analyzed in depth, or will a number of domains be studied less intensively? After making this decision, a **taxonomy**—a system of classifying and organizing terms—is developed to illustrate the internal organization of a domain and the relationship among the subcategories of the domain.

In *componential analysis*, multiple relationships among terms in the domains are examined. The ethnographer analyzes data for similarities and differences among cultural terms in a domain. Finally, in *theme analysis*, cultural themes are uncovered. Domains are connected in cultural themes, which helps to provide a holistic view of the culture being studied. The discovery of cultural meaning is the outcome.

Example using Spradley's method:
Tzeng and Lipson (2004) investigated experiences of patients and family members after a suicide attempt within the cultural context of Taiwan. Data from interviews and participant observations were analyzed in an ongoing fashion. The analysis began with the coding of categories and terms, which they "associated into higher order domains" (p. 348). They also undertook a componential analysis by conducting "a back and forth process to establish different categories: searching for contrasts among these domains, grouping some together as dimensions, and combining related dimensions" (p. 348). The postsuicide stigma suffered by patients and their families was based on such cultural themes as "Suicide is bu-hsiao" (non-filial piety).

Other approaches to ethnographic analysis have also been developed. For example, in their ethnonursing research method, Leininger and McFarland (2006) provided ethnographers with a four-phase ethnonursing data analysis guide. In the first phase, ethnographers collect, describe, and record data. The second phase involves identifying and categorizing descriptors. In phase 3, data are analyzed to discover repetitive patterns in their context. The fourth and final phase involves abstracting major themes and presenting findings.

Example using Leininger's method:
DeOliveira and Hoga (2005) studied the process of seeking and undergoing surgical contraception by low-income Brazilian women. Using Leininger's ethnonursing research method, the researchers interviewed 7 key informants and 11 additional informants. The cultural theme was that "being *operada* was the realization of a great dream" (p. 5).

Phenomenological Analysis

Schools of phenomenology have developed different approaches to data analysis. Three frequently used methods for descriptive phenomenology are the methods of Colaizzi (1978), Giorgi (1985), and Van Kaam (1966), all of whom are from the Duquesne school of phenomenology, based on Husserl's philosophy. Table 17.1 presents a comparison of these three methods of analysis. The basic outcome of all three methods is the description of the meaning of an experience, often through the identification of essential themes.

Phenomenologists search for common patterns shared by particular instances. There are, however, some important differences among these three approaches. Colaizzi's method, for example, is the only one that calls for a validation of results by returning to study participants. Giorgi's analysis relies solely on researchers. His view is that it is inappropriate either to return to participants to validate findings or to use external judges to review the analysis. Van Kaam's method requires that intersubjective agreement be reached with other expert judges.

TABLE 17.1 ▶ COMPARISON OF THREE PHENOMENOLOGICAL METHODS

COLAIZZI (1978)	GIORGI (1985)	VAN KAAM (1966)
1. Read all protocols to acquire a feeling for them.	1. Read the entire set of protocols to get a sense of the whole.	1. List and group preliminarily the descriptive expressions, which must be agreed upon by expert judges. Final listing presents percentages of these categories in that particular sample.
2. Review each protocol and extract significant statements.	2. Discriminate units from participants' description of phenomenon being studied.	2. Reduce the concrete, vague, and overlapping expressions of the participants to more descriptive terms. (Inter-subjective agreement among judges needed.)
3. Spell out the meaning of each significant statement (i.e., formulate meanings).	3. Articulate the psychological insight in each of the *meaning units*.	3. Eliminate elements not inherent in the phenomenon being studied or that represent blending of two related phenomena.
4. Organize the formulated meanings into clusters of themes. a. Refer these clusters back to the original protocols to validate them. b. Note discrepancies among or between the various clusters, avoiding the temptation of ignoring data or themes that do not fit.	4. Synthesize all of the transformed meaning units into a consistent statement regarding participants' experiences (referred to as the "structure of the experience"); can be expressed on a specific or general level.	4. Write a hypothetical identification and description of the phenomenon being studied.
5. Integrate results into an exhaustive description of the phenomenon under study.		5. Apply hypothetical description to randomly selected cases from the sample. If necessary, revise the hypothesized description, which must then be tested again on a new sample.
6. Formulate an exhaustive description of the phenomenon under study in as unequivocal a statement of identification as possible.		6. Consider the hypothesized identification as a valid identification and description once preceding operations have been carried out successfully.
7. Ask participants about the findings thus far as a final validating step.		

Example of a study using Colaizzi's method:
Tanyi and Werner (2008) explored women's experience of spirituality within end-stage renal disease. Transcribed interviews with 16 women who attended a dialysis center were analyzed using Colaizzi's method. The two researchers independently reviewed transcripts line-by-line and extracted significant statements relating to spirituality. These statements led to formulated meanings (shown in their Table 1), and four themes emerged pertaining to the women's spiritual experience within their illness: Acceptance, understanding, fortification, and emotion modulation.

A second school of phenomenology is the Utrecht School. Phenomenologists using this Dutch approach combine characteristics of descriptive and interpretive phenomenology. Van Manen's (1997) method is an example of this combined approach in which researchers try to grasp the essential meaning of the experience being studied. Van Manen's approach involves six activities: (1) turning to the nature of the lived experience; (2) exploring the experience as we live it; (3) reflecting on essential themes; (4) describing the phenomenon through the art of writing and rewriting; (5) maintaining a strong relation to the phenomenon; and (6) balancing the research context by considering parts and whole. According to Van Manen, thematic aspects of experience can be uncovered or isolated from participants' descriptions of the experience by three methods: the holistic, selective, or detailed approach. In the **holistic approach**, researchers view the text as a whole and try to capture its meanings. In the **selective** (or highlighting) **approach,** researchers highlight or pull out statements or phrases that seem essential to the experience under study. In the **detailed** (or line-by-line) **approach**, researchers analyze every sentence. Once themes have been identified, they become the objects of reflection and interpretation through follow-up interviews with participants. Through this process, essential themes are discovered.

Example of a study using Van Manen's method:
Enns and Gregory (2007) studied expressions of caring by surgical nurses using Van Manen's approach. They noted that, "Thematic statements were isolated using Van Manen's highlighting approach, while the six interrelated research activities of the phenomenological process were concomitantly applied." The major theme of *lamentation and loss* was identified in their analysis.

In addition to identifying themes from participants' descriptions, Van Manen also called for gleaning thematic descriptions from artistic sources. Van Manen urged qualitative researchers to keep in mind that literature, music, painting, and other art forms can provide a wealth of experiential information that can increase insights in efforts to interpret and grasp the essential meaning of the experience being studied.

Example of a phenomenological analysis using artistic expressions:
Lauterbach (2007) investigated mothers' experiences with the death of a wished-for baby. Poetry, literature, and art helped Lauterbach's interpretation of the mothers' experiences. For instance, Herbert Mason's poem "The Memory of Death," in which he reflected on the death of his child, and Robert Frost's poem "Home Burial," in which Frost described gender differences in the experience of infant death, were used in data analysis. Memorial art in cemeteries and funeral photographs also provided insight.

A third school of phenomenology is an interpretive approach called Heideggerian hermeneutics. Central to analyzing data in a hermeneutic study is the notion of the **hermeneutic circle**. The circle signifies a methodologic process in which, to reach understanding, there is continual movement between the parts and the whole of the text being analyzed. Gadamer (1975) stressed that, to interpret a text, researchers cannot separate themselves from the meanings of the text and must strive to understand possibilities that the text can reveal. Ricoeur (1981) broadened this notion of text to include not just the written text but any human action or situation.

Example of Gadamerian hermeneutics:
Annells (2006) sought to interpret and present possible meanings in the stories of people with bowel ostomies about their experience of the effect of flatus incontinence on their lives. Her study, which involved videotaped interviews with six participants with a bowel ostomy, was guided by Gadamer's writings: "I wanted to become immersed in generated text and remain open to intuitive construction, with freedom about process and style, this being guided by flow of interpretation" (p. 519).

Diekelmann and colleagues (1989) proposed a seven-stage process of data analysis in hermeneutics that involves collaborative effort by a *team* of researchers. The goal of this process is to describe common meanings. Diekelmann and colleagues' stages include the following:

1. All the interviews or texts are read for an overall understanding.

2. Interpretive summaries of each interview are written.

3. A team of researchers analyzes selected transcribed interviews or texts.

4. Any disagreements on interpretation are resolved by going back to the text.

5. Common meanings and shared practices are identified by comparing and contrasting the text.

6. Relationships among themes emerge.

7. A draft of the themes and exemplars from texts are presented to the team. Responses or suggestions are incorporated into the final draft.

According to Diekelmann and colleagues, the discovery in stage 6 of a **constitutive pattern**—a pattern that expresses the relationships among relational themes and is present in all the interviews or texts—forms the highest level of hermeneutical analysis. A situation is constitutive when it gives actual content to a person's self-understanding or to a person's way of being in the world.

Example of a Diekelmann's hermeneutical analysis:
Parsons-Suhl and co-researchers (2008) used Diekelman's seven-stage analytic method in their study of the experience of memory loss in individuals with early Alzheimer's disease. First, all four researchers read each text independently and reflected on the descriptions to get an overall sense of the meaning. Themes were then identified by the lead researcher, in consultation with other members of the team. The primary researcher wrote interpretive summaries of each interview and identified relational themes. Constitutive patterns were identified and shared with the team.

Benner (1994) offered another analytic approach for hermeneutic phenomenology. Her interpretive analysis consists of three interrelated processes: the search for paradigm cases, thematic analysis, and analysis of exemplars. **Paradigm cases** are "strong instances of concerns or ways of being in the world" (Benner, 1994, p. 113). Paradigm cases are used early in the analytic process as a strategy for gaining understanding. Thematic analysis is done to compare and contrast similarities across cases. Lastly, paradigm cases and thematic analysis can be enhanced by *exemplars* that illuminate aspects of a paradigm case or theme. The presentation of paradigm cases and exemplars in research reports allows readers to play a role in consensual validation of the results by deciding whether the cases support the researchers' conclusions.

Example using Benner's hermeneutical analysis:
Mauleon and co-researchers (2007) conducted an interpretive phenomenological study of patients receiving local anesthesia and remaining awake during surgery. They used Benner's approach to extract the experience of what it means to be in local anesthesia and surgery. A paradigm case was used to illustrate the results that showed that the well-being of patients may be compromised by challenges such as severe pain and long waits.

Grounded Theory Analysis

The grounded theory method emerged in the 1960s in connection with research that focused on dying in hospitals by two sociologists, Glaser and Strauss (1967). The two co-originators eventually split and developed divergent schools of thought, which have been called the "Glaserian" and "Straussian" versions of grounded theory.

Glaser and Strauss' Grounded Theory Method
Grounded theory in both analytic systems uses **constant comparison,** a method that involves comparing elements present in one data source (e.g., in one interview) with those in another. The process is continued until the content of each source has been compared with the content in all sources. In this fashion, commonalities are identified.

The concept of fit is an important element in Glaserian grounded theory analysis. **Fit** has to do with how closely emerging concepts fit with the incidents they are representing, which in turn is related to how thoroughly the constant comparison of incidents to concepts was done. *Fit* is also an important issue when a grounded theory is applied in new contexts: The theory must closely "fit" the substantive area where it will be used.

Coding in the Glaserian grounded theory approach is used to conceptualize data into patterns. Coding helps the researcher to discover the *basic social psychological problem* with which study participants must contend. The substance of the topic under study is conceptualized through **substantive codes**, whereas **theoretical codes** provide insights into how substantive codes relate to each other. There are two types of substantive codes: open and selective. **Open coding**, used in the first stage of the constant comparative analysis, captures what is going on in the data.

TABLE 17.2 · COLLAPSING LEVEL I CODES INTO THE LEVEL II CODE OF *"REAPING THE BLESSINGS"* (BECK, 2002)

EXCERPT	LEVEL I CODE
I enjoy just watching the twins interact so much. Especially now that they are mobile. They are not walking yet but they are crawling. I will tell you they are already playing. Like one will go around the corner and kind of peek around and they play hide and seek. They crawl after each other.	Enjoying Twins
With twins it's amazing. She was sick and she had a fever. He was the one acting sick. She didn't seem like she was sick at all. He was. We watched him for like 6–8 hours. We gave her the medicine and he started calming down. Like WOW! That is so weird. 'Cause you read about it but it's like, Oh come on! It's really neat to see.	Amazing
These days it's really neat 'cause you go to the store or you go out and people are like, "Oh, they are twins, how nice." And I say, "Yeah they are. Look, look at my kids."	Getting Attention
I just feel blessed to have two. I just feel like I am twice as lucky as a mom who has one baby. I mean that's the best part. It's just that instead of having one baby to watch grow and change and develop and become a toddler and school age child you have two.	Feeling Blessed
It's very exciting. It's interesting and it's fun to see them and how the twin bond really is. There really is a twin bond. You read about it and you hear about it but until you experience it, you just don't understand. One time they were both crying and they were fed. They were changed and burped. There was nothing wrong. I couldn't figure out what was wrong. So I said to myself, "I am just going to put them together and close the door." I put them in my bed together and they patty caked their hands and put their noses together and just looked at each other and went right to sleep.	Twin Bonding

Open codes may be the actual words used by the participants. Through open coding, data are broken down into incidents and their similarities and differences are examined.

There are three different levels of open coding that vary in degree of abstraction. **Level I codes** (or *in vivo codes*) are derived directly from the language of the substantive area. They have vivid imagery and "grab." Table 17.2 presents five level I codes from interviews in Beck's (2002) grounded theory study on mothering twins, and excerpts associated with those codes.

As researchers constantly compare new level I codes with previously identified ones, they condense them into broader **level II codes**. For example, in Table 17.2, Beck's five level I codes were collapsed into the level II code, "Reaping the Blessings." **Level III codes** (or theoretical constructs) are the most abstract. Collapsing level II codes aids in identifying constructs.

Example of open coding in Glaserian grounded theory analysis:
Knobf (2002) studied responses to chemotherapy-induced premature menopause in women with early stage breast cancer. Her report included an excellent figure that showed how 20 level I codes were collapsed into three level II codes (Relying on Self, Structured Silence, and Being Prepared). These, in turn, were integrated in the theoretical construct (level III code), Facing Uncertainty. Because this figure is highly illuminating, we have included it in the Toolkit on the accompanying CD-ROM. ✖

Open coding ends when the core category is discovered, and then selective coding begins. The **core category** is a pattern of behavior that is relevant, problematic, or both for study participants. In **selective coding** (which can also have three levels of abstraction), researchers code only those data that are related to the core category. One kind of core category is a **basic social process (BSP)** that evolves over time in two or more phases. All BSPs are core variables, but not all core variables have to be BSPs.

Glaser (1978) provided nine criteria to help researchers decide on a core category:

1. It must be central, meaning that it is related to many categories.
2. It must reoccur frequently in the data.
3. It takes more time to saturate than other categories.
4. It relates meaningfully and easily to other categories.
5. It has clear and grabbing implications for formal theory.
6. It has considerable carry-through.
7. It is completely variable.
8. It is a dimension of the problem.
9. It can be any kind of theoretical code.

Theoretical codes help grounded theorists to weave the broken pieces of data back together again. Glaser (1978) proposed 18 families of theoretical codes that researchers can use to conceptualize how substantive codes relate to each other (although he subsequently expanded possibilities in 2005). Four examples of his families of theoretical codes include the following:

➤ Process: stages, phases, passages, transitions
➤ Strategy: tactics, techniques, maneuverings
➤ Cutting point: boundaries, critical junctures, turning points
➤ The six C's: causes, contexts, contingencies, consequences, covariances, and conditions

Throughout coding and analysis, grounded theory analysts document their ideas about the data, themes, and emerging conceptual scheme in **memos**. Memos preserve ideas that may initially not seem productive but may later prove valuable once further developed. Memos also encourage researchers to reflect on (and describe) patterns in the data, relationships between categories, and emergent conceptualizations.

Glaser's grounded theory method is concerned with the *generation* of categories and hypotheses rather than testing them. The product of the typical grounded theory analysis is a theoretical model that endeavors to explain a pattern of behavior that is both relevant and problematic for study participants. Once the basic problem emerges, the grounded theorist goes on to discover the process these participants experience in coping with or resolving this problem.

Example of Glaser and Strauss grounded theory analysis:
Figure 17.2 presents Beck's (2002) model from a grounded theory study that conceptualized "Releasing the Pause Button" as the core category and process through which mothers of twins progressed as they attempted to resume their lives after giving birth. In this model, the process involves four phases: Draining Power, Pausing Own Life, Striving to Reset, and Resuming Own Life. Beck used 10 coding families in her theoretical coding for the Releasing the Pause Button process. The family *cutting point* provides an illustration. Three months seemed to be the turning point for mothers, when life started to become more manageable. Here is an excerpt from an interview that Beck coded as a cutting point: "Three months came around and the twins sort of slept through the night and it made a huge, huge difference."

Although Glaser and Straus cautioned against consulting the literature before a basic theoretical framework is stabilized, they also viewed grounded theory as a process that could benefit from scrutiny of other work. Glaser discussed the evolution of grounded theories through the process of **emergent fit**, to prevent individual substantive theories from being "respected little islands of knowledge" (1978, p. 148). As he noted, generating grounded theory does not necessarily require discovering all new categories or ignoring ones previously identified in the literature. Through constant comparison, researchers can compare concepts emerging from

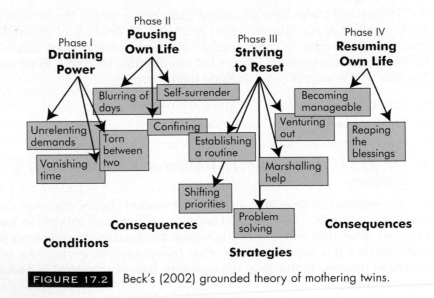

FIGURE 17.2 Beck's (2002) grounded theory of mothering twins.

TABLE 17.3	COMPARISON OF GLASER'S AND STRAUSS/CORBIN'S METHODS	
	GLASER	STRAUSS & CORBIN
Initial data analysis	Breaking down and conceptualizing data involves comparison of incident to incident so patterns emerge	Breaking down and conceptualizing data includes taking apart a single sentence, observation, and incident
Types of coding	Open, selective, theoretical	Open, axial, selective
Connections between categories	18 coding families (plus others added subsequently)	Paradigm model (conditions, contexts, action/interactional strategies, and consequences)
Outcome	Emergent theory (discovery)	Conceptual description (verification)

the data with similar concepts from existing theory or research to determine which parts have emergent fit with the theory being generated.

Strauss and Corbin's Approach

The Strauss and Corbin (1998) approach to grounded theory analysis differs from the original Glaser and Strauss method with regard to method, processes, and outcomes. Table 17.3 summarizes major analytic differences between these two grounded theory analysis methods.

Glaser (1978) stressed that to generate a grounded theory, the basic problem must emerge from the data—it must be discovered. The theory is, from the very start, grounded in the data, rather than starting with a preconceived problem. Strauss and Corbin, however, stated that the research itself is only one of four possible sources of a research problem. Research problems can, for example, come from the literature or a researcher's personal and professional experience.

The Strauss and Corbin method involves three types of coding: open, axial, and selective coding. In open coding, data are broken down into parts and compared for similarities and differences. Similar actions, events, and objects are grouped together as more abstract concepts, which are called categories. In open coding, the researcher focuses on generating categories and their properties and dimensions. In **axial coding**, the analyst systematically develops categories and links them with subcategories. Strauss and Corbin (1998) term this process of relating categories and their subcategories as "axial because coding occurs around the axis of a category, linking categories at the level of properties and dimensions" (p. 123). What is called the *paradigm* is used to help identify linkages among categories. The basic components of the paradigm include conditions, actions or interactions, and consequences. Selective coding is the process in which the findings are integrated and refined. The first step in integrating the findings is to decide on the **central category** (sometimes called the *core category*), which is the main category of the research. Recommended techniques to facilitate identifying the central category are writing the storyline, using diagrams, and reviewing and organizing memos.

The outcome of the Strauss and Corbin approach is a full conceptual description. The original grounded theory method, by contrast, generates a theory that explains how a basic social problem that emerged from the data is processed in a social setting.

Example of Strauss and Corbin grounded theory analysis:

Meadus (2007) used Strauss and Corbin's methods in a grounded theory study of coping among adolescents with a mood disorder. Data from interviews with nine adolescents were coded and analyzed. Open coding involved looking for similarities and differences. Then, axial coding "was used to put the data back together by identifying connections between the categories and subcategories. The last phase of the analysis involved . . . selective coding, leading to a descriptive narrative about the central phenomenon. This process served to identify the core category" (p. 212).

CRITIQUING QUALITATIVE ANALYSIS

Evaluating a qualitative analysis is not easy, even for experienced researchers. The main problem is that readers do not have access to the information they would need to determine whether researchers exercised good judgment and critical insight in coding the narrative materials, developing a thematic analysis, and integrating materials into a meaningful whole. Researchers are seldom able to include more than a handful of examples of actual data in a journal article. Moreover, the process they used to inductively abstract meaning from the data is difficult to describe and illustrate.

In a critique of qualitative analysis, a primary task usually is determining whether researchers took sufficient steps to validate inferences and conclusions. A major focus of a critique of qualitative analyses, then, is whether the researchers have adequately documented the analytic process. The report should provide information about the approach used to analyze the data. For example, a report for a grounded theory study should indicate whether the researchers used the Glaser and Strauss or the Strauss and Corbin method.

Critiquing analytic decisions is substantially less clear-cut in a qualitative than in a quantitative study. For example, it would be inappropriate to critique a phenomenological analysis that followed Giorgi's approach rather than Colaizzi's approach. Both are respected methods of conducting a phenomenological study— although phenomenologists themselves may have cogent reasons for preferring one approach over the other.

One aspect of a qualitative analysis that *can* be critiqued, however, is whether the researchers have documented that they have used one approach consistently and have been faithful to the integrity of its procedures. Thus, for example, if researchers say they are using the Glaser and Strauss approach to grounded theory analysis, they should not also include elements from the Strauss and Corbin method. An even more serious problem occurs when, as sometimes happens, the researchers "muddle" traditions. For example, researchers who describe their study as a grounded theory study should not present *themes*, because grounded theory analysis does not yield themes. Furthermore, researchers who attempt to blend elements from two traditions may not have a clear grasp of the analytic precepts of

---

BOX 17.2 GUIDELINES FOR CRITIQUING QUALITATIVE DESIGNS

1. Given the nature of the data, was the data analysis approach appropriate for the research design?

2. Is the category scheme described? If so, does the scheme appear logical and complete? Does there seem to be unnecessary overlap or redundancy in the categories?

3. Were manual methods used to index and organize the data, or was a computer program used?

4. Does the report adequately describe the process by which the actual analysis was performed? Does the report indicate whose approach to data analysis was used (e.g., Glaserian or Straussian, in grounded theory studies)? Was this method consistently and appropriately applied?

5. What major themes or processes emerged? If excerpts from the data are provided, do the themes appear to capture the meaning of the narratives—that is, does it appear that the researcher adequately interpreted the data and conceptualized the themes? Is the analysis parsimonious—could two or more themes be collapsed into a broader and perhaps more useful conceptualization?

6. What evidence does the report provide that the analysis is accurate and replicable? Were data displayed in a manner that allows you to verify the researcher's conclusions?

7. Was a conceptual map, model, or diagram effectively displayed to communicate important processes?

8. Was the context of the phenomenon adequately described? Does the report give you a clear picture of the social or emotional world of study participants?

9. Did the analysis yield a meaningful and insightful picture of the phenomenon under study? Is the resulting theory or description trivial or obvious?

---

either one. For example, a researcher who claims to have undertaken an ethnography using a grounded theory approach to analysis may not be well-informed about the underlying goals and philosophies of these two traditions.

Some further guidelines that may be helpful in evaluating qualitative analyses are presented in Box 17.2. ⊗

RESEARCH EXAMPLES AND CRITICAL THINKING ACTIVITIES

EXAMPLE 1 ■ A Grounded Theory Analysis

Study

Moral reckoning in nursing (Nathaniel, 2006).

Statement of Purpose

The purpose of this study was to elucidate the experiences and consequences of professional nurses' moral distress, and to formulate an explanatory theory of moral distress and its consequences.

Method

This grounded theory study involved in-depth interviews with 21 registered nurses. Informants were highly educated (most had graduate degrees) and experienced (80% had over 10 years of experience). All participants had been involved in a troubling patient care situation that caused distress. The study began with a broad research question: What transpires in morally laden situations in which nurses experience distress? The initial question was narrowed and redirected as the research progressed. Because the nature of the information was considered sensitive, Nathaniel did not tape record the interviews. She made brief, contemporaneous notes, and then wrote detailed field notes immediately following the interviews.

Analysis

Interview data were analyzed using the classic Glaserian method. Analysis began with the first episode of data gathering. Using constant comparison, data were analyzed sentence by sentence as they were coded. Nathaniel began with open coding, which led to theoretical sampling and the generation of memos. As analysis proceeded, core social psychological processes began to emerge which, in turn, furnished the foundation for subsequent theoretical sampling, coding, and memoing around the core category of *moral reckoning in nursing*. As the interviews were coded and compared, moral distress—which was the original focus of the study—failed to emerge as a major category. "The core variable, moral reckoning, was identified when it emerged as the one to which all others were related . . . As categories became saturated and the relationships among them became clear, the substantive grounded theory of moral reckoning in nursing emerged" (p. 423).

Key Findings

- Moral distress occurred in nurses who were in the midst of the moral reckoning process; moral reckoning is broader, both temporally and psychosocially, than moral distress.
- Moral reckoning was conceptualized as a three-stage process that begins with a stage of ease, which is then interrupted by a situational bind that challenges the nurse's core beliefs. This compels the nurses into the stage of resolution, in which he or she either gives up or makes a stand. The final stage is the stage of reflection. Nathaniel's paper includes a good figure (Figure 2) that graphically portrays the grounded theory of moral reckoning in nursing (p. 426).

CRITICAL THINKING SUGGESTIONS*:

*See the Student Resource CD-ROM for a discussion of these questions. 💿

1. Answer the relevant questions from Box 17.2 regarding this study.
2. Also, consider the following targeted questions, which may further sharpen your critical thinking skills and assist you in understanding this study:
   a. Which families of theoretical codes might have been relevant in this study?
   b. Nathaniel wrote that ". . . the theory itself emerged from the interviews and also other forms of data, including the extant literature on moral distress" (p. 424). Comment on this statement.
3. What might be some of the uses to which the findings could be put in clinical practice?

EXAMPLE 2 ■ A Phenomenological Analysis in Appendix B

1. Read the method and results sections from Beck's phenomenological study ("Anniversary of birth trauma") in Appendix B of this book, and then answer the relevant questions from Box 17.2 regarding this study.

2. Also, consider the following targeted questions, which may further sharpen your critical thinking skills and assist you in understanding this study:
   a. Comment of the amount of data that had to be analyzed in this study.
   b. Refer to Table 2 in the article, which presents a list of 10 significant statements made by study participants. Cover up the right panel of this table, which shows Beck's *formulated meanings* for each statement. Try to develop your own *formulated meanings*, and then compare your answers to those of Beck.

CHAPTER REVIEW

Key new terms introduced in the chapter, together with a summary of major points, are presented in this section. In addition, Chapter 17 of the *Study Guide for Essentials of Nursing Research*, 7th edition offers various exercises and study suggestions for reinforcing concepts presented in this chapter. For additional review, see the Student Self-Study Review Questions section of the Student Resource CD-ROM provided with this book. 💿

Key New Terms

Axial coding	Content analysis	Paradigm case
Basic social process (BSP)	Core category	Quasi-statistics
Category scheme	Domain	Selective coding
Central category	Emergent fit	Substantive coding
Conceptual file	Hermeneutic circle	Taxonomy
Constant comparison	Level I, II, and III codes	Theme
Constitutive pattern	Open coding	Theoretical coding

Summary Points

➤ Qualitative analysis is a challenging, labor-intensive activity, guided by few standardized rules.

➤ Although there are no universal strategies, three prototypical analytic styles are as follows: (1) a *template analysis style* that involves the development of an analysis guide (**template**) to sort the data; (2) an *editing analysis style* that involves an interpretation of the data on which a **category scheme** is based; and (3) an *immersion/crystallization style* that is characterized by the analyst's total immersion in and reflection of text materials.

➤ The first major step in analyzing qualitative data is to organize and index the materials for easy retrieval, typically by coding the content of the data according to a category scheme.

➤ Traditionally, researchers have organized their data by developing **conceptual files**, which are physical files in which coded excerpts of data relevant to specific categories are placed. Now, however, computer programs (CAQDAS) are widely used to perform basic indexing functions, and to facilitate data analysis.

➤ The actual analysis of data begins with a search for patterns and **themes**, which involves the discovery not only of commonalities across subjects, but also of natural variation in the data. Some qualitative analysts use **metaphors** or figurative comparisons to evoke a visual and symbolic analogy.

➤ The next analytic step usually involves a validation of the thematic analysis. Some researchers use **quasi-statistics**, a tabulation of the frequency with which certain themes or relations are supported by the data.

➤ In a final analytic step, the analyst tries to weave the thematic strands together into an integrated picture of the phenomenon under investigation.

➤ Some researchers identify neither a specific approach nor a specific research tradition; those whose goal is qualitative description often say they used **qualitative content analysis** as their analytic method.

➤ In ethnographies, analysis begins as the researcher enters the field. Ethnographers continually search for *patterns* in the behavior and expressions of study participants.

➤ One approach to analyzing ethnographic data is Spradley's method, which involves four levels of data analysis: *domain analysis* (identifying **domains**, or units of cultural knowledge); *taxonomic analysis* (selecting key domains and constructing **taxonomies** or systems of classification); *componential analysis* (comparing and contrasting terms in a domain); and a *theme analysis* (to uncover cultural themes).

➤ Leininger's method to ethnonursing research involves four phases: collecting and recording data; categorizing descriptors; searching for repetitive patterns; and abstracting major themes.

➤ There are numerous approaches to phenomenological analysis, including the descriptive methods of Colaizzi, Giorgi, and Van Kaam, in which the goal is to find common patterns of experiences shared by particular instances.

➤ In Van Manen's approach, which involves efforts to grasp the essential meaning of the experience being studied, researchers search for themes, using either a **holistic approach** (viewing text as a whole); a **selective approach** (pulling out key statements and phrases); or a **detailed approach** (analyzing every sentence).

➤ Central to analyzing data in a hermeneutic study is the notion of the **hermeneutic circle**, which signifies a methodologic process in which there is continual movement between the parts and the whole of the text under analysis.

➤ In hermeneutics there are several choices for data analysis. Diekelmann's method calls for the discovery of a **constitutive pattern** that expresses the relationships among themes. Benner's approach consists of three processes: searching for **paradigm cases**, thematic analysis, and analysis of *exemplars*.

➤ Grounded theory uses the **constant comparative** method of data analysis, a method that involves comparing elements present in one data source (e.g., in one interview) with those in another. **Fit** has to do with how closely concepts fit with incidents they represent, which is related to how thoroughly constant comparison was done.

➤ One approach to grounded theory is the Glaser and Strauss (Glaserian) method, in which there are two broad types of codes: **substantive codes** (in which the empirical substance of the topic is conceptualized) and **theoretical codes** (in which the relationships among the substantive codes are conceptualized).

➤ Substantive coding involves **open coding** to capture what is going on in the data, and then **selective coding**, in which only variables relating to a core category are coded. The **core category**, a behavior pattern that has relevance for participants, is sometimes a **basic social process (BSP)** that involves an evolutionary process of coping or adaptation.

➤ In the Glaser and Strauss method, open codes begin with **level I (in vivo) codes**, which are collapsed into a higher level of abstraction in **level II codes.** Level II codes are then used to formulate **level III codes**, which are theoretical constructs.

➤ Through constant comparison, the researcher compares concepts emerging from the data with similar concepts from existing theory or research to determine which parts have **emergent fit** with the theory being generated.

➤ The Strauss and Corbin (Straussian) method is an alternative grounded theory method whose outcome is a full conceptual description. This approach to grounded theory analysis involves three types of coding: open (in which categories are generated), **axial coding** (where categories are linked with subcategories), and selective (in which the findings are integrated and refined).

STUDIES CITED IN CHAPTER 17

Annells, M. (2006). The experience of flatus incontinence from a bowel ostomy: A hermeneutic phenomenology. *Journal of Wound, Ostomy, & Continence Nursing, 33,* 518–524.

Bakitas, M. (2007). Background noise: The experience of chemotherapy-induced peripheral neuropathy. *Nursing Research, 56,* 323–331.

Barnes, D., & Aguilar, R. (2007), Community social support for Cuban refugees in Texas. *Qualitative Health Research,17,* 225–237.

Beck, C. T. (2002). Releasing the pause button: Mothering twins during the first year of life. *Qualitative Health Research, 12,* 593–608.

Beck, C.T. (2006). Anniversary of birth trauma: Failure to rescue. *Nursing Research, 55,* 381–390.

DeOliveira, E. A., & Hoga, L. A. (2005). The process of seeking and undergoing surgical contraception: An ethnographic study in a Brazilian community. *Journal of Transcultural Nursing, 16,* 5–14.

Enns, C., & Gregory, D. (2007). Lamentation and loss: Expressions of caring by contemporary surgical nurses. *Journal of Advanced Nursing, 58,* 339–347.

Feely, M., Sines, D., & Long, A. (2007). Early life experiences and their impact on our understanding of depression. *Journal of Psychiatric & Mental Health Nursing, 14,* 393–402.

Knobf, M. T. (2002). Carrying on: The experience of premature menopause in women with early stage breast cancer. *Nursing Research, 51,* 9–17.

Lauterbach, S. (2007). Meanings in mothers' experience with infant death (pp. 211–238). In P.L. Munhall (Ed.), *Nursing research: A qualitative perspective,* 2nd ed. Sudbury, MA: Jones & Bartlett Publishers.

Mauleon, A., Palo-Bengtsson, L., & Ekman, S. (2007). Patients experiencing local anesthesia and hip surgery. *Journal of Clinical Nursing, 16,* 892–899.

Meadus, R. (2007). Adolescents coping with mood disorder: A grounded theory study. *Journal of Psychiatric and Mental Health Nursing, 14,* 209–217.

Nathaniel, A. K. (2006). Moral reckoning in nursing. *Western Journal of Nursing Research, 28,* 419–438.

Parsons-Suhl, K., Johnson, M. E., McCann, J., & Solberg, S. (2008). Losing one's memory in early Alzheimer's disease. *Qualitative Health Research, 18,* 31–42.

Perry, C., Rosenfeld, A., & Kendall, J. (2008). Rural women walking for health. *Western Journal of Nursing Research, 30,* 295–316.

Polit, D. F., London, A., & Martinez, J. M. (2000). Food security and hunger in poor, mother-headed families in four U.S. cities. New York: MDRC.

Roulin, M. J., Hurst, S., & Spirig, R. (2007). Diaries written for ICU patients. *Qualitative Health Research, 17,* 893–901.

Strang, V., Koop, P., Dupuis-Blanchard, S., Nordstrom, M., & Thompson, B. (2006). Family caregivers and transition to long-term care. *Clinical Nursing Research, 15,* 27–45.

Tanyi, R., & Werner, J. S. (2008). Women's experience of spirituality within end-stage renal disease and hemodialyis. *Clinical Nursing Research, 17,* 32–49.

Tzeng, W., & Lipson, J. G. (2004). The cultural context of suicide stigma in Taiwan. *Qualitative Health Research, 14,* 345–358.

Zanchetta, M., Perreault, M., Kaszap, M., & Viens, C. (2007). Patterns in information strategies used by older men to understand and deal with prostate cancer. *International Journal of Nursing Studies, 44,* 961–972.

18 Trustworthiness and Integrity in Qualitative Research

STUDENT OBJECTIVES

On completing this chapter, you will be able to:

➤ Discuss some controversies relating to the issue of quality in qualitative research

➤ Identify the quality criteria proposed in two frameworks for evaluating quality and integrity in qualitative research

➤ Discuss strategies for enhancing quality in qualitative research

➤ Describe different dimensions relating to the interpretation of qualitative results

➤ Define new terms in the chapter

Integrity in qualitative research is an issue of concern throughout the course of a study. For those learning to critique qualitative research, we consider this a particularly important chapter.

PERSPECTIVES ON QUALITY IN QUALITATIVE RESEARCH

Qualitative researchers agree on the importance of doing high-quality research, yet few issues in qualitative inquiry have been more controversial than efforts to define what is meant by "high-quality." Although it is beyond the scope of this book to explain arguments of the debate in detail, we provide a brief overview.

Debates About Rigor and Validity

One of the most contentious issues in debates about quality concerns the use of the terms *rigor* and *validity*—terms some people shun because they are associated with the positivist paradigm and viewed as inappropriate goals for research within the naturalistic or critical paradigms. Those who advocate different criteria and terms for evaluating quality in qualitative research argue that the issues at stake in alternative paradigms are fundamentally divergent and require altogether different terminology. For these critics, the concept of rigor is by its nature an empirical analytic term that does not fit into an interpretive approach that values insight and creativity.

Others disagree with those opposing the term *validity*. Whittemore and colleagues (2001), for example, argued that validity is an appropriate term in all paradigms, noting that the dictionary definition of validity (the state or quality of being sound, just, and well-founded) lends itself equally to qualitative and quantitative research. Similarly, Morse and colleagues (2002) posited that "the broad and abstract concepts of reliability and validity can be applied to all research because the goal of finding plausible and credible outcome explanations is central to all research" (p. 3). Another, more pragmatic, argument favoring the use of "mainstream" terms such as validity and rigor is precisely that they *are* mainstream. In a world dominated by quantitative researchers whose evidence hierarchies place qualitative studies on a low rung, and whose quality criteria are used to make decisions about research funding, some people believe that it is useful to use terms and criteria that are recognizable and widely accepted.

The debate is complex and has given rise to a variety of positions. At one extreme are those who think that validity is an appropriate criterion for assessing quality in both qualitative and quantitative studies, although qualitative researchers must use different procedures to achieve it. At the opposite extreme are those who have berated the "absurdity" of validity. Perhaps the most widely adopted stance is what has been called a *parallel perspective*. This position was adopted by Lincoln and Guba (1985), who promulgated standards for the **trustworthiness** of qualitative research that parallel the standards of reliability and validity in quantitative research.

Generic Versus Specific Standards

Another issue in the controversy about quality criteria for qualitative inquiry concerns whether there should be a generic set of standards, or whether specific standards are needed for different types of inquiry—for example, for ethnographers and grounded theory researchers. Many writers subscribe to the idea that research conducted within different qualitative traditions must attend to different concerns, and that techniques for enhancing and demonstrating research integrity vary. Watson and Girard (2004), for example, proposed that quality standards should be reflective of the research method used, and that they must be "congruent with the philosophical underpinnings supporting the research tradition endorsed" (p. 875). Reflecting this viewpoint of having criteria aligned with tradition, many writers have offered standards for specific forms of qualitative inquiry, such as grounded theory, phenomenology and hermeneutics, ethnography, and critical research.

Other writers believe, however, that some quality criteria are fairly universal within the naturalistic paradigm. In their synthesis of criteria for developing evidence of validity in qualitative studies, Whittemore and associates (2001) proposed four primary criteria that they viewed as essential to all qualitative inquiry.

Terminology Proliferation and Confusion

The result of these controversies is that no common vocabulary exists for quality criteria in qualitative research—nor, for that matter, for quality goals. Terms such as *goodness, integrity, truth value, rigor, trustworthiness*, and so on abound and, for each proposed term, several writers have published papers refuting it as appropriate.

With regard to actual *criteria* for evaluating quality in qualitative research, dozens (if not hundreds) of terms have been suggested. Establishing a consensus on what the quality criteria for qualitative inquiry should be, and what they should be named, remains elusive, and it is unlikely that a consensus will be achieved in the near future, if ever. Some feel that the ongoing debate is productive, whereas others feel that "the situation is confusing and has resulted in a deteriorating ability to actually discern rigor" (Morse et al., 2002, p. 5).

Given the lack of consensus, and the heated arguments supporting and contesting various frameworks, it is difficult to provide guidance about quality standards. We present information about *criteria* from two frameworks in the section that follows, and then describe *strategies* that researchers use to diminish threats to integrity in qualitative research. These frameworks and strategies should be viewed as points of departure for considering whether a qualitative study is sufficiently rigorous, trustworthy, insightful, or valid.

FRAMEWORKS OF QUALITY CRITERIA

Although not without critics, the criteria often thought of as the "gold standard" for qualitative research are those outlined by Lincoln and Guba (1985), and later augmented by Guba and Lincoln (1994). The second framework described here is the synthesis proposed by Whittemore and colleagues (2001).

An important point in thinking about criteria for qualitative inquiry is that attention needs to be paid to both "art" and "science," and to interpretation and description. Creativity and insightfulness need to be attained, but not at the expense of scientific excellence. And the quest for rigor cannot sacrifice inspiration and elegant abstractions, or else the results are likely to be "perfectly healthy but dead" (Morse, 2006, p. 6). Good qualitative work is both descriptively accurate and explicit, and interpretively rich and innovative.

Lincoln and Guba's Framework

Lincoln and Guba (1985) suggested four criteria for developing the *trustworthiness* of a qualitative inquiry: credibility, dependability, confirmability, and transferability. These four criteria for trustworthiness represent parallels to the positivists' criteria of internal validity, reliability, objectivity, and external validity, respectively. The Lincoln-Guba framework provided the initial platform upon which much of the current controversy on rigor emerged. In their later writings, responding to numerous criticisms and to their own evolving conceptualizations, a fifth criterion that is more distinctively within the naturalistic paradigm was added: authenticity (Guba & Lincoln, 1994).

Credibility

Credibility is viewed by Lincoln and Guba as an overriding goal of qualitative research. **Credibility** refers to confidence in the truth of the data and interpretations of them. Qualitative researchers must strive to establish confidence in the truth of the findings for the particular participants and contexts in the research. Lincoln and Guba pointed out that credibility involves two aspects: first, carrying out the study in a way that enhances the believability of the findings, and second, taking steps to *demonstrate* credibility to external readers.

Dependability

The second criterion in the Lincoln and Guba framework is **dependability**, which refers to the stability (reliability) of data over time and over conditions. The dependability question is: "Would the study findings be repeated if the inquiry were replicated with the same (or similar) participants in the same (or similar) context?" Credibility cannot be attained in the absence of dependability, just as validity in quantitative research cannot be achieved in the absence of reliability.

Confirmability

Confirmability refers to objectivity, that is, the potential for congruence between two or more independent people about the data's accuracy, relevance, or meaning. This criterion is concerned with establishing that the data represent the information participants provided, and that the interpretations of those data are not figments of the inquirer's imagination. For this criterion to be achieved, the findings must reflect the participants' voice and the conditions of the inquiry, and not the biases, motivations, or perspectives of the researcher.

Transferability

Transferability, analogous to generalizability, refers to the extent to which qualitative findings can be transferred to (or have applicability in) other settings or groups.

As Lincoln and Guba noted, the responsibility of the investigator is to provide sufficient descriptive data in the research report so that consumers can evaluate the applicability of the data to other contexts: "Thus the naturalist cannot specify the external validity of an inquiry; he or she can provide only the thick description necessary to enable someone interested in making a transfer to reach a conclusion about whether transfer can be contemplated as a possibility" (p. 316).

> **TIP**
>
> You may run across the term *fittingness,* a term used in earlier writings of Guba and Lincoln to refer to the degree to which research findings have meaning to others in similar situations. In later work, however, they used the term *transferability.* Similarly, in their early discussions of quality criteria, they used the term *auditability,* which was later refined and called *dependability.*

Authenticity

Authenticity refers to the extent to which researchers fairly and faithfully show a range of different realities. Authenticity emerges in a report when it conveys the feeling tone of participants' lives as they are lived. A text has authenticity if it invites readers into a vicarious experience of the lives being described, and enables readers to develop a heightened sensitivity to the issues being depicted. When a text achieves authenticity, readers are better able to understand the lives being portrayed "in the round," with some sense of the mood, feeling, experience, language, and context of those lives.

Whittemore and Colleagues' Framework

Whittemore and colleagues (2001), in their synthesis of qualitative criteria from 10 prominent systems (including that of Lincoln and Guba), used the term *validity* as the overarching goal. In their view, four primary criteria are essential to all qualitative inquiry, whereas six secondary criteria provide supplementary benchmarks and are not relevant to every study.

The primary criteria are credibility, authenticity, criticality, and integrity. The six secondary criteria include explicitness, vividness, creativity, thoroughness, congruence, and sensitivity. Thus, the terminology overlaps with that of Lincoln and Guba's framework with regard to two criteria (credibility and authenticity), whereas the other eight represent concepts either not captured in the Lincoln and Guba framework or are nuanced variations. We briefly define each of these eight terms, and then offer questions relating to the attainment of these criteria.

Criticality refers to the researcher's critical appraisal of every decision made throughout the research process. **Integrity** is demonstrated by on-going self-reflection and self-scrutiny to ensure that interpretations are valid and grounded in the data. Criticality and integrity are strongly interrelated and are sometimes considered jointly.

In terms of secondary criteria, **explicitness** (similar to auditability) is the ability to follow the researcher's decisions and interpretive efforts by means of carefully maintained records and explicitly presented results. **Vividness** involves the presentation of rich, vivid, faithful, and artful descriptions that highlight salient themes in the data. **Creativity** reflects challenges to traditional ways of thinking and is demonstrated through innovative approaches to collecting, analyzing, and interpreting data. **Thoroughness** refers to adequacy of the data as a result of sound sampling and data collection decisions (saturation), as well as to the full development of ideas. **Congruence** refers to interconnectedness between (1) methods and question, (2) the current study and earlier ones, and (3) theory and approach; it also refers to connections between study findings and contexts outside the study situation. Finally, **sensitivity** refers to the degree to which the research was implemented in a manner that reflects respectful sensitivity to (and concern for) the people, groups, and communities being studied.

Table 18.1 presents these 10 criteria, together with a set of relevant questions. Consumers of a qualitative report can apply these questions in evaluating both the process and the product of qualitative inquiry. ✖

STRATEGIES TO ENHANCE QUALITY IN QUALITATIVE INQUIRY

The criteria for establishing integrity in a qualitative study are complex and challenging—regardless of the names people attach to them. A variety of strategies have been proposed to address these challenges. This section describes some of them in the hope that they will prompt a more careful and critical assessment of steps researchers take or do not take to enhance integrity.

Some quality-enhancement strategies are linked to a specific criterion—for example, maintaining records to document methodologic decisions is a strategy that addresses the *explicitness* criterion in the Whittemore framework. Many strategies, however, simultaneously address multiple criteria. For this reason, we have not organized strategies according to quality criteria—for example, strategies researchers can use to enhance *credibility*. Instead, we have organized strategies according to different phases of a study, namely data generation, coding and analysis, and report preparation. This organization is imperfect, because of the nonlinear nature of research activities in qualitative studies, and so we acknowledge upfront that some activities described for one aspect of a study are likely to have relevance for another.

Table 18.2 offers some guidance about how various quality-enhancement strategies map onto the criteria in the Lincoln and Guba and the Whittemore frameworks.

Quality-Enhancement Strategies During Data Collection

Qualitative researchers use many strategies to enrich and strengthen their studies, some of which are difficult to discern in a report. For example, intensive listening during an interview, careful probing to obtain rich and comprehensive data, and taking pains to gain people's trust during data collection are all strategies to

TABLE 18.1 ▶	PRIMARY AND SECONDARY QUALITATIVE VALIDITY CRITERIA: WHITTEMORE ET AL. FRAMEWORK*
CRITERIA	RELEVANT QUESTIONS FOR ASSESSING THE STUDY
Primary Criteria	
Credibility	Do the research results reflect participants' experiences and context in a believable way? Were adequate verification procedures used?
Authenticity	Has the researcher adequately represented the multiple realities of those being studied? Has an emic perspective been portrayed?
Criticality	Is there evidence that the inquiry involved critical appraisal of key decisions and critical self-reflection? Does the report demonstrate the researcher's responsiveness to the data?
Integrity	Does the research reflect ongoing, repetitive checks on the many aspects of validity? Are the findings humbly presented?
Secondary Criteria	
Explicitness	Have methodologic decisions been explained and justified? Have biases been identified? Is evidence presented in support of conclusions and interpretations?
Vividness	Have rich, evocative, and compelling descriptions been presented?
Creativity	Do the findings illuminate the phenomenon in an insightful and original way? Are new perspectives and rich imagination brought to bear on the inquiry?
Thoroughness	Has sufficient attention been paid to sampling adequacy, information richness, data saturation, and contextual completeness?
Congruence	Is there congruity between the questions and methods, the methods and participants, the data and categories? Do themes fit together coherently? Is there adequate information for determining the fit with other contexts?
Sensitivity	Has the research been undertaken in a way that is sensitive to the cultural, social, and political contexts of those being studied?

*Criteria are from Whittemore and colleagues' (2001) synthesis of qualitative validity criteria. Questions reflect the thinking of Whittemore et al., and other sources.

enhance data quality that cannot easily be communicated in a report. In this section, we focus on some strategies that can be described to readers to increase their confidence in the integrity of the study results.

Prolonged Engagement and Persistent Observation

An important step in establishing rigor and integrity in qualitative studies is **prolonged engagement** (Lincoln & Guba, 1985)—the investment of sufficient time collecting data to have an in-depth understanding of the culture, language, or views of the people or group under study, to test for misinformation and distortions, and

TABLE 18.2 — QUALITY ENHANCEMENT STRATEGIES IN RELATION TO QUALITY CRITERIA FOR QUALITATIVE INQUIRY

STRATEGY	CRITERIA: GUBA & LINCOLN[a]					CRITERIA: WHITTEMORE et al.[b]							
	Dep.	Conf.	Trans.	Cred.	Auth.	Crit.	Integ.	Explic.	Viv.	Creat.	Thor.	Congr.	Sens.
Throughout the Inquiry													
Reflexivity/reflective journaling				X	X		X					X	
Careful documentation, decision trail	X	X				X	X	X					
Data Generation													
Prolonged engagement				X	X						X		X
Persistent observation				X	X		X				X		X
Comprehensive field notes			X	X			X		X		X		
Theoretically driven sampling											X		
Audiotaping & verbatim transcription				X	X				X	X			
Triangulation (data, method)	X			X							X	X	
Saturation of data			X	X							X		
Member checking	X			X		X							
Data Coding/Analysis													
Transcription rigor/data cleaning				X		X							
Intercoder checks; development of a codebook		X		X		X							
Quasi-statistics				X		X							
Triangulation (investigator, theory, analysis)	X	X		X		X						X	
Stepwise replication	X	X				X							
Search for disconfirming evidence/negative case analysis				X		X	X				X		
Peer review/debriefing		X		X		X							
Inquiry audit	X	X				X	X	X				X	
Presentation of Findings													
Documentation of enhancement quality efforts			X	X			X	X			X		
Thick, vivid description			X		X		X		X			X	X
Impactful, evocative writing					X				X	X			X
Documentation of researcher credentials, background				X			X				X		
Documentation of reflexivity				X		X	X				X		

[a] The criteria from the Lincoln and Guba (1985, 1996) framework include dependability (Dep.), confirmability (Conf.), transferability (Trans.), credibility (Cred.), and authenticity (Auth.); the last two criteria are identical to two primary criteria in the Whittemore et al. (2001) framework.

[b] The criteria from the Whittemore et al. (2001) framework include, in addition to credibility and authenticity, criticality (Crit.), integrity (Integ.), explicitness (Expl.), vividness (Viv.), creativity (Creat.), thoroughness (Thor.), congruence (Congr.), and sensitivity (Sens.)

to ensure saturation of important categories. Prolonged engagement is also essential for building trust and rapport with informants, which in turn makes it more likely that useful, accurate, and rich information will be obtained. Thus, in evaluating a qualitative study, readers often can judge whether researchers engaged in field work for a sufficiently long period of time.

Example of prolonged engagement:
Lyndon (2008) conducted a study of the social and environmental conditions affecting the agency for safety (willingness to take a stand on a safety issue) in academic birth centers. Observational and interview data were gathered in two teaching hospitals over a 16-month period.

High-quality data collection in naturalistic inquiries also involves **persistent observation**, which concerns the salience of the data being gathered and recorded. Persistent observation refers to the researchers' focus on the characteristics or aspects of a situation or a conversation that are relevant to the phenomena being studied. As Lincoln and Guba (1985) noted, "If prolonged engagement provides scope, persistent observation provides depth" (p. 304).

Example of persistent observation:
Jacelon (2004) conducted a grounded theory study to examine the process of hospitalization for elders. She became immersed in the everyday life of hospitalized elders through participant observation. She spent at least 2 hours in the hospital at each observational session, and she staggered her participant observations throughout the day and night.

Data and Method Triangulation
Triangulation refers to the use of multiple referents to draw conclusions about what constitutes truth. Triangulation aims to "overcome the intrinsic bias that comes from single-method, single-observer, and single-theory studies" (Denzin, 1989, p. 313). Triangulation can also help to capture a more complete and contextualized portrait of the phenomenon under study. Denzin identified four types of triangulation (data, investigator, method, and theory), and many other types have been proposed. Two types are described here because of their relevance to data collection.

Data triangulation involves the use of multiple data sources to validate conclusions. The three types of data triangulation are time, space, and person. **Time triangulation** involves collecting data on the same phenomenon or about the same people at different points in time. Time triangulation can involve gathering data at different times of the day, or at different times in the year. This concept is similar to test–retest reliability assessment—the point is not to study a phenomenon longitudinally to determine how it changes, but to establish the congruence of the phenomenon across time. **Space triangulation** involves collecting data on the same phenomenon in multiple sites, to test for cross-site consistency. Finally, **person triangulation** involves collecting data from different types or levels of people (e.g., individuals, groups, such as families, and collectives, such as communities), to validate data through multiple perspectives on the phenomenon.

Example of data (person/time) triangulation:
Verhaeghe and colleagues (2007) studied the process and meaning of hope for family members of traumatic coma patients. Data were gathered from a variety of family members (partners, children, parents, siblings) of ICU patients. Interviews were conducted shortly after admission and then again, for some, shortly after the patient had regained consciousness or had died.

Method triangulation involves using multiple methods of data collection about the same phenomenon. In qualitative studies, researchers often use a rich blend of unstructured data collection methods (e.g., interviews, observations, documents) to develop a comprehensive understanding of a phenomenon. Multiple data collection methods provide an opportunity to evaluate the extent to which a consistent and coherent picture of the phenomenon emerges.

Example of method triangulation:
Gillespie and colleagues (2008), in their ethnographic study of operating theater culture, gathered data through participant observations (70 observations were recorded) and in-depth interviews—both formal and informal—with 27 staff members, including surgeons, anesthetists, nurses, and support staff. The authors noted that "a triangulated approach using multiple sources of data enabled a broad range of issues to be cross-checked, thus achieving . . . confirmation of the data" (p. 266.)

Comprehensive and Vivid Recording of Information

In addition to taking steps to record data from interviews accurately (e.g., via carefully transcriptions of audiotaped interviews), researchers should thoughtfully prepare field notes that are rich with descriptions of what transpired in the field. Even if interviews are the only source of data, researchers should record descriptions of the participants' demeanor and behaviors during the interactions, and they should thoroughly describe the interview context. Other record-keeping activities are also important. A log of decisions needs to be maintained, and reflective journals help to enhance rigor. Thoroughness in record-keeping helps readers to develop confidence in the data.

Researchers sometimes specifically develop an **audit trail**, that is, a systematic collection of materials and documentation that would allow an independent auditor to come to conclusions about the data. Six classes of records are useful in creating an adequate audit trail: (1) the raw data (e.g., interview transcripts); (2) data reduction and analysis products (e.g., theoretical notes, working hypotheses); (3) process notes (e.g., methodologic notes); (4) materials relating to researchers' intentions and dispositions (e.g., reflexive notes); (5) instrument development information (e.g., pilot forms); and (6) data reconstruction products (e.g., drafts of the final report). Similarly, the maintenance of a *decision trail* that articulates the researcher's decision rules for categorizing data and making analytic inferences is a useful way to enhance the auditability (explicitness) of the study. When researchers can share some decision trail information in their reports, readers can better evaluate the soundness of the decisions and draw conclusions about the trustworthiness of the findings.

Example of an audit trail:

In her in-depth study of lesbian body image perceptions, Kelly (2007) maintained on ongoing audit trail. "In this study the process of data collection and analysis was recorded explicitly so that other researchers could clearly understand the methodological and analytic decisions made. The audit trail also assisted me in formulating new questions for my interviews" (p. 876).

Member Checking

Lincoln and Guba considered member checking a particularly important technique for establishing the credibility of qualitative data. In a **member check**, researchers provide feedback to study participants about emerging interpretations, and obtain participants' reactions. The argument is that to assess whether researchers' interpretations are good representations of participants' realities, participants should be given an opportunity to validate them. Member checking with participants can be carried out in an ongoing way as data are being collected (e.g., through deliberate probing to ensure that interviewers have understood participants' meanings), and more formally after data have been fully analyzed in a follow-up conversation.

Despite the potential contribution that member checking can make to a study's credibility, several issues need to be kept in mind in evaluating its contribution. One issue is that member checks can lead to misleading conclusions of credibility if participants "share some common myth or front, or conspire to mislead or cover up" (Lincoln & Guba, 1985, p. 315). Also, some participants might not express disagreement with researchers' interpretations either out of politeness or in the belief that researchers are "smarter" or more knowledgeable than they themselves are. Thorne and Darbyshire (2005), in fact, cautioned against what they irreverently called *adulatory validity*, "a mutual stroking ritual that satisfies the agendas of both researcher and researched" (p. 1110). They noted that member checking tends to privilege interpretations that place study participants in the most charitable light.

> **TIP**
>
> It is important to assess methodologic congruence with regard to member checking. For example, if Giorgi's phenomenological methods were used, member checking would not be undertaken, but member checking *is* called for in studies following Colaizzi's approach (see Table 17.1).

Example of member checking:

Hawley and Jensen (2007) conducted a hermeneutic inquiry that explored critical care nurses' lived experiences of making a difference in their practice. A sample of 16 critical care nurses were interviewed and then the researchers negotiated further conversations "to discuss and reflect on the evolving analysis and the interpretive description" (p. 665). The researchers believed that they had achieved adequate "validity of the interpretive-descriptive text...when, after we had discussed the evolving text with the participants, they responded with such statements as 'Yes, that's it. You've really captured it.'" (p. 665).

Few strategies for enhancing data quality are as controversial as member checking. Nevertheless, it is a strategy that has the potential to enhance credibility if it is done in a manner that encourages candor and critical appraisal by participants.

Strategies Relating to Coding and Analysis

Excellent qualitative inquiry is likely to involve the simultaneous collection and analysis of data, and so several of the strategies described in the preceding section are relevant to ensuring high-quality data *and* analytic integrity. Member checking, for example, can occur in an ongoing fashion as part of the data collection process, but typically also involves participants' review of preliminary analytic constructions. Also, some validation procedures, such as the calculation of quasi-statistics, were described in Chapter 17. In this section we introduce a few additional quality-enhancement strategies associated with the coding, analysis, and interpretation of qualitative data.

Investigator and Theory Triangulation

Triangulation offers opportunities to sort out "true" information from irrelevant or erroneous information by using multiple methods and perspectives. During analysis, several types of triangulation are pertinent. **Investigator triangulation** refers to the use of two or more researchers to make data collection, coding, and analytic decisions. The underlying premise is that through collaboration, investigators can reduce the possibility of biased decisions and idiosyncratic interpretations of the data.

Conceptually, investigator triangulation is analogous to interrater reliability in quantitative studies, and is a strategy that is often used in coding qualitative data. Some researchers take formal steps to compare two or more independent category schemes or independent coding decisions.

Example of independent coding:
Butt and colleagues (2008) studied how people live with the stigma of chronic hepatitis C and make self-care decisions. Data were obtained from interviews with (and daily recorded thoughts of) 26 participants. Transcripts were reviewed and coded by members of the research team who "reviewed each other's coding and discussed any discrepancies to arrive at consensus" (p. 210).

If investigators bring to the analysis task a complementary blend of skills and expertise, the analysis and interpretation can potentially benefit from divergent perspectives. Blending diverse methodologic, disciplinary, and clinical skills also can contribute to other types of triangulation.

Example of investigator triangulation:
Snethen and a team of co-researchers (2006) studied family decision-making relating to children's participation in pediatric clinical trials. The team was composed of specialists in the fields of cultural diversity, ethics, pediatrics, and women's health. Each team member took responsibility for developing a case summary of families after examining transcripts relating to the full family unit (mothers, fathers, affected children, and siblings). Data matrices were developed to assist in comparing both within and across 14 family units. The team then met over a 2-day period to review, discuss, analyze and interpret the case summaries.

One form of investigator triangulation is called **stepwise replication**, a strategy most often mentioned in connection with Lincoln and Guba's dependability criterion. This technique involves having a research team that can be divided into two groups. These groups deal with data sources separately and conduct, essentially, independent inquiries through which data can be compared. Ongoing, regular communication between the groups is essential for the success of this procedure.

With **theory triangulation**, researchers use competing theories or hypotheses in the analysis and interpretation of their data. Qualitative researchers who develop alternative hypotheses while still in the field can test the validity of each because the flexible design of qualitative studies provides ongoing opportunities to direct the inquiry. Theory triangulation can help researchers to rule out rival hypotheses and to prevent premature conceptualizations.

Searching for Disconfirming Evidence and Competing Explanations

A powerful verification procedure that occurs at the intersection of data collection and data analysis involves a systematic search for data that will challenge a categorization or explanation that has emerged early in the analysis. The search for **disconfirming evidence** occurs through purposive or theoretical sampling methods. Clearly, this strategy depends on concurrent data collection and data analysis: researchers cannot look for disconfirming data unless they have a sense of what they need to know. Indeed, Morse and colleagues (2002) consider the iterative interaction between data and analysis essential to verification in qualitative inquiry.

Example of searching for disconfirming evidence:
Enarsson and colleagues (2007) conducted a grounded theory study to examine common approaches among staff toward patients in long-term psychiatric care. The researchers found that all the categories they were discovering were negative in nature. To assess the integrity of their categories, the researchers performed a specific search for data reflecting common staff approaches that related to positive experiences. No such positive episodes could be found either in interviews or observations.

Lincoln and Guba (1985) discussed the related activity of **negative case analysis**. This strategy (sometimes called *deviant case analysis*) is a process by which researchers revise their interpretations by including cases that appear to disconfirm earlier hypotheses. The goal of this procedure is the continuous refinement of a hypothesis or theory until it accounts for *all* cases. Patton (1999) similarly encouraged a systematic exploration for rival themes and explanations during the analysis.

He noted that "failure to find strong supporting evidence for alternative ways of presenting the data or contrary explanations helps increase confidence in the original, principal explanation generated by the analyst" (p. 1191).

Example of a search for rival explanations:
Fleury and Sedikides (2007) studied the role of self-knowledge as a factor in cardiovascular risk modification among patients undergoing cardiac rehabilitation. They analyzed data from interviews with 24 patients and explicitly explored alternative explanations for their emerging findings with both cardiac rehabilitation staff and study participants.

Peer Review and Debriefing

Another quality-enhancement strategy involves external validation. **Peer debriefing** involves sessions with peers to review and explore various aspects of the inquiry. Peer debriefing exposes researchers to the searching questions of others who are experienced in either the methods of naturalistic inquiry, the phenomenon being studied, or both.

In a peer debriefing session, researchers might present written or oral summaries of the data that have been gathered, categories and themes that are emerging, and researchers' interpretations of the data. In some cases, taped interviews might be played. Among the questions that peer debriefers might address are the following:

➤ Is there evidence of researcher bias?

➤ Have the researchers been sufficiently reflexive?

➤ Do the gathered data adequately portray the phenomenon?

➤ If there are important omissions, what strategies might remedy this problem?

➤ Are there any apparent errors of fact?

➤ Are there possible errors of interpretation?

➤ Are there competing interpretations or more parsimonious interpretations?

➤ Have all important themes been identified?

➤ Are the themes and interpretations knit together into a cogent, useful, and creative conceptualization of the phenomenon?

Example of peer debriefing:
Clabo (2008) conducted an ethnography of nurses' pain assessment in two postoperative units. Field notes from the observations and transcripts from interviews with nurses were reviewed by two nurse researchers, who concurred with Clabo's analysis and interpretation.

Inquiry Audits

A similar, but more formal, approach is to undertake an inquiry audit, a procedure that is a means of enhancing a study's dependability and confirmability. An **inquiry audit** involves scrutiny of the data and relevant supporting documents by an external reviewer. Such an audit requires careful documentation of all aspects of the inquiry. Once the audit trail materials are assembled, the inquiry auditor proceeds to audit, in a fashion analogous to a financial audit, the trustworthiness of the data and the meanings attached to them. Although the auditing task is complex, it is a good tool for persuading others that qualitative data are worthy of confidence. Relatively few comprehensive inquiry audits have been reported in the literature, but some studies report partial audits or the assembling of auditable materials.

Example of an inquiry audit:
Erwin and colleagues (2005) provided a detailed account of how they used an audit to address issues of trustworthiness in their study of violence in the lives of high-risk urban teenagers. The audit involved a five-phase process that unfolded over a 6-week period: engagement of the auditor, familiarization with the study, evaluation of the strengths and weaknesses of the study, articulation of the audit findings, and presentation of the audit report to the entire research team. The researchers concluded that "Positioning the audit before producing final results allows researchers to address many study limitations, uncover potential sources of bias in the thematic structure, and systematically plan subsequent steps in an emerging design" (p. 707).

Strategies Relating to Presentation

This section describes some aspects of the qualitative report itself that can help to persuade readers of the high quality of the inquiry.

Thick and Contextualized Description

Thick description, as noted in previous chapters, refers to a rich, thorough, and vivid description of the research context, the people who participated in the study, and the experiences and processes observed during the inquiry. The prevailing sentiment is that if findings are to be transferable, the burden rests with the investigator to provide sufficient information to permit judgments about contextual similarity. Lucid and textured descriptions, with the judicious inclusion of verbatim quotes from study participants, also contribute to other quality criteria, including the authenticity and vividness of a qualitative study.

TIP

Sandelowski (2004) cautioned as follows: " . . . the phrase *thick description* likely ought not to appear in write-ups of qualitative research at all, as it among those qualitative research words that should be seen but not written" (p. 215).

Example of thick description:
Some of the context of Beck's (2004) birth trauma study that could not be shared in the written report but that is imparted in oral presentations comes from powerful photographs that some mothers sent Beck to help bring alive their written stories. For example, one mother sent three photos of herself because she said she wanted to vividly show the immediate impact of birth trauma. The first photo was of the mother smiling before the traumatic delivery of her twins. The next two pictures were of the mother with her newborn twins in the delivery room. She wrote in her email, "Cheryl, focus on my eyes. There is nobody home!" Her eyes were vacant. When Beck showed these pictures (with the mother's permission) at a nursing research conference, one attendee said that the mother looked as if she had lost her soul during the birth of her twins.

In high-quality qualitative studies, descriptions typically need to go beyond a faithful and thorough rendering of information. Powerful description often has an evocative quality and the capacity for emotional impact. Qualitative researchers should, however, avoid misrepresenting their findings by sharing only the most dramatic or sensational stories. Thorne and Darbyshire (2005) cautioned against what they called *lachrymal validity*, a criterion for evaluating research according to the extent to which the report can wring tears from its readers! At the same time, they noted that the opposite problem with some reports is that they are "bloodless." Bloodless findings are characterized by a tendency of some researchers to "play it safe in writing up the research, reporting the obvious . . . (and) failing to apply any inductive analytic spin to the sequence, structure, or form of the findings" (p. 1109).

Researcher Credibility

An aspect of credibility discussed by Patton (1999, 2002) is *researcher credibility*. In qualitative studies, researchers *are* the data collecting instruments—as well as creators of the analytic process. Therefore, researcher qualifications, experience, and reflexivity are relevant in establishing confidence in the data. Patton has argued that trustworthiness of the inquiry is enhanced if the report contains information about the researchers, including information about credentials. In addition, the report may need to make clear the personal connections the researchers had to the people, topic, or community under study. For example, it is relevant for a reader of a report on the coping mechanisms of AIDS patients to know that the researcher is HIV positive. Patton (2002) recommended that researchers report "any personal and professional information that may have affected data collection, analysis and interpretation—either negatively or positively . . ." (p. 566).

Example of researcher credibility:
Gabrielle and co-researchers (2008) undertook a feminist study of older women nurses to explore their concerns about aging and their self-care strategies. The authors (three female nurses) wrote this: "Motivation for this study came from first authors' concern for her own health as a practicing older nurse. This led to concern about other ageing working nurses, and to adopting a feminist qualitative perspective . . . This shared view between participants and researcher added to the study's 'authenticity' and honesty" (p. 317).

Researcher credibility is also enhanced when research reports describe the researchers' efforts to be self-reflective and to take their own prejudices and perspectives into account.

INTERPRETATION OF QUALITATIVE FINDINGS

It is difficult to describe the interpretive process in qualitative studies, but there is considerable agreement that the ability to "make meaning" from qualitative texts depends on researchers' immersion in (and closeness to) the data. **Incubation** is the process of *living* the data, a process in which researchers must try to understand their meanings, find their essential patterns, and draw well-grounded, insightful conclusions. Another key ingredient in interpretation and meaning-making is researchers' self-awareness and the ability to reflect on their own world view and perspectives—that is, reflexivity. Creativity also plays an important role in uncovering meaning in the data. Researchers need to give themselves sufficient time to achieve the *aha* that comes with making meaning beyond the facts.

For *readers* of qualitative reports, interpretation is hampered by having limited access to the data and no opportunity to "live" the data. Researchers are necessarily selective in the amount and types of information to include in their reports. Nevertheless, you should strive to at least consider some of the same interpretive dimensions for qualitative studies as for quantitative ones. Next, we discuss five dimensions, omitting issues relating to precision, which is not relevant in qualitative studies.

The Credibility of Qualitative Results

As was true for quantitative reports, you should consider whether the results of a qualitative inquiry are believable. It is reasonable to expect authors of qualitative reports to provide *evidence* of the credibility of the findings. Because readers of qualitative reports are exposed to only a portion of the data, they must rely on researchers' efforts to corroborate findings through such mechanisms as peer debriefings, member checks, audits, triangulation, and negative cases analysis. They must also rely on researchers' honesty in acknowledging known limitations.

In thinking about the believability of qualitative results—as with quantitative results—it is advisable to adopt the posture of a person who needs to be persuaded about the researcher's conceptualization and to expect the researcher to marshal evidence with which to persuade you. It is also appropriate to consider whether the researcher's conceptualization of the phenomenon is consistent with common experiences and with your own clinical insights.

The Meaning of Qualitative Results

From the point of view of researchers themselves, interpretation and analysis of qualitative data occur virtually simultaneously, in an iterative process. That is, researchers interpret the data as they read and re-read them, categorize and code them, inductively discern themes and patterns, and go back in search of new data to flesh out the emerging conceptualization. Efforts to validate the qualitative analysis are necessarily efforts to validate interpretations as well. Thus, unlike quantitative analyses, the meaning of the data flows directly from qualitative analysis.

Nevertheless, prudent qualitative researchers hold their interpretations up for closer scrutiny—self-scrutiny as well as review by peers and outside reviewers. Even when researchers have undertaken peer debriefings and other strategies described in this chapter, these procedures do not constitute proof that interpretations are correct. For both qualitative and quantitative researchers, it is important to consider possible alternative explanations for the findings and to take into account methodologic or other limitations that could have affected study results.

TIP

Interpretation in qualitative studies often yields hypotheses that can be put to further tests, sometimes in more controlled quantitative studies. Thus, it is not uncommon to find that qualitative researchers attribute causal mechanisms relating to key phenomena under scrutiny. Qualitative studies are well suited to generating causal hypotheses, but not to testing them.

The Importance of Qualitative Results

Qualitative research is especially productive when it is used to describe and explain poorly understood phenomena. The scantiness of prior research on a topic is not, however, a sufficient barometer for deciding whether the findings can contribute to nursing knowledge. The phenomenon must be one that merits scrutiny. For example, some people prefer the color green and others like red. Color preference may not, however, be a sufficiently important topic for an in-depth inquiry. Thus, you must judge whether the topic under study is important or trivial.

You should also consider whether the findings themselves are trivial. Perhaps the topic is worthwhile, but you may feel after reading the report that nothing has been learned beyond what is common sense or everyday knowledge—which can result when the data are too "thin" or when the conceptualization is shallow. Readers, like researchers, want to have an *aha* experience when they read about the lives and concerns of clients and their families. Qualitative researchers often attach catchy labels to their themes and processes, but you should ask yourself whether the labels have really captured an insightful construct.

The Transferability of Qualitative Results

Although qualitative researchers do not strive for generalizability, the application of the results to other settings and contexts must be considered. If the findings are only relevant to the people who participated in the study, they cannot be useful to nursing practice. Thus, in interpreting qualitative results, you should consider how transferable the findings are. In what other types of settings and contexts would you expect the phenomena under study to be manifested in a similar fashion? Of course, to make such an assessment, the author of the report must have described in sufficient detail the participants and the context in which the data were collected. Because qualitative studies are context bound, it is only through a careful analysis of the key parameters of the study context that the transferability of results can be assessed.

The Implications of Qualitative Results

If the findings are judged to be believable and important, and if you are satisfied with the interpretation of the meaning of the results, you can begin to consider what the implications of the findings might be. As with quantitative studies, the implications can be multidimensional. First, you can consider the implications for further research: Should a similar study be undertaken in a new setting? Can the study be expanded (or circumscribed) in meaningful or productive ways? Has an important construct been identified that merits the development of a formal measuring instrument—or an important intervention? Does the emerging theory suggest hypotheses that could be tested through controlled quantitative research? Second, do the findings have implications for nursing practice? For example, could the health care needs of a subculture (e.g., the homeless) be identified and addressed more effectively as a result of the study? Finally, do the findings shed light on fundamental processes that could play a role in nursing theories?

CRITIQUING INTEGRITY AND INTERPRETATIONS IN QUALITATIVE STUDIES

For qualitative research to be judged trustworthy, investigators must *earn* the trust of their readers. Many qualitative reports do not provide much information about the researchers' efforts to ensure that their research is strong with respect to the quality criteria described in this chapter, but there appears to be a promising trend toward greater transparency and forthrightness about quality issues. In a world that is very conscious about the quality of research evidence, qualitative researchers need to be proactive in performing high-quality research. They also need to share their quality-enhancement strategies with readers so that readers can draw their own conclusions about the quality of the evidence and its relevance to their own practice.

A large part of demonstrating integrity to others in a research report involves providing a good description of the quality-enhancement activities that were undertaken. Yet, some qualitative reports do not address the subject of rigor, validity, integrity, or trustworthiness at all. Others pay lip service to validity concerns, simply noting, for example, that reflexive journals or an audit trail were maintained. Just as clinicians seek *evidence* relating to the health care needs of clients, readers of reports need evidence that the findings are believable and true. Researchers should include sufficient information about their quality-enhancement strategies for readers to draw conclusions about study quality. The research example at the end of this chapter is exemplary with regard to the level of information provided to readers.

Part of the difficulty that qualitative researchers face in demonstrating trustworthiness and authenticity is that page constraints in journals impose conflicting demands. It takes a precious amount of space to describe quality-enhancement strategies adequately and convincingly. Using space for such documentation means that there is less space for the thick description of context and rich verbatim accounts that support authenticity and vividness. Qualitative research is often characterized by the need for critical compromises. It is well to keep such compromises in mind in critiquing qualitative research reports.

Table 18.1 offered questions that are useful in considering whether researchers have attended important quality criteria. As noted earlier, not all questions are equally relevant for all types of qualitative inquiry. Reports that explicitly state which criteria guided the inquiry demonstrate sensitivity to readers' needs. Some further guidelines that may be helpful in evaluating qualitative methods and analyses are presented in Box 18.1, and these guidelines include several borrowed from Chapter 16 concerning the interpretive aspects of a study. ⊗

BOX 18.1   GUIDELINES FOR EVALUATING TRUSTWORTHINESS AND INTEGRITY IN QUALITATIVE STUDIES

1. Does the report discuss efforts to enhance or evaluate the quality of the data and the overall inquiry? If so, is the description sufficiently detailed and clear? If not, is there other information that allows you to draw inferences about the quality of the data, the analysis, and the interpretations?

2. Which specific techniques (if any) did the researcher use to enhance the trustworthiness and integrity of the inquiry? Were these strategies used judiciously and to good effect?

3. What quality-enhancement strategies were *not* used? Would supplementary strategies have strengthened your confidence in the study and its evidence?

4. Which specific quality criteria (e.g. credibility, authenticity, and so on) were addressed through quality-enhancement efforts, and which were not addressed?

5. Given the efforts to enhance data quality, what can you conclude about the study's validity/integrity/rigor/trustworthiness?

6. Does the report adequately address the transferability of the findings?

7. Did the report discuss any study limitations and their possible effects on the credibility of the results or on interpretations of the data? Were results interpreted in light of findings from other studies?

8. Did the researchers discuss the study's implications for clinical practice or future research? Were the implications well grounded in the study evidence, and in evidence from earlier research?

RESEARCH EXAMPLES AND CRITICAL THINKING ACTIVITIES

EXAMPLE 1 ■ Trustworthiness in an Ethnographic Study

Study

A context of uncertainty: How context shapes nurses' research utilization behaviors (Scott et al., 2008).

Statement of Purpose

This ethnographic study explored the context and organizational culture that helped to shape the utilization of research by nurses in a pediatric intensive care unit.

Method

The study was conducted in a 16-bed pediatric critical care unit in an urban tertiary care hospital. Data were collected through in-depth, unstructured observation and through interviews with unit nurses, managers, and other health care professionals. Observations were conducted three to four times per week over a 7-month period, with observational sessions averaging about 2 hours. Observations were done on all nursing shifts and every day of the week, and were recorded in field notes. Interviews lasting 1 to 4 hours were conducted with 29 unit members. All interviews were tape recorded and transcribed for analysis.

Quality Enhancement Strategies

Scott and colleagues' report provided abundant detail about the efforts the researchers made to enhance the trustworthiness and integrity of their study. Their report noted specific strategies to enhance the credibility, confirmability, dependability, and transferability of their data. Triangulation was an important quality-enhancement strategy. Data were collected from different perspectives (person triangulation), using multiple methods— personal interviews and extensive observation— (method triangulation), and at different times of the day and week (time triangulation). The report carefully described how method triangulation was operationalized in the analysis: "Data were constantly triangulated, meaning that one source of information (e.g., observational data) was tested against another source of information . . ." (p. 349). The researchers noted that person triangulation ". . . allowed for multiple and diverse perspectives in the data and ensured that data did not reflect an elite bias" (p. 349). The investigators' strategies included both prolonged engagement (7 months of intensive work in the field) and persistent observation, which entailed extensive periods of observation of patient rounds, communication patterns, and unit routines. The report noted that prolonged engagement was a strategy designed to limit the potential from the biases of a more narrow observation, and compensated for the effects of unusual events. Detailed record-keeping and memo writing resulted in the creation of a comprehensive audit trail that documented all conclusions, interpretations, and recommendations. Analytic memos were recorded after each observation sessions and yielded 596 pages of memos. Moreover, Scott (who was responsible for collecting the data) documented all of her personal bias and expectations in a reflexive journal before entering the field. The researchers also noted efforts to test and rule out competing explanations during data analysis. Transferability was enhanced "through the purposive sampling of events to observe, and unit members to interview" (p. 349), as well as through the thick description of the nursing unit studied. Finally, the researchers shared information in their report to strengthen credibility—for example, their Table 1 provided actual interview excerpts to illustrate sources of uncertainty identified in their analysis.

Key Findings

The researchers found that the primary characteristic of the nursing unit was *uncertainty*, and that a climate of uncertainty shaped nurses' behavior in such a way that research use was not relevant. The four major sources of uncertainty were (1) the precarious state of serious ill children; (2) the inherent unpredictability of nurses' work; (3) the complexity of teamwork in a highly sophisticated health care environment; and (4) a changing management.

CRITICAL THINKING SUGGESTIONS*:

*See the Student Resource CD-ROM for a discussion of these questions.

1. Answer the relevant questions from Box 18.1 regarding this study.
2. Also, consider the following targeted questions, which may further sharpen your critical thinking skills and assist you in understanding this study:
   a. Which quality-enhancement strategy used by Scott and co-researchers gave you the *most* confidence in the integrity and trustworthiness of their study? Why?
   b. Think of an additional type of triangulation that the researchers could have used in their study and describe how this could have been operationalized.
3. What might be some of the uses to which the findings could be put in clinical practice?

EXAMPLE 2 ■ Trustworthiness in the Phenomenologic Study in Appendix B

1. Read the method and results sections from Beck's phenomenological study ("Anniversary of birth trauma") in Appendix B of this book, and then answer the relevant questions from Box 18.1 regarding this study.
2. Also consider the following targeted questions, which may further sharpen your critical thinking skills and assist you in understanding this study:
   a. Beck is the mother of two children. She herself has not experienced birth trauma—although she has interacted with pregnant women and new mothers extensively, both clinically and in her research, for over two decades. What are the implications of this information for researcher credibility in this study?
   b. Which quality-enhancement strategy used by Beck gave you the *most* confidence in the integrity and trustworthiness of her study? Why?

EXAMPLE 3 ■ Ethnographic Study in Appendix D

Read Walsh's (2006) study ("Beliefs and Rituals in Traditional Birth Attendant Practice in Guatemala.") in Appendix D (on the accompanying Student Resource CD-ROM) and then address the following suggested activities or questions.

1. Before reading our critique, which accompanies the full report on the CD-ROM, either write your own critique or prepare a list of what you think are the major strengths and weaknesses of the study. Pay particular attention to issues relating to the integrity, quality, and trustworthiness of the study. Then contrast your critique with ours. Remember that you (or your instructor) do not necessarily have to agree with all of the points made in our critique, and that you may identify strengths and weaknesses that we overlooked. You may find the broad critiquing guidelines in Table 4.2 helpful.
2. Write a short summary of how credible, important, and transferable you find the study results to be. Your summary should conclude with your interpretation of what the results mean, and what their implications are for nursing practice. Contrast your summary with the discussion section in the report itself.
3. In selecting studies to include with this textbook, we avoided choosing a poor-quality study, which would have been easier to critique. We did not, however, wish to create a publicly embarrassing situation for any nurse researchers. In the questions below, we offer some "pretend" scenarios in which the researchers for the study in Appendix D made different methodologic decisions than the ones they in fact did make. Write a paragraph or

two critiquing these "pretend" decisions, pointing out how these alternatives would have affected the trustworthiness of the study and the inferences that could be made.

a. Pretend that Walsh had used structured rather than unstructured methods of data collection (e.g., formal structured interviews, structured observation).

b. Pretend that Walsh had only spent a month or two in the Guatemalan community.

CHAPTER REVIEW
● ●

Key new terms introduced in the chapter, together with a summary of major points, are presented in this section. In addition, Chapter 18 of the accompanying *Study Guide for Essentials of Nursing Research,* 7th edition offers various exercises and study suggestions for reinforcing concepts presented in this chapter. For additional review, see the Student Self-Study Review Questions section of the Student Resource CD-ROM provided with this book. 💿

Key New Terms
● ●

Audit trail	Disconfirming evidence	Prolonged engagement
Authenticity	Inquiry audit	Researcher credibility
Confirmability	Member check	Transferability
Credibility	Negative case analysis	Triangulation
Criticality	Peer debriefing	Trustworthiness
Dependability	Persistent observation	

Summary Points
● ●

➤ Several controversies surround the issue of *quality* in qualitative studies; one involves terminology. Some argue that *rigor* and *validity* are quantitative terms that are not suitable as goals in qualitative inquiry, but others believe these terms are appropriate. Other controversies involve what criteria to use as indicators of integrity and whether there should be generic or study-specific criteria.

➤ A prominent evaluative framework is that of Lincoln and Guba, who identified criteria for evaluating **trustworthiness** in qualitative inquiries: credibility, dependability, confirmability, transferability, and authenticity.

➤ **Credibility**, which refers to confidence in the truth value of the findings, has been viewed as the qualitative equivalent of internal validity. **Dependability**, the stability of data over time and over conditions, is somewhat analogous to reliability in quantitative studies. **Confirmability** refers to the objectivity of the data. **Transferability**, the analog of external validity, is the extent to which findings can be transferred to other settings or groups. **Authenticity** is the extent to which researchers faithfully show a range of different realities and convey the feeling tone of lives as they are lived.

➤ Whittemore and colleagues proposed an alternative framework, representing a synthesis of 10 qualitative validity schemes: four primary criteria (credibility, authenticity, criticality, and integrity) and six secondary criteria (explicitness, vividness, creativity, thoroughness, congruence, and sensitivity). The primary criteria can be applied to any qualitative inquiry; the secondary criteria can be given different weight depending on study goals.

➤ **Criticality** is the researcher's critical appraisal of every research decision. **Integrity** is demonstrated by on-going self-scrutiny to ensure that interpretations are valid and grounded in the data.

➤ **Explicitness** is the ability to follow the researcher's decisions, reflecting careful documentation. **Vividness** involves rich and vivid descriptions. **Creativity** reflects challenges to traditional ways of thinking. **Throroughness** refers to comprehensive data and the full development of ideas. **Congruence** is interconnectedness between parts of the inquiry and the whole, and between study findings and external contexts. **Sensitivity**, the sixth secondary criterion in the Whittemore et al. framework, is the degree to which an inquiry reflects respect for those being studied.

➤ Strategies for enhancing quality during qualitative data collection include **prolonged engagement**, which strives for adequate scope of data coverage; **persistent observation**, which is aimed at achieving adequate depth; comprehensive recording of information (including maintenance of an **audit trail**); triangulation, and **member checks** (asking study participants to review and react to study data and emerging themes and conceptualizations).

➤ **Triangulation** is the process of using multiple referents to draw conclusions about what constitutes the truth. This includes **data triangulation** (using multiple data sources to validate conclusions) and **method triangulation** (using multiple methods to collect data about the same phenomenon.

➤ Strategies for enhancing quality during the coding and analysis of qualitative data include **investigator triangulation** (independent coding and analysis of some of the data by two or more researchers); **theory triangulation** (use of competing theories or hypotheses in the analysis and interpretation of data); **stepwise replication** (dividing the research team into two groups that conduct independent inquiries that can be compared and merged); searching for **disconfirming evidence**; searching for rival explanations and undertaking a **negative case analysis** (revising interpretations to account for cases that appear to disconfirm early conclusions); external validation through **peer debriefings** (exposing the inquiry to the searching questions of peers); and launching an **inquiry audit** (a formal scrutiny of audit trail documents by an independent auditor).

➤ Strategies that can be used to convince readers of reports of the high quality of qualitative inquiries include using *thick description* to vividly portray contextualized information about study participants and the central phenomenon, and making efforts to be transparent about researcher credentials and reflexivity so that **researcher credibility** can be established.

❧ Interpretation in qualitative research involves "making meaning"—a process that is difficult to describe or critique. Yet interpretations in qualitative inquiry need to be reviewed in terms of credibility, importance, transferability, and implications.

STUDIES CITED IN CHAPTER 18

Beck, C.T. (2004). Birth trauma: In the eye of the beholder. *Nursing Research, 53,* 28–35.

Butt, G., Paterson, B., & McGuinness, L. (2008). Living with the stigma of hepatitis C. *Western Journal of Nursing Research, 30,* 204–221.

Clabo, L. L. (2008). An ethnography of pain assessment and the role of social context on two postoperative units. *Journal of Advanced Nursing, 61,* 531–539.

Enarsson, P., Sandman, P-O., & Hellzen, O. (2007). The preservation of order: The use of common approaches among staff toward clients in long-term psychiatric care. *Qualitative Health Research, 17,* 718–729.

Erwin, E., Meyer, A., & McClain, N. (2005). Use of an audit in violence prevention research. *Qualitative Health Research, 15,* 707–718.

Fleury, J., & Sedikides, C. (2007). Wellness motivation in cardiac rehabilitation: The role of self-knowledge in cardiovascular risk modification. *Research in Nursing & Health, 30,* 373–384.

Gabrielle, S., Jackson, D., & Mannix, J. (2008). Older women nurses: Health, ageing concerns and self-care strategies. *Journal of Advanced Nursing, 61,* 316–325.

Gillespie, B., Wallis, M., & Chaboyer, W. (2008). Operating theater culture: Implications for nurse retention. *Western Journal of Nursing Research, 30,* 259–277.

Hawley, M. P., & Jensen, L. (2007). Making a difference in critical care nursing practice. *Qualitative Health Research, 17,* 663–674.

Jacelon, C.S. (2004). Managing personal integrity: The process of hospitalization for elders. *Journal of Advanced Nursing, 46,* 549–557.

Kelly, L. (2007). Lesbian body image perceptions: The context of body silence. *Qualitative Health Research, 17,* 873–883.

Lyndon, A. (2008). Social and environmental conditions creating fluctuating agency for safety in two urban academic birth centers. *Journal of Obstetric, Gynecologic & Neonatal Nursing, 37,* 13–23.

Scott, S., Estabrooks, C., Allen, M., & Pollock, C. (2008). A context of uncertainty: How context shapes nurses' research utilization behaviors. *Qualitative Health Research, 18,* 347–357.

Snethen, J., Broome, M., Knafl, K., Deatrick, J., & Angst, D. (2006). Family patterns of decision making in pediatric clinical trials. *Research in Nursing & Health, 29,* 223–232.

Verhaeghe, S., van Zuuren, F., Defloor, T., Duijnstee, M., & Grypdonck, M. (2007). The process and the meaning of hope for family members of traumatic coma patients in intensive care. *Qualitative Health Research, 17,* 730–743.

CHAPTER

19 Systematic Reviews: Meta-Analysis and Metasynthesis

STUDENT OBJECTIVES

On completing this chapter, you will be able to:

⇨ Discuss alternative approaches to integrating research evidence, and advantages to using systemetic methods

⇨ Describe key decisions and steps in doing a meta-analysis and metasynthesis

⇨ Critique key aspects of a written systematic review

⇨ Define new terms in the chapter

In Chapter 7 we described major steps in conducting a literature review. This chapter also discusses reviews of existing evidence, but focuses on integration projects that are in themselves considered research—**systematic reviews** (sometimes called *integrative reviews)* in the form of meta-analyses and metasyntheses.

RESEARCH INTEGRATION AND SYNTHESIS

Evidence-based practice relies (EBP) on meticulous integration of research evidence on a topic. Nurses seeking to adopt best practices from research findings must take into account as much of the evidence as possible, organized and synthesized in a diligent manner. Indeed, many consider systematic reviews a cornerstone of EBP. Systematic reviews are inquiries that follow many of the same rules as those for **primary studies** (i.e., original research investigations). This chapter provides some guidance in helping you to understand and evaluate systematic research integration.

Until fairly recently, the most common type of systematic review was narrative integration, using nonstatistical methods to synthesize research findings. Such reviews continue to be published in the nursing literature. More recently, however, meta-analytic techniques that use a common metric for combining study results statistically are being increasingly used to integrate quantitative evidence. Most reviews in the Cochrane Collaboration, for example, are meta-analyses. Statistical integration, however, is not always appropriate, as we shall see.

Qualitative researchers also are developing techniques to integrate findings across studies. Many terms exist for such endeavors (e.g., meta-study, meta-method, meta-summary, meta-ethnography, qualitative meta-analysis, formal grounded theory), but the one that appears to be emerging as the leading term among nurses researchers is *metasynthesis*.

In this chapter, we focus primarily on meta-analysis as a method for synthesizing quantitative findings, and metasynthesis as an approach to integrating qualitative findings. The field of research integration is expanding at a rapid pace, both in terms of the number of integration studies being conducted and in the techniques used to perform them. This chapter provides a brief introduction to this extremely important and complex topic.

UNDERSTANDING META-ANALYSES

Meta-analyses of randomized clinical trials (RCTs) are at the pinnacle of traditional evidence hierarchies (see Figure 2.1). The essence of a **meta-analysis** is that information from various studies is used to develop a common metric, an *effect size*. Effect sizes are averaged across studies, yielding information about both the *existence* of a relationship between variables in many studies and an estimate of its *magnitude*.

Advantages of Meta-Analyses

Meta-analysis offers a simple yet powerful advantage as a method of integration: *objectivity*. It is often difficult to draw objective conclusions about a body of evidence using narrative methods when results are disparate, as they often are. Narrative reviewers make subjective decisions about how much weight to give findings from different studies, and thus different reviewers may come to different conclusions about the state of the evidence in reviewing the same set of studies. Meta-analysts also make decisions—sometimes based on personal preferences—but in a meta-analysis these decisions are explicit, and readers of the report can evaluate the impact of the decisions. Moreover, the integration itself is objective because it relies on statistical formulas. Readers of a meta-analysis can be confident that another analyst using the same data set and making the same analytic decisions would come to the same conclusions.

Another advantage of meta-analysis concerns *power*, which, it may be recalled from Chapter 15, is the probability of detecting a true relationship between variables. By combining results across multiple studies, power is increased. Indeed, in a meta-analysis it is possible to conclude, with a given probability, that a relationship is real (e.g., an intervention is effective), even when a series of small studies have yielded ambiguous nonsignificant findings. In a narrative review, 10 nonsignificant findings would almost surely be interpreted as lack of evidence of a true relationship, which could be an erroneous conclusion.

Another benefit of meta-analysis involves precision. Meta-analysts can draw conclusions about how big an effect an intervention has, with a specified probability that the results are accurate. Estimates of effect size across multiple studies yield smaller confidence intervals than individual studies, and thus precision is enhanced. Both power and precision are enticing qualities in EBP, as suggested by the EBP questions for appraising evidence described in Chapter 2 (see Box 2.1).

Despite these strengths, meta-analysis is not always appropriate. Indiscriminate use has led critics to warn against potential abuses.

Criteria for Using Meta-Analytic Techniques in a Systematic Review

In doing a synthesis project, reviewers need to decide whether it is appropriate to use statistical integration. One basic criterion is that the research question being addressed or hypothesis being tested across studies should be nearly identical. This means that the independent and the dependent variables, and the study populations, are sufficiently similar to merit integration. The variables may be operationalized differently, to be sure. A nurse-led intervention to promote weight loss among diabetics could be a 4-week clinic-based program in one study and a 6-week home-based intervention in another, for example, and the dependent variable (weight) could be operationalized differently across studies. However, a study of the effects of a 1-hour lecture to discourage eating "junk food" among overweight adolescents would be a poor candidate to include in this meta-analysis. This is frequently referred to as the "apples and oranges" or "fruit" problem. Meta-analyses should not be about *fruit* (i.e., a broad and encompassing category), but rather about specific questions that have been addressed in multiple studies (i.e., "apples," or, even better, "Granny Smith apples").

A second criterion concerns whether there is a sufficient base of knowledge for statistical integration. If there are only a few studies, or if all of the studies are weakly designed and harbor extensive bias, it usually would not make sense to compute an "average" effect.

One final issue concerns the consistency of the evidence. When the same hypothesis has been tested in multiple studies and the results are highly conflicting, meta-analysis is likely not appropriate. As an extreme example, if half the studies testing an intervention found benefits for those in the intervention group, but the other half found benefits for the controls, it would be misleading to compute an average effect. In this situation, it would be better to do an in-depth narrative analysis of *why* the results are conflicting. Reviewers can use diagnostic techniques to test formally whether differences across studies are merely chance differences.

Example of inability to conduct a meta-analysis:
Berry and colleagues (2007) did a systematic review of oral hygiene interventions for intensive care patients receiving mechanical ventilation. They determined that, although there were many relevant studies, there was too much diversity to undertake a meta-analysis.

Steps In a Meta-Analysis

In this section, we describe major steps in the conduct of a meta-analysis. Our intent is not to guide you in *doing* a meta-analysis, but in helping you understand the kinds of decisions a meta-analyst makes—decisions that affect the quality of the review and therefore need to be evaluated when reading a review.

Problem Formulation

As with any scientific endeavor, a systematic review begins with a problem statement and a research question or hypothesis. Data cannot be meaningfully collected and integrated until there is a clear sense of what question is being addressed. As with a primary study, the reviewers should take care to develop a problem statement and research questions that are clearly worded and specific. Key constructs should be conceptually defined, and the definitions should indicate the boundaries of the inquiry. The definitions are critical for deciding whether a primary study qualifies for the synthesis.

Example of research question from a systematic review:
Conn and colleagues (2008) conducted a meta-analysis that addressed the following question: "What is the effect of patient education to increase physical activity (PA) on post-intervention PA among chronically ill adults?" In this example, receipt versus nonreceipt of a patient education intervention was the independent variable, physical activity was the dependent variable, and adults with chronic illness constituted the population.

As indicated previously, questions for a meta-analysis are usually narrow, focusing, for example, on a particular type of intervention and specific outcomes. Forbes (2003) described a systematic review guided by the question, "What strategies, within the scope of nursing, are effective in managing the behavioral symptoms associated with Alzheimer's disease?" She noted that "in retrospect, selecting specific interventions would have made the review more manageable" (p. 182). In fact, Forbes found it was not possible to use meta-analysis in her systematic review.

The Design of a Meta-Analysis

Meta-analysts, as do other researchers, make many decisions that affect the rigor and validity of the study findings. Ideally, these decisions are made in a conscious, planned manner before the study gets underway, and are communicated to readers of the review. We identify a few of the major design decisions in this section.

Sampling is a critical design issue. In a systematic review, the sample consists of the primary studies that have addressed the research question. Reviewers must formulate exclusion or inclusion criteria for the search, which typically encompass substantive, methodologic, and practical elements. Substantively, the criteria stipulate key variables and the population. For example, if the reviewer is integrating material about the effectiveness of a nursing intervention, which outcomes (dependent variables) *must* the researchers have studied? With regard to the study population, will, for example, certain age groups be excluded? Methodologically, the criteria might specify that only studies that used a true experimental design will be included. From a practical standpoint, the criteria might exclude, for example, reports written in a language other than English, or reports published before a certain date. Another decision is whether both published and unpublished reports will be included in the review, a topic we discuss in the next section.

Example of sampling criteria:
Coussement and colleagues (2008) did a meta-analysis of studies that tested interventions to prevent falls in hospitals. Included studies met the following criteria: (1) primary study of a hospital-based fall prevention intervention; (2) outcomes included number of falls or fallers; (3) design was either experimental or quasi-experimental; and (4) report was published in English, French, or Dutch.

A related issue concerns the quality of the primary studies, a topic that has stirred some controversy. Researchers sometimes use quality as a sampling criterion, either directly or indirectly. Screening out studies of lower quality can occur indirectly if the meta-analyst excludes studies that did not use a randomized design, or studies that were not published in a peer-reviewed journal. More directly, each potential primary study can be rated for quality, and excluded if the quality score falls below a certain threshold. Alternatives to handling study quality are discussed in a later section. Suffice it to say, however, that evaluations of study quality are inevitably part of the integration process, and so analysts need to decide how to assess quality and what to do with the assessment information.

Another design issue concerns the **statistical heterogeneity** of results in the primary studies. For each study, meta-analysts compute an index to summarize the strength and direction of the relationship between an independent variable and a dependent variable. Just as there is inevitably variation *within* studies (not all people in a study have identical scores on the outcome measures), so there is inevitably variation in effects *across* studies. If the results are highly variable (e.g., results are conflicting across studies), a meta-analysis may be inappropriate. But, if the results are modestly variable, an important design decision concerns steps that will be taken to explore the source of the variation. For example, the effects of an intervention might be systematically different for men and women, or for different periods of follow-up. If such subgroup effects are anticipated, researchers need to plan for subgroup analyses during the design phase of the project.

The Search for Data in the Literature

Before a search for primary studies begins, reviewers must decide whether the review will cover both published and unpublished results. Some disagree about whether reviewers should limit their sample to published studies, or should cast as wide a net as possible and include **grey literature**—that is, studies with a more limited distribution, such as dissertations, unpublished reports, and so on. Some people restrict their sample to reports in peer-reviewed journals, arguing that the peer review system is an important, tried-and-true screen for findings worthy of consideration as evidence.

The limitations of excluding nonpublished findings, however, have increasingly been noted in the literature on systematic reviews (e.g., Conn et al., 2003; Ciliska & Guyatt, 2005). The primary issue concerns **publication bias**—the tendency for published studies to systematically over-represent statistically significant findings (this bias is sometimes referred to as the *bias against the null hypothesis*). Explorations of this bias have revealed that the bias is widespread: authors tend to refrain from submitting manuscripts with nonsignificant findings; reviewers and editors tend to reject such reports when they are submitted; and users of evidence tend to ignore the findings when they are published. The exclusion of grey literature in a systematic review can lead to bias, notably the overestimation of effects.

Meta-analysts can use various aggressive search strategies to locate grey literature, in addition to the usual tactics used in a literature review. These include *hand searching* journals known to publish relevant content, contacting key researchers in the field to see if they have done studies that have not (yet) been published or if they know of such studies, and contacting funders of relevant research.

Example of a search strategy from a systematic review:

Wagg and Bunn (2007) systematically reviewed research on the effect of unassisted pelvic floor exercises on postnatal stress incontinence. Their comprehensive search strategy, nicely summarized in a table, included a search of nine electronic databases (one of which was specifically for grey literature), perusal of four evidence-based journals, a search of government documents, and contact with the Continence Foundation. Their report included a flow diagram that showed the results of their search results.

Evaluations of Study Quality

In systematic reviews, the evidence from primary studies needs to be evaluated to determine how much confidence to place in the findings. Strong studies clearly should be given more weight than weaker ones in coming to conclusions about a body of evidence. In meta-analyses, evaluations of study quality often involve quantitative ratings of each study in terms of the strength of evidence it yields. Literally hundreds of rating instruments and systems have been developed. The Agency for Healthcare Research and Quality or AHRQ (2002) published a guide that described and evaluated various systems and instruments to rate the strength of evidence in quantitative studies. The report identified 19 of 121 systems reviewed that fully address essential quality domains.

Example of a quality assessment tool:
One of the 19 systems considered to be of especially high quality in the AHRQ report was developed by a team working at the Royal College of Nursing Institute at the University of Oxford (Sindhu et al., 1997). The instrument, developed by an expert panel of researchers for assessing reports of randomized clinical trials, consists of 53 items on 15 dimensions (e.g., appropriateness of controls, measurement of outcomes, blinding of treatments). Those using the instrument assign scores for each dimension and then total the points, which can range from 0 to 100.

Despite the availability of many quality assessment instruments, little consensus is found about which ones are especially useful for nurse researchers. As Conn and Rantz (2003) have noted, one major obstacle is that no "gold standard" exists for determining the scientific rigor and validity of primary studies, and so it is difficult to validate the assessment instruments. Quality criteria vary widely from instrument to instrument, and the result is that study quality can be rated quite differently with two different assessment tools.

Some meta-analysts use an alternative—or supplementary—strategy of identifying individual methodologic features that they judge to be of critical importance for the type of question begin addressed in the review—a component approach, as opposed to a scale approach. So, for example, a researcher might code for such design elements as whether randomization was used, the extent of attrition from the study, and so on.

Quality assessments of primary studies, whether they are assessments of individual study features or overall ratings, should be done by two or more qualified individuals. If the raters disagree, there should be a discussion until a consensus has been reached or other raters should be asked to help resolve the difference. Indexes of interrater reliability are often calculated to demonstrate to readers that rater agreement on study quality was adequate.

Extraction and Encoding of Data for Analysis

The next step in a systematic review is to extract and record relevant information about the findings, methods, and study characteristics. The goal of these tasks is to produce a data set amenable to statistical analysis.

Basic source information must be recorded, including year of publication, country where data were collected, and so on. In terms of methodologic information, the most critical element across all studies is sample size. Other important attributes that should be recorded vary by study question. Examples of features likely to be important include whether subjects were randomly assigned to treatments, whether subjects, agents, or data collectors were blinded, and the response or attrition rates. Information about the timing of the measurements (i.e., the period of follow-up) is also likely to be critical. Characteristics of study participants must be encoded as well (e.g., the percentage of the sample that was female, the mean age of participants). Finally, information about findings must be extracted. Reviewers must either calculate effect sizes (discussed in the next section) or must enter sufficient statistical information that the computer program can compute them.

As with other decisions, extraction and coding of information should be completed by two or more people, at least for a portion of the studies in the sample. This allows for an assessment of interrater agreement, which should be sufficiently high to persuade readers of the review that the recorded information is accurate.

Example of intercoder agreement:

Mahon and colleagues (2006) used a complex system of coding checks in their meta-analysis of factors that predicted loneliness in adolescents. Two teams with two researchers per team independently coded half the 95 studies in the analyses. Initial interrater agreement between pairs ranged from 95% to 100%; disagreements were then resolved through discussions. Then one member of each team reviewed a sample of the others' coding, and 100% agreement was achieved.

Calculation of Effects

Meta-analyses depend on the calculation of an index that encapsulates the relationship between the independent and dependent variable in each study. Because effects are captured differently depending on the level of measurement of variables, there is no single formula for calculating an effect size. In nursing, the three most common scenarios for meta-analysis involve comparisons of two groups, such as an experimental versus a control group on a continuous outcome (e.g., the body mass index or BMI), comparisons of two groups on a dichotomous outcome (e.g., stopped smoking versus continued smoking), or correlations between two continuous variables (e.g., the correlation between body mass index (BMI) and scores on a depression scale).

The first scenario, comparison of two group means, is especially common in nursing studies. When the outcomes across studies are on identical scales (e.g., all outcomes are measures of weight in pounds), the effect is captured by simply subtracting the mean for one group from the mean for the other. For example, if the mean postintervention weight in an intervention group were 182.0 pounds and that for a control group were 194.0 pounds, the effect would be −8.0. More typically, however, outcomes are measured on different scales (e.g., different scales to measure stress). Mean differences across studies cannot be combined and averaged in such situations—researchers need an index that is neutral to the original metric.

Cohen's *d*, described in Chapter 15, is the effect size index most often used. This effect size index transforms all effects to standard deviation units. That is, if *d* were computed to be .50, it means that the group mean for one group was one-half a standard deviation higher than the mean for the other group—regardless of the original measurement scale.

> **TIP**
>
> The term *effect size* is widely used for *d* in the nursing literature, but the preferred term for Cochrane reviews is **standardized mean difference** or SMD. Other writers have referred to *d* as **Hedges' g**.

When the outcomes in the primary studies are dichotomous, meta-analysts have a choice of effect index, including the odds ratio (OR), relative risk (RR), and absolute risk reduction (ARR). Sometimes, especially for nonexperimental studies, the most common statistic used to express the relationship between independent and dependent variables is Pearson's *r*. In such cases, the *r* itself serves as the indicator of the magnitude and direction of effect.

Data Analysis

Meta-analysis is often described as a two-step analytic process. In the first step, a summary statistic that captures an effect is computed for each study, as just described. In the second step, a pooled effect estimate is computed as a *weighted average* of the individual effects. The bigger the weight given to any study, the more that study will contribute to the weighted average. Thus, weights should reflect the amount of information that each study provides. One widely used approach in meta-analysis is called the *inverse variance method*, which involves using the standard error to calculate the weight. Larger studies, which have smaller standard errors, are given greater weight than smaller ones.

In formulating an analytic strategy, meta-analysts must make many decisions. In this brief overview, we touch on a few of them. One concerns the heterogeneity of findings (i.e., differences from one study to another in the magnitude and direction of the effect size). As discussed earlier, heterogeneity across studies may rule out the possibility that a meta-analysis can be done. Unless it is obvious that effects are consistent in magnitude and direction based on a subjective perusal, heterogeneity should be formally tested and meta-analysts should report their results in their reports.

Visual inspection of heterogeneity can most readily be accomplished by constructing forest plots, which are sometimes included in reports. **A forest plot** graphs the estimated effect size for each study, together with the 95% confidence interval (CI) around each estimate. Figure 19.1 illustrates forest plots for situations in which there is low heterogeneity (A) and high heterogeneity (B) for five studies in which the effect size index was the odds ratio. In panel A, all effect size estimates favor the intervention group; the CI information indicates the effect is statistically significant (does not encompass 0.0) for three of them, studies 2, 4, and 5. In panel B, by contrast, the results are "all over the map." Two studies favor

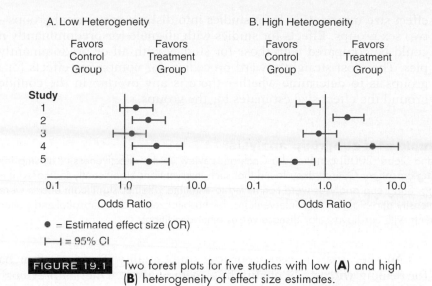

FIGURE 19.1 Two forest plots for five studies with low (**A**) and high (**B**) heterogeneity of effect size estimates.

controls at significant levels (studies 1 and 5) and two favor the treatment group (studies 2 and 4). Meta-analysis is not appropriate for the situation in panel B. Heterogeneity can be evaluated using statistical methods that test the null hypothesis that heterogeneity across studies represents random fluctuations. The test yields a *p* value that indicates the probability of obtaining effect size differences as large as those observed if the null hypothesis were true.

Heterogencity affects not only whether a meta-analysis is appropriate, but also which of two statistical models should be used in the analysis. Although this is too complex a topic for this book, suffice it to say that when heterogeneity is fairly low, the researchers may use a *fixed effects model*. When study results are more varied, it is usually better to use what is called a *random effects model*. Some argue that a random effects model is almost always more tenable. One solution is to perform a **sensitivity analysis**—which, in general, refers to an effort to test how sensitive the results of an analysis are to changes in the way the analysis was done. In this case, it would involve using *both* statistical models to determine how the results are affected. If the results differ, estimates from the random effects model would be preferred.

A random effects meta-analysis is intended primarily to address study-by-study variation that cannot be explained. Many meta-analysts seek to understand the determinants of effect size heterogeneity through formal analyses. Variation across studies could reflect systematic differences with regard to important clinical or methodologic characteristics. For example, in intervention studies, variation in effects could reflect who the agents were (e.g., nurses versus others), how long the intervention lasted, and whether or not the intervention was individualized. Or, variation in results could be explained by differences in participant characteristics (e.g., men versus women).

One strategy for exploring moderating effects on effect size is to perform subgroup analyses. **Subgroup analyses** (or *moderator analyses*) involve splitting the effect size information from studies into distinct categorical groups—for example, two sex groups. Effects for studies with all-male (or predominantly male) samples could be compared with those for studies with all or predominantly female samples. The most straightforward procedure for comparing effects for different subgroups is to determine whether there is any overlap in the confidence intervals around the effect size estimates for the groups.

Example of a subgroup analysis:

Rice and Stead (2008) conducted a Cochrane review on the effectiveness of nursing interventions for smoking cessation. Overall, they found that such interventions significantly increased the likelihood of quitting. Subgroup analyses were conducted to examine whether significant effects were observed for low-intensity and high-intensity interventions, for hospitalized and nonhospitalized patients, and for inpatients with cardiovascular disease versus other conditions.

Another analytic issue concerns study quality. There are four basic strategies for dealing with study quality in a meta-analysis. One, as previously noted, is to establish a quality threshold for study inclusion (e.g., totally omitting studies with a low score on a quality assessment scale).

Example of excluding low-quality studies:

Peacock and Forbes (2003) systematically reviewed interventions for caregivers of persons with dementia. A total of 36 relevant studies were rated using various methodologic criteria, and then the scores were used to categorize studies as strong, moderate, weak, or poor. Only the 11 studies in the *strong* category were included in the review.

A second strategy is to undertake sensitivity analyses to determine whether the exclusion of lower-quality studies changes the results of analyses based only on the most rigorous studies. Another approach is to consider quality as the basis for exploring variation in effects. For example, do randomized designs yield different average effect size estimates than quasi-experimental designs? Do effects vary as a function of the study's score on a quality assessment scale? A fourth strategy is to *weight* studies according to quality criteria. Most meta-analyses routinely give more weight to larger studies, but effect sizes can also be weighted by quality scores, thereby placing more weight on the estimates from rigorous studies. A mix of strategies, together with appropriate sensitivity analyses, is probably the most prudent approach to dealing with variation in study quality.

Example of a quality-related sensitivity analysis:

Choi and colleagues (2007) performed a meta-analysis of RCTs that tested the efficacy of pelvic floor muscle training for incontinent women. They examined whether the inclusion of low-quality studies affected their conclusions by computing effect sizes separately for six studies rated highly and four studies with low-quality ratings. The average effect size for both groups of studies was statistically significant (in both cases *d* was greater than .50), and the difference between effect sizes was not significant.

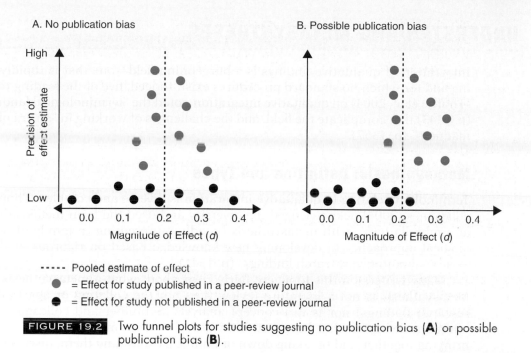

FIGURE 19.2 Two funnel plots for studies suggesting no publication bias (**A**) or possible publication bias (**B**).

One final analytic issue concerns publication biases. Even a strong commitment to a comprehensive search for reports on a given research question is unlikely to result in the identification of all studies. Some researchers, therefore, use strategies to assess publication bias, and to make adjustments for them. One way to examine the possibility of publication bias among studies in the meta-analysis is to construct a **funnel plot**. Figure 19.2 illustrates two hypothetical funnel plots for a meta-analysis of a nursing intervention in which the pooled average effect size estimate (d) for 20 studies (10 published and 10 unpublished) is .2. In the funnel plot on the left (A), the effects are fairly symmetric around the pooled effect size for both published and unpublished studies. In the asymmetric plot on the right (B), however, unpublished studies have consistently lower effect size estimates, suggesting the possibility that the pooled effect size has been overestimated. One strategy for *addressing* publication bias is to compute a **fail-safe number** that estimates the number of studies with an effect size of zero that would be needed to reverse the conclusion of a significant effect in a meta-analysis. The fail-safe number is compared with a *tolerance level* ($5k + 10$), where k is the number of studies included in the analysis.

Example of calculating a fail-safe number:
Zangaro and Soeken (2007) performed a meta-analysis of factors associated with nurses' job satisfaction. Their computed fail-safe numbers suggested that publication bias was unlikely. For example, the fail-safe number for the variable job stress was 234, which far exceeded their tolerance level of 95 for 17 studies in this analysis.

UNDERSTANDING METASYNTHESES

Integration of qualitative findings is a burgeoning field—one that is rapidly evolving and for which no standard procedures exist. Indeed, five of the leading thinkers (Thorne et al, 2004) on qualitative integration noted the "terminological landmines" (p. 1343) that complicate the field, and the challenges of working in "an era of meta-madness" (p. 1357).

Metasynthesis: Definition and Types

Terminology relating to qualitative integration is diverse and complex. Thorne and colleagues (2004) acknowledged the diversity and used the term metasynthesis as an umbrella term, with metasynthesis broadly representing "a family of methodological approaches to developing new knowledge based on rigorous analysis of existing qualitative research findings" (p. 1343).

Many writers on this topic are fairly clear about what a metasynthesis is *not*. Metasynthesis is not a literature review (i.e., not the collating or aggregation of research findings) nor is it a concept analysis. Schreiber and colleagues (1997) offered a definition that has often been used for what metasynthesis *is*, ". . . the bringing together and breaking down of findings, examining them, discovering the essential features and, in some way, combining phenomena into a transformed whole" (p. 314). Consistent with this definition, Sandelowski (in Thorne et al., 2004) suggested that Metasyntheses "are integrations that are more than the sum of parts, in that they offer novel interpretations of findings" (p. 1358).

Schreiber and colleagues described a three-category typology of metasyntheses that puts the role of theory at center stage. *Theory-building metasyntheses* are inquiries that extend the level of theory beyond what could be achieved in individual investigations. In *theory explication metasyntheses*, researchers "flesh out" and reconceptualize abstract concepts. Finally, *descriptive metasynthesis* involves a comprehensive analysis of a phenomenon based on a synthesis of qualitative findings; findings are not typically deconstructed and then reconstructed as they are in theory-related inquiries.

Metasynthesis has had its share of controversies, one of which concerns whether to integrate studies based on different research traditions and methods. Some researchers have argued against combining studies from different epistemologic perspectives, and have recommended separate analyses using groupings from different traditions. Others, however, advocate combining findings across traditions and methodologies. Which path to follow is likely to depend on several factors, including the focus of the inquiry, its intent vis-à-vis theory development, and the nature of the available evidence at the time the metasynthesis is undertaken.

Steps in a Metasynthesis

Many of the steps in a metasynthesis are similar to ones we described in connection with a meta-analysis, and so many details will not be repeated here. However, we point out some distinctive issues relating to qualitative integration that are relevant in the various steps.

Problem Formulation

In metasynthesis, researchers begin with a research question or a focus of investigation, and a key issue concerns the scope of the inquiry. Finfgeld (2003) recommended a strategy that balances breadth and utility. She advised that the scope be broad enough to fully capture the phenomenon of interest, but focused enough to yield findings that are meaningful to clinicians, other researchers, and public policy makers.

Example of a research question in a metasynthesis:

Noyes and Popay (2007) undertook a metasynthesis that addressed the following question: "What does qualitative research tell us about the facilitators of and barriers to accessing and complying with tuberculosis treatment?"

The Design of a Metasynthesis

Like a quantitative systematic review, a metasynthesis requires considerable advance planning. Having a team of at least two researchers to design and implement the study is often advantageous because of the highly subjective nature of interpretive efforts. Just as in a primary study, the design of a qualitative metasynthesis should involve efforts to enhance integrity and rigor, and investigator triangulation is one such strategy.

> **TIP**
>
> Meta-analyses often are undertaken by researchers who did not do one of the primary studies in the review. Metasyntheses, by contrast, are often done by researchers whose area of interest has led them to do both original studies and metasyntheses on the same topic. Prior work in an area offers obvious advantages in terms of researchers' ability to grasp subtle nuances and to think abstractly about a topic, but a disadvantage may be a certain degree of partiality about one's own work.

Like meta-analysts, metasynthesists must also make upfront decisions about sampling, and they face the same issue of deciding whether to include only findings from peer-reviewed journals in the analysis. One advantage of including alternative sources, in addition to wanting a more comprehensive analysis, is that journal articles tend to be constrained by space limitations. Finfgeld (2003) noted that in her metasynthesis on *courage*, she used dissertations even when a peer-reviewed journal article was available from the same study because the dissertation offered richer information and many more excerpts. Another sampling decision, as previously noted, involves whether to search for qualitative studies about a phenomenon in multiple traditions.

Example of sampling decisions:

Xu (2007) conducted a metasynthesis of studies on the experiences of immigrant Asian nurses working in Western countries. He noted that "types of qualitative research design had no effect on selection. For a qualified study using a mixed method design or an overall quantitative design with a qualitative component, only data from the qualitative portion of the study were included for synthesis" (p. 247). (Note: Xu's study is reprinted in its entirety in the accompanying *Study Guide*).

Decisions relating to study quality and how to assess it are also needed early in the project. Finfgeld (2003), who did not advocate using peer review as a screen for quality, did, however, suggest two basic quality criteria. The first is that the report provide sufficient assurance that the study used "widely accepted qualitative methods" (p. 899). The second is that the findings be well supported by the raw data (i.e., quotes from study participants).

The Search for Data in the Literature

It is generally more difficult to find qualitative than quantitative studies using mainstream approaches such as searching electronic databases. For example, "qualitative" is not a MeSH (medical subject heading) term in MEDLINE—although "qualitative studies" *is* used in the controlled vocabulary of CINAHL. This means that a searcher typically has to try many different terms (e.g., "grounded theory," phenomenolog*, ethnograph*, "case study," and so on), and hope that one of these terms was used in the abstract or title of relevant studies.

TIP

Sample sizes in nursing metasyntheses are highly variable, ranging from a very small number—e.g., three primary studies on health care relationships in the meta-ethnography of Varcoe and colleagues (2003)—to nearly 300 in Paterson's (2001) synthesis of qualitative studies on chronic illness. Sample size is likely to vary as a function of scope of the inquiry, the extent of prior research, and type of metasynthesis undertaken. As with primary studies, one guideline for sampling adequacy is whether categories in the metasynthesis are saturated.

Evaluations of Study Quality

Formal evaluations of primary study quality are not as common in metasynthesis as in meta-analysis, and developing quality criteria about which there would be widespread agreement is likely to prove challenging. One available instrument, developed by Paterson and colleagues (2001), is the Primary Research Appraisal Tool, which covers such aspects of a qualitative study as the sampling procedure, data analysis, researcher credentials, and researcher reflexivity. The tool was designed to be used to screen primary studies for inclusion in a metasynthesis.

Not everyone agrees, however, that quality ought to be a criterion for eliminating studies for a metasynthesis. Sandelowski and Barroso (2003b), for example, advocated a certain degree of inclusiveness: "Excluding reports of qualitative studies because of inadequacies in reporting . . . , or because of what some reviewers might perceive as methodological mistakes, will result in the exclusion of reports with findings valuable to practice that are not necessarily invalidated by these errors" (p. 155).

Example of study quality decisions:

Briggs and Flemming (2007) synthesized qualitative findings on living with leg ulceration. Although they completed quality appraisals of the 12 studies in their metasynthesis "to provide us with a formal baseline assessment of quality" (p. 321), they elected not to reject any paper on grounds of quality.

Extraction of Data for Analysis

Information about various features of the study need to be abstracted and coded as part of the project. Just as in quantitative integration, the metasynthesist records features of the data source (e.g., year of publication, country), characteristics of the sample (e.g., age, sex, number of participants), and methodologic features (e.g., research tradition). Most important, of course, information about the study findings must be extracted and recorded. Sandelowski and Barroso (2003a) have defined *findings* as the "data-based and integrated discoveries, conclusions, judgments, or pronouncements researchers offered regarding the events, experiences, or cases under investigation (i.e., their interpretations, no matter the extent of the data transformation involved)" (p. 228). Others characterize findings as the key themes, metaphors, or categories from each study.

As Sandelowski and Barroso (2002) have noted, however, *finding* the findings is not always easy. Qualitative researchers intermingle data with interpretation, and findings from other studies with their own. Noblit and Hare (1988) advised that, just as primary study researchers must read and re-read their data before they can proceed with a meaningful analysis, metasynthesists must read the primary studies multiple times to fully grasp the categories or metaphors being explicated. In essence, a metasynthesis becomes "another 'reading' of data, an opportunity to reflect on the data in new ways" (McCormick et al., 2003, p. 936).

Data Analysis

Strategies for metasynthesis diverge most markedly at the analysis stage. We briefly describe three approaches. Regardless of approach, metasynthesis is a complex interpretive task that involves "carefully peeling away the surface layers of studies to find their hearts and souls in a way that does the least damage to them" (Sandelowski et al., 1997, p.370).

The Noblit and Hare Approach

Noblit and Hare's (1988) methods of integration have been highly influential among nurse researchers. Noblit and Hare, who referred to their approach as meta-ethnography, argued that the integration should be interpretive and not aggregative (i.e., that the synthesis should focus on constructing interpretations rather than descriptions). Their approach for synthesizing qualitative studies includes seven phases that overlap and repeat as the metasynthesis progresses, the first three of which are preanalytic: (1) deciding on the phenomenon, (2) deciding which studies are relevant for the synthesis, and (3) reading and re-reading each study. Phases 4 through 6 concern the analysis:

➤ *Phase 4*: Deciding how the studies are related. In this phase, the researcher makes a list of the key metaphors (or themes/concepts) in each study and their relation to each other. Studies can be related in three ways: *reciprocal* (directly comparable), *refutational* (in opposition to each other), and in a line of argument rather than either reciprocal or refutational.

➤ *Phase 5*: Translating the qualitative studies into one another. Noblit and Hare noted that "translations are especially unique syntheses because they protect the particular, respect holism, and enable comparison. An adequate translation maintains the central metaphors and/or concepts of each account in their relation to other key metaphors or concepts in that account" (p. 28).

➤ *Phase 6:* Synthesizing translations. Here the challenge for the researcher is to make a whole into more than the individual parts imply.

The final phase (Phase 7) is to express the synthesis in a written or oral report.

Example of Noblit and Hare's approach:

Goodman (2005) used Noblit and Hare's approach in her metasynthesis of ten published articles from seven qualitative studies on becoming an involved father of an infant. Key metaphors from each study were compared and translated into one another by applying each metaphor to that in all other studies. The translations were then synthesized into a whole that depicted a four-phase process and experience of being an involved father of an infant.

The Paterson, Thorne, Canam, and Jillings Approach

The method developed by Paterson and a team of Canadian colleagues (2001) involves three components: meta-data analysis, meta-method, and meta-theory. These components often are conducted concurrently, and the metasynthesis results from the integration of findings from these three analytic components. Paterson and colleagues define **meta-data analysis** as the study of results of reported research in a specific substantive area of investigation by means of analyzing the "processed data." **Meta-method** is the study of the methodologic rigor of the studies included in the metasynthesis. Lastly, **metatheory** refers to the analysis of the theoretical underpinnings on which the studies are grounded. The end product is a metasynthesis that results from bringing back together the findings of these three meta-study components.

Example of the Paterson et al. approach:

Berterö and Chamberlain-Wilmoth (2007) used the Paterson approach in their metasynthesis of 30 qualitative studies on the impact of a breast cancer diagnosis on the self. Their meta-data analysis revealed four aspects of the self that are affected by breast cancer and its treatment. These researchers presented a useful table summarizing meta-findings, meta-method, and meta-theory aspects of the 30 studies.

The Sandelowski and Barroso Approach

The strategies developed by Sandelowski and Barroso (2006) are likely to inspire metasynthesis efforts in the years ahead. In their multiyear, methodologic project, they dichotomized integration studies based on level of synthesis and interpretation. Reports are called *summaries* if the findings are descriptive synopses of the qualitative data, usually with lists and frequencies of themes, without any conceptual reframing. *Syntheses,* by contrast, are findings that are more interpretive and that involve conceptual or metaphoric reframing. Sandelowski and Barroso have argued that only findings that are syntheses should be used in a metasynthesis.

Both summaries and syntheses can, however, be used in a **meta-summary**, which can lay a good foundation for a metasynthesis. Sandelowski and Barroso (2003a) provided an example of a meta-summary, using studies of mothering within the context of HIV infection. The first step, extracting findings, resulted in almost 800 complete sentences from 45 reports and represented a comprehensive inventory of findings. The 800 sentences were then reduced to 93 thematic statements, or abstracted findings.

The next step was to calculate **manifest effect sizes** (i.e., effect sizes calculated from the manifest content pertaining to mothering in the context of HIV, as represented in the 93 abstracted findings). Qualitative effect sizes are not to be confused with treatment effects, but the ". . . calculation of effect sizes constitutes a quantitative transformation of qualitative data in the service of extracting more meaning from those data and verifying the presence of a pattern or theme" (Sandelowski & Barroso, 2003a, p 231). They argued that by calculating effect sizes, integration that avoids the possibility of over- or underweighting findings can be achieved.

Two types of effect size can be created from the abstracted findings. **A frequency effect size**, which indicates the magnitude of the findings, is the number of reports that contain a given finding, divided by all reports (excluding reports with duplicated findings from the same data set). For example, Sandelowski and Barroso (2003a) calculated an overall frequency effect size of 60% for the finding about a mother's struggle about whether or not to disclose her HIV status to her children. In other words, 60% of the 45 reports had a finding of this nature. Such effect size information can be calculated for subgroups of reports (e.g., for published versus unpublished reports, for reports from different research traditions, and so on).

An **intensity effect size** indicates the concentration of findings *within* each report. It is calculated by calculating the number of different findings in a given report, divided by the total number of findings in all reports. As an example, one primary study had 29 of the 93 total findings, for an intensity effect size of 31% (Sandelowski & Barroso, 2003a).

Metasyntheses can build upon meta-summaries, but require findings that are more interpretive (i.e., from reports that are characterized as syntheses). The purpose of a metasynthesis is not to summarize, but to offer novel interpretations of interpretive findings. Such interpretive integrations require metasynthesists to piece the individual syntheses together to craft a new coherent explanation of a target event or experience. An array of quantitative analytic methods can be used to achieve this goal, including, ". . . for example, constant comparison, taxonomic analysis, the reciprocal translation of *in vivo* concepts, and the use of imported concepts to frame data" (Sandelowski in Thorne et al., 2004, p. 1358).

Example of Sandelowski and Barroso's approach:

Sandelowski and Barroso (2005) applied their procedures to qualitative studies of expectant parents receiving positive prenatal diagnosis. Meta-summary techniques were used to aggregate findings from 17 reports, and metasynthesis techniques, including constant comparative analysis, were used to interpret the findings. A total of 39 meta-findings were abstracted, with frequency effect sizes ranging from 100% to 6%. The thematic emphasis was on the dilemmas of choice and decision-making. Positive prenatal diagnosis was an experience of chosen losses and lost choices.

WRITTEN REPORTS OF SYSTEMATIC REVIEWS

Reports for systematic reviews typically follow much the same format as for a research report for a primary study. That is, there is usually an introduction, method section, results section, and discussion. In most cases, there are full citations for the entire sample of studies included in the review. Often these are identified separately from other citations—for example, by noting them with asterisks.

In reading a review, particular attention should be paid to the method section. Readers of the review need to assess the validity of the findings, and so methodologic and statistical strategies, and their rationales, should be adequately described. For example, if reviewers of quantitative studies decided that a meta-analysis was not justified, the rationale for this decision must be made clear.

Tables and figures typically play a key role in reports of systematic reviews. For meta-analyses, forest plots are often presented, showing effect size and 95% CI information for each study, as well as for the overall pooled result. Typically, there is also a table showing the characteristics of studies included in the review.

Metasynthesis reports are similar in many respects to meta-analytic reports—except that the results section contains the new interpretations rather than quantitative findings. Of course, when a meta-summary has been done, the meta-findings would typically be presented in a table. The method section of a metasynthesis report should contain a detailed description of the sampling criteria, the search procedures, and efforts made to enhance the integrity and rigor of the integration. The sample of selected studies should also be described; key features are often summarized in a table.

A thorough discussion section is also crucial in systematic reviews. The discussion should include an overall summary of the findings, the reviewers' assessment about the strength and limitations of the body of evidence, what further research should be undertaken to improve the evidence base, and what the implications of the review are for clinicians and patients. The review should also discuss the consistency of findings across studies and provide an interpretation of why there might be inconsistency. Did the samples, research designs, or data collection strategies in the studies differ in important ways? Or, do differences reflect substantive differences, such as variation in the interventions or outcomes themselves?

CRITIQUING SYSTEMATIC REVIEWS

Like all studies, systematic reviews should be thoroughly critiqued before the findings are deemed trustworthy and relevant to clinicians. Box 19.1 offers guidelines for evaluating systematic reviews.

Although these guidelines are fairly broad, not all questions apply equally well to all types of systematic reviews. In particular, we have distinguished questions about analysis separately for meta-analyses and metasyntheses. The list of questions in Box 19.1 is not necessarily comprehensive. Supplementary questions might be needed for particular types of review.

In drawing conclusions about a research synthesis, one issue is to evaluate whether reviewers did a good job in pulling together and summarizing the evidence. Another aspect, however, is inferences about how *you* might use the evidence in clinical practice. It is not the reviewers' job, for example, to consider such issues as barriers to making use of the evidence, acceptability of an innovation, costs and benefits of change in various settings, and so on. These are issues for practicing nurses seeking to maximize the effectiveness of their actions and decisions.

BOX 19.1 GUIDELINES FOR CRITIQUING SYSTEMATIC REVIEWS

The Problem

- Did the report clearly state the research problem and/or research questions? Is the scope of the project appropriate?
- Is the topic of the integration important for nursing?
- Were concepts, variables, or phenomena adequately defined?
- Was the approach to integration adequately described, and was the approach appropriate?

Search Strategy

- Did the report clearly describe criteria for selecting primary studies, and are those criteria defensible?
- Were the databases used by the reviewers identified, and are they appropriate and comprehensive? Were key words identified, and are they exhaustive?
- Did the reviewers use adequate supplementary efforts to identify relevant studies?

The Sample

- Did the search strategy yield a strong and comprehensive sample of studies? Were strengths and limitations of the sample identified?
- If an original report was lacking key information, did reviewers attempt to contact the original researchers for additional information—or did the study have to be excluded?
- If studies were excluded for reasons other than insufficient information, did the reviewers provide a rationale for the decision?

Quality Appraisal

- Did the reviewers appraise the quality of the primary studies? Did they use a defensible and well-defined set of criteria, or a well-validated quality appraisal scale?
- Did two or more people do the appraisals, and was inter-rater agreement reported?
- Was quality appraisal information used in an appropriate manner in the selection of studies, or in the analysis of results?

Data Extraction

- Was adequate information extracted about methodologic and administrative aspects of the study? Was adequate information about sample characteristics extracted?
- Was sufficient information extracted about study findings?
- Were steps taken to enhance the integrity of the dataset (e.g., were two or more people used to extract and record information for analysis)?

Data Analysis—General

■ Did the reviewers explain their method of pooling and integrating the data?

■ Was the analysis of data thorough and credible?

■ Were tables, figures, and text used effectively to summarize findings?

Data Analysis—Quantitative

■ If a meta-analysis was not performed, was there adequate justification for using a narrative integration method? If a meta-analysis *was* performed, was this justifiable?

■ For meta-analyses, did the report describe how effect sizes were computed? Were appropriate procedures followed for computing effect size estimates for all relevant outcomes?

■ Was heterogeneity of effects adequately dealt with? Was the decision to use a random effects model versus a fixed effects model sound? Were appropriate subgroup analyses undertaken—or was the absence of subgroup analyses justified?

■ Was the issue of publication bias adequately addressed?

Data Analysis—Qualitative

■ In a metasynthesis, did the reviewers describe the techniques they used to compare the findings of each study, and do they explain their method of interpreting their data?

■ If a meta-summary was undertaken, did the abstracted findings seem appropriate and convincing? Were appropriate methods used to compute effect sizes? Was information presented effectively?

■ In a metasynthesis, did the synthesis achieve a fuller understanding of the phenomenon to advance knowledge? Do the interpretations seem well-grounded? Was there a sufficient amount of data included to support the interpretations?

Conclusions

■ Did the reviewers draw reasonable conclusions about the quality, quantity, and consistency of evidence relating to the research question?

■ Are limitations of the review/synthesis noted?

■ Are implications for nursing practice and further research clearly stated?

     All systematic reviews
     Systematic reviews of quantitative studies
     Metasyntheses

We conclude this chapter with a description two systematic reviews. We note also that two synthesis reports (a meta-analysis and a metasynthesis) appear in their entirety in the *Study Guide* for this book.

EXAMPLE 1 ■ A Meta-Analysis

Study

Effects of acculturation on smoking behavior in Asian Americans: A meta-analysis (Choi et al., 2008).

Purpose

The purposes of the study were to undertake a meta-analysis to (1) examine the extent to which acculturation (the process by which foreign-born people adopt the values, customs, and behaviors of the mainstream culture) affects smoking behavior in Asian immigrants to the United States and (2) examine whether acculturation had different effects on subgroups of immigrants, specifically men, women, and adolescents.

Eligibility Criteria

A study was included if it examined the relationship between acculturation and smoking, involved Asian American study participants, and was published in English or Korean. Studies were excluded if they used qualitative methods, focused on Pacific Islander populations, or duplicated a dataset already in the analysis.

Search Strategy

The strategy involved a search of four databases: MEDLINE (via PubMed), CINAHL, the Cochrane Library, and PsychInfo. The search terms included acculturation; smoking; tobacco; and Asian, Asian American, and Asian immigrants.

Sample

The initial search yielded 21 studies, of which 11 met the eligibility criteria. Two of the 11 studies were subsequently excluded because the researchers were unable to calculate effect sizes with the data provided. Thus, nine studies, all of which were cross-sectional, nonexperimental studies, were included in the meta-analysis. The nine studies involved a total of nearly 17,000 study participants who had immigrated to the United States from Korea, China, Japan, Vietnam, Cambodia, and other Asian countries.

Data Extraction

Using a data extraction form developed for the study, data were extracted to record sample characteristics, acculturation, smoking rate or prevalence, and methodologic characteristics of the study.

Quality Assessments

The quality of the study methods was assessed by the first author using a quality assessment scale that was adapted from an existing instrument. Ten criteria were appraised on a 4-point scale and then added to form a total quality score. Total possible scores could range from 0 to 30. Any study with a score of less than 20 was eliminated from the analysis. Actual quality scores ranged from 23 to 28, and thus no studies were eliminated based on quality.

Effect Size Calculation

The odds ratio (OR) was selected as the effect size measure in this study, with the OR representing the ratio of the odds of smoking in the acculturated group relative to the odds of smoking in the traditional (nonacculturated) group. Although researchers in the primary studies used different means of measuring acculturated versus traditional, Choi and colleagues used the operational definitions or cutpoints adopted in the original studies. For adult samples, a smoker was defined as someone who had smoked at least 100 cigarettes in his or her lifetime and was currently smoking. For adolescents, smoking was defined as ever smoked a cigarette.

Statistical Analyses

Both random effects and fixed effects models were used to estimate pooled effect sizes in this study but, because of considerable heterogeneity, random effects results were reported. Subgroup analyses were performed to examine whether the effect size results varied by population subgroups. Publication bias was not formally assessed.

Key Findings

The overall average weighted effect size (OR) was .98, with the 95% CI = .53, 1.81. If the 95% CI around an OR includes 1, the OR is not statistically significant, and so there was no overall difference in the prevalence of smoking between acculturated and traditional groups in this meta-analysis. The subgroup analyses, however, suggested that acculturated men were .53 times less likely to smoke than traditional men (OR = .53, 95% CI = .28, .99). By contrast, acculturated women were found to be 5 times *more* likely to smoke than traditional women (OR = 5.26, 95% CI = 2.75, 10.05). Adolescent Asian Americans who were acculturated were about twice as likely to smoke as their traditional counterparts (OR = 1.92, 95% CI = 1.22, 3.01).

Discussion

The researchers concluded that acculturation may have a protective effect for Asian American men, but a harmful effect for women and adolescents, which in turn suggests special opportunities for smoking cessation programs—and the need to take acculturation into account.

CRITICAL THINKING SUGGESTIONS*:

*See the Student Resource CD-ROM for a discussion of these questions.

1. Answer the relevant questions from Box 19.1 regarding this study.
2. Also, consider the following targeted questions, which may further sharpen your critical thinking skills and assist you in understanding this study:
   a. Comment on the fact that the review included articles published in both English and Korean.
   b. Comment on the reviewers' definition of their independent variable (i.e., acculturation).
3. What might be some of the uses to which the findings could be put in clinical practice?

EXAMPLE 2 ■ A Metasynthesis

Study

Adolescent depression: A metasynthesis (Dundon, 2006).

Purpose

The purpose of the study was to synthesize qualitative studies on the experience of adolescent depression. Dundon wrote, "The aim of this study was to unify the voices of the adolescents who have participated in qualitative research in order to contribute to the theoretic base of the experience of adolescent depression, affect future research, and guide clinical practice" (p. 384).

Eligibility Criteria

The only inclusion criteria noted in the report were that the study design of a primary study had to be qualitative and that the study had to focus on adolescent depression. (Presumably, studies not reported in English-language publications were excluded.)

Search Strategy

Dundon did an interdisciplinary online search of the following databases for studies published between 1970 and January, 2005: CINAHL, Psychlit, MEDLINE, Sociological Abstracts, and Dissertation Abstracts. Search terms included adolescent depression, teen depression, child depression, qualitative research, theme, grounded theory, and phenomenology.

Sample

The sample for the metasynthesis included four articles and two dissertations published between 2002 and 2004. All studies were conducted in the United States or Canada. The disciplinary roots of the six studies included nursing, psychology, public health, preventive medicine, and social work. The research traditions of the primary studies included grounded theory, discourse analysis, narrative therapy, participatory action research, and phenomenology

Data Extraction and Analysis

Noblit and Hare's approach was used to compare and integrate study findings. The original metaphors, themes, concepts, and phrases from each of the six studies were organized and reciprocally translated. Dundon noted the special challenges involved in integrating findings from such a wide array of qualitative traditions. For example, findings from the study that used discourse analysis were not arranged thematically but rather as significant statements from which meanings and themes had to be formulated.

Key Findings

Dundon's metasynthesis revealed six themes that outline the course of adolescents struggling with depression: (1) beyond the blues; (2) spiraling down and within; (3) breaking points; (4) seeing and being seen; (5) seeking solutions; and (6) taking control.

Discussion

Dundon concluded that the metasynthesis provides practitioners with a more detailed understanding of the experience of adolescent depression, and can serve to guide efforts to recognize the symptoms and to intervene with appropriate help.

CRITICAL THINKING SUGGESTIONS*:

*See the Student Resource CD-ROM for a discussion of these questions.

1. Answer the relevant questions from Box 19.1 regarding this study.
2. Also, consider the following targeted questions, which may further sharpen your critical thinking skills and assist you in understanding this study:
   a. Do you think it would have been possible for Dundon to compute frequency and intensity effect sizes with her sample of studies?
   b. Do you think Dundon should have searched for studies done in other countries and written in other languages? Why or why not?
3. What might be some of the uses to which the findings could be put in clinical practice?

CHAPTER REVIEW
....

Key new terms introduced in the chapter, together with a summary of major points, are presented in this section. In addition, Chapter 19 of the accompanying *Study Guide for Essentials of Nursing Research*, 7th edition offers various exercises and study suggestions for reinforcing concepts presented in this chapter. For additional review, see the Student Self-Study Review Questions section of the Student Resource CD-ROM provided with this book.

Key New Terms
....

Forest plot	Meta-analysis	Primary study
Funnel plot	Meta-summary	Publication bias
Manifest effect size	Metasynthesis	Statistical heterogeneity

Summary Points
....

➤ Evidence-based practice relies on rigorous integration of research evidence on a topic through **systematic reviews** of quantitative findings and metasyntheses of qualitative findings.

➤ Systematic reviews often involve statistical integration of findings through meta-analysis, a procedure whose advantages include objectivity, enhanced power, and precision; **meta-analysis** is not appropriate, however, for broad questions or when there is substantial inconsistency of findings.

➤ The steps in both quantitative and qualitative integration are similar and involve: formulating the problem, designing the study (including establishing sampling criteria), searching the literature for a sample of **primary studies** to be included in the review, evaluating study quality, extracting and encoding data for analysis, analyzing the data, and reporting the findings.

➤ There is no consensus on whether integrations should include the **grey literature** (i.e., unpublished reports); in quantitative studies, a concern is that there is a *bias against the null hypothesis*, a **publication bias** stemming from the underrepresentation of nonsignificant findings in the published literature.

➤ In meta-analysis, findings from primary studies are represented by an **effect size** index that quantifies the magnitude and direction of relationship between the independent and dependent variables. The most common effect size indexes in nursing are *d* (the *standardized mean difference*) and the odds ratio.

➤ Effects from individual studies are pooled to yield an estimate of the population effect size by calculating a weighted average of effects, often using the *inverse variance* as the weight—which gives greater weight to larger studies

❧ **Statistical heterogeneity** (diversity in effects across studies) is a major issue in meta-analysis, and affects decisions about using a **fixed effects model** (which assumes a single true effect size) or a **random effects model** (which assumes a distribution of effects). Heterogeneity can be examined using a **forest plot**.

❧ Nonrandom heterogeneity can be explored through **subgroup analyses** (*moderator analyses*), the purpose of which is to identify clinical or methodologic features systematically related to variation in effects.

❧ Quality assessments (which may involve formal quantitative ratings of methodologic rigor) are sometimes used to exclude weak studies from the analysis, but they can also be used to differentially weight studies or in **sensitivity analyses** to determine if including or excluding weaker studies changes conclusions.

❧ Publication bias can be examined by constructing a **funnel plot**, and can be partially addressed by calculating a **fail-safe number** that estimates the number of studies with a zero effect size that would be needed to reverse the conclusion of a significant effect.

❧ Metasyntheses are more than just summaries of prior qualitative findings; they involve a discovery of essential features of a body of findings and a transformation that yields new interpretations.

❧ Numerous approaches to metasynthesis (and many terms related to qualitative integration) have been proposed. Metasynthesists grapple with such issues as whether to combine findings from different research traditions, and whether to exclude poor quality studies.

❧ One approach to qualitative integration, proposed by Noblit and Hare, involves listing key themes or metaphors across studies and then translating them into each other.

❧ Paterson and colleagues' meta-study method integrates three components: (1) **meta-data analysis**, the study of results in a specific substantive area through analysis of the "processed data;" (2) **meta-method**, the study of the studies' methodologic rigor; and (3) **meta-theory**, the analysis of the theoretical underpinnings on which the studies are grounded.

❧ A **meta-summary**, a method developed by Sandelowski and Barroso, involves listing abstracted findings from the primary studies and calculating **manifest effect sizes**. A **frequency effect size** is the percentage of reports that contain a given findings. An **intensity effect size** indicates the percentage of all findings that are contained in any given report.

❧ In the Sandelowski and Barroso approach, a meta-summary can lay the foundation for a metasynthesis, which can use a variety of qualitative approaches to analysis and interpretations (e.g., constant comparison).

STUDIES CITED IN CHAPTER 19

Berry, A., Davidson, P., Masters, J., & Rolls, K. (2007). Systematic literature review of oral hygiene practices for intensive care patients. *American Journal of Critical Care, 16,* 552–562.

Berterö, C., & Chamberlain-Wilmoth, M. (2007). Breast cancer diagnosis and its treatment affecting the self: A metasynthesis. *Cancer Nursing, 30,* 194–202.

Briggs, M., & Flemming, K. (2007). Living with leg ulceration: A synthesis of qualitative research. *Journal of Advanced Nursing, 59*, 319–328.

Choi, H., Palmer, M., & Park, J. (2007). Meta-analysis of pelvic floor muscle training. *Nursing Research, 56*, 226–234.

Choi, S., Rankin, S., Stewart, A., & Oka, R. (2008). Effects of acculturation on smoking behavior in Asian Americans: A meta-analysis. *Journal of Cardiovascular Nursing, 23*, 67–73.

Conn, V., Hafdahl, A., Brown, S., & Brown, L. (2008). Meta-analysis of patient education interventions to increase physical activity among chronically ill adults. *Patient Education and Counseling, 70*, 57–172.

Coussement, J., De Paepe, L., Schwendimann, R., Denhaerynck, E., Dejaeger, E., & Milisen, K. (2008). Interventions for preventing falls in acute- and chronic-care hospitals: A systematic review and meta-analysis. *Journal of the American Geriatrics Society, 56*, 29–36.

Dundon, E. (2006). Adolescent depression: A metasynthesis. *Journal of Pediatric Health Care, 20*, 384–392.

Forbes, D. A. (2003). An example of the use of systematic reviews to answer an effectiveness question. *Western Journal of Nursing Research, 25*, 179–192.

Goodman, J. H. (2005). Becoming an involved father of an infant. *Journal of Obstetric, Gynecologic, & Neonatal Nursing, 34*, 190–200.

Mahon, N., Yarcheski, A., Yarcheski, T., Cannella, B., & Hanks, M. (2006). A meta-analytic study of predictors for loneliness during adolescence. *Nursing Research, 55*, 308–315.

Noyes, J., & Popay, J. (2007). Directly observed therapy and tuberculosis: How can a systematic review of qualitative research contribute to improving services? A qualitative metasynthesis. *Journal of Advanced Nursing, 57*, 227–243.

Paterson, B. (2001). The shifting perspectives model of chronic illness. *Journal of Nursing Scholarship, 33*, 57–62.

Peacock, S. C., & Forbes, D. A. (2003). Interventions for caregivers of persons with dementia: A systematic review. *Canadian Journal of Nursing Research, 35*, 88–107.

Rice, V., & Stead, L. (2008). Nursing interventions for smoking cessation. *Cochrane Database of Systematic Reviews*, Issue 1, Art. No: CD001188.

Sandelowski, M., & Barroso, J. (2005). The travesty of choosing after positive prenatal diagnosis. *Journal of Obstetric, Gynecologic, & Neonatal Nursing, 34*, 307–318.

Varcoe, C., Rodney, P., & McCormick, J. (2003). Health care relationships in context: An analysis of three ethnographies. *Qualitative Health Research, 13*(7), 957–973.

Wagg, A., & Bunn, F. (2007). Unassisted pelvic floor exercises for postnatal women: A systematic review. *Journal of Advanced Nursing, 58*, 407–417.

Xu, Y. (2007). Strangers in strange lands: A metasynthesis of lived experiences of immigrant Asian nurses working in western countries. *Advances in Nursing Science, 30*, 246–265.

Zangaro, G., & Soeken, K. (2007). A meta-analysis of studies of nurses' job satisfaction. *Research in Nursing & Health, 30*, 445–458.

Methodologic and Theoretical References

Agency for Healthcare Research and Quality. (2002). *Systems to rate the strength of scientific evidence.* Washington, DC: AHRQ.

AGREE Collaboration. (2001). *Appraisal of guidelines for research and evaluation (AGREE instrument).* Retrieved January 11, 2008 from http://www.agree collaboration.org.

Ajzen, I. (2005). *Attitudes, personality, and behavior.* (2nd ed.). Milton Keynes, United Kingdom: Open University Press/McGraw Hill.

Allen, F. M., & Warner, M. (2002). A developmental model of health and nursing. *Journal of Family Issues, 8,* 96–135.

Bandura, A. (1985). *Social foundations of thought and action: A social cognitive theory.* Englewood Cliffs, NJ: Prentice Hall.

Becker, M. (1976). *Health Belief Model and personal health behavior.* Thorofare, NJ: Slack, Inc.

Becker, H. S. (1970). *Sociological work.* Chicago: Aldine.

Benner, P. (1994). The tradition and skill of interpretive phenomenology in studying health, illness, and caring practices (pp. 99–127) in P. Benner (ed). *Interpretive phenomenology.* Thousand Oaks, Ca: Sage.

Blumer, H. (1986). *Symbolic interactionism: Perspective and method.* Berkeley: University of California Press.

Bradford-Hill, A. (1971). *Principles of medical statistics* (9th ed.). New York: Oxford University Press.

Bulecheck G., Butcher, H., & Dochterman, J. M. (2007). *Nursing interventions classification (NIC)* (5th ed.). St. Louis: Mosby.

Burke, K. (1969). *A grammar of motives.* Berkley, Ca: University of California Press.

Chinn, P. L., & Kramer, M. K. (2003). *Integrated knowledge development in nursing.* St. Louis: C. V. Mosby.

Ciliska, D., & Guyatt, G. (2005). Publication bias. In DiCenso, A., Guyatt, G., & Ciliska, D. *Evidence-based nursing: A guide to clinical practice.* St. Louis: Elsevier Mosby.

Cohen, J. (1988). *Statistical power analysis for the behavioral sciences* (2nd ed.). Mahwah, NJ: Erlbaum.

Colaizzi, P. (1978). Psychological research as the phenomenologist views it. In R. Valle & M. King (Eds.), *Existential phenomenological alternatives for psychology* (pp. 48–71). New York: Oxford University Press.

Conn, V., & Rantz, M. (2003). Research methods: Managing primary study quality in meta-analyses. *Research in Nursing & Health, 26,* 322–333.

Conn, V., Valentine, J., Cooper, H., & Rantz, M. (2003). Grey literature in meta-analyses. *Nursing Research, 52,* 256–261.

Cook, K. E. (2005). Using critical ethnography to explore issues in health promotion. *Qualitative Health Research, 15*(1), 129–138.

Cooper, H. (1998). *Synthesizing research* (3rd ed.). Thousand Oaks, CA: Sage Publications.

Crabtree, B. F., & Miller, W. L. (Eds.). (1999). *Doing qualitative research* (2nd ed.). Newbury Park, CA: Sage.

Denzin, N. K. (1989). *The research act* (3rd ed.). New York: McGraw-Hill.

Denzin, N. K., & Lincoln, Y. S. (Eds.). (2000). *Handbook of qualitative research* (2nd ed.). Thousand Oaks, CA: Sage.

DeSantis, L., & Ugarriza, D. N. (2000). The concept of theme as used in qualitative nursing research. *Western Journal of Nursing Research, 22,* 351–372.

DiCenso, A., Guyatt, G., & Ciliska, D. (2005). *Evidence-based nursing: A guide to clinical practice.* St. Louis, MO: Elsevier Mosby.

Diekelmann, N. L., Allen, D., & Tanner, C. (1989). *The NLN criteria for appraisal of baccalaureate programs. A critical hermeneutic analysis.* New York: NLN Press.

Dodd, M., Janson, S., Facione, N., Fawcett, J., Froelicher, E.S., Humphreys, J., et al. (2001). Advancing the science of symptom management. *Journal of Advanced Nursing, 33,* 668–676.

Donabedian, A. (1987). Some basic issues in evaluating the quality of health care. In L. T. Rinke (Ed.), *Outcome measures in home care* (Vol. I, pp. 3–28). New York: National League for Nursing.

Donaldson, S. K. (2000). Breakthroughs in scientific research: The discipline of nursing, 1960–1999. *Annual Review of Nursing Research, 18,* 247–311.

Fawcett, J. (2005). *Contemporary nursing knowledge: Analysis and evaluation of nursing models and theories.* Philadelphia: F. A. Davis.

Fawcett, J. (1999). *The relationship between theory and research* (3rd ed.). Philadelphia: F. A. Davis.

Fetterman, D. M. (1997). *Ethnography*: *Step by step* (2nd ed.). Newbury Park, CA: Sage.

Fineout-Overholt, E., & Johnston, L. (2005). Teaching EBP: Asking searchable, answerable clinical questions. *Worldviews on Evidence-Based Nursing, 2,* 157–160.

Finfgeld, D. (2003). Metasynthesis: The state of the art—so far. *Qualitative Health Research, 13,* 893–904.

Fink, A. (2005). *Conducting research literature reviews: From paper to the Internet* (2nd ed.). Thousand Oaks, CA: Sage.

Gadamer, H. G. (1975). *Truth and method.* G. Borden & J. Cumming (trans). London: Sheed and Ward.

Galvan, J. L. (2003). *Writing literature reviews: A guide for students of the social and behavioral sciences* (2nd ed.). Los Angeles: Pyrczak Pub.

Garrard, J. (2004). Health sciences literature review made easy: The matrix method. Boston: Jones and Bartlett Publishers.

Gee, J. P. (1996). *Social linguistics and literacies: Ideology in discourses* (2nd ed.). London: Taylor & Francis.

Gennaro, S., Hodnett, E., & Kearney, M. (2001). Making evidence-based practice a reality in your institution. *MCN: The American Journal of Maternal/ Child Nursing, 26,* 236–244.

Giorgi, A. (1985). *Phenomenology and psychological research.* Pittsburgh, PA: Duquesne University Press.

Glaser, B. G. (2005). *The grounded theory perspective III: Theoretical coding.* Mill Valley: Sociology Press.

Glaser, B. G. (1998). *Doing grounded theory: Issues and discussions.* Mill Valley, CA: Sociology Press.

Glaser, B. G. (1992). *Emergence versus forcing: Basics of grounded theory analysis.* Mill Valley, CA.: Sociology Press.

Glaser, B. G. (1978). *Theoretical sensitivity.* Mill Valley, CA: Sociology Press.

Glaser, B. G., & Strauss, A. L. (1967). *The discovery of grounded theory: Strategies for qualitative research.* Chicago: Aldine.

Guba, E., & Lincoln, Y. (1994). Competing paradigms in qualitative research. In N. Denzin & Y. Lincoln (Eds.). *Handbook of qualitative research,* pp. 105–117. Thousand Oaks, CA: Sage.

Guyatt, G., & Rennie, D. (2002). *Users' guide to the medical literature: Essentials of evidence-based clinical practice.* Chicago: American Medical Association Press.

Horsley, J. A., Crane, J., & Bingle, J. D. (1978). Research utilization as an organizational process. *Journal of Nursing Administration, 8,* 4–6.

Huberman, A. M., & Miles, M. (1994). Data management and analysis methods. In Denzin, N. K., & Lincoln, Y. S. (Eds.). *Handbook of qualitative research.* (1st ed.). Thousand Oaks, CA: Sage.

Johnson, J. E. (1999). Self-Regulation Theory and coping with physical illness. *Research in Nursing & Health, 22,* 435–448.

Kerlinger, F. N., & Lee, H. B. (2000). *Foundations of behavioral research* (4th ed.). Orlando, FL: Harcourt College Publishers.

Kolcaba, K. (2003). *Comfort theory and practice.* New York: Springer Publishing Co.

Lazarus, R., & Folkman, S. (1984). *Stress, appraisal, and coping.* New York: Springer Publishing Co.

Leininger, M. & McFarland, M. (2006). *Culture care diversity and universality: A worldwide nursing theory* (2nd ed.). Sudbury, Ma: Jones and Bartlett Publishers.

Lenz, E. R., Pugh, L. C., Milligan, R. A., Gift, A., & Suppe, F. (1997). The middle-range theory of unpleasant symptoms. *Advances in Nursing Science, 19,* 14–27.

Levine, M. E. (1973). *Introduction to clinical nursing* (2nd ed.). Philadelphia: F. A. Davis.

Lewis, S. (2001). Further disquiet on the guidelines front. *Canadian Medical Association Journal, 154,* 180–181.

Lincoln, Y. S., & Guba, E. G. (1985). *Naturalistic inquiry.* Newbury Park, CA: Sage.

Logan, J., & Graham, I. (1998). Toward a comprehensive interdisciplinary model of health care research use. *Science Communication, 20,* 227–246.

McCormick, J., Rodney, P., & Varcoe, C. (2003). Reinterpretations across studies: An approach to meta-analysis. *Qualitative Health Research, 13,* 933–944.

Meleis, A., I., Sawyer, L. M., Im, E., Hilfinger, Messias, D., & Schumacher, K. (2000). Experiencing transitions: An emerging middle-range theory. *Advances in Nursing Science, 23,* 12–28.

Melnyk, B. M., & Fineout-Overhold, E. (2005). *Evidence-based practice in nursing and healthcare: A guide to best practice.* Philadelphia: Lippincott Williams & Wilkins.

Millenson, M. L. (1997). *Demanding medical evidence.* Chicago: University of Chicago Press.

Mishel, M. H. (1990). Reconceptualization of the Uncertainty in Illness Theory. *Image: Journal of Nursing Scholarship, 22*(4), 256–262.

Mitchell, P., Ferketich, S., & Jennings, B. (1998). Quality health outcomes model. *Image: The Journal of Nursing Scholarship, 30,* 43–46.

Moorhead, S., Johnson, M., Maas, M., & Swanson, E. (2007). *Nursing outcomes classification (NOC)* (4th ed.). St. Louis: Mosby.

Morse, J. (2005). Beyond the clinical trial: Expanding criteria for evidence. *Qualitative Health Resaerch, 15,* 3–4.

Morse, J. M. (2006). Insight, inference, evidence, and verification: Creating a legitimate discipline. *International Journal of Qualitative Methods, 5*(1), Article 8. Retrieved January 12, 2007 from http://www.ualberta.ca/ijqm/.

Morse, J. M. (2006). The scope of qualitatively derived clinical interventions. *Qualitative Health Research, 16*(5), 591–593.

Morse, J. M. (2004). Qualitative comparison: Appropriateness, equivalence, and fit. *Qualitative Health Research, 14*(10), 1323–1325

Morse, J. M. (2000). Determining sample size. *Qualitative Health Research, 10,* 3–5.

Morse, J. M. (1991). Strategies for sampling. In J. M. Morse (Ed.), *Qualitative nursing research: A contemporary dialogue.* Newbury Park, CA: Sage.

Morse, J. M., Barrett, M., Mayan, M., Olson, K., & Spiers, J. (2002). Verification strategies for establishing reliability and validity in qualitative research. *International Journal of Qualitative Methods, 1*(2), Article 2. Retrieved January 12, 2007 from http://www.ualberta.ca/ijqm/.

Morse, J. M., & Field, P. A. (1995). *Qualitative research methods for health professionals* (2nd ed.). Thousand Oaks, CA: Sage Publications.

Morse, J. M., Solberg, S. M., Neander, W. L., Bottorff, J. L., & Johnson, J. L. (1990). Concepts of caring and caring as a concept. *Advances in Nursing Science, 13,* 1–14.

Munro, B. H. (Ed.). (2004). *Statistical methods for health-care research* (5th ed.). Philadelphia: Lippincott Williams & Wilkins.

NANDA International. (2008). *Nursing Diagnoses: Definitions and Classification, 2007–2008.* Philadelphia: Author.

National Institute for Nursing Research (2006). *Changing practice, changing lives: Ten landmark nursing research studies.* Washington, DC: NINR.

Neuman, B. & Fawcett, J. (2001). *The Neuman Systems Model* (4th ed.). Englewood, NJ: Prentice Hall.

Newhouse, R., Dearholt, S., Poe, S., Pugh, L. C., & White, K. M. (2005). Evidence-based practice: A practical approach to implementation. *Journal of Nursing Administration, 35,* 35–40.

Newman, M. (1994). *Health as expanding consciousness* (2nd ed.). New York: National League for Nursing.

Noblit, G., & Hare, R. D. (1988). *Meta-ethnography: Synthesizing qualitative studies.* Newbury Park, CA: Sage.

Olesen, V. (2000). Feminisms and qualitative research at and into the millennium. In N. K. Denzin & Y. S. Lincoln (Eds.), *Handbook of qualitative research* (2nd ed., pp. 215–255). Thousand Oaks, CA: Sage.

Orem, D. E., Taylor, S. G., Renpenning, K. M., & Eisenhandler, S. A. (2003). *Self-care theory in nursing: Selected papers of Dorothea Orem.* New York: Springer Publishing Co.

Parse, R. R. (1999). *Illuminations: The human becoming theory in practice and research.* Sudbury, MA: Jones & Bartlett.

Paterson, B. L., Thorne, S. E., Canam, C., & Jillings, C. (2001). *Meta-study of qualitative health research.* Thousand Oaks, CA: Sage.

Patton, M. (1999). Enhancing the quality and credibility of qualitative analysis. *Health Services Research, 34*(5 Part 2), 1189–1208.

Patton, M. Q. (2002). *Qualitative evaluation and research methods* (3rd ed.). Thousand Oaks, CA: Sage.

Pender, N. J., Murdaugh, C., & Parsons, M. A. (2006). *Health promotion in nursing practice* (5th ed.). Upper Saddle River, NJ: Prentice Hall.

Polit, D. F. (1996). *Data analysis and statistics for nursing research.* Stamford, CT: Appleton & Lange.

Polit, D., & Beck, C. (2008). *Nursing research: Generating and appraising evidence for nursing practice* (8th ed.) Philadelphia: Lippincott Williams & Wilkins.

Polit, D., & Beck, C. (2006). The content validity index: Are you sure you know what's being reported? *Research in Nursing & Health, 29,*489–497.

Prochaska, J. O., Redding, C. A., & Evers, K. E. (2002). The Transtheoretical Model and stages of changes. In F. M. Lewis (Ed.) *Health behavior and health education: Theory, research and practice* (pp. 99–120). San Francisco: Jossey Bass.

Reed, P. G. (1991). Toward a nursing theory of self-transcendence. *Advances in Nursing Science, 13*(4), 64–77.

Ricoeur, P. (1981). *Hermeneutics and the social sciences.* (J. Thompson, trans. & ed). New York: Cambridge University Press.

Riessman, C. K. (1993). *Narrative analysis.* Newbury Park, CA: Sage.

Rogers, E. M. (1995). *Diffusion of innovations* (4th ed.). New York: Free Press.

Rogers, M. E. (1986). Science of unitary human beings. In V. Malinski (Ed.), *Explorations on Martha Rogers' science of unitary human beings.* Norwalk, CT: Appleton-Century-Crofts.

Rosenstock, I., Stretcher, V., & Becker, M. (1988). Social learning theory and the Health Belief Model. *Health Education Quarterly, 15,* 175–183.

Roy, C. Sr., & Andrews, H. (1999). *The Roy Adaptation Model.* (2nd ed.). Norwalk, CT: Appleton & Lange.

Rycroft-Malone, J. (2007). Theory and knowledge translation, *Nursing Research, 56,* S78–S85.

Rycroft-Malone, J., Seers, K., Titchen, A., Harvey, G., Kitson, A., & McCormack, B. (2002). Getting evidence into practice: Ingredients for change. *Nursing Standard, 16,* 38–43.

Sackett, D. L., Straus, S. E., Richardson, W. S., Rosenberg, W., & Haynes, R. B. (2000). *Evidence-based medicine: How to practice and teach EBM* (2nd ed.). Edinburgh: Churchill Livingstone.

Sandelowski, M. (2000). Combining qualitative and quantitative sampling, data collection, and analysis techniques in mixed-method studies. *Research in Nursing & Health, 23,* 246–255.

Sandelowski, M. (2004). Counting cats in Zanzibar. *Research in Nursing & Health, 27,* 215–216.

Sandelowski, M. (1993). Theory unmasked: The uses and guises of theory in qualitative research. *Research in Nursing & Health, 16,* 213–218.

Sandelowski, M., & Barroso, J. (2006). *Synthesizing qualitative research.* York: Springer Publishing Company.

Sandelowski, M., & Barroso, J. (2003a). Creating metasummaries of qualitative findings. *Nursing Research, 52,* 226–233.

Sandelowski, M., & Barroso, J. (2003b). Toward a metasynthesis of qualitative findings on motherhood in HIV-positive women. *Research in Nursing & Health, 26,* 153–170.

Sandelowski, M., & Barroso, J. (2002). Finding the findings in qualitative studies. *Journal of Nursing Scholarship, 34,* 213–219.

Sandelowski, M., Docherty, S., & Emden, C. (1997). Qualitative metasynthesis: Issues and techniques. *Research in Nursing & Health, 20,* 365–377.

Schreiber, R., Crooks, D., & Stern, P. N. (1997). Qualitative meta-analysis. In J. M. Morse (Ed.), *Completing a qualitative project* (pp. 311–326). Thousand Oaks, CA: Sage.

Shadish, W. R., Cook, T. D., & Campbell, D. T. (2002). *Experimental and quasi-experimental designs for generalized causal inference.* Boston: Houghton Mifflin Co.

Sidani, S., & Braden, C. J. (1998). *Evaluating nursing interventions: A theory driven approach.* Thousand Oaks, CA: Sage.

Sindhu, F., Carpenter, L., & Seers, K. (1997). Development of a tool to rate the quality assessment of randomized controlled trials using a Delphi technique. *Journal of Advanced Nursing, 25,* 1262–1268.

Sigma Theta Tau International. (2005). Resource paper on global health and nursing research priorities. Accessed January 7, 2008 at http://www2.nursingsociety.org/about/position_GHNRPRP.doc .

Silva, M. C. (1986). Research testing nursing theory: State of the art. *Advances in Nursing Science, 9,* 1–11.

Smith, M. J., & Liehr, P. (2003). *Middle-range theory for nursing.* New York, NY: Springer Publishing Co.

Spradley, J. P. (1979). *The ethnographic interview.* New York: Holt, Rinehart, and Winston.

Stetler, C. B. (2001). Updating the Stetler model of research utilization to facilitate evidence-based practice. *Nursing Outlook, 49,* 272–279.

Stetler, C. B., & Marram, G. (1976). Evaluating research findings for applicability in practice. *Nursing Outlook, 24,* 559–563.

Strauss, A., & Corbin, J. (1998). Basics of qualitative research: Grounded theory procedures and techniques (2nd ed.). Thousand Oaks, CA: Sage.

Strauss, A. L., & Corbin, J. M. (1998). *Basics of qualitative research: Techniques and procedures for developing grounded theory* (2nd ed.) Thousand Oaks, CA: Sage.

Tashakkori, A., & Teddlie, C. (2003). *Handbook of mixed methods in social and behavioral research* (2nd ed.). Thousand Oaks, CA: Sage.

Taylor, S. G., Geden, E., Isaramalai, S., & Wong-vatunyu, S. (2000). Orem's Self-Care Deficit Nursing Theory: Its philosophic foundation and the state of the science. *Nursing Science Quarterly, 13*(2), 104–110.

Thorne, S. (1994). Secondary analysis in qualitative research: Issues and implications. In J. M. Morse (Ed.), *Critical issues in qualitative research methods.* Thousand Oaks, CA: Sage.

Thorne, S. & Darbyshire, P. (2005). Land mines in the field: A modest proposal for improving the craft of qualitative health research. *Qualitative Health Research, 15*(8), 1105–1113.

Titler, M. G., & Everett, L. Q. (2001). Translating research into practice. Considerations for critical care investigators. *Critical Care Nursing Clinics of North America, 13,* 587–604.

Titler, M. G., Kleiber, C., Steelman, V., Rakel, B., Budreau, G., Everett, L., Buckwalter, K., Tripp-Reimer, T., & Goode, C. (2001). The Iowa model of evidence-based practice to promote quality care. *Critical Care Nursing Clinics of North America, 13,* 497–509.

Tomey, A., & Alligood, M. (2006). *Nursing theorists and their work.* (6th ed.). St. Louis: Mosby.

Turkel, M. C., Reidinger, G., Ferket, K., & Reno, K. (2005). An essential component of the magnet journey: Fostering an environment for evidence-based practice and nursing research. *Nursing Administration Quarterly, 29,* 254–262.

Van Kaam, A. (1966). *Existential foundations of psychology.* Pittsburgh, PA: Duquesne University Press.

Van Manen, M. (1997). *Researching lived experience* (2nd ed.). London, ON: The Althouse Press.

Walker, L., & Avant, K. (2004). *Strategies for theory construction in nursing* (4th ed.). Upper Saddle River, NJ: Prentice-Hall.

Waltz, C. F., Strickland, O. L., & Lenz, E. R. (2005). *Measurement in nursing and health research.* (3rd ed.). New York: Springer Publishing Co.

Watson, J. (2005). *Caring science as sacred science.* Philadelphia: F. A. Davis.

Watson, L., & Girard, F. (2004). Establishing integrity and avoiding methodological misunderstanding. *Qualitative Health Research, 14,* 875–881.

Whittemore, R., Chase, S. K., & Mandle, C. L. (2001). Validity in qualitative research. *Qualitative Health Research, 11*(4), 522–537.

Whittemore, R., & Grey, M. (2002). The systematic development of nursing interventions. *Journal of Nursing Scholarship, 34,* 115–120.

Glossary

*Entries preceded by an asterisk (*) are terms that were not explained in this book, but they are included here because you might come across them in the research literature. For further explanation of these terms, please refer to Polit and Beck (2008) *Nursing Research: Generating and Assessing Evidence for Nursing Practice*, 8th edition. Philadelphia, PA: Lippincott Williams & Wilkins.

absolute risk The proportion of people in a group who experienced an undesirable outcome.

absolute risk reduction (ARR) The difference between the absolute risk in one group (e.g., those exposed to an intervention) and the absolute risk in another group (e.g., those not exposed).

abstract A brief description of a study, usually located at the beginning of a report.

accessible population The population of people available for a particular study—often, a nonrandom subset of the target population.

acquiescence response set A bias in self-report instruments, especially in psychosocial scales, created when participants characteristically agree with statements ("yea-say"), independent of content.

after-only design An experimental design in which data are collected from participants only after an intervention has been introduced.

***allocation concealment** The process used to ensure that those enrolling participants into a clinical trial are unaware of upcoming assignments (i.e., the treatment group to which new enrollees will be assigned).

alpha (α) (1) In tests of statistical significance, the level indicating the probability of a Type I error; (2) in assessments of internal consistency reliability, a reliability coefficient, Cronbach's alpha.

analysis The process of organizing and synthesizing data so as to answer research questions and test hypotheses.

analysis of covariance (ANCOVA) A statistical procedure used to test mean differences among groups on a dependent variable, while controlling for one or more covariates.

analysis of variance (ANOVA) A statistical procedure for testing mean differences among three or more groups by comparing variability between groups to variability within groups.

ancestry approach In literature searches, using citations from relevant studies to track down earlier research on which the studies are based (the "ancestors").

anonymity Protection of participants' confidentiality such that even the researcher cannot link individuals with data provided.

applied research Research designed to find a solution to an immediate practical problem.

***arm** A group of participants, allocated a particular treatment condition (e.g., the control *arm* or treatment *arm*).

assent The affirmative agreement of a vulnerable subject (e.g., a child) to participate in a study.

associative relationship An association between two variables that cannot be described as causal (i.e., one variable *causing* the other).

assumption A principle that is accepted as being true based on logic or reason, without proof.

asymmetric distribution A distribution of data values that is skewed, with two halves that are not mirror images of each other.

attention control group A control group that gets a similar amount of attention to those in the intervention group, without the "active ingredients" of the treatment.

attrition The loss of participants over the course of a study, which can create bias by changing the composition of the sample initially drawn.

audit trail The systematic documentation of material that allows an independent auditor of a qualitative study to draw conclusions about trustworthiness.

authenticity The extent to which qualitative researchers fairly and faithfully show a range of different realities in the analysis and interpretation of their data.

autoethnography An ethnographic study in which a researcher studies his or her own culture or group.

axial coding The second level of coding in a grounded theory study using the Strauss and Corbin approach, involving the process of categorizing, recategorizing, and condensing first level codes by connecting a category and its subcategories.

baseline data Data collected before an intervention, including pretreatment measures of the outcomes.

basic research Research designed to extend the base of knowledge in a discipline for the sake of knowledge production or theory construction, rather than for solving an immediate problem.

basic social process (BSP) The central social process emerging through an analysis of grounded theory data.

before-after design An experimental design in which data are collected from subjects both before and after the introduction of an intervention.

beneficence A fundamental ethical principle that seeks to maximize benefits for study participants, and prevent harm.

beta (β) (1) In multiple regression, the standardized coefficients indicating the relative weights of the predictor variables in the equation; (2) in statistical testing, the probability of a Type II error.

between-subjects design A research design in which there are separate groups of people being compared (e.g., smokers and nonsmokers).

bias Any influence that distorts the results of a study and undermines validity.

bimodal distribution A distribution of data values with two peaks (high frequencies).

bivariate statistics Statistics derived from analyzing two variables simultaneously to assess the empirical relationship between them.

blind review The review of a manuscript or proposal such that neither the author nor the reviewer is identified to the other party.

blinding The process of preventing those involved in a study (participants, intervention agents, or data collectors) from having information that could lead to a bias (e.g., knowledge of which treatment group a participant is in); also called *masking.*

*Bonferroni correction An adjustment made to establish a more conservative alpha level when multiple statistical tests are being run from the same data set; the correction is computed by dividing the desired $α$ by the number of tests (e.g., .05/3 = .017).

bracketing In phenomenological inquiries, the process of identifying and holding in abeyance any preconceived beliefs and opinions about the phenomena under study.

*canonical analysis A statistical procedure for examining the relationship between two or more independent variables *and* two or more dependent variables.

carry-over effect The influence that one treatment can have on subsequent treatments.

case-control design A nonexperimental research design involving the comparison of "cases" (i.e., people with the condition under scrutiny, such as having had a fall) and matched controls (similar people without the condition).

case study A research method involving a thorough, in-depth analysis of an individual, group, or other social unit.

categorical variable A variable with discrete values (e.g., sex) rather than values along a continuum (e.g., weight).

category system (1) In studies involving observation, the prespecified plan for recording the behaviors and events under observation; (2) in qualitative studies, a system used to sort and organize the data.

causal modeling The development and statistical testing of an explanatory model of hypothesized causal relationships among phenomena.

causal (cause-and-effect) relationship A relationship between two variables such that the presence or absence of one variable (the "cause") determines the presence or absence (or value) of the other (the "effect").

cell (1) The intersection of a row and column in a table with two or more dimensions; (2) in an experimental design, the representation of an experimental condition in a schematic diagram.

central (core) category The main category or pattern of behavior in grounded theory analysis using the Strauss and Corbin approach.

central tendency A statistical index of the "typicalness" of a set of scores, derived from the center of the score distribution; indices of central tendency include the mode, median, and mean.

chi-squared test A statistical test used to assess group differences in proportions; symbolized as χ^2.

clinical research Research designed to generate knowledge to guide nursing practice.

clinical trial A study designed to assess the safety, efficacy, and effectiveness of a new clinical intervention, sometimes involving several phases, one of which (phase III) is a *randomized clinical trial* (RCT) using an experimental design.

closed-ended question A question that offers respondents a set of mutually exclusive response options.

***cluster analysis** A statistical procedure used to cluster people or things (rather than variables, as in a factor analysis) based on patterns of association.

***cluster randomization** The random assignment of intact groups of participants—rather than individual participants—to treatment conditions.

cluster sampling A form of sampling in which large groupings ("clusters") are selected first (e.g., nursing schools), with successive subsampling of smaller units (e.g., nursing students).

Cochrane Collaboration An international organization that aims to facilitate well-informed decisions about health care by preparing and disseminating systematic reviews of the effects of health care interventions.

code of ethics The fundamental ethical principles established by a discipline or institution to guide researchers' conduct in research with human (or animal) study participants.

coding The process of transforming raw data into standardized form for data processing and analysis; in quantitative research, the process of attaching numbers to categories; in qualitative research, the process of identifying recurring words, themes, or concepts within the data.

coefficient alpha (Cronbach's alpha) A reliability index that estimates the internal consistency (homogeneity) of a measure composed of several items or subparts.

coercion In a research context, the explicit or implicit use of threats (or excessive rewards) to gain people's cooperation in a study.

***cognitive questioning** A method sometimes used during a pretest of an instrument in which respondents are asked to verbalize what comes to mind when they hear a question.

Cohen's *d* An effect size for comparing two group means, computed by subtracting one mean from the other and dividing by the pooled standard deviation; also called *standardized mean difference*.

cohort design A nonexperimental design in which a defined group of people (a cohort) is followed over time to study outcomes for subsets of the cohorts; also called a *prospective design*.

comparison group A group of study participants whose scores on a dependent variable are used to evaluate the outcomes of the group of primary interest (e.g., nonsmokers as a comparison group for smokers); term often used in lieu of *control group* when the study design is not a true experiment.

component design A study design for a mixed-method study in which qualitative and quantitative aspects are implemented as discrete components of the overall inquiry.

concealment A tactic involving the unobtrusive collection of research data without participants' knowledge or consent, used to obtain an accurate view of naturalistic behavior when the known presence of an observer would distort the behavior of interest.

concept An abstraction based on observations of behaviors or characteristics (e.g., fatigue, pain).

conceptual definition The abstract or theoretical meaning of a concept being studied.

conceptual file A manual method of organizing qualitative data, by creating file folders for each category in the category scheme, and inserting relevant excerpts from the data.

conceptual map A schematic representation of a theory or conceptual model that graphically represents key concepts and linkages among them.

conceptual model Interrelated concepts or abstractions assembled together in a rational scheme by virtue of their relevance to a common theme; sometimes called *conceptual framework*.

conceptual utilization The use of research findings in a general, conceptual way to broaden one's thinking about an issue, without putting the knowledge to any specific use.

concurrent validity The degree to which scores on an instrument are correlated with scores on an external criterion, measured at the same time.

confidence interval (CI) The range of values within which a population parameter is estimated to lie, at a specified probability of accuracy (e.g., 95% CI).

confidence limit The upper limit (UL) or lower limit (LL) of a confidence interval.

confidentiality Protection of study participants so that data provided are never publicly divulged.

confirmability A criterion for integrity in a qualitative inquiry, referring to the objectivity or neutrality of the data and interpretations.

*confirmatory factor analysis (CFA) A factor analysis designed to confirm a hypothesized measurement model, using a form of estimation called maximum likelihood estimation.

consecutive sampling The recruitment of *all* people from an accessible population who meet the eligibility criteria over a specific time interval or for a specified sample size.

consent form A written agreement signed by a study participant and a researcher concerning the terms and conditions of voluntary participation in a study.

CONSORT guidelines Widely used guidelines (Consolidated Standards of Reporting Trials) for reporting information on clinical trials, including a flow chart for tracking participants through a trial.

constant comparison A procedure used in a grounded theory analysis wherein newly collected data are compared in an ongoing fashion with data obtained earlier, to refine theoretically relevant categories.

constitutive pattern In hermeneutic analysis, a pattern that expresses the relationships among relational themes and is present in all the interviews or texts.

construct An abstraction or concept that is deliberately invented (constructed) by researchers for a scientific purpose (e.g., health locus of control).

construct validity The validity of inferences from *observed* persons, settings, and interventions in a study to the constructs that these instances might represent; for an instrument, the degree to which it measures the construct under investigation.

contamination The inadvertent, undesirable influence of one treatment condition on another treatment condition.

content analysis The process of organizing and integrating narrative, qualitative information according to emerging themes and concepts.

content validity The degree to which the items in an instrument adequately represent the universe of content for the concept being measured.

content validity index (CVI) An index of the degree to which an instrument is content valid, based on aggregated ratings of a panel of experts; content validity for individual items and the overall scale can be calculated.

contingency table A two-dimensional table in which the frequencies of two categorical variables are cross-tabulated.

continuous variable A variable that can take on an infinite range of values along a specified continuum (e.g., height).

control The process of holding constant confounding influences on the dependent variable under study.

control group Subjects in an experiment who do not receive the experimental treatment and whose performance provides a baseline against which the effects of the treatment can be measured (see also *comparison group*).

*controlled trial A test of an intervention using a design that includes a control group, with or without randomization.

convenience sampling Selection of the most readily available persons as participants in a study.

*convergent validity An approach to construct validation that involves assessing the degree to which two methods of measuring a construct are similar (i.e., converge).

core variable (category) In a grounded theory study, the central phenomenon that is used to integrate all categories of the data.

correlation A bond or association between variables, with variation in one variable systematically related to variation in another.

correlation coefficient An index summarizing the degree of relationship between variables, typically ranging from +1.00 (for a perfect positive relationship) through .00 (for no relationship) to −1.00 (for a perfect negative relationship).

correlation matrix A two-dimensional display showing the correlation coefficients between all pairs of a set of variables.

correlational research Research that explores the interrelationships among variables of interest, without researcher intervention.

cost analysis An analysis of the relationship between costs and outcomes of alternative nursing or other health care interventions.

*cost–benefit analysis An economic analysis in which both costs and outcomes of a program or intervention are expressed in monetary terms, and compared.

*cost-effectiveness analysis An economic analysis in which costs of an intervention are measured in monetary terms, but outcomes are expressed in natural units (e.g., the costs per added year of life).

*cost-utility analysis An economic analysis that expresses the effects of an intervention as overall health improvement and describes costs for some additional utility gain—usually in relation to gains in quality-adjusted life years (QALY).

counterbalancing The process of systematically varying the order of presentation of stimuli or treatments to control for ordering effects, especially in a crossover design.

counterfactual The condition or group used as a basis of comparison in a study, embodying what would have happened *to the same people* exposed to a causal factor if they *simultaneously* were *not* exposed to the causal factor.

covariate A variable that is statistically controlled (held constant) in ANCOVA, typically a confounding influence on the outcome (dependent) variable, or a preintervention measure of the outcome.

*Cramér's *V* An index describing the magnitude of relationship between nominal-level data, used when the contingency table to which it is applied is larger than 2 × 2.

credibility A criterion for evaluating integrity and quality in qualitative studies, referring to confidence in the truth of the data; analogous to internal validity in quantitative research.

criterion-related validity The degree to which scores on an instrument are correlated with some external criterion.

*critical case sampling A sampling approach used by qualitative researchers involving the purposeful selection of cases that are especially important or illustrative.

critical ethnography An ethnography that focuses on raising consciousness in the group or culture under study in the hope of effecting social change.

critical incident technique A method of obtaining data from study participants by in-depth exploration of specific incidents and behaviors related to the topic under study.

*critical region The area in a sampling distribution representing values that are "improbable" if the null hypothesis is true.

critical theory An approach to viewing the world that involves a critique of society, with the goal of envisioning new possibilities and effecting social change.

critically appraised topic (CAT) A quick summary of a clinical question and an appraisal of the best evidence that typically begins with a clinical bottom line (i.e., best-practice recommendation).

critique A critical, balanced appraisal of a research report or proposal.

Cronbach's alpha A widely used reliability index that estimates the internal consistency of a measure composed of several subparts; also called *coefficient alpha*.

crossover design An experimental design in which one group of subjects is exposed to more than one condition or treatment, in random order.

cross-sectional design A study design in which data are collected at one point in time; sometimes used to infer change over time when data are collected from different age or developmental groups.

crosstabulation A calculation of frequencies for two variables considered simultaneously (e.g., sex [male/female]) crosstabulated with smoking status (smoker/nonsmoker).

cut-off point The score on a screening or diagnostic instrument used to distinguish *cases* (e.g., people with depression) and *noncases* (people without it).

d See *Cohen's d*.

data The pieces of information obtained in a study (singular is *datum*).

data analysis The systematic organization and synthesis of research data and, in quantitative studies, the testing of hypotheses using those data.

data collection protocols The formal guidelines researchers develop to give direction to the collection of data in a standardized fashion.

data saturation See *saturation*.

data set The total collection of data on all variables for all study participants.

data triangulation The use of multiple data sources for the purpose of validating conclusions.

debriefing Communication with study participants after participation has concluded regarding aspects of the study (e.g., explaining the study purpose more fully).

deception The deliberate withholding of information, or the provision of false information, to study participants, usually to reduce potential biases.

deductive reasoning The process of developing specific predictions from general principles (see also *inductive reasoning*).

degrees of freedom (*df*) A statistical concept referring to the number of sample values free to vary (e.g., with a given sample mean, all but one value would be free to vary).

***Delphi survey** A technique for obtaining judgments from an expert panel about an issue of concern; experts are questioned individually in several rounds, with a summary of the panel's views circulated between rounds, to foster consensus.

dependability A criterion for evaluating integrity in qualitative studies, referring to the stability of data over time and over conditions; analogous to reliability in quantitative research.

dependent variable The variable hypothesized to depend on or be caused by another variable (the *independent variable*); the outcome variable of interest.

descendancy approach In literature searches, finding a pivotal early study and searching forward in citation indexes to find more recent studies ("descendants") that cited the key study.

descriptive research Research that has as its main objective the accurate portrayal of the characteristics of persons, situations, or groups, and/or the frequency with which certain phenomena occur.

descriptive statistics Statistics used to describe and summarize data (e.g., means, percentages).

descriptive theory A broad characterization that thoroughly accounts for a phenomenon.

determinism The belief that phenomena are not haphazard or random, but rather have antecedent causes; an assumption in the positivist paradigm.

***deviation score** A score computed by subtracting an individual score from the mean of all scores.

dichotomous variable A variable having only two values or categories (e.g., sex).

directional hypothesis A hypothesis that makes a specific prediction about the direction of the relationship between two variables.

discourse analysis A qualitative tradition, from the discipline of sociolinguistics, that seeks to understand the rules, mechanisms, and structure of conversations.

***discrete variable** A variable with a finite number of values between two points.

***discriminant function analysis** A statistical procedure used to predict group membership or status on a categorical (nominal level) variable on the basis of two or more independent variables.

***discriminant validity** A construct validation approach that involves assessing the degree to which a single method of measuring two constructs yields different results (i.e., discriminates the two).

disproportionate sample A sample in which the researcher samples varying proportions of subjects from different population strata to ensure adequate representation from smaller strata.

domain In ethnographic analysis, a unit or broad category of cultural knowledge.

*__dose-response analysis__ An analysis to assess whether larger doses of an intervention are associated with greater benefits, usually in a quasi-experimental framework.

double-blind experiment An experiment in which neither the subjects nor those who administer the treatment know who is in the experimental or control group.

*__dummy variable__ Dichotomous variables created for use in many multivariate statistical analyses, typically using codes of 0 and 1 (e.g., female = 1, male = 0).

ecologic psychology A qualitative tradition that focuses on the environment's influence on human behavior and attempts to identify principles that explain the interdependence of humans and their environmental context.

*__ecologic validity__ The extent to which study designs and findings have relevance and meaning in a variety of real-world contexts.

economic analysis An analysis of the relationship between costs and outcomes of alternative health care interventions.

editing analysis style An approach to the analysis of qualitative data in which researchers read through texts in search of meaningful segments, and develop a categorization scheme that is used to sort and organize the data.

effect size A statistical expression of the magnitude of the relationship between two variables, or the magnitude of the difference between groups on an attribute of interest; also used in metasynthesis to characterize the salience of a theme or category.

effectiveness study A clinical trial designed to shed light on effectiveness of an intervention under ordinary conditions, with an intervention that already has been found to be efficacious in an efficacy study.

efficacy study A tightly controlled clinical trial designed to establish the efficacy of an intervention under ideal conditions, using a design that stresses internal validity.

*__eigenvalue__ In factor analysis, the value equal to the sum of the squared weights for each factor.

element The most basic unit of a population for sampling purposes, typically a human being.

eligibility criteria The criteria designating the specific attributes of the target population, by which people are selected for inclusion in a study.

emergent design A design that unfolds in the course of a qualitative study as the researcher makes ongoing design decisions reflecting what has already been learned.

*__emergent fit__ A concept in grounded theory that involves comparing new data and new categories with previously existing conceptualizations.

emic perspective A ethnographic term referring to the way members of a culture themselves view their world; the "insider's view."

empirical evidence Evidence rooted in objective reality and gathered using one's senses as the basis for generating knowledge.

*__endogenous variable__ In causal modeling, a variable whose variation is determined by other variables within the model.

error of measurement The deviation between true scores and obtained scores of a measured characteristic.

*__error term__ The mathematic expression (e.g., in a regression analysis) that represents all unknown or unmeasured attributes that can affect the dependent variable.

estimation procedures Statistical procedures that estimate population parameters based on sample statistics.

*__eta squared__ In ANOVA, a statistic calculated to indicate the proportion of variance in the dependent variable explained by the independent variables, analogous to R^2 in multiple regression.

ethics A system of moral values that is concerned with the degree to which research procedures adhere to professional, legal, and social obligations to the study participants.

ethnography A branch of human inquiry, associated with anthropology, that focuses on the culture of a group of people, with an effort to understand the world view of those under study.

ethnomethodology A branch of human inquiry, associated with sociology, that focuses on the way in which people make sense of their everyday activities and come to behave in socially acceptable ways.

ethnonursing research The study of human cultures, with a focus on a group's beliefs and practices relating to nursing care and related health behaviors.

etic perspective An ethnographic term referring to the "outsider's" view of the experiences of a cultural group.

evaluation research Research aimed at learning how well a program, practice, or policy is working.

event sampling A sampling plan that involves the selection of integral behaviors or events to be observed.

evidence-based practice (EBP) A practice that involves making clinical decisions on the best available evidence, with an emphasis on evidence from disciplined research.

evidence hierarchy A ranked arrangement of the validity and dependability of evidence of causality based on the rigor of the method that produced it.

exclusion criteria The criteria specifying characteristics that a study population does *not* have.

***exogenous variable** In causal modeling, a variable whose determinants lie outside the model.

experiment A study in which the researcher controls (manipulates) the independent variable and randomly assigns subjects to different conditions.

experimental group The study participants who receive the experimental treatment or intervention.

***exploratory factor analysis (EFA)** A factor analysis undertaken to explore the underlying dimensionality of a set of variables.

***external criticism** In historical research, the systematic evaluation of the authenticity and genuineness of data.

external validity The degree to which study results can be generalized to settings or samples other than the one studied.

extraneous variable A variable that confounds the relationship between the independent and dependent variables and that needs to be controlled either statistically or in the research design.

extreme case sampling A qualitative sampling approach that involves the purposeful selection of the most extreme or unusual cases.

extreme response set A bias in psychosocial scales created when participants select extreme response alternatives (e.g., "strongly agree"), independent of the item's content.

F-ratio The statistic obtained in several statistical tests (e.g., ANOVA) in which score variation attributable to different sources (e.g., between groups and within groups) is compared.

face validity The extent to which an instrument looks as though it is measuring what it purports to measure.

factor analysis A statistical procedure for reducing a large set of variables into a smaller set of variables with common underlying dimensions.

***factor extraction** The first phase of a factor analysis, which involves the extraction of as much variance as possible through the successive creation of linear combinations of the variables in the data set.

***factor loading** In factor analysis, the weight associated with a variable on a given factor.

***factor rotation** The second phase of factor analysis, during which the reference axes for the factors are moved to more clearly align variables with a single factor.

***factor score** A person's score on a latent variable (factor).

factorial design An experimental design in which two or more independent variables are simultaneously manipulated, permitting a separate analysis of the main effects of the independent variables and their interaction.

fail-safe number In meta-analysis, an estimate of the number of studies with nonsignificant results that would be needed to reverse the conclusion of a significant effect.

feminist research Research that seeks to understand, typically through qualitative approaches, how gender and a gendered social order shape women's lives and their consciousness.

field diary A daily record of events and conversations in the field; also called a log.

field notes The notes taken by researchers to record the unstructured observations made in the field, and the interpretation of those observations.

field research Research in which the data are collected "in the field" from individuals in their normal roles, with the aim of understanding the practices, behaviors, and beliefs of individuals or groups as they normally function in real life.

fieldwork The activities undertaken by qualitative researchers to collect data out in the field (i.e., in natural settings).

findings The results of the analysis of research data.

*****Fisher's exact test** A statistical procedure used to test the significance of the difference in proportions; it is used when the sample size is small or cells in the contingency table have no observations.

fit In grounded theory analysis, the process of identifying characteristics of one piece of data and comparing them with the characteristics of another datum to assess similarity.

fittingness The degree of congruence between a research sample in a qualitative study and another group or setting of interest, a concept often referred to as *transferability*.

fixed alternative question A question that offers respondents a set of prespecified response options.

fixed effects model In meta-analysis, a model in which studies are assumed to be measuring the same overall effect; a pooled effect estimate is calculated under the assumption that observed variation between studies is attributable to chance.

focus group interview An interview with a group of individuals assembled to answer questions on a given topic.

focused interview A loosely structured interview in which an interviewer guides the respondent through a set of questions using a topic guide.

follow-up study A study undertaken to determine the outcomes of individuals with a specified condition or who have received a specified treatment.

forest plot A graphic representation of effects across studies in a meta-analysis, permitting an assessment of heterogeneity.

formal grounded theory A theory developed at a more abstract level of theory by integrating several substantive grounded theories.

framework The conceptual underpinnings of a study (e.g., a *theoretical framework* in theory-based studies, or *conceptual framework* in studies based on a specific conceptual model).

frequency distribution A systematic array of numeric values from the lowest to the highest, together with a count of the number of times each value was obtained.

frequency effect size In a metasynthesis, the percentage of reports that contain a given thematic finding.

frequency polygon Graphic display of a frequency distribution, in which dots connected by a straight line indicate the number of times score values occur in a data set.

*****Friedman test** A nonparametric analog of ANOVA, used with paired-groups or repeated measures situations.

full disclosure The communication of complete, accurate information about the study to potential study participants.

functional relationship A relationship between two variables in which it cannot be assumed that one variable caused the other.

funnel plot In a meta-analysis, a graphic display of some measure of study precision (e.g., sample size) plotted against effect size that can be used to explore relationships that might reflect publication bias.

gaining entrée The process of gaining access to study participants through the cooperation of key actors in the selected community or site.

generalizability The degree to which the research methods justify the inference that the findings are true for a broader group than study participants; in particular, the inference that the findings can be generalized from the sample to the population.

*****"going native"** A pitfall in ethnographic research wherein a researcher becomes too emotionally involved with participants and, therefore, loses the ability to observe objectively.

grand theory A broad theory aimed at describing large segments of the physical, social, or behavioral world; also called a *macrotheory*.

grand tour question A broad question asked in an unstructured interview to gain a general overview of a phenomenon, on the basis of which more focused questions are subsequently asked.

*****graphic rating scale** A scale in which respondents are asked to rate a concept along an ordered bipolar continuum (e.g., "excellent" to "very poor").

grey literature Unpublished, and thus less readily accessible, research reports.

grounded theory An approach to collecting and analyzing qualitative data that aims to develop theories grounded in real-world observations.

hand searching The planned searching of a journal "by hand," to identify all relevant reports that might be missed by electronic searching.

Hawthorne effect The effect on the dependent variable resulting from subjects' awareness that they are participants under study.

hermeneutic circle In hermeneutics, the methodologic process in which, to reach understanding, there is continual movement between the parts and the whole of the text being analyzed.

hermeneutics A qualitative research tradition, drawing on interpretive phenomenology, which focuses on the lived experiences of humans, and on how they interpret those experiences.

heterogeneity The degree to which objects are dissimilar (i.e., characterized by variability) on some attribute.

*****hierarchical multiple regression** A multiple regression analysis in which predictor variables are entered into the equation in steps that are prespecified by the analyst.

historical research Systematic studies designed to discover facts and relationships about past events.

history threat The occurrence of events external to an intervention but concurrent with it, which can affect the dependent variable and threaten the study's internal validity.

homogeneity (1) In terms of the reliability of an instrument, the degree to which its subparts are internally consistent (i.e., are measuring the same critical attribute); (2) more generally, the degree to which objects are similar (i.e., characterized by low variability).

hypothesis A statement of predicted relationships between variables or predicted outcomes.

impact analysis An evaluation of the effects of a program or intervention on outcomes of interest, net of other factors influencing those outcomes.

*****impact factor** An annual measure of citation frequency for an average article in a given journal (i.e., the ratio between citations and recent citable items published in the journal).

implementation analysis In evaluations, a description of the process by which a program or intervention was implemented in practice.

implementation potential The extent to which an innovation is amenable to implementation in a new setting, an assessment of which is often made in an evidence-based practice project.

implied consent Consent to participate in a study that a researcher assumes has been given based on participants' actions, such as returning a completed questionnaire.

IMRAD format The organization of a research report into four main sections: the Introduction, Method, Results, and Discussion sections.

*****incidence rate** The rate of new cases with a specified condition, determined by dividing the number of new cases over a given period of time by the number at risk of becoming a new case (i.e., free of the condition at the outset of the time period).

independent variable The variable that is believed to cause or influence the dependent variable; in experimental research, the manipulated treatment variable.

inductive reasoning The process of reasoning from specific observations to more general rules (see also *deductive reasoning*).

inferential statistics Statistics that permit inferences about whether results observed in a sample are likely to occur in the larger population.

informant An individual who provides information to researchers about a phenomenon under study, usually in qualitative studies.

informed consent An ethical principle that requires researchers to obtain people's voluntary participation in a study, after informing them of possible risks and benefits.

inquiry audit An independent scrutiny of qualitative data and relevant supporting documents by an external reviewer, to determine the dependability and confirmability of qualitative data.

insider research Research on a group or culture—usually in an ethnography—by a member of that group or culture.

Institutional Review Board (IRB) In the United States, a group of people affiliated with an institution who convene to review proposed and ongoing studies with respect to ethical considerations.

instrument The device used to collect data (e.g., a questionnaire, test, observation schedule).

instrumental utilization Clearly identifiable attempts to base some specific action or intervention on the results of research findings.

***instrumentation threat** The threat to the internal validity of the study that can arise if the researcher changes the measuring instrument between two points of data collection.

integrated design A mixed method design in which there is integration of the method types throughout the project.

intensity effect size In a metasynthesis, the percentage of all thematic findings that are contained in any given report.

***intensity sampling** A sampling approach used by qualitative researchers involving the purposeful selection of intense (but not extreme) cases.

***intention to treat** A strategy for analyzing data in an intervention study that includes participants with the group to which they were assigned, whether or not they received or completed the treatment associated with the group.

interaction effect The effect of two or more independent variables acting in combination (interactively) on a dependent variable.

intercoder reliability The degree to which two coders, operating independently, agree on coding decisions.

internal consistency The degree to which the subparts of an instrument are measuring the same attribute or dimension, as a measure of the instrument's reliability.

***internal criticism** In historical research, an evaluation of the worth of the historical evidence.

internal validity The degree to which it can be inferred that the experimental treatment (independent variable), rather than uncontrolled, confounding factors, caused the observed effects.

interrater (interobserver) reliability The degree to which two raters or observers, operating independently, assign the same ratings or values for an attribute being measured or observed.

***interrupted time series design.** See *time series design*.

interval estimation A statistical estimation approach in which the researcher establishes a range of values that are likely, within a given level of confidence, to contain the true population parameter.

interval measurement A measurement level in which an attribute of a variable is rank ordered on a scale that has equal distances between points on that scale (e.g., Fahrenheit degrees).

intervention In experimental research, the experimental treatment or manipulation.

intervention fidelity The extent to which the implementation of a treatment is faithful to its plan.

intervention protocol The specification of exactly what an intervention and alternative treatment conditions will be, and how they are to be administered.

intervention research Research involving the development, implementation, and testing of an intervention.

intervention theory The conceptual underpinning of a health care intervention, providing the theoretical basis for what must be done to achieve desired outcomes.

interview A data collection method in which an interviewer asks questions of a respondent, either face-to-face, by telephone, or over the Internet.

interview schedule The formal instrument that specifies the wording of all questions to be asked of respondents in structured self-report studies.

intuiting The second step in descriptive phenomenology, which occurs when researchers remain open to the meaning attributed to the phenomenon by those who experienced it.

inverse relationship A relationship characterized by the tendency of high values on one variable to be associated with low values on the second variable; also called a *negative relationship*.

inverse variance method In meta-analysis, a method that uses the inverse of the variance of the effect estimate (one divided by the square of its standard error) as the weight to calculate a weighted average of effects.

investigator triangulation The use of two or more researchers to analyze and interpret a data set, to enhance validity.

item A single question on an instrument, or a single statement on a scale.

journal article A report appearing in professional journals such as *Nursing Research*.

journal club A group that meets regularly in clinical settings to discuss and critique research reports appearing in journals.

judgmental sampling A type of nonprobability sampling method in which the researcher selects study participants based on personal judgment about who will be most representative or informative; also called *purposive sampling*.

*kappa An index used to measure interrater agreement, which summarizes the extent of agreement beyond the level expected to occur by chance.

*Kendall's tau A correlation coefficient used to indicate the magnitude of a relationship between ordinal-level variables.

key informant A person well-versed in the phenomenon or culture of interest and who is willing to share the information and insight with the researcher.

keyword An important term used to search for references on a topic in a bibliographic database.

known-groups technique A technique for estimating the construct validity of an instrument through an analysis of the degree to which the instrument separates groups predicted to differ based on known characteristics or theory.

*Kruskal-Wallis test A nonparametric test used to test the difference between three or more independent groups, based on ranked scores.

*latent variable An unmeasured variable that represents an underlying, abstract construct (usually in the context of a structural equations analysis or confirmatory factor analysis).

*least-squares estimation A method of statistical estimation in which the solution minimizes the sums of squares of error terms; also called OLS (ordinary least squares).

level of measurement A system of classifying measurements according to the nature of the measurement and the type of permissible mathematical operations; the levels are nominal, ordinal, interval, and ratio.

level of significance The risk of making a Type I error in a statistical analysis, established by the researcher beforehand (e.g., the .05 level).

life history A narrative self-report about a person's life experiences vis-à-vis a theme of interest.

likelihood ratio (LR) For a screening or diagnostic instrument, the relative likelihood that a given result is expected in a person with (as opposed to one without) the target attribute; LR indexes summarize the relationship between specificity and sensitivity in a single number.

Likert scale A composite measure of an attribute involving the summation of scores on a set of items that respondents typically rate for their degree of agreement or disagreement.

linear regression An analysis for predicting the value of a dependent variable from one or more independent (predictor) variables by determining a straight-line fit to the data that minimizes deviations from the line.

*LISREL An acronym for linear structural relation analysis, used for testing causal models.

literature review A critical summary of research on a topic, often prepared to put a research problem in context or to summarize existing evidence.

log In participant observation studies, the observer's daily record of events and conversations.

logical positivism The philosophy underlying the traditional scientific approach; see also *positivist paradigm.*

logistic regression A multivariate regression procedure that analyzes relationships between one or more independent variables and categorical dependent variables and yields an odds ratio.

longitudinal study A study designed to collect data at more than one point in time, in contrast to a cross-sectional study.

macrotheory A broad theory aimed at describing large segments of the physical, social, or behavioral world; also called a *grand theory.*

main effects In a study with multiple independent variables, the noninteractive effects of each independent variable on the dependent variable.

*manifest variable An observed, measured variable that serves as an indicator of an underlying construct (i.e., a latent variable).

manipulation The introduction of an intervention or treatment in an experimental or quasi-experimental study to assess its impact on the dependent variable.

*manipulation check In experimental studies, a test to determine whether the manipulation was implemented as intended.

*Mann-Whitney *U* test A nonparametric statistic used to test the difference between two independent groups, based on ranked scores.

MANOVA See *multivariate analysis of variance.*

masking See *blinding.*

matching The pairing of subjects in one group with those in a comparison group based on their similarity on one or more dimension, to enhance group comparability.

maturation threat A threat to the internal validity of a study that results when changes to the outcome (dependent) variable result from the passage of time.

*maximum likelihood estimation An estimation approach in which the estimators are ones that estimate the parameters most likely to have generated the observed measurements.

maximum variation sampling A sampling approach used by qualitative researchers involving the purposeful selection of cases with a wide range of variation.

*McNemar test A statistical test for comparing differences in proportions when values are derived from paired (nonindependent) groups.

mean A measure of central tendency, computed by summing all scores and dividing by the number of subjects.

measurement The assignment of numbers to objects according to specified rules to characterize quantities of some attribute.

*measurement model In structural equations modeling, the model that stipulates the hypothesized relationships among the manifest and latent variables.

median A descriptive statistic that is a measure of central tendency, representing the exact middle value in a score distribution; the value above and below which 50% of the scores lie.

*median test A nonparametric statistical test involving the comparison of median values of two independent groups to determine if the groups are from populations with different medians.

mediating variable A variable that mediates or acts like a "go-between" in a causal chain linking two other variables.

member check A method of enhancing credibility in qualitative data analysis through debriefings and discussions with informants.

meta-analysis A technique for quantitatively integrating the results of multiple studies addressing the same or similar research question.

*metamatrix A device sometimes used in a mixed method study that permits researchers to recognize important patterns and themes across data sources and to develop hypotheses.

*meta-regression In meta-analyses, an analytic approach for exploring clinical and methodologic factors contributing to variation in effect size.

meta-summary A process that lays the foundation for a metasynthesis, involving the development of a list of abstracted findings from primary studies and calculating manifest effect sizes (frequency and intensity effect size).

metasynthesis The grand narratives or interpretive translations produced from the integration or comparison of findings from qualitative studies.

method triangulation The use of multiple methods of data collection about the same phenomenon, to enhance validity.

methodologic notes In observational field studies, the researcher's notes about the methods used in collecting data.

methodologic research Research designed to develop or refine methods of obtaining, organizing, or analyzing data.

methods (research) The steps, procedures, and strategies for gathering and analyzing data in a study.

middle-range theory A theory that focuses on a limited segment of reality or human experience, involving a selected number of concepts (e.g., a theory of stress).

minimal risk Anticipated risks that are no greater than those ordinarily encountered in daily life or during the performance of routine tests or procedures.

*****missing values** Values missing from a data set for some study participants; for example, due to refusals, errors, or skip patterns.

mixed method research Research in which both qualitative and quantitative data are collected and analyzed.

modality A characteristic of a frequency distribution describing the number of peaks (i.e., values with high frequencies).

moderator variable A variable that affects (moderates) the relationship between the independent and dependant variables.

mode A measure of central tendency; the score value that occurs most frequently in a distribution of scores.

model A symbolic representation of concepts or variables and interrelationships among them.

mortality threat A threat to the internal validity of a study, referring to the differential loss of participants (attrition) from different groups.

*****multicollinearity** A problem that can occur in multiple regression when predictor variables are too highly intercorrelated, which can lead to unstable estimates of the regression coefficients.

multimodal distribution A distribution of values with more than one peak (high frequency).

multiple comparison procedures Statistical tests, normally applied after an ANOVA indicates statistically significant group differences, that compare different pairs of groups; also called *post hoc tests*.

multiple correlation coefficient An index that summarizes the degree of relationship between two or more independent variables and a dependent variable; symbolized as R.

multiple regression analysis A statistical procedure for understanding the effects of two or more independent (predictor) variables on a dependent variable.

multistage sampling A sampling strategy that proceeds through a set of stages from larger to smaller sampling units (e.g., from states, to census tracts, to households).

*****multitrait–multimethod matrix method** A method of assessing an instrument's construct validity using multiple measures for a set of subjects; the target instrument is valid to the extent that there is a strong relationship between it and other measures of the same attribute (convergence) and a weak relationship between it and measures purporting to measure a different attribute (discriminability).

multivariate analysis of variance (MANOVA) A statistical procedure used to test the significance of differences between the means of two or more groups on two or more dependent variables, considered simultaneously.

multivariate statistics Statistical procedures designed to analyze the relationships among three or more variables (e.g., multiple regression, ANCOVA).

N The symbol designating the total number of subjects (e.g., "the total N was 500").

n The symbol designating the number of subjects in a subgroup or cell of a study (e.g., "each of the four groups had an n of 125, for a total N of 500").

narrative analysis A type of qualitative approach that focuses on the story as the object of the inquiry.

*****natural experiment** A nonexperimental study that takes advantage of a naturally occurring event (e.g., an earthquake) that is explored for its effect on people's behavior or condition, typically by comparing people exposed to the event with those not exposed.

naturalistic paradigm An alternative paradigm to the traditional positivist paradigm that holds that there are multiple interpretations of reality, and that the goal of research is to understand how individuals construct reality within their context; often associated with qualitative research.

naturalistic setting A study setting that is natural to those being studied (e.g., homes, places of work, and so on).

*needs assessment A study designed to describe the needs of a group, community, or organization, usually as a guide to policy planning and resource allocation.

negative case analysis The refinement of a theory or description in a qualitative study through the inclusion of cases that appear to disconfirm earlier hypotheses.

*negative predictive value (NPV) A measure of the usefulness of a screening/diagnostic test that can be interpreted as the probability that a negative test result is correct; calculated by dividing the number with a negative test who do not have disease by the number with a negative test.

negative relationship A relationship between two variables in which there is a tendency for high values on one variable to be associated with low values on the other (e.g., as stress increases, emotional well-being decreases); also called an *inverse relationship*.

negative results Results that fail to support the researcher's hypotheses.

negatively skewed distribution An asymmetric distribution of data values with a disproportionately high number of cases at the upper end; when displayed graphically, the tail points to the left.

net effect The effect of an independent variable on a dependent variable, after controlling for the effect of one or more covariates through multiple regression or ANCOVA.

network sampling The sampling of participants based on referrals from others already in the sample; also called *snowball sampling*.

*nocebo effect Adverse side effect experienced by those receiving a placebo treatment.

nominal measurement The lowest level of measurement involving the assignment of

characteristics into categories (e.g., males, category 1; females, category 2).

nominated sampling A sampling method in which researchers ask early informants to make referrals to other potential participants.

nondirectional hypothesis A research hypothesis that does not stipulate the expected direction of the relationship between variables.

nonequivalent control group design A quasi-experimental design involving a comparison group that was not created through random assignment.

nonexperimental research Studies in which the researcher collects data without introducing an intervention; also called *observational research*.

nonparametric tests A class of statistical tests that do not involve stringent assumptions about the distribution of variables in the analysis.

nonprobability sampling The selection of sampling units (e.g., people) from a population using nonrandom procedures (e.g., convenience and quota sampling).

*nonrecursive model A causal model that predicts reciprocal effects (i.e., a variable can be both the cause of—and an effect of—another variable).

nonresponse bias A bias that can result when a nonrandom subset of people invited to participate in a study decline to participate.

nonsignificant result The result of a statistical test indicating that group differences or an observed relationship could have occurred by chance, at a given level of significance; sometimes abbreviated as NS.

normal distribution A theoretical distribution that is bell-shaped and symmetrical; also called a *bell-shaped curve* or *Gaussian distribution*.

norms Test-performance standards, based on test score information from a large, representative sample.

null hypothesis A hypothesis stating no relationship between the variables under study; used primarily in statistical testing as the hypothesis to be rejected.

*number needed to treat (NNT) An estimate of how many people would need to receive an intervention to prevent one undesirable outcome, computed by dividing 1 by the value of the absolute risk reduction.

nursing research Systematic inquiry designed to develop knowledge about issues of importance to the nursing profession.

objectivity The extent to which two independent researchers would arrive at similar judgments or conclusions (i.e., judgments not biased by personal values or beliefs).

*oblique rotation In factor analysis, a rotation of factors such that the reference axes are allowed to move to acute or oblique angles and hence the factors are allowed to be correlated.

observational notes An observer's in-depth descriptions about events and conversations observed in naturalistic settings.

observational research Studies that do not involve an experimental intervention (i.e., nonexperimental research; also, research in which data are collected through direct observation).

observed (obtained) score The actual score or numerical value assigned to a person on a measure.

odds A way of expressing the chance of an event—the probability of an event occurring to the probability that it will not occur, calculated by dividing the number of people who experienced an event by the number for whom it did not occur.

odds ratio (OR) The ratio of one odds to another odds (e.g., the ratio of the odds of an event in one group to the odds of an event in another group); an odds ratio of one indicates no difference between groups.

*on-protocol analysis A principle for analyzing data that includes data only from those members of a treatment group who actually received the treatment; distinct from an intention-to-treat analysis.

*one-tailed test A statistical test in which only values in one tail of a distribution are considered in determining significance; sometimes used when the researcher states a directional hypothesis.

open-ended question A question in an interview or questionnaire that does not restrict respondents' answers to preestablished response alternatives.

open coding The first level of coding in a grounded theory study, referring to the basic descriptive coding of the content of narrative materials.

operational definition The definition of a concept or variable in terms of the procedures by which it is to be measured.

operationalization The translation of research concepts into measurable phenomena.

*oral history An unstructured, self-report technique used to gather personal recollections of events and their perceived causes and consequences.

ordinal measurement A measurement level that rank orders phenomena along some dimension.

*ordinary least squares (OLS) regression Regression analysis that uses the least-squares criterion for estimating the parameters in the regression equation.

*orthogonal rotation In factor analysis, a rotation of factors such that the reference axes are kept at right angles, and hence the factors remain uncorrelated.

outcome analysis An evaluation of what happens to outcomes of interest after implementing a program or intervention, typically using a one group before-after design.

outcome measure A term sometimes used to refer to the dependent variable (i.e., the measure that captures the outcome of an intervention).

outcomes research Research designed to document the effectiveness of health care services and the end results of patient care.

*outliers Values that lie outside the normal range of values for other cases for a variable in a data set.

_p_ value In statistical testing, the probability that the obtained results are due to chance alone; the probability of a Type I error.

pair matching See _matching_.

panel study A longitudinal survey study in which data are collected from the same people (_a panel_) at two or more points in time.

paradigm A way of looking at natural phenomena that encompasses a set of philosophical assumptions and that guides one's approach to inquiry.

paradigm case In a hermeneutic analysis following the precepts of Benner, a strong exemplar of the phenomenon under study, often used early in the analysis to gain understanding of the phenomenon.

parameter A characteristic of a population (e.g., the mean age of all U.S. citizens).

parametric tests A class of statistical tests that involve assumptions about the distribution of the variables and the estimation of a parameter.

participant See *study participant*.

participant observation A method of collecting data through the participation in (and observation of) a group or culture.

participatory action research (PAR) A research approach based on the premise that the use and production of knowledge can be political and used to exert power.

path analysis A regression-based procedure for testing causal models, typically using correlational data.

***path coefficient** The weight representing the effect of one variable on another in a path analytic model.

***path diagram** A graphic representation of the hypothesized interrelationships and causal flow among variables.

Pearson's *r* A correlation coefficient designating the magnitude of relationship between two interval- or ratio-level variables; also called the *product-moment correlation*.

peer debriefing Meetings with peers to review and explore various aspects of a study, used to enhance trustworthiness in a qualitative study.

peer reviewer A researcher who reviews and critiques a research report or proposal, and who makes a recommendation about publishing or funding the research.

pentadic dramatism An approach for analyzing narratives, developed by Burke, that focuses on five key elements of a story: act (what was done), scene (when and where it was done), agent (who did it), agency (how it was done), and purpose (why it was done).

perfect relationship A correlation between two variables such that the values of one variable can perfectly predict the values of the other; designated as 1.00 or −1.00.

***permuted block randomization** Randomization that occurs for blocks of subjects of even size (e.g., six or eight at a time), to ensure that, at any given time, roughly equal numbers of subjects have been allocated to all treatment groups.

persistent observation A qualitative researcher's intense focus on the aspects of a situation that are relevant to the phenomena being studied.

person triangulation The collection of data from different levels of persons, with the aim of validating data through multiple perspectives on the phenomenon.

personal interview An in-person, face-to-face interview between an interviewer and a respondent.

personal notes In field studies, written comments about the observer's own feelings during the research process.

phenomenology A qualitative research tradition, with roots in philosophy, that focuses on the lived experience of humans.

phenomenon The abstract concept under study; a term sometimes used by qualitative researchers in lieu of *variable*.

***phi coefficient** A statistical index describing the magnitude of relationship between two dichotomous variables.

***photo elicitation** An interview stimulated and guided by photographic images.

pilot study A small-scale version, or trial run, done in preparation for a major study.

placebo A sham or pseudo intervention, often used as a control group condition.

placebo effect Changes in the dependant variable attributable to the placebo.

point estimation A statistical procedure that uses information from a sample (a statistic) to estimate the single value that best represents the population parameter.

***point prevalence rate** The number of people with a condition or disease divided by the total number at risk, multiplied by the total number for whom the rate is being established (e.g., per 1,000 population).

population The entire set of individuals or objects having some common characteristics (e.g., all RNs in New York); sometimes called *universe*.

***positive predictive value (PPV)** A measure of the usefulness of a screening/diagnostic test that can be interpreted as the probability that a positive test result is correct; calculated by dividing the number with a positive test who have disease by the number with a positive test.

positive relationship A relationship between two variables in which high values on one variable tend to be associated with high values on the other (e.g., as physical activity increases, pulse rate increases).

positive results Research results that are consistent with the researcher's hypotheses.

positively skewed distribution An asymmetric distribution of values with a disproportionately high number of cases at the lower end; when displayed graphically, the tail points to the right.

positivist paradigm The paradigm underlying the traditional scientific approach, which assumes that there is an orderly reality that can be objectively studied; often associated with quantitative research.

***post hoc* test** A test for comparing all possible pairs of groups following a significant test of overall group differences (e.g., in an ANOVA).

poster session A session at a professional conference in which several researchers simultaneously present visual displays summarizing their studies, while conference attendees circulate around the room perusing the displays.

posttest The collection of data after introducing an intervention.

posttest-only design An experimental design in which data are collected from subjects only after the intervention has been introduced; also called an *after-only design*.

power A research design's ability to detect relationships that exist among variables.

power analysis A procedure for estimating either the needed sample size for a study or the likelihood of committing a Type II error.

***practical (pragmatic) clinical trial** Trials that address practical questions about the benefits, risks, and costs of an intervention as they would unfold in routine clinical practice, using less rigid controls than in typical efficacy trials.

precision In statistics, the extent to which random errors have been reduced, usually expressed in terms of the width of the confidence interval around an estimate.

prediction The use of empirical evidence to make forecasts about how variables will behave with a new group of people.

predictive validity The degree to which an instrument can predict a criterion observed at a future time.

pretest (1) The collection of data before the experimental intervention; sometimes called baseline data. (2) The trial administration of a newly developed instrument to identify potential weaknesses.

pretest-posttest design An experimental design in which data are collected from research subjects both before and after introducing an intervention; also called a *before-after design*.

***prevalence study** A cross-sectional study undertaken to estimate the proportion of a population having a particular condition (e.g., fibromyalgia) at a given point in time.

primary source First-hand reports of facts or findings; in research, the original report prepared by the investigator who conducted the study.

probability sampling The selection of sampling units (e.g., participants) from a population using random procedures (e.g., simple random sampling).

probing Eliciting more useful or detailed information from a respondent in an interview than was volunteered in the first reply.

problem statement An expression of a dilemma or disturbing situation that needs investigation.

process analysis A descriptive analysis of the process by which a program or intervention gets implemented and used in practice.

process consent In a qualitative study, an ongoing, transactional process of negotiating consent with participants, allowing them to collaborate in the decision-making about their continued participation.

product moment correlation coefficient (r) An index designating the magnitude and direction of the relationship between two variables measured on at least an interval scale; also called *Pearson's r*.

***projective technique** A method of measuring psychological attributes (values, attitudes, personality) by providing respondents with unstructured stimuli to which to respond (e.g., a Rorschach test).

prolonged engagement In qualitative research, the investment of sufficient time during data collection to have an in-depth understanding of the group under study, thereby enhancing credibility.

*proportional hazards model A model in which independent variables are used to predict the risk (hazard) of experiencing an event at a given point in time.

proportionate sample A sample that results when the researcher samples from different strata of the population in proportion to their representation in the population.

proposal A document communicating a research problem, proposed procedures for solving the problem, and, when funding is sought, how much the study will cost.

prospective design A study design that begins by measuring a presumed cause (e.g., cigarette smoking) and then goes forward in time to measure presumed effects (e.g., lung cancer); also called a *cohort design*.

psychometric assessment An evaluation of the quality of an instrument, primarily in terms of its reliability and validity.

psychometrics The theory underlying principles of measurement and the application of the theory in the development of measuring tools.

publication bias The tendency for published studies to systematically over represent statistically significant findings, reflecting the tendency of researchers, reviewers, and editors not to publish nonsignificant results; also called a *bias against the null hypothesis*.

purposive (purposeful) sampling A nonprobability sampling method in which the researcher selects participants based on personal judgment about who will be most informative; also called *judgmental sampling*.

Q sort A data collection method in which participants sort statements into piles (usually 9 or 11) according to some bipolar dimension (e.g., most helpful/least helpful).

qualitative analysis The organization and interpretation of narrative data for the purpose of discovering important underlying themes, categories, and patterns.

qualitative data Information collected in narrative (nonnumeric) form, such as the transcript of an unstructured interview.

qualitative research The investigation of phenomena, typically in an in-depth and holistic fashion, through the collection of rich narrative materials using a flexible research design.

quantitative analysis The statistical manipulation of numeric data for the purpose of describing phenomena or making inferences about how phenomena are related.

quantitative data Information collected in a quantified (numeric) form.

quantitative research The investigation of phenomena that lend themselves to precise measurement and quantification, often involving a rigorous and controlled design.

quasi-experimental design A design for testing an intervention in which participants are not randomly assigned to treatment conditions; also called a *nonrandomized trial* or a *controlled trial without randomization*.

quasi-statistics An "accounting" system used to assess the validity of conclusions derived from qualitative analysis.

questionnaire A document used to gather self-report data via self-administration of questions.

quota sampling A nonrandom sampling method in which "quotas" for certain sample characteristics are established to increase the representativeness of the sample.

r The symbol for a bivariate correlation coefficient, summarizing the magnitude and direction of a relationship between two variables measured on an interval or ratio scale.

R The symbol for the multiple correlation coefficient, indicating the magnitude (but not direction) of the relationship between the dependent variable and multiple independent variables, taken together.

R^2 The squared multiple correlation coefficient, indicating the proportion of variance in the dependent variable explained by a group of independent variables.

random assignment The assignment of participants to treatment conditions in a random manner (i.e., in a manner determined by chance alone); also called *randomization*.

random effects model In meta-analysis, a model in which studies are not assumed to be measuring the same overall effect, but rather reflect a distribution of effects; often preferred to a fixed effect model when there is extensive variation of effects across studies.

random number table A table displaying hundreds of digits (from 0 to 9) in random order; each number is equally likely to follow any other.

random sampling The selection of a sample such that each member of a population has an equal probability of being selected.

randomization The assignment of subjects to treatment conditions in a random manner (i.e., in a manner determined by chance alone); also called *random assignment*.

*randomized block design An experimental design involving two or more factors (independent variables), some of which are not experimentally manipulated.

randomized controlled trial (RCT) A full experimental test of an intervention, involving random assignment to treatment groups; often, an RCT is phase III of a full clinical trial.

randomness An important concept in quantitative research, involving having certain features of the study established by chance rather than by design or personal preference.

range A measure of variability, computed by subtracting the lowest value from the highest value in a distribution of scores.

rating scale A scale that requires ratings of an object or concept along a continuum.

ratio measurement A measurement level with equal distances between scores and a true meaningful zero point (e.g., weight).

raw data Data in the form in which they were collected, without being coded or analyzed.

reactivity A measurement distortion arising from the study participant's awareness of being observed, or, more generally, from the effect of the measurement procedure itself.

readability The ease with which materials (e.g., a questionnaire) can be read by people with varying reading skills, often determined through readability formulas.

*receiver operating characteristic curve (ROC curve) A method used in developing and refining a screening instrument to determine the best cut-off point for "caseness."

*recursive model A path model in which the causal flow is unidirectional, without any feedback loops; opposite of a nonrecursive model.

refereed journal A journal in which decisions about the acceptance of manuscripts are made based on recommendations from peer reviewers.

reflexive notes Notes that document a qualitative researcher's personal experiences, reflections, and progress in the field.

reflexivity In qualitative studies, critical self-reflection about one's own biases, preferences, and preconceptions.

regression analysis A statistical procedure for predicting values of a dependent variable based on one or more independent variables.

relationship A bond or a connection between two or more variables.

*relative risk (RR) An estimate of risk of "caseness" in one group compared with another, computed by dividing the absolute risk for one group (e.g., an exposed group) by the absolute risk for another (e.g., the nonexposed); also called the *risk ratio*.

*relative risk reduction (RRR) The estimated proportion of baseline (untreated) risk that is reduced through exposure to the intervention, computed by dividing the absolute risk reduction (ARR) by the absolute risk for the control group.

reliability The degree of consistency or dependability with which an instrument measures an attribute.

reliability coefficient A quantitative index, usually ranging in value from .00 to 1.00, that provides an estimate of how reliable an instrument is (e.g., Cronbach's alpha).

repeated-measures ANOVA An analysis of variance used when there are multiple measurements of the dependent variable over time.

replication The deliberate repetition of research procedures in a second investigation for the purpose of determining if earlier results can be confirmed.

representative sample A sample whose characteristics are comparable to those of the population from which it is drawn.

research Systematic inquiry that uses orderly methods to answer questions or solve problems.

research control See *control*.

research design The overall plan for addressing a research question, including strategies for enhancing the study's integrity.

research hypothesis The actual hypothesis a researcher wishes to test (as opposed to the *null hypothesis*), stating the anticipated relationship between two or more variables.

research methods The techniques used to structure a study and to gather and analyze information in a systematic fashion.

research misconduct Fabrication, falsification, plagiarism, or other practices that deviate from those that are commonly accepted within the scientific community for conducting or reporting research.

research problem A disturbing or perplexing condition that can be investigated through disciplined inquiry.

research proposal See *proposal*.

research question A specific query the researcher wants to answer to address a research problem.

research report A document summarizing the main features of a study, including the research question, the methods used to address it, the findings, and the interpretation of the findings.

research utilization The use of some aspect of a study in an application unrelated to the original research.

researcher credibility The faith that can be put in a researcher, based on his or her training, qualifications, and experience.

respondent In a self-report study, the participant responding to questions posed by the researcher.

response rate The rate of participation in a study, calculated by dividing the number of persons participating by the number of persons sampled.

response set bias The measurement error resulting from the tendency of some individuals to respond to items in characteristic ways (e.g., always agreeing), independently of item content.

results The answers to research questions, obtained through an analysis of the collected data.

retrospective design A study design that begins with the manifestation of the dependent variable in the present (e.g., lung cancer), followed by a search for a presumed cause occurring in the past (e.g., cigarette smoking).

risk–benefit ratio The relative costs and benefits, to an individual subject and to society at large, of participation in a study; also, the relative costs and benefits of implementing an innovation.

*risk ratio See *relative risk*.

rival hypothesis An alternative explanation, competing with the researcher's hypothesis, for interpreting the results of a study.

*ROC curve See *receiver operating characteristic curve*.

sample A subset of a population, selected to participate in a study.

sampling The process of selecting a portion of the population to represent the entire population.

sampling bias Distortions that arise when a sample is not representative of the population from which it was drawn.

sampling distribution A theoretical distribution of a statistic, using the values of the statistic computed from an infinite number of samples as the data points.

sampling error The fluctuation of the value of a statistic from one sample to another drawn from the same population.

sampling frame A list of all the elements in the population, from which a sample is drawn.

sampling plan The formal plan specifying a sampling method, a sample size, and procedures for recruiting subjects.

saturation The collection of qualitative data to the point where a sense of closure is attained because new data yield redundant information.

scale A composite measure of an attribute, involving the combination of several related items, resulting in the assignment of a score to place people on a continuum with respect to the attribute.

*scatter plot A graphic representation of the relationship between two variables.

scientific method A set of orderly, systematic, controlled procedures for acquiring dependable, empirical—and typically quantitative—information; the methodologic approach associated with the positivist paradigm.

scientific merit The degree to which a study is methodologically and conceptually sound.

screening instrument An instrument used to determine whether potential subjects for a study meet eligibility criteria, or for determining whether a person tests positive for a specified condition.

secondary analysis A form of research in which the data collected by one researcher are reanalyzed by another investigator to answer new questions.

secondary source Second-hand accounts of events or facts; in research, a description of a study prepared by someone other than the original researcher.

selection threat (self-selection) A threat to a study's internal validity resulting from preexisting differences between groups under study; the differences affect the dependent variable in ways extraneous to the effect of the independent variable.

selective coding A level of coding in a grounded theory study that involves selecting the core category, systematically integrating relationships between the core category and other categories, and validating those relationships.

self-determination A person's ability to voluntarily decide whether or not to participate in a study.

self-report A data collection method that involves a direct verbal report by a person being studied (e.g., by interview or questionnaire).

semantic differential A technique used to measure attitudes in which respondents rate concepts of interest on a series of bipolar rating scales.

semistructured interview An open-ended interview in which the researcher is guided by a list of specific topics to cover.

sensitivity The ability of a screening instrument to correctly identify a "case" (i.e., to diagnose a condition correctly).

sensitivity analysis An effort to test how sensitive the results of a statistical analysis are to changes in assumptions or in the way the analysis was done (e.g., in a meta-analysis, used to assess whether conclusions are sensitive to the quality of the studies included).

setting The physical location and conditions in which data collection takes place in a study.

significance level The probability that an observed statistical result could be caused by chance; significance at the .05 level indicates the probability that a relationship of the observed magnitude would be found by chance only 5 of 100 times.

simple random sampling Basic probability sampling involving the selection of sample members from a sampling frame through completely random procedures.

*simultaneous multiple regression A multiple regression analysis in which all predictor variables are entered into the equation simultaneously.

site The overall location where a study is undertaken.

skewed distribution The asymmetric distribution of a set of data values around a central point.

snowball sampling The selection of participants through referrals from earlier participants; also called *network sampling*.

social desirability response set A bias in self-report instruments created when participants have a tendency to misrepresent their opinions in the direction of answers consistent with prevailing social norms.

space triangulation The collection of data on the same phenomenon in multiple sites, to enhance the validity of the findings.

Spearman's rank-order correlation (Spearman's rho) A correlation coefficient indicating the magnitude of a relationship between variables measured on the ordinal scale.

specificity The ability of a screening instrument to identify noncases correctly.

standard deviation The most frequently used statistic for measuring the degree of variability in a set of scores.

standard error The standard deviation of a sampling distribution, such as the sampling distribution of the mean.

*standard scores Scores expressed in terms of standard deviations from the mean, with raw scores transformed to have a mean of 0 and a standard deviation of 1; also called *z* scores.

standardized mean difference (SMD) In meta-analysis, the effect size for comparing two group means, computed by subtracting one mean from the other and dividing by the pooled standard deviation; also called Cohen's *d*.

statement of purpose A declarative statement of the overall goals of a study.

statistic An estimate of a parameter, calculated from sample data.

statistical analysis The organization and analysis of quantitative data using statistical procedures, including both descriptive and inferential statistics.

statistical conclusion validity The degree to which inferences about relationships and differences from a statistical analysis of the data are accurate.

statistical control The use of statistical procedures to control confounding influences on the dependent variable.

statistical inference The process of inferring attributes about the population based on information from a sample, using laws of probability.

statistical power The ability of the research design or analytic strategy to detect true relationships among variables.

statistical significance A term indicating that the results from an analysis of sample data are unlikely to have been caused by chance, at a specified level of probability.

statistical test An analytic tool that estimates the probability that obtained results from a sample reflect true population values.

*stepwise multiple regression A multiple regression analysis in which predictor variables are entered into the equation in steps, in the order in which the increment to R is greatest.

stipend A monetary payment to individuals participating in a study to serve as an incentive for participation and/or to compensate for time and expenses.

strata Subdivisions of the population according to some characteristic (e.g., males and females); singular is *stratum*.

stratified random sampling The random selection of study participants from two or more strata of the population independently.

structural equations Equations representing the magnitude and nature of hypothesized relations among sets of variables, typically based on theoretical predictions.

structured data collection An approach to collecting data from participants, either through self-report or observations, in which response categories are specified in advance.

study participant An individual who participates and provides information in a study.

subgroup effect The differential effect of the independent variable on the dependent variable for subsets of the sample, as detected in subgroup analyses.

subject An individual who participates and provides data in a study; term used primarily in quantitative research.

summated rating scale See *Likert scale*.

survey research Nonexperimental research in which information about people's activities, beliefs, preferences, and attitudes is obtained via direct questioning.

symmetric distribution A distribution of values with two halves that are mirror images of each other.

systematic review A rigorous and systematic synthesis of research findings on a research question.

systematic sampling The selection of sample members such that every *kth* (e.g., every 10th) person or element in a sampling frame is chosen.

tacit knowledge Information about a culture that is so deeply embedded that members do not talk about it or may not even be consciously aware of it.

target population The entire population in which a researcher is interested and to which he or she would like to generalize the study results.

taxonomy In an ethnographic analysis, a system of classifying and organizing terms and concepts, developed to illuminate a domain's organization and the relationship among the categories of the domain.

template analysis style An approach to qualitative analysis in which a preliminary template or coding scheme is used to sort the narrative data.

test statistic A statistic computed to assess the statistical reliability of relationships between variables (e.g., chi-squared, t); the sampling distributions of test statistics are known for circumstances in which the null hypothesis is true.

test–retest reliability Assessment of the stability of an instrument by correlating the scores obtained on two administrations with the same people.

*testing threat A threat to a study's internal validity that occurs when the administration of a baseline measure of a dependent variable results in changes on the variable, apart from the effect of the independent variable.

theme A recurring regularity emerging from an analysis of qualitative data.

theoretical notes In field studies, notes detailing the researcher's interpretations of observed behavior.

theoretical sampling In qualitative studies, the selection of sample members based on emerging findings to ensure adequate representation of important theoretical categories.

theory An abstract generalization that presents a systematic explanation about relationships among phenomena.

theory triangulation The use of competing theories or hypotheses in the analysis and interpretation of data.

thick description A rich and thorough description of the research context and participants in a qualitative study.

think aloud method A qualitative method used to collect data about cognitive processes (e.g., decision-making), in which people's reflections on decisions or problem-solving are captured as they are being made.

time sampling In structured observations, the sampling of time periods during which observations will take place.

time series design A quasi-experimental design involving the collection of data over an extended time period, with multiple data collection points both before and after an intervention.

time triangulation The collection of data on the same phenomenon or about the same people at different points in time, to enhance validity.

topic guide A list of broad question areas to be covered in a semistructured interview or focus group interview.

*tracing Procedures used to relocate subjects to avoid attrition in a longitudinal study.

transferability The extent to which qualitative findings can be transferred to other settings or groups; analogous to generalizability.

treatment The experimental intervention under study; the condition being manipulated.

treatment group The group receiving the intervention being tested; the experimental group.

trend study A form of longitudinal research in which different samples from a population are studied over time with respect to some phenomenon (e.g., annual Gallup polls on abortion attitudes).

triangulation The use of multiple methods to collect and interpret data about a phenomenon, so as to converge on an accurate representation of reality.

true score A hypothetical score that would be obtained if a measure were infallible.

trustworthiness The degree of confidence qualitative researchers have in their data, assessed using the criteria of credibility, transferability, dependability, confirmability, and authenticity.

t-test A parametric statistical test for analyzing the difference between two group means.

*two-tailed tests Statistical tests in which both ends of the sampling distribution are used to determine improbable values.

Type I error An error created by rejecting the null hypothesis when it is true (i.e., the researcher concludes that a relationship exists when in fact it does not—a false–positive finding).

Type II error An error created by accepting the null hypothesis when it is false (i.e., the researcher concludes that *no* relationship exists when in fact it does—a false–negative finding).

unimodal distribution A distribution of values with one peak (high frequency).

unit of analysis The basic unit or focus of a researcher's analysis—typically individual study participants.

univariate statistics Statistical analysis of a single variable for descriptive purposes (e.g., computing a mean).

unstructured interview An interview in which the researcher asks respondents questions without having a predetermined plan regarding the content or flow of information to be gathered.

unstructured observation The collection of descriptive data through direct observation that is not guided by a formal, prespecified plan for observing or recording the information.

validity A quality criterion referring to the degree to which inferences made in a study are accurate and well-founded; in measurement, the degree to which an instrument measures what it is intended to measure.

validity coefficient An index, usually ranging from .00 to 1.00, yielding an estimate of how valid an instrument is.

variability The degree to which values on a set of scores are dispersed.

variable An attribute that varies, that is, takes on different values (e.g., body temperature, heart rate).

variance A measure of variability or dispersion, equal to the standard deviation squared.

vignette A brief description of an event, person, or situation to which respondents are asked to express their reactions.

visual analog scale (VAS) A scaling procedure used to measure certain clinical symptoms (e.g., pain, fatigue) by having people indicate on a straight line the intensity of the symptom.

vulnerable subjects Special groups of people whose rights in studies need special protection because of their inability to provide meaningful informed consent or because their circumstances place them at higher-than-average-risk of adverse effects (e.g., children, unconscious patients).

*web-based survey The administration of a self-administered questionnaire over the Internet on a dedicated survey website.

*weighting A correction procedure used to estimate population values when a disproportionate sampling design has been used.

*Wilcoxon signed ranks test A nonparametric statistical test for comparing two paired groups, based on the relative ranking of values between the pairs.

within-subjects design A research design in which a single group of subjects is compared under different conditions or at different points in time (e.g., before and after surgery).

*z score A standard score, expressed in terms of standard deviations from the mean.

GLOSSARY OF SELECTED STATISTICAL SYMBOLS

This list contains some commonly used symbols in statistics. The list is in approximate alphabetical order, with English and Greek letters intermixed. Nonletter symbols have been placed at the end.

a	Regression constant, the intercept
α	Greek alpha; significance level in hypothesis testing, probability of Type I error; also, a reliability coefficient
b	Regression coefficient, slope of the line
β	Greek beta, probability of a Type II error; also, a standardized regression coefficient (beta weight)
χ^2	Greek chi squared, a test statistic for several nonparametric tests
CI	Confidence interval around estimate of a population parameter
d	An effect size index, a standardized mean difference
df	Degrees of freedom
η^2	Greek eta squared, index of variance accounted for in ANOVA context
f	Frequency (count) for a score value
F	Test statistic used in ANOVA, ANCOVA, and other tests
H_O	Null hypothesis
H_A	Alternative hypothesis; research hypothesis
λ	Greek lambda, a test statistic used in several multivariate analyses (Wilks' lambda)
μ	Greek mu, the population mean
M	Sample mean (alternative symbol for $\bar{X}$)
MS	Mean square, variance estimate in ANOVA
n	Number of cases in a subgroup of the sample
N	Total number of cases or sample members
NNT	Number needed to treat
OR	Odds ratio
p	Probability that observed data are consistent with null hypothesis
r	Pearson's product–moment correlation coefficient for a sample
r_s	Spearman's rank-order correlation coefficient
R	Multiple correlation coefficient
R^2	Coefficient of determination, proportion of variance in *dependent variable* attributable to *independent variables*
R_c	Canonical correlation coefficient
RR	Relative risk
ρ	Greek rho, population correlation coefficient
SD	Sample standard deviation
SEM	Standard error of the mean
σ	Greek sigma (lowercase), population standard deviation
Σ	Greek sigma (uppercase), sum of
SS	Sum of squares
t	Test statistics used in *t*-tests (sometimes called Student's *t*)
U	Test statistic for the Mann-Whitney U-test
$\bar{X}$	Sample mean
x	Deviation score
Y'	Predicted value of Y, dependent variable in regression analysis
z	Standard score in a normal distribution
$||$	Absolute value
$\leq$	Less than or equal to
$\geq$	Greater than or equal to
$\neq$	Not equal to

APPENDIX A

ELSEVIER

Applied Nursing Research 20 (2007) 17–23

Applied
Nursing
Research

www.elsevier.com/locate/apnr

Original article

The relationships among anxiety, anger, and blood pressure in children

Carol C. Howell, PhD, APRN-BC[a],[*], Marti H. Rice, PhD, RN[b],
Myra Carmon, EdD, RN, CPNP[a], Roxanne Pickett Hauber, PhD, CNRN[c]

[a]Byrdine F. Lewis School of Nursing, Georgia State University, PO Box 4019, Atlanta, Georgia 30302-4019, USA
[b]School of Nursing, University of Alabama at Birmingham, Birmingham, Alabama 35294-1210, USA
[c]Department of Nursing, University of Tampa, Tampa, FL 33615, USA

Received 15 July 2005; accepted 23 October 2005

Abstract

Relationships between anger and anxiety have been examined in adults but less frequently in children. This investigation explored relationships among trait anxiety, trait anger, anger expression patterns, and blood pressure in children. The participants were 264 third- through sixth-grade children from five elementary schools who completed Jacob's Pediatric Anger and Anxiety Scale and Jacob's Pediatric Anger Expression Scale and had their blood pressure measured. Data were analyzed using descriptive and correlational statistics and hierarchical regression. Results have implications for the way in which anxiety and anger are perceived in children and the importance of teaching children to deal with emotions.
© 2007 Elsevier Inc. All rights reserved.

1. Introduction

Hypertension affects over 50 million Americans aged 6 and over and is a recognized risk factor for the development of cardiovascular disease (American Heart Association, 2004). Although few children have hypertension or cardiovascular disease, biological and psychosocial risk factors for the development of hypertension in adulthood are estimated to be present in children by the age of 8 (Solomon & Matthews, 1999). With the large number of individuals with hypertension and the progressive nature of cardiovascular disease, it is important to identify and modify risk factors early in life. Although some risk factors are not modifiable, others, such as anger and anxiety, are more amenable to change. The identification and modification of risk factors at an early age might reduce the incidence of hypertension in adulthood (Ewart & Kolodner 1994; Hauber, Rice, Howell, & Carmon, 1998; Meininger, Liehr, Chan, Smith, & Mueller, 2004).

2. Review of the literature

Trait anger (Johnson, 1989, 1990; Siegel, 1984), patterns of anger expression (Johnson, 1989; Muller, Grunbaum, & Labarthe, 2001; Seigel, 1984), and trait anxiety (Ewert & Kolodner, 1994; Johnson, 1989; Meininger et al., 2004) are psychological factors that have been associated with high blood pressure in adolescents. Biological factors such as sex, height, and weight have also been significantly associated with high blood pressure (Johnson, 1984, 1989; Meininger et al., 2004; Muller et al., 2001). Although the contribution of these factors to the development of hypertension has been investigated in adults and adolescents (Ewart & Kolodner, 1994; Harburg, Gkeuberman, Russell, & Cooper, 1991; Meininger et al., 2004), much less research has been done with children (Hauber et al., 1998). It is the intent of this study to investigate relationships among psychosocial factors, biological factors, and blood pressure in children.

2.1. Psychosocial factors

2.1.1. Trait anger

Trait anger is defined as an emotion that can vary from mild displeasure to rage and reflects a more permanent characteristic than state anger (Speilberger et al., 1985). Anger is thought to lead to an increase in blood pressure through its effect on the sympathetic nervous system (Meininger et al., 2004; Muller

* Corresponding author. Tel.: +1 404 651 3645 (home); +1 404 255 5453; fax: +1 404 255 1086.

E-mail addresses: chowell@gsu.edu (C.C. Howell), schauf@uab.edu (M.H. Rice), mcarmon@gsu.edu (M. Carmon), rhauber@ut.edu (R.P. Hauber).

et al., 2001; Taylor, Repetti, & Seeman, 1997; Williams & Williams, 1993). Repeated episodes of anger arousal may lead to a chronic state of elevated blood pressure or hypertension (Muller et al., 2001; Williams & Williams, 1993). Researchers have noted an association between anger scores and blood pressure (Hauber et al., 1998; Johnson, 1989, 1990; Siegel, 1984; Siegel & Leitch, 1981).

2.1.2. Anger expression patterns

Anger expression patterns include anger out, which implies that anger is openly expressed. Anger suppression or anger in implies that the anger is denied and held in. Anger reflection control involves a cognitive approach to resolving anger (Speilberger et al., 1985).

Siegel (1984) found that subjects who had higher scores on the Frequent Anger Directed Outward factor also had higher systolic (SBP) and diastolic blood pressure (DBP). In contrast, Johnson (1984, 1989) found significant positive correlations between anger suppression and high blood pressures in male and female adolescents. In one of the few studies with children, Hauber et al. (1998), in a study of 230 third-grade children, found significant inverse relationships between anger suppression and DBP and anger reflection/control for both SBP and DBP. Muller et al. (2001) found that anger expression predicted blood pressure in 167 11 year olds or after controlling ethnicity, height, weight, percent body fat, and maturity. However, the instrument used in this study did not differentiate between anger in and anger out.

2.1.3. Trait anxiety

Trait anxiety is defined as a subjective feeling of apprehension, tension, and worry, which is thought to be a relatively stable personality characteristic (Speilberger, Edwards, Lushene, Montuori, & Platzek, 1973). Jonas, Franks, and Ingram (1997) suggested that anxiety contributes to the development of hypertension in two ways. Anxiety has been shown to directly stimulate acute autonomic arousal (Russek, King, Russek, & Russek, 1990) and blood pressure reactivity (Krantz & Manuck, 1984; Suls & Wan, 1993; Waked & Jutai, 1990). Responding to stress or anxiety-provoking experiences with anger has been shown to contribute to cardiovascular disease (Chang, Ford, Meoni, Wang & Klag, 2002; Wascher, 2002). The presence of anxiety has been associated with high-risk health behaviors such as smoking, drinking, low levels of physical activity, and noncompliance with prescribed medical treatments, which in turn have been associated with elevations in blood pressure (Jonas et al., 1997). In addition, Heker, Whalen, Jamner, and Delfino (2002) found that high-anxiety teenagers expressed higher levels of anger when compared with low-anxiety teenagers.

2.2. Biological factors

2.2.1. Gender

Research with children and adolescents has shown a differential association between anger, anger expression, and blood pressure when gender is considered (Hauber et al., 1998; Johnson, 1984, 1989; Muller et al., 2001; Weinrich et al., 2000). In a study with third graders, Hauber et al. (1998) identified a positive correlation between anger reflection/control and SBP in female third graders. In male third graders, however, there was a positive correlation between anger reflection/control and DBP. Starner and Peters (2004) found a significant correlation between anger in and SBP and between anger out and SBP.

2.2.2. Height and weight

Among the factors known to influence blood pressure in children are height and weight. Normative tables published by the National Heart, Lung, and Blood Institute (1996) (Task Force Report of High Blood Pressure in Children and Adolescents) list blood pressure standards based on height, weight, and sex in order to include body size to more accurately classify blood pressure norms. However, a more recent report no longer used weight as a factor for calculating normal blood pressure (National High Blood Pressure Education Program Working Group on High Blood Pressure in Children and Adolescents, 2004). However, the increasing occurrence of hypertension in children has been linked to the increase in weight (Couch & Daniels, 2005; Davis et al., 2005; Wyllie, 2005). Overall, the literature supports height and weight as factors that affect blood pressure (Couch & Daniels, 2005; Markovitz, Matthews, Wing, Kuller, & Meilahn, 1991, Muller et al., 2001; Muller, Wiechmann, Helms, Wulff, & Kolenda, 2000).

3. Purpose

The purpose of this study was to determine the relationships between trait anxiety, trait anger, height, weight, patterns of anger expression, and blood pressure in a group of elementary school children.

4. Research questions

Specific research questions addressed were as follows:

1. What are the bivariate relationships between SBP and DBP and height, weight, and sex, trait anger and patterns of anger expression, and trait anxiety in elementary school children?
2. What is the contribution of height, weight, trait anger, anger expression patterns, and trait anxiety to SBP and DBP in elementary school boys and girls?

5. Method

5.1. Design

A descriptive correlational design was used in this study.

5.2. Sample and setting

A convenience sample of 264 children was recruited from the third through the sixth grades in five public elementary schools serving kindergarten through sixth grade in a large metropolitan city in the southeastern United States. These schools served communities of varying socioeconomic levels in urban and suburban locations.

5.3. Instruments

5.3.1. Trait anger

Trait anger was measured by the Trait Anger subscale of the Jacobs Pediatric Anger Scale (Jacobs & Blumer, 1984) (PANG Forms PPS-1 and PPS-2). The PANG is a 10-item self-report inventory developed for use with children. Reliability coefficients for the PANG range from .77 to .84 (Jacobs & Mehlhaff, 1994). A more recent study found the reliability to be .89 (M. Rice, personal communication, November 2004). Items included in the scale are in a Likert format with responses of 1, *hardly ever*; 2, *sometimes*; and 3, *often*. Scores on the PANG range from 10 to 30 and the higher the score, the greater the trait anger.

5.3.2. Anger expression

The 15-item Jacobs Pediatric Anger Expression Scale (PAES) (Jacobs, Phelps, & Rohrs, 1989) was used to measure patterns of anger expression. The instrument contains three scales that have five items each and measure anger-out, anger suppression, and anger reflection/control. Each item is in the form of declarative statements with choices for responses of 1 for *hardly ever*, 2 for *sometimes*, and 3 for *often*. Possible scores for each scale range from 5 to 15. Alpha coefficients for the entire PAES ranged from .57 to .79 (Jacobs et al., 1989). Coefficients for anger out ranged from .66 to .78, for anger suppression from .57 to .76, and for the anger reflection/control scale from .36 to .62 (Jacobs & Mehlhaff, 1994). A more recent study found reliability measure of internal consistency for anger out to be .85, for anger suppression to be .76, and for anger reflection/control to be .70 (M. Rice, personal communication, November 2004).

5.3.3. Trait anxiety

Measurement of trait anxiety was accomplished through use of the Jacob's Pediatric Anxiety Scale (PANX) (Jacobs & Blumer, 1984), a 10-item self-report inventory designed for use with young children. Item to total correlations range from .37 to .53 with an alpha reliability score of .78 for the total scale. A Likert format with three responses was used with a 1 for *hardly ever*, 2 for *sometimes*, and 3 for *often*. Scale scores are calculated by summing the responses on all items so that scores can range from 10 to 30. The higher the score the greater the anxiety. Alpha coefficients on the scale range from .77 to .84 (Jacobs & Mehlhaff, 1994). A more recent study found the reliability to be .80 (M. Rice, personal communication, November 2004).

5.3.4. Blood pressure

The Hawksley's Random Zero sphygmomanometer (W. A. Braum Company Inc., Copiagne, NY), a conventional mercury sphygmomanometer with calibrations 0 to 300 mmHg, was used to obtain blood pressure. This sphygmomanometer is designed to eliminate error variance due to operator and technique by using a shifting zero device. This allows random halting of the mercury between 0 and 20 mmHg so that the operator cannot automatically assume a value. Mercury values must be subtracted from both systolic and diastolic readings to obtain correct blood pressure. The researchers for the study reported here were trained to use the Hawksley. Independent blood pressures on the same participant were taken until a 100% agreement rate was achieved in order to assure interrater reliability. The suggested protocol for measurement of children, including choice of correct cuff size and use of the first reading for nondiagnostic purposes, was followed (National Heart, Lung, and Blood Institute, 1996). Because blood pressure readings were not obtained for the purpose of diagnosing hypertension but for determining the relationships of blood pressure to anger and anxiety scores, only one blood pressure reading was obtained.

5.3.5. Height and weight

Height and weight were measured by a balanced beam scale and the height rod of the balanced beam scale, respectively.

5.4. Procedures

The human assurance committee of the university and the research committee of the county school district approved the proposal. A letter explaining the project and requesting consent for the child to participate was sent home to each child's legally designated caregiver 1 month prior to data collection at each school. On the day of data collection, children with returned completed forms were requested to sign assent forms. The assent form was read aloud to the children before they were requested to sign the form. After assent forms were signed by the children, the PANG, PAES, and the PANX instruments were administered. All instruments were administered by the same investigator. Directions were read aloud, and then the children responded.

Every child read and completed the scales independently. Special effort was taken to stress to the children that this was not a test and that there were no "right" or "wrong" answers. When the scales were completed, the children walked to an adjoining room where a blood pressure reading was obtained for each child.

6. Results

6.1. Sample characteristics

Of the 264 participants enrolled in the study who indicated gender and ethnicity, 107 were boys, 155 were girls; 189 were Black, 58 were White, and 17 were other ethnicities.

6.2. Scale scores

Table 1 shows scores on the study variables for the entire group and then separately for girls and boys. Boys had

Table 1
Scale scores

Variable	Total		Boys		Girls	
	M	SD	M	SD	M	SD
Trait anxiety	18.66	4.16	18.13	4.23	19.0	4.11
Trait anger	17.87	4.84	18.72	4.74	17.34	4.84
Anger out	9.00	2.61	9.50	2.62	8.69	2.57
Anger suppression	9.28	2.27	9.30	2.23	9.29	2.31
Anger reflection	9.98	2.42	9.55	2.22	10.32	2.47
Systolic BP	102.58	10.96	104.66	11.03	101.16	10.75
Diastolic BP	63.28	9.83	64.30	8.72	62.55	10.50

higher mean anger scores but lower mean anxiety scores than the girls. The girl participants had higher SBP and DBP readings, lower anger out, lower anger suppression, and higher anger reflection/control scores than the boys.

6.3. Research Question 1: bivariate correlations

Pearson's product–moment correlations were done in order to address Research Question 1. Table 2 shows correlation results for the children as a group and then separately for boys and girls. For the group as a whole, significant although weak correlations were found between anger reflection/control scores and DBP. Significant and moderately strong correlations were found between height and weight and both SBP and DBP. In addition, there was a significant inverse correlation between height and anger/reflection control scores. Moderate to strong correlations between height and weight and both SBP and DBP were noted for boys and girls.

When correlation analyses were restricted to boys and then girls, different results were obtained. Significant although weak correlations were noted in the boys between DBP and trait anger. A moderate significant correlation was noted between weight and DBP, and a significant although weak correlation was noted between height and DBP in the boys. When girls were considered, a significant although weak negative correlation was found between DBP and anger reflection/control scores.

6.4. Research Question 2: hierarchical multiple regression

In order to answer Research Question 2, six separate hierarchical regression analyses were performed. Two regressions were tested with the entire group, for SBP and DBP in turn, followed by two regressions restricted to sample boys and sample girls, again for SBP then DBP. The variables of height, weight, and sex were entered first as a block as these variables were correlated with blood pressure in this study. The next block included the variables of trait anger, anger out, anger reflection control, and anger suppression because links between blood pressure and anger have been widely documented. The anxiety variable was entered last. When SBP was the dependent variable, 24% of the variance was accounted for in the entire group. Only the first block contributed significantly ($p < .001$; $F = 22.58$).

When DBP was the dependent variable, sex, height, and weight together accounted for 12.4% of the variance ($F = 10.21$; $p < .001$). Only the first block contributed significantly to the model.

6.4.1. Gender

In the next two multiple regression equations, the contribution of study variables to SBP and DBP was restricted to the boys in the study group. Thirty percent of the variance in SBP was accounted for by height and weight ($F = 18.05$; $p < .001$). Height and weight also accounted for 8% of the variance in DBP in the boys ($F = 3.90$; $p < .001$). In the last two multiple regression equations, the contribution of study variables to SBP and DBP was restricted to the girls in the study group. Here, the first block, sex, height, and weight, accounted for 18% of the variance in SBP ($F = 14.53$; $p < .001$). Neither the anger variables nor the anxiety variable that was added in the next block contributed significantly to the model. Height and

Table 2
Correlation table for the entire group, boys, and girls

Variable	Trait anger	Anger out	Anger suppression	Anger reflection	Trait anxiety	Height	Weight
SBP							
Entire group	−.02	−.04	−.04	−.08	−.07	.30***	.46***
Boys	−.04	−.03	−.14	−.13	−.02	.45***	.57***
Girls	−.00	−.06	−.04	−.20*	−.13	.27**	.45***
DPB							
Entire group	−.06	−.07	−.04	−.12*	−.04	.21**	.34***
Boys	−.19*	.08	−.07	−.07	−.04	.20	.27**
Girls	−.04	.07	−.10	−.19	−.05	.24**	.37***

* $p \le .05$.
** $p \le .01$.
*** $p \le .001$.

weight accounted for 13% of the variance in DBP ($F =$ 10.09; $p < .001$). Again, neither anger nor anxiety variables made significant contributions to the model.

7. Discussion

In this study, support was found for the relationships of some of the identified psychosocial and biological factors and blood pressure in children. Children in the group as a whole who indicated more use of anger reflection/control had lower DBP readings. This is consistent with earlier research reporting an association between anger reflection/control and lower blood pressures in adults and children (Harburg, Blakelock, Roeper, 1979; Harburg et al., 1991; Hauber et al., 1998; Muller et al., 2001).

There were no significant relationships between trait anxiety and blood pressure. Much of the research linking anxiety to blood pressure has been conducted with adult samples. Anxiety is thought to contribute to hypertension through repeated autonomic arousal (Jonas et al., 1997; Russek et al., 1990), blood pressure reactivity (Suls & Wan, 1993; Waked & Jutai, 1990), or through the association of anxiety and high-risk health behaviors. The findings in the current study are consistent with the work of Johnson (1989) who found that anxiety was not a predictor of blood pressure in a group of older adolescents. Perhaps the young participants in the current study, as well as Johnson's study, had not yet experienced the long-term negative effects of anxiety on blood pressure.

In this study, height and weight were significantly correlated with SBP and DBP for the entire group. In boys, height and weight were significantly correlated with SBP but not with DBP. In girls, height and weight were significantly correlated with both SBP and DBP. As noted earlier, this relationship is widely acknowledged. Blood pressure has been found to vary with the height, weight, sex, age, and fitness of an individual (Task Force Report of High Blood Pressure in Children and Adolescents, National Heart, Lung, & Blood Institute, 1996). Although weight is no longer used as a factor for calculating normal blood pressure (National High Blood Pressure Education Program Working Group on High Blood Pressure in Children and Adolescents, 2004), the results of this research strongly suggest a relationship.

A bivariate correlation between height and anger reflection control was found in this study. This implies that the taller the individual, the less anger reflection control is used. Perhaps taller children feel less inhibited about expressing their anger in more aggressive ways because their size protects them somewhat from reprisal.

Boys had significant correlations between trait anger scores and DBP. Similar findings have been reported between trait anger and higher blood pressure in both adolescents and adults (Markovitz et al., 1991; Siegel & Leitch, 1981). Girls in the present study showed negative correlations between both SBP and DBP and anger reflection/control. Similar findings were obtained in an earlier study with children (Hauber et al., 1998) where an inverse relationship was noted between anger reflection/control and SBP in girls. These findings suggest the importance of gender-specific research in the area of hypertension and cardiovascular disease. In her study of gender and gender-role identity and expression of anger, Thomas (1997) found that gender was an important factor in anger expression. She suggested that masculine sex-role identity was associated with being more anger prone, expressing anger in an outward manner, and being less likely to control anger expression. Female sex role types were less likely to express anger outwardly or to suppress anger and more likely to attempt anger control. Fabes and Eisenberg (1992) found that female preschoolers vented their anger less than their male counterparts. Fuchs and Thelen (1988) suggested that girls were socialized to hide their anger where boys were taught to hide their sadness or any other feeling such as anxiety that could be interpreted as a sign of weakness. Perhaps, even at this young age, anger reflection is a less acceptable choice for males and does not translate into lower blood pressure in male children in this sample. It may be that no particular expression pattern is associated with blood pressure with boys, although the characteristic of trait anger is related.

In the regression models, neither trait anxiety nor any of the other anger expression patterns accounted for any of the variance in blood pressure. Muller et al. (2001) also found that anger variables did not account for any of the variance in blood pressure in a group of 167 adolescents. In their longitudinal study with 541 normotensive middle-aged women, Raikkonen, Matthews, and Kuller (2001) found that baseline levels of anxiety and anger did not predict subsequent hypertension. However, in the 75 women who became hypertensive during this 9-year study, increases in anger and anxiety during follow-up significantly predicted the incidence of hypertension.

When separate analyses were done for boys and girls after controlling for height and weight, no additional variance in SBP or DBP was explained by trait anger, patterns of anger expression, or trait anxiety. These findings were similar to those of Johnson (1990), who identified no overall relationship between anger variables and SBP.

Although neither the anger variables nor anxiety contributed significantly to the regression model in this study, it should be recognized that factors considered in this study are thought to influence blood pressure in adulthood and are risk factors in children for the future development of hypertension. As children with these risk factors move into adulthood, they may develop hypertension due to repeated episodes of anger and anxiety, which continually stimulate the sympathetic–adrenal–medullary system. The end result is damage to cardiovascular health (Muller et al., 2001). It is important to know that these risk factors, if identified as early as childhood, can be modified before hypertension develops (Meininger et al., 2004; Solomon & Matthews, 1999).

8. Limitations

Blood pressure readings and anger instruments were administered only once per subject. Multiple measurements could provide a pattern of blood pressure, and tracking participants for a longer period could aid in the identification of patterns across developmental periods.

9. Implications and recommendations

Because anger and anxiety are associated with hypertension in adults, a longitudinal study would help identify when anger and anxiety begin to contribute to the explanation of hypertension.

Current results indicate that anger reflection/control patterns are associated with lower levels of blood pressure in girls of this age. This finding is consistent with results of an earlier study with 230 third-grade boys and girls (Hauber et al., 1998) and suggests that children may benefit from anger management interventions aimed at anger control strategies. Identification of factors that influence a child's choice of anger expression patterns, the effect on blood pressure, and the contributions of gender would be helpful when designing intervention programs. The school nurse could be involved in identifying and recommending interventions for children who have frequent anger problems in the classroom or whose parents report frequent angry outbursts in the home environment.

Future research should investigate whether these findings remain consistent across younger age groups, different socioeconomic groups, varying regions of the country, and more varied ethnic groups (Rice & Howell, 2006).

This study supports the belief that certain modifiable risk factors for hypertension are present at an early age. It has been recommended that BP should be monitored by the age of 3 for every child during every scheduled physical examination (National High Blood Pressure Education Program Working Group on High Blood Pressure in Children and Adolescents, 2004). It is important to monitor BP across a period of time to determine any elevations or pattern of BP (Cook, Gillman, Rosner, Taylor, & Hennekens, 2000). This type of assessment is most often performed by a nurse (Hauber et al., 1998). According to Moran, Panzarino, Darden, and Reigart (2003) although the rate of BP screening during well-child checkups has increased, it does not meet current recommendations. If the BP reading is normal (less than 90th percentile for sex, age, and height) it should be rechecked at the next scheduled physical exam and the nurse should encourage adequate sleep and an active lifestyle with healthy meals. A prehypertensive reading is the 90th percentile to less than the 95th percentile. This reading should be rechecked in 6 months. In this instance the nurse should counsel the parents and the child about active lifestyle and diet changes and weight reduction if

the child is overweight (National High Blood Pressure Education Program Working Group on High Blood Pressure in Children and Adolescents, 2004). If hypertensive (95th–99th percentile with the addition of 5 mmHg) the reading should be checked again on at least two occasions, usually within a few weeks to confirm the diagnosis of hypertension (National High Blood Pressure Education Program Working Group on High Blood Pressure in Children and Adolescents, 2004).

The nurse may also be the first health care professional to recognize unhealthy patterns of anger and anger expression. The nurse may be able to teach healthier means of expressing anger, such as anger reflection control, physical activity, or cognitive behavioral interventions (Rice & Howell, 2006). It is important to intervene in unhealthy lifestyles early rather than later when the disease becomes evident (Meininger et al., 2004; Solomon & Matthews, 1999). Lifestyle changes are more easily accomplished at early ages before behavior patterns become ingrained. If risk factors for cardiovascular disease are reduced early enough, cardiovascular disease will be delayed or avoided altogether. Early anger management training for children holds promise for preventing the translation of anger into medical and behavioral problems.

Acknowledgment

This research was supported by grants from the College of Health Sciences, Georgia State University, Atlanta, Georgia.

References

American Heart Association. (2004). Statistical supplement. Retrieved August 10, 2004, from http://www.americanheart.org.

Chang, P., Ford, D., Meoni, L., Wang, N., & Klag, M. (2002, Apr). Anger in young men and subsequent premature cardiovascular disease. *Archives of Internal Medicine, 162*(8), 901–906.

Cook, N., Gillman, M., Rosner, B., Taylor, J., & Hennekens, C. (2000). Combining annual blood pressure measurements in childhood to improve prediction of young adult blood pressure. *Statistics in Medicine, 19*(19), 2625–2640.

Couch, S., & Daniels, S. (2005). Diet and blood pressure in children. *Current Opinions in Pediatrics, 17*(5), 642–647

Davis, C., Flickinger, B., Moore, D., Bassali, R., Domel Baxter, S., & Yin, Z. (2005, Aug). Prevalence of cardiovascular risk factors in schoolchildren in a rural Georgia community. *American Journal of Medicine and Science, 330*(2), 53–59.

Ewart, C., & Kolodner, K. (1994). Negative affect, gender and expressive style predict elevated ambulatory blood pressure in adolescents. *Journal of Personality and Social Psychology, 66*(3), 596–605.

Fabes, R., & Eisenberg, N. (1992). Young children's coping with interpersonal anger. *Child Development, 63*, 116–128.

Fuchs, D., & Thelen, M. (1988). Children's expected interpersonal consequences of communicating their affective state and reported likelihood of expression. *Childhood Development, 59*, 1314–1322.

Harburg, E., Blakelock, E., & Roeper, P. (1979). Resentful and reflective coping with arbitrary authority and blood pressure: Detroit. *Psychosomatic Medicine, 41*, 189–202.

Harburg, E., Gleiberman, L., Russell, M., & Cooper, M. (1991). Anger-coping styles and blood pressure in Black and White males: Buffalo, New York. *Psychosomatic Medicine, 41*, 189–202.

Hauber, R., Rice, M., Howell, C., & Carmon, M. (1998). Anger and blood pressure readings in children. *Psychosomatic Medicine, 11*(1), 2–11.

Heker, B., Whalen, C., Jamner, L., & Delfino, R. (2002, June). Anxiety, affect, and activity teenagers: Monitoring daily life with electronic diaries. *Journal of American Academy of Child and Adolescent Psychiatry, 41*(6), 660–670.

Jacobs, G., & Blumer, C. (1984). *The pediatric anger scale.* Vermillion: University of South Dakota, Department of Psychology.

Jacobs, G., & Mehlhaff, C. (1994). *Children's stress and the expression and experience and experience of anger.* Unpublished manuscript, University of South Dakota, Vermillion.

Jacobs, G., Phelps, M., & Rhors, B. (1989). Assessment of anger in children: The pediatric anger scale. *Personality and Individual Differences, 10*, 59–65.

Johnson, E. (1984). *Anger and anxiety as determinants of elevated blood pressure in adolescents: The Tampa study.* Unpublished doctoral dissertation, University of South Florida, Tampa.

Johnson, E. (1989). The role of the experience and expression of anger and anxiety in elevated blood pressure among black and white adolescents. *Journal of the National Medical Association, 81*(5), 573–584.

Johnson, E. (1990). Interrelationships between psychological factors, overweight, and blood pressure in adolescents. *Journal of Adolescent Healthcare, 11*, 310–318.

Jonas, B., Franks, P., & Ingram, D. (1997). Are symptoms of anxiety and depression risk factors for hypertension? *Archives of Family Medicine, 6*, 43–49.

Krantz, D., & Manuck, S. (1984). Acute psychophysiologic reactivity and risk of cardiovascular disease: A review and methodological critique. *Psychological Bulletin, 96*, 535–564.

Markovitz, J. H., Matthews, K., Wing, R. R., Kuller, L. H., & Meilahn, E. N. (1991). Psychological, biological and health behavior predictors of blood pressure changes in middle-aged women. *Journal of Hypertension, 9*, 399–406.

Meinginger, J., Liehr, P., Chan, W., Smith, G., & Muller, W. (2004). Developmental, gender, and ethic group differences in moods and ambulatory blood pressure in adolescents. *Annals of Behavioral Medicine, 28*(1), 10–19.

Moran, C., Panzarino, V., Darden, P., & Reigart, J. (2003). Preventive services: Blood pressure checks at well child visits. *Clinical Pediatrics, 42*(7), 627–634.

Muller, W., Grunbaum, J., & Labarthe, D. (2001, Jul–Aug). Anger expression, body fat, and blood pressure in adolescents: Project HeartBeat. *American Journal of Human Biology, 13*(4), 531–538.

Muller, M., Wiechmann, M., Helms, C., Wulff, C., & Kolenda, K. (2000, May). Nutrient intake with low-fat diets in rehabilitation of patients with coronary heart disease. *Zeitschrift fur Kardiologie, 89*(5), 454–464.

National Heart, Lung, and Blood Institute. National Institutes of Health. (1996). *Update on the task force report on high blood pressure in children and adolescents: A working group report from the National High Blood Pressure Education Program (SDHSS Publication No. NIH 96-3790).* Washington, DC: U.S. Government Printing Office. Children and Adolescents.

National High Blood Pressure Education Program Working Group on High Blood Pressure in Children and Adolescents. (2004). The fourth report on the diagnosis, evaluation, and treatment of high blood pressure in children and adolescents. *Pediatrics, 114*(2), 555–576.

Raikkonen, K., Matthews, K., & Kuller, L. (2001). Trajectory of psychological risk and incident of hypertension in middle-aged women. *Hypertension, 38*(4), 798–802.

Rice, M., & Howell, C. (2006). Differences in trait anger among children with varying levels of anger expression patterns. *Journal of Child and Adolescent Psychiatric Nursing, 19*(2), 51–61.

Russek, L., King, S., Russek, S., & Russek, H. (1990). The Harvard Mastery of Stress Study 35-year follow-up: Prognostic significance of patterns of psychophysiological arousal and adaptation. *Psychosomatic Medicine, 52*, 271–285.

Siegel, J. (1984). Anger and cardiovascular risk in adolescents. *Health Psychology, 3*, 293–313.

Siegel, J., & Leitch, C. (1981). Behavioral factors and blood pressure in adolescence: The Tacoma study. *American Journal of Epidemiology, 113*, 171–181.

Solomon, K., Matthews, K. (1999, March). *Paper presented at the American Psychosomatic Society Annual Meeting.* Vancouver, British Columbia, Canada.

Speilberger, C., Edwards, C., Lushene, R., Montuori, J., & Platzek, D. (1973). *State-trait anxiety inventory for children.* Palo Alto, CA: Consulting Psychologists Press.

Speilberger, C., Johnson, E., Russell, S., Crane, R., Jacobs, G., & Worden, T. (1985). The experience and expression of anger: Construction and validation of an anger expression scale. In M. Chesney, R. Rosenman, (Eds.), *Anger and hostility in cardiovascular and behavioral disorders* (pp. 5–30). Washington, DC: Hemisphere.

Starner, T., & Peters, R. (2004). Anger expression and blood pressure in adolescents. *Journal of School Nursing, 20*(6), 335–342.

Suls, J., & Wan, C. (1993). The relationship between trait hostility and cardiovascular reactivity: A quantitative review and analysis. *Psychophysiology, 30*, 615–626 http://www.nhlbi.nih.gov/meetings/ish/stamler.htm.

Taylor, S., Repetti, R., & Seeman, T. (1997). Health psychology: What is an unhealthy environment and how does it get under the skin? *Annual Review of Psychology, 48*, 411–447.

Thomas, S. (1997). Women's anger: Relationship of suppression to blood pressure. *Nursing Research, 46*(6), 324–330.

Waked, E., & Jutai, J. (1990). Baseline and reactivity measures of blood pressure and negative affect in borderline hypertension. *Physiological Behavior, 47*, 266–271.

Wascher, R. (2002, April). Stay at home dads and risk of cardiovascular disease. *Jewish World Review* 2002, April.

Weinrich, S., Weinrich, M., Hardin, S., Gleaton, J., Pesut, D., & Garrison, C. (2000). Effects of psychological distress on blood pressure in adolescents. *Holistic Nurse Practitioner, 5*(1), 57–65.

Williams, R., & Williams, V. (1993). *Anger kills.* New York: Harper Collins Publishers.

Wyllie, R. (2005). Obesity in childhood: An overview. *Current Opinions Pediatrics, 17*(5), 632–635.

APPENDIX B

Nursing Research • November/December 2006 • Vol 55, No 6, 381–390

The Anniversary of Birth Trauma

Failure to Rescue

Cheryl Tatano Beck

Editor's Note

Materials documenting the review process for this article are posted at http://www.nursing-research-editor.com.

▶ **Background:** The reported prevalence of posttraumatic stress disorder secondary to birth trauma ranges from 1.5% to 5.6%. Serious ramifications of birth trauma are beginning to be recognized, such as impaired mother-infant interaction.

▶ **Objective:** The aim of this study was to determine the essence of mothers' experiences regarding the anniversary of their birth trauma.

▶ **Methods:** Colaizzi's method of phenomenology was used to guide the study. Participants were recruited via the Internet through a charitable trust located in New Zealand called Trauma and Birth Stress. Thirty-seven women sent attachment stories describing their experiences of the anniversary of their traumatic childbirths.

▶ **Results:** Four themes revealed the essence of women's experiences of the anniversary of their birth trauma: (a) The prologue: An agonizing time; (b) The actual day: A celebration of a birthday or the torment of an anniversary; (c) The epilogue: A fragile state; and (d) Subsequent anniversaries: For better or worse.

▶ **Discussion:** Based on the findings of this study on the anniversary of traumatic childbirths, the time seems right to broaden the use of the term *failure to rescue* to these childbearing women. Not only clinicians but also family and friends failed to rescue mothers during the period surrounding the anniversary of their birth trauma.

▶ **Key Words:** birth trauma · failure to rescue · posttraumatic stress disorder

In the words of one mother, "Every birthday is no longer the celebration of the child but is really an anniversary for the rape. Rape day. My son was conceived from love and born out of rape." The reported prevalence of posttraumatic stress disorder (PTSD) secondary to child-birth ranges from 1.5% (Ayers & Pickering, 2001) to 5.6% (Creedy, Shochet, & Horsfall, 2000). This PTSD has been reported recently after stillbirths (Turton, Hughes, Evans, & Fainman, 2001), after pregnancy complicated by severe preeclampsia (van Pampus, Wolf, Weijmar Schultz, Neeleman, & Aarnoudse, 2004), and after birth of very low birth weight infants (Kersting et al., 2004). In other studies, although no formal diagnosis of PTSD was made, the percentage of women reporting traumatic births ranged from 34% (Soet, Brack, & Dilorio, 2003) to 55% (Ryding, Wijma, & Wijma, 1998).

The long-term effects of PTSD secondary to birth trauma on women and their families can include mother–infant attachment difficulties and related parenting problems (Bailham & Joseph, 2003; Beck, 2004a, 2004b). Sexual avoidance and fear of childbirth are two other effects (Fones, 1996; Goldbeck-Wood, 1996). Serious ramifications of just the perception of delivery as a negative experience are now being recognized. For example, in Sweden, women who reported a very negative experience of their first birth had fewer subsequent children and a larger time interval to the second baby as compared with women who reported positive birth experiences (Gottvall & Waldenstrom, 2002).

In their recent literature review, Olde, van der Hart, Kleber, and van Son (2006) concluded that more attention needs to be focused on birth trauma and PTSD as serious mental health problems. Olde et al. called for investigation of the chronic nature of birth trauma, particularly to examine childbirth-related posttraumatic stress lasting for more than 6 months postpartum.

Literature Review

Persons with PTSD, no matter what the original traumatic event was (i.e., rape, domestic violence, war, motor vehicle accidents, burns), experience a trio of distressing symptom

Cheryl Tatano Beck, DNSc, CNM, FAAN, is Professor, School of Nursing, University of Connecticut, Storrs.

behaviors. These symptoms are (a) reexperiencing the traumatic event through flashbacks, nightmare, or distressing recollections; (b) avoidance of stimuli or triggers (thoughts or activities related to the original trauma); and (c) hyperarousal or hypervigilance, such as exaggerated startle response, anger, or sleep disturbance (American Psychiatric Association [APA], 2000).

Repeatedly confirmed in the literature is that triggering events that resemble an aspect of the traumatic event can result in distress, heightened arousal, or both. For example, a trigger for a military returnee from Afghanistan and Iraq is driving along a highway (Friedman, 2006). His original traumatic event had been the explosion of a roadside bomb. Since being back in the United States, at times, when he is a passenger in a car, he will reach over suddenly and grab the steering wheel because he saw something he thought was a roadside bomb. Another example of a trigger comes from a motor vehicle accident victim (Ehlers, Hackmann, & Michael, 2004). After her car accident, she had been trapped in her car and a paramedic had touched her shoulder as he inquired if she was all right. She reexperiences a flashback to her accident when someone touches her shoulder.

In the *Diagnostic and Statistical Manual for Mental Disorders* (*DSM-IV*; APA, 2000), the anniversary of a traumatic event is identified as one possible trigger for intense psychological distress. The anniversary of birth trauma, however, has a complicating factor that other anniversaries do not have. The day of the anniversary is also the day of an event that should be cause for celebration: the birthday of the child who was born on the day of the original traumatic event.

The limited studies that have been published on birth trauma and the resulting PTSD have been concentrated on identifying prevalence and risk factors. Reported predictors include high degree of obstetric intervention, dissatisfaction with care received during labor and delivery, feelings of powerlessness, history of psychological problems, anxiety sensitivity, and previous birth trauma (Creedy et al., 2000; Czarnocka & Slade, 2000; Keogh, Ayers, & Francis, 2002; Skari et al., 2002; Soet et al., 2003).

Recently, a couple of interventions aimed at decreasing the risk of developing psychological trauma have been tested with new mothers. In Italy, 64 women with an uncomplicated pregnancy and no history of diagnosed psychopathology were assigned randomly to either an experimental or control group. Prior to the intervention, women did not report that their births had been traumatic. Examined was the impact of written expression of negative emotions connected to labor and delivery on the occurrence of stress symptoms (DiBlasio & Ionio, 2002). Two days after delivery, women in the experimental group were asked to write a brief account of their childbirth experience, including their personal thoughts and feelings. Women completed the Perinatal PTSD Questionnaire (DeMier, Hynan, Harris, & Manniello, 1996) 2 days after delivery and again at 2 months postpartum. The experimental group reported significantly less stress symptoms in all three categories of avoidance, hyperarousal, and reexperiencing the unpleasant event than did the control group at 2 months postpartum. The authors concluded that it was not possible to understand completely whether these differences were due to the narrative accounts written by the mothers or environmental factors, such as social networks or family environment.

In Australia, Gamble et al. (2005) assessed the impact of a midwife-led brief counseling intervention for postpartum women at risk of developing psychological trauma symptoms. The sample of 103 mothers who had experienced a traumatic delivery were assigned randomly to either an experimental group or control group. The intervention consisted of face-to-face counseling within 72 hours of birth and again by telephone at 4 to 6 weeks postpartum. At 3 months postpartum, the intervention group mothers reported a significant decrease in trauma symptoms.

Only three qualitative studies were found in which traumatic births or PTSD secondary to birth trauma were examined. Allen, Nicholson, and Woollett (1998) interviewed 20 mothers 10 months after their delivery that they perceived as being traumatic. Using a grounded theory design, Allen et al. revealed that the core category associated with birth trauma was the women's feelings of loss of control of events or their own behavior.

Beck (2004a) examined the meaning of women's birth trauma experiences using a phenomenological design. Analysis of the stories of 40 women revealed four themes: (a) To care for me: Was that too much to ask?; (b) To communicate with me: Why was this neglected?; (c) To provide safe care: You betrayed my trust and I felt powerless; and (d) The end justifies the means: At whose expense? At what price?

Beck (2004b) went on to investigate the effect of birth trauma on 38 mothers, namely, PTSD due to the traumatic births. In this phenomenological study, five themes emerged: (a) Going to the movies: Please don't make me go; (b) A shadow of myself: Too numb to try and change; (c) Seeking to have questions answered and wanting to talk, talk, talk; (d) The dangerous trio of anger, anxiety, and depression: spiraling downward; and (e) Isolation from the world of motherhood: dreams shattered.

No research was found to show what mothers who perceive they have had traumatic childbirths experience each year as the anniversary of their birth trauma occurs. The purpose of this study was to describe the essence of women's experiences regarding the anniversary of their birth trauma.

Methods

Sample

Criteria for sample eligibility included the following: (a) a woman perceived her childbirth had been traumatic, (b) she had experienced at least one anniversary of that birth trauma, (c) she was 18 years of age or older, and (d) she could articulate her experience. The Internet-based sample consisted of 37 women who perceived their labor and delivery as traumatic. Eighteen women (49%) reported having been diagnosed with PTSD due to childbirth. Twelve of those mothers are currently undergoing therapy for their PTSD. Approximately half of the sample was from the United States. Age ranged from 24 to 54 years old, with a mean of 32 years. The demographic and obstetrical characteristics of the sample are located in Table 1.

Mothers described having endured various birth traumas. Examples of some of the more frequently cited traumatic

TABLE 1. Demographic and Obstetrical Characteristics of the Sample

Characteristic	n	%
Marital status (n = 33)		
Married	31	94
Single	1	3
Divorced	1	3
Education (n = 29)		
High school	7	25
Some college	1	3
Associate degree	2	7
College	12	41
Masters	6	21
PhD	1	3
Country (n = 37)		
United States	20	54
New Zealand	8	22
Australia	4	11
United Kingdom	4	11
Canada	1	2
Parity (n = 33)		
Primipara	19	58
Multipara	14	42
Delivery (n = 31)		
Vaginal	18	58
Cesarean	13	42

births included preterm delivery, shoulder dystocia, excruciating pain, and emergency cesarean deliveries. Amniotic fluid embolism, cardiac arrest, and prolapsed cord are examples of birth traumas that were cited by only one woman each.

Research Design and Data Analysis

Colaizzi's (1973, 1978) method of phenomenological psychology was used to guide this study. He offered four sources of descriptive data for a phenomenological study: written descriptions, dialogal interviews, observation of lived events, and imaginative presence. Each source of descriptive data has a corresponding descriptive method for analysis. Written descriptions were the source of data selected for this anniversary of birth trauma study because mothers would send their stories via attachments over the Internet. Protocol analysis is Colaizzi's (1978) method for the analysis of written descriptions of the phenomenon being studied.

The researcher began by examining her presuppositions about the phenomenon under study. Here, the researcher asked, "Why am I involved with this phenomenon?" (Colaizzi, 1978, p. 55). This inquiry included reviewing two previous studies the researcher had conducted on birth trauma and the resulting PTSD, where some mothers had touched briefly on the anniversary of their traumatic childbirths (Beck, 2004a, 2004b).

Colaizzi's (1978) method of data analysis calls for seven procedural steps.

1. Read the participants' written descriptions (protocols) of the phenomenon under study to obtain a feel for them and to make sense of them.
2. From each protocol, extract significant phrases or sentences that pertain to the phenomenon being studied. If protocols include the same or nearly the same statements, repetitions can be eliminated.
3. Formulate meanings for each significant statement. Creative insight, according to Colaizzi (1978), is needed for this precarious leap from what the participants said to what they mean. In this step, the researcher does not sever ties to the original protocols but attempts to discover hidden meanings.
4. Organize the formulated meanings into clusters of themes. Formulated meanings are grouped into clusters to allow for themes that are common to the participants' protocols to emerge. The clusters of themes are referred back to the original protocols to validate them. At this stage in data analysis, Colaizzi (1978) warns the researcher to "rely upon tolerance for ambiguity" (p. 61) and not to give in to temptation to ignore data or themes that do not seem to fit.
5. All the findings from the data analysis so far are combined into an exhaustive description of the phenomenon under study.
6. The exhaustive description is tightened up into "as unequivocal a statement of identification of its fundamental structure as possible" (Colaizzi, 1978, p. 61).
7. The final step is validation, when the researcher can return to participants and ask them to review the results thus far. The researcher can inquire, for example, if any aspects of their experience have been left out. Any new, relevant data offered as participants validate the results should be integrated into the final product of the research.

Procedure

After approval was obtained from the university's institutional review board, data collection began. This phase of the research extended over a 15-month period. Mothers were recruited via the Internet through a charitable trust located in New Zealand called Trauma and Birth Stress (TABS). Their Web site is www.tabs.org.nz and e-mail is ptsdtabs@ihug.co.nz. With TABS, support is provided to women who have suffered from traumatic births and provides education to healthcare providers and the public regarding PTSD due to childbirth.

A recruitment notice was placed on the Web site of TABS and also in their newsletter. For the 15-month period of data collection, the average number of hits to the Web site was 2,126 per month. A link was provided directly to the researcher's e-mail address at the University for any mothers interested in participating in the study. In addition to recruitment from TABS, a few mothers learned about the study from two other Web sites: one for mothers who had preterm infants and one for women whose infants had a brachial plexus injury. Women who visited these Web sites and participated in this study notified other mothers of this research.

Response rates for Internet research are based on the number of persons who initially contact the researcher for details of the study and then agree to participate (Hamilton & Bowers, 2006). In this anniversary of birth trauma study, 62 women initially responded to the Internet recruitment notice and requested additional information about the study. Of these 62 women, 37 mothers participated in the study, for a response rate of 60%.

Informed consent and directions for the research were sent via e-mail attachment to prospective participants. The women had the opportunity to e-mail the researcher if they had any questions regarding the study. The participants electronically signed the informed consent and returned it to the researcher via attachment. Participation in the study entailed the woman describing her experience of the anniversary of her birth trauma in as much detail as she wished to share. The women sent their anniversary stories to the researcher over the Internet as e-mail attachments. The length of time it took mothers to send their stories after they had signed the informed consent ranged from as short as a few days to over 6 months. A benefit of e-mail interviews is that participants can take as much time as needed to reflect on the questions (Hamilton & Bowers, 2006). The e-mail interviews that the women sent to the researcher were in such rich detail and depth that rarely did the researcher need to contact the participants for any additional information. If contact was needed at all, it was just to ask a mother to clarify a point she had made or to provide a specific example.

Trustworthiness

Rigor was achieved by addressing credibility, confirmability, dependability, and transferability. In regard to credibility and confirmability, member checking was conducted as per Colaizzi's (1978) method of analysis. The findings were reviewed by two women who had experienced multiple anniversaries of their birth trauma and also by one of their husbands. Their reactions to the themes can be summarized by a segment from one of these mothers' e-mails after she had read the manuscript: "This is superb and I love every word of it." Saturation of data was achieved much earlier than the final sample size of 37 mothers. Because the women were eager to have their stories help to prevent other women from suffering from birth trauma, the researcher made a decision not to turn away these participants and to include their additional e-mail interviews.

Credibility was enhanced also by keeping a reflexive journal throughout the 15-month data collection phase and during the data analysis phase. Efforts were made to avoid what Thorne and Darbyshire (2005) call *lachrymal validity*. The concern with this type of validity is the misrepresentation of findings by including only the most dramatic or poignant stories that bring tears to the eyes of its readers. For example, positive aspects of subsequent anniversaries of birth trauma were included purposely in the results so as not to give a false impression that mothers' experiences never improved as the years passed from the original traumatic event.

Transferability of the results was enhanced by using the Internet to recruit the sample, which represented five different countries from around the world. A thick description of rich, vivid quotes was included in the findings to increase also the study's transferability. The dependability of the study was enhanced by adding Hycner's (1985) suggestion of listing for each theme its subsumed significant statements and their original numeration (Table 2). E-mail interviewing also allows for an easily maintained audit trail (Hamilton & Bowers, 2006). Intersubjective agreement among expert judges was not assessed in this study. Unlike Van Kaam's (1966) phenomenological analysis, Colaizzi's (1978) method does not include such a step for intersubjective agreement.

This Internet sampling method, however, can be viewed as a possible limitation of the study. A disadvantage of Internet recruitment is that the population typically is skewed toward those with a higher income and higher level of education (Hamilton & Bowers, 2006). Only women who had access to the Internet participated in the study. These women also used the resource of TABS, the charitable trust providing support to mothers who have suffered traumatic childbirths. It is not known whether women who have neither Internet access nor support from TABS would describe their experiences of the anniversary of their birth trauma differently than what emerged from the current study.

Results

Birthdays—what do they mean to you? For me a birthday prior to my son's birth meant joy, presents, relaxation and celebration. Now it has a darker side to it. A profound depth that I never could have imagined was possible. So what changed? Well, everything and all in the space of some 24 hours during my labor and delivery. This is my story of how birthdays became the BIRTH day!

From the 37 stories of the anniversary of birth trauma, 231 significant statements, including the paragraph above, were extracted. Analysis of these significant statements revealed four clusters of themes that captured the essence of this phenomenon of the anniversary of the BIRTH day. A portion of the audit trail is illustrated in Table 2.

Cluster of Themes I—The Prologue: An Agonizing Time

During the weeks and months leading up to the anniversary of traumatic births, women were plagued by an array of distressing thoughts and emotions. For some women, the approaching anniversary also took a toll on them physically. Clocks, calendars, and seasons all play key roles as the anniversary of birth trauma approaches. Clock watching consumed some mothers' days and nights. As one woman shared,

The entire 2 days before the anniversary I watch the clock and relive all the hell I know that a year or two or three now ago for the first 30 plus hours of labor I was hanging in there suffering but dealing with the pain virtually alone.

TABLE 2. Partial Audit Trail for Two Themes Included Under the Cluster of Themes 2—The Actual Day: A Celebration of a Birthday or the Torment of an Anniversary

Significant Statements	Formulated Meanings
1. Various ways to make it through the day	
A. "I knew I didn't want to be home on birthday or I would have been crying all day. That's why we planned a vacation to Disneyland." (68)	Going away on vacation/holiday to make certain the mother would not be home for the actual birthday.
B. "I have always held a birthday party for my son but usually delay it until about a week after. This year, I held it 3 weeks after his actual birthday as I couldn't deal with it at the time and became ill probably due to the stress of wanting to avoid his birthday." (100)	Delaying the celebration of the child's birthday for a week or so after the actual anniversary of the birth trauma.
C. "There were times when I could tell I was overanalyzing details of the party (decorations, food) to numb out the feelings of the trauma. When I was obsessed with trivial details, I embraced it as a sign of self-protection." (199)	Focusing on the birthday party being a technical success so as to avoid concentrating on the meaning of the day.
D. "I still remember feeling like a total faker with my feigned excitement and smile just trying to appear happy for my son as he opened up his presents and played with the cake." (15)	Feigning excitement and happiness at the child's birthday celebration.
E. "There is sooo much emphasis on time in the birthing process. So this seemed to carry and surface on his birthday. I found myself linking the time of day to what happened that day driving to the hospital, number of dilation to the minute, and when my water broke." (141)	Clock watching as mothers retraced the trauma they had to endure on the actual day of the birth year(s) ago.
2. Difficult emotions mothers had to contend with.	
A. "I felt full of rage at the selfish people who stole the birth of my son from me and now manage to steal the fun of his birthday from me each year." (211)	Consumed with rage at the clinicians who not only stole her son's birth from her but also the joy of celebrating his birthday every year.
B. "My self esteem was really low that day. I felt like a complete failure as a mother." (4)	Self-esteem plummeted due to feeling like such a failure as a mother on her daughter's birthday.
C. "I felt overwhelmed with sadness and grief over what I had to endure that day." (32)	Grief stricken as she relived what she had endured the year before on this day.
D. "I felt such guilt because I wasn't truly 'there'—mind, body, or spirit on her birthday." (155)	Filled with guilt because the mother knew she was not fully present for her daughter on her birthday.
E. "I was angry when my family and friends didn't mention the birth or my hospital experience at all. I had hoped that my 'support' around me would break out of their denial and happy faces and suddenly acknowledge the trauma and its affect on me." (124)	Anger replaced the woman's hope as her family and friends failed to acknowledge the trauma she had endured during the birth and the hold it still had on her.

The numbers in parentheses indicate significant statement's original numeration.

As the season of the year approached when the traumatic birth had occurred, the change in the weather or an upcoming holiday triggered fear and "bad memories" in some women. For one mother, autumn was the difficult season,

There is also a distinct smell of dead leaves in the air that screams, "October!" Hearing the word, October, and seeing the word in writing gives me chills. When I would see decorations for Halloween, fear rushed through my body.

In the days approaching the birth trauma anniversaries, women kept ruminating about the day their babies had been born. As one mother reflected on her fourth anniversary,

I still after 4 years find that before her birthday I go back over that night again and again thinking about the things

I could/should have done to change things (although in reality there was almost nothing I could have done). I kept going over in my head all of the details but I just couldn't stop thinking about her birth.

Dread, anxiety, stress, sadness, grief, loss, fear, and guilt were some of the distressing emotions that came to the forefront as women's birth trauma anniversaries loomed near. One mother remembered feeling extremely anxious and frightened the 2 months leading up to her baby's first birthday. Terrifying flashbacks would come without any warning during this 2-month period.

Complicating these distressing emotions as the anniversary drew near was the harsh reality that the anniversary day was also the birthday of their children. Mothers struggled not to let their children know what they were feeling. This battle within the mother is clearly seen in the next excerpt.

I'm filled with an overwhelming sense of dread of the upcoming occasion and my nightmares are more ferocious. I am locked in a battle of will at not letting my daughter sense or become aware of my problem. I never want her to know the reason for my problem/behavior. The birth trauma and her injury has taken soooo much from my child and our entire family for that matter but I don't want it to continue to impact her special day, her BIRTHDAY, as well.

Oftentimes, mothers were grateful that their children were too young to know the significance of the day. As the first birthday approached, this mom revealed,

I anxiously opened birthday cards for my son during the week prior. I passed them to him with a plastic smile and that was all I could muster. I was pleased when he chewed them and tore them to shreds with his new teeth. I didn't have to display the cards and I tossed them in the recycling bin before anyone else saw them.

The traumatic deliveries left some mothers feeling like they were not "a real mommy" and that the emotional bonding with their infants was missing. One woman shared,

I continually tell myself that I am "over" the birth and a real mommy but each year as my daughter's birthday approaches I feel more and more anxious. I have a strong belief that her real parents will turn up and demand to know why I had been so bad at looking after their child.

For another mother, as her daughter's first birthday approached, she painfully shared that

I wanted to die. I felt nothing for her and found it hard to celebrate the joy of this child that meant so little to me. I took excellent care of her but it was if I was babysitting, the emotional bond just wasn't there.

The struggles surrounding the looming anniversary physically took a toll on some women. For example, one woman revealed that "my asthma and psoriasis flared up, my digestive problems became debilitating at least 3 weeks before my daughter's birthday." Exhaustion becomes a problem due to disturbed sleep patterns: "I found it very difficult to sleep for several weeks before the birthday. I could not sleep at all the night before her birthday (she was born at 7:15 am so labor was overnight)."

A couple of nights before her baby's first birthday a mother recalled,

I went to bed and experienced a nightmare linked to my c-section which took on the form of an assault. I woke up as the doctor was wielding a weapon (a chainsaw I think) and everything turned to white. I went back to sleep and then woke up in the morning with pains in my upper legs. I was convinced that something was wrong and that I was going to die because these pains were fatal, i.e. thrombosis.

As the anniversary of their birth trauma lurked on the horizon, some women restricted their food intake. The reasoning of one mother was as follows:

I tried to fast for 52 hours (the length of my labor and delivery ordeal) and retrace and re-script every humiliat-

ing, dehumanizing, torturous detail of the trauma in an attempt to reclaim some semblance of personal power but I made it for only 36 hours into the fast before I was sick from dehydration and hypoglycemia.

Cluster of Themes 2—The Actual Day: A Celebration of a Birthday or the Torment of an Anniversary

When the anniversary day finally arrived, it was all the women had dreaded and more. What added an extra layer of difficulty was the fact that the day was also supposed to be the celebration of their children's birthdays. Just as in the period leading up to the anniversary, the concept of time took center stage during the actual day itself. Hard as mothers would try to avoid clock-watching, the inevitable would happen. As one woman recalled during her first anniversary, "I relived every moment synchronized to the clock. Even today a clock reading 8:46 will turn my stomach upside down." Relief was experienced by some of the women as they looked at the clock and saw that the time their children had been born had passed.

Some women who have experienced birth trauma do not know how to celebrate their child's birthday,

I can't stop seeing images of a woman drugged and strapped down and being gutted like a fish. I can't get those or my own images out of my mind. I didn't know how to celebrate my daughter's birthday.

The powerful emotions that surfaced and tormented the mothers during the anniversary day added yet another layer of burden that they had to contend with while trying their best to celebrate their child's birthday. Reflecting over four birthdays, one mother shared that

It breaks my heart because the very day when I should be honoring the precious life of my child and just truly enjoying his birthday, I often feel overwhelmed with sadness and grief over the loss we all endured.

During the birthday itself, for some women, anxiety heightened to panic. One woman who had "celebrated" 23 years of anniversaries of her birth trauma revealed that "on my son's birthdays I would always feel a bit 'funny' trying not to remember my stress and panic attacks would be worse."

Guilt was pervasive. Recalling her daughter's first birthday, one mother said,

I look at her first birthday as a loss and with guilt. My whole being continued to center around the hospital events. I craved "speed healing." I questioned why do I bother going on as I am a worthless mom and I will never be good enough for my baby.

For some women, all they recalled about their child's birthday was feeling empty inside, like a "total faker." During the party, one mother described, "I was really empty inside. It felt as though I was looking in at the party from a window. Again I think I was hoping for someone to take me aside and to acknowledge the birth trauma!" Other mothers confirmed this wish that at least their traumatic births would be recognized by family and friends at some point during the day's celebration. As the day ended, women's unmet hopes for the much needed acknowledgment turned to anger.

For those mothers who did celebrate their child's birthday on the actual day, there were varying approaches they used to make it through the day and try to protect themselves. Being consumed with the technical aspects and details of the birthday party was one way women coped. Other mothers needed to get away physically and so vacations were planned so that the anniversary occurred while they were away from home. The following quote illustrates this:

> I thought that I would re-experience many of the memories and feelings on my son's birthday. I wanted us to be alone as we had been alone on the day. I wanted to be able to have time to think. I didn't want to share the day with people who had been unsupportive at the time. I wanted my son to have a great day but I knew if we stayed at home, it would be all about him and my experience would once again be treated like it meant nothing.

Tears often made an appearance at some point during the actual day of the anniversary. For some mothers, the day began with tears. "I had a good cry in the morning with my husband and daughter and we just sat for an hour holding each other. Then I threw myself face first into making it the happiest day of my daughter's life." For 10 long years, one woman painfully shared that "my tears for myself remain internal. I carry this alone. How else do I get through the birthday and care for my previous children."

The following excerpt illustrates how some women manage to hold their emotions together until the end of the anniversary day but then the tears finally were allowed to emerge.

> Yesterday was my daughter's second birthday. We did our best to make her feel very special and it was fun watching her open presents and blow out her candles. But underneath that I felt a need to "mourn" something. After everyone had gone to bed, I lit a candle and read my doula's write-up about the birth. I couldn't get through it without crying. Imagine it's been 2 years!

To survive the actual anniversary day, frequently, mothers scheduled the birthday party on a different day or week. Fearing the actual birthday would become too triggering, a date that did not hold such traumatic memories would be chosen for the birthday celebration. For 3 years now, one woman chooses a random day to hold her son's birthday. As she described,

> We made a cake on a random day. I never told my son it was coming up. I bought him things and wrapped them but he doesn't know what they are for. I kissed him and told him before I went to work Happy Birthday but only when he was asleep.

Cluster of Themes 3—The Epilogue: A Fragile State

Surviving the actual anniversary of their birth trauma took a heavy toll on the women. After the anniversary, women needed time to recuperate and heal their raw wounds that had been freshly reopened.

> As hard as I try to move away from the trauma, at birthday anniversary time I am pulled straight back as if on a giant rubber band into the midst of it all and spend

MONTHS AFTER trying to pull myself away from it again.

The crippling emotions of stress, anxiety, fear, grief, loss, and depression lingered in the postanniversary period. Ten years later, one mother revealed that once her daughter's birthday celebration is over each year, it leaves her "emotionally fragile and struggling to cope with even the basics. The need for self care and not punishment becomes a priority." Another woman recalled that after her daughter's birthday party was finished, she came home and was physically ill almost immediately. She was ill for 3 days and slept a great deal of that time.

One primipara shared that her traumatic birth "was as close to a sense of rape without being physically raped. These feelings were vividly present not only before my anniversary but afterward too. They were heightened and lingered." After the birthday is over, her "nerves are definitely raw right now."

Other factors that occurred in the postanniversary phase involved exaggerated reactions to "mundane items or activities that link to the traumatic experience. Some of them include: hearing birth stories, hospital or dental offices, cramps and body feelings related to labor, seeing pregnant women or women with newborns and shopping for baby supplies."

One mother became extremely distraught after she experienced her first anniversary.

> I thought that maybe I had the thing beat, but once the birthday was over all hell broke loose; crying jags, shaking, insomnia and repetitive thoughts. I felt as if all the work I had done all year to overcome the trauma had been for naught. For days I would sit for hours sobbing and comatose on the living room floor after I took my son to day care.

Relief was yet another emotion experienced afterward.

> Today I have a sense of relief. I survived another birthday. I know the tiredness that all this causes will go and that I'll feel like smiling again. I know the emails from friends can now be answered and that they'll understand when I tell them why I haven't been in touch. The price is still too high.

Cluster of Themes 4—Subsequent Anniversaries: For Better or Worse

Once a woman has survived the first anniversary of her birth trauma, what of subsequent anniversaries? Is each successive anniversary easier or more difficult for women? No consistent pattern was reported by the mothers who had experienced more than one anniversary of their birth trauma. Twenty-three anniversaries were the most any mother in the study had experienced. For some women "each birthday the memories become slightly easier to cope with, less intense in memory but they are still there, deep inside."

A woman celebrating her son's fourth birthday painfully revealed,

> His birthday sits as a permanent barrier both in my relationship with my husband and in my sense of attachment to my child. Although this is getting better year by year, I

am not sure it will ever really disappear. The reawakening of the birth each birthday does mean I think again about what happened, my role in it, what I would have done to prevent it from happening and my sadness at what was taken away from me. The decisions I made that led down the path to the birth trauma haunt me.

For some fortunate women, the second anniversary was much different than the first one had been.

A year on, life is very different, my daughter turned two and that day was the most joyful time I've ever had. My husband and I threw a fairy party for our daughter and 14 other little fairies. The actual party was a virtual sea of pink and fairies and I felt a sort of magic coming from the children. That night when our little fairy was tucked in bed, we lay on the sofas and I remember a feeling of joy and peace. We had our beautiful daughter and no memory, however painful, could take that from us anymore.

Women who are not as fortunate as this mother worry about what will happen as their children get older and figure out what birthdays are all about.

For some women, the improvement from one anniversary to the next one could only be measured in the smallest of increments.

On my son's first birthday I had such a feeling of dread, I only invited three couples that we are friends with because I couldn't face planning a big party. The day of the party, I went upstairs to my dressing room and crawled underneath my dressing table, which sits against the wall. I pulled the bench in front of me so that I was enclosed on all sides in a very small space. I just wanted to stay huddled in there and never leave. I cried for awhile, but knew that I had to pull myself together somehow. I did manage to make it downstairs for the party though I secretly counted the minutes until it was over.

This same mother then described her second anniversary.

We cooked hamburgers and this time I made the cake (my husband had make it the year before). I was determined not to fall apart again. Sadly it was not to be. Although I didn't crawl under the table this time, I again headed to my dressing room. It is the smallest, most private room for me in the house—and sat hunched against the wall shivering under a blanket. A while later I managed to pull myself together and get on with the party preparations. I am more conscious of what went on this time and did enjoy most of it.

As this mother shared,

Each anniversary is a lottery. A real time bomb really. One is at the mercy of one's emotions, one's memories and of course other people and daily life, which of course are the indefinable triggers, the worst of all! Each year has its challenges and are different. None have ever been as intense as the first year. So PTSD can be like an octopus and its tentacles can take hold at any time. Its punishment is weird, wily and crippling. Your life is NEVER the same again. It can take hold at any time.

For other mothers, they did not experience any improvement with subsequent anniversaries. Writing about her fifth anniversary day a woman shared,

I can't believe 5 years later that I feel such strong emotions and that my body responds physically. It is like the birthing trauma and the anxiety, loss and pain associated with it seem to reside in every cell of my being, with a memory capacity that serves to never let me forget.

Discussion

Failure to rescue refers to a "clinician's inability to save a hospitalized patient's life when he experiences a complication (a condition not present on admission)" (Clarke & Aiken, 2003, p. 42–43). The term was first used to evaluate medical care (Silber, Williams, Krakauer, & Schwartz, 1992) but now has been suggested for use as a nursing outcome measure (Clarke & Aiken, 2003). Failure to rescue is based on the premise that, in hospitals, deaths are at times unavoidable, but there are many deaths that could have been prevented. Clarke and Aiken (2003) cite that this concept has been used rarely with any persons but surgical patients and not at all in settings outside the hospital.

Because of the invisibility of the phenomenon of birth trauma anniversaries, the time seemed right to broaden the use of "failure to rescue" to these childbearing women. Failure to rescue was one of the themes (difficult emotions mothers had to contend with) under Cluster of Themes 2— The actual day: A celebration of a birthday or the torment of an anniversary. Application of the term to this phenomenon will hopefully help bring some attention to the yearly ordeal that mothers suffer so covertly. Not only clinicians, but also family and friends, failed to rescue the women during the period surrounding the anniversary of their birth trauma. One of the themes of Beck's (2004a) birth trauma study seemed to still be operating 1 year or many years after the traumatic birth. The theme was, "The end justifies the means; At whose expense? At what price?" (p. 34). The mother's birth trauma was glossed over again and pushed into the background as the celebration of the child's birthday took center stage.

Clinicians need to be vigilant around children's birthdays for early signs of distress in mothers who perceived that they had experienced birth trauma. Interventions can be put in motion before a potential crisis occurs. Clinicians cannot be lulled into a false sense of security that, because a year or even many years have passed since a traumatic childbirth, mothers are not still struggling around their yearly anniversary.

If a woman is a multipara, even though she is not having a problem with the anniversary of the birth of one of her children, clinicians cannot assume that the anniversaries of the births of her other children are not problematic for her. This implication for clinical practice is illustrated vividly by one of the multiparas in this study who has had three deliveries.

I have had one (okay but unnecessary c/s), one awful, dreadful VBAC and a fantastic homebirth. I feel very differently over all of their birthdays. One I celebrate but don't think about. Another I cry all day long—and have his party on the day before! And one makes me want to drink champagne, put Alf on my shoulders and parade the streets screaming "We did it."

Some practical suggestions for providers to assess for the risk of PTSD related to birth trauma can include screening for traumatic stress symptoms. Reliable and valid instruments are available for use, such as the Perinatal PTSD Questionnaire (DeMier et al., 1996). Clinicians need to have a heightened awareness for women who share that they are experiencing any of the clinical symptoms consistent with the *DSM-IV* criteria for PTSD, namely, avoidance, reexperiencing, and increased arousal (APA, 2000). These women may need to be referred for mental healthcare follow-up.

Some of the mothers' heart-wrenching descriptions of their feelings about their children are disturbing and warrant further study. Research has confirmed the negative effects that postpartum depression has on mother–infant interactions (Beck, 1995) and on the children's cognitive and emotional development (Grace, Evindar, & Stewart, 2003; Hay, Pawlby, Angold, Harold, & Sharp, 2003). Future research needs to focus on examining if birth trauma and PTSD due to childbirth have similar disruptions in maternal–child relationships.

Also important to consider for future studies is the question of comorbidity with PTSD due to birth trauma. Research with PTSD not related to childbirth indicates that comorbid depression and other anxiety disorders are common (Schnurr, Friedman, & Bernardy, 2002). A recent study of low-income pregnant women diagnosed with PTSD also revealed comorbid depression and panic disorder (Smith, Poschman, Cavaleri, Howell, & Yonkers, 2006). Comorbidity makes the diagnosis of each disorder more difficult.

Lastly, additional studies are needed to determine if women who do not have the outlet or ability to talk about their experiences as those in this study, who had access to the Internet and TABS, are different in their experiences regarding the anniversary of their traumatic births.

The outcome of the original term *failure to rescue* (Silber et al., 1992) was an unnecessary death that occurred as a complication of surgery. The failure to rescue of women who are experiencing the anniversary of their birth trauma was not an unnecessary death but instead unnecessary emotional and physical suffering. Mothers' quality of life took a sharp decline during the period surrounding the anniversary of their birth trauma. Knowledge generated in this study emphasizes the critical importance of addressing both the vital psychosocial needs and the physical needs of the women during birth. ▼

Accepted for publication July 25, 2006.

Thank you to Sue Watson, the chairperson of TABS, a charitable trust located in New Zealand, for her invaluable assistance in recruitment and her continual support for this research. Thank you also to Debra Lajoie, MSN, Assistant Professor of Nursing at Western Connecticut State University, for her insightful suggestion to apply the term failure to rescue to the discussion of the findings. Lastly, words do not seem enough to thank the women from around the world who so willingly shared their painful and vivid stories with me in the hopes of helping other mothers who have experienced birth trauma.

Corresponding author: Cheryl Tatano Beck, DNSc, CNM, FAAN, School of Nursing, University of Connecticut, 231 Glenbrook Road, Storrs, CT 06269-2026 (e-mail: Cheryl.beck@uconn.edu).

References

Allen, S., Nicholson, P., & Woollett, A. (1998). A qualitative analysis of the process, mediating variables and impact of traumatic childbirth. *Journal of Reproductive and Infant Psychology, 16,* 107–131.

American Psychiatric Association. (2000). *Diagnostic and statistical manual of mental disorders.* (4th ed.). Washington, DC: Author.

Ayers, S., & Pickering, A. (2001). Do women get post-traumatic stress disorder as a result of childbirth? A prospective study of incidence. *Birth, 28,* 111–118.

Bailham, D., & Joseph, S. (2003). Post-traumatic stress following childbirth: A review of the emerging literature and directions for research and practice. *Psychology, Health, & Medicine, 8,* 159–168.

Beck, C. T. (1995). The effects of postpartum depression on maternal–infant interaction: A meta-analysis. *Nursing Research, 44,* 298–304.

Beck, C. T. (2004a). Birth trauma: In the eye of the beholder. *Nursing Research, 53,* 28–35.

Beck, C. T. (2004b). Post-traumatic stress disorder due to childbirth: The aftermath. *Nursing Research, 53,* 216–224.

Clarke, S. P., & Aiken, L. H. (2003). Failure to rescue. *American Journal of Nursing, 103,* 42–47.

Colaizzi, P. F. (1973). *Reflection and research in psychology: A phenomenological study of learning.* Dubuque, IA: Kendall/Hunt Publishing Company.

Colaizzi, P. F. (1978). Psychological research as the phenomenologist views it. In R. Valle & M. King (Eds.), *Existential phenomenological alternatives for psychology* (pp. 48–71). New York: Oxford University Press.

Creedy, D. K., Shochet, I. M., & Horsfall, J. (2000). Childbirth and the development of acute trauma symptoms: Incidence and contributing factors. *Birth, 27,* 104–111.

Czarnocka, J., & Slade, P. (2000). Prevalence and predictors of post-traumatic stress symptoms following childbirth. *British Journal of Clinical Psychology, 39,* 35–51.

DeMier, R. L., Hynan, M. T., Harris, H. B., & Manniello, R. L. (1996). Perinatal stressors as predictors of symptoms of posttraumatic stress in mothers and infants at high risk. *Journal of Perinatology, 16,* 276–280.

DiBlasio, P., & Ionio, C. (2002). Childbirth and narratives: How do mothers deal with their child's birth? *Journal of Prenatal and Perinatal Psychology and Health, 17,* 143–151.

Ehlers, A., Hackmann, A., & Michael, T. (2004). Intrusive re-experiencing in post-traumatic stress disorder: Phenomenology, theory, and therapy. *Memory, 12,* 403–415.

Fones, C. (1996). Posttraumatic stress disorder occurring after painful childbirth. *Journal of Nervous and Mental Disease, 184,* 195–196.

Friedman, M. J. (2006). Posttraumatic stress disorder among military returnees from Afghanistan and Iraq. *American Journal of Psychiatry, 163,* 586–593.

Gamble, J., Creedy, D., Moyle, W., Webster, J., McAllister, M., & Dickson, P. (2005). Effectiveness of a counseling intervention after a traumatic childbirth; A randomized controlled trial. *Birth, 32,* 11–19.

Goldbeck-Wood, S. (1996). PTSD may follow childbirth. *British Medical Journal, 313,* 774.

Gottvall, K., & Waldenstrom, U. (2002). Does a traumatic birth experience have an impact on future reproduction? *BJOG: An*

International Journal of Obstetrics and Gynecology, 109, 254–260.

Grace, S. L., Evindar, A., & Stewart, D. E. (2003). The effect of postpartum depression on child cognitive development and behavior: A review and critical analysis of the literature. *Archives of Women's Mental Health, 6,* 263–274.

Hamilton, R. J., & Bowers, B. J. (2006). Internet recruitment and E-mail interviews in qualitative studies. *Qualitative Health Research, 16,* 821–835.

Hay, D. F., Pawlby, S., Angold, A., Harold, G. T., & Sharp, D. (2003). Pathways to violence in the children of mothers who were depressed postpartum. *Developmental Psychology, 39,* 1083–1094.

Hycner, R. (1985). Some guidelines for the phenomenological analysis of interview data. *Human Studies, 8,* 279–303.

Keogh, E., Ayers, S., & Francis, H. (2002). Does anxiety sensitivity predict post-traumatic stress symptoms following childbirth? A preliminary report. *Cognitive Behaviour Therapy, 31,* 145–155.

Kersting, A., Dorsch, M., Wesselmann, U., Ludorff, K., Witthaut, J., Ohrmann, P., et al. (2004). Maternal posttraumatic stress response after the birth of a very low-birth-weight infant. *Journal of Psychosomatic Research, 57,* 473–476.

Olde, E., van der Hart, O., Kleber, R., & van Son, M. (2006). Posttraumatic stress following childbirth: A review. *Clinical Psychology Review, 26,* 1–16.

Ryding, E. L., Wijma, K., & Wijma, B. (1998). Experiences of emergency cesarean section: A phenomenological study of 53 women. *Birth, 25,* 246–251.

Schnurr, P. P., Friedman, M. J., & Bernardy, N. C. (2002). Research on posttraumatic stress disorder: Epidemiology, pathophysiology, and assessment. *Journal of Clinical Psychology, 58,* 877–889.

Silber, J. H., Williams, S. V., Krakauer, H., & Schwartz, J. S. (1992). Hospital and patient characteristics associated with death after surgery. A study of adverse occurrence and failure to rescue. *Medical Care, 30,* 615–629.

Skari, H., Skreden, M., Malt, U. F., Dalholt, M., Ostensen A. B., Egeland, T., et al. (2002). Comparative levels of psychological distress, stress symptoms, depression and anxiety after childbirth—a prospective population based study of mothers and fathers. *BJOG, 109,* 1154–1163.

Smith, M. V., Poschman, K., Cavaleri, M. A., Howell, H. B., & Yonkers, K. A. (2006). Symptoms of posttraumatic stress disorder in a community sample of low-income pregnant women. *American Journal of Psychiatry, 163,* 881–884.

Soet, J. E., Brack, G. A., & DiIorio, C. (2003). Prevalence and predictors of women's experience of psychological trauma during childbirth. *Birth, 30,* 36–46.

Thorne, S., & Darbyshire, P. (2005). Land mines in the field: A modest proposal for improving the craft of qualitative health research. *Qualitative Health Research, 15,* 1105–1113.

Turton, P., Hughes, P., Evans, C. D., & Fainman, D. (2001). Incidence, correlates and predictors of post-traumatic stress disorder in the pregnancy after stillbirth. *British Journal of Psychiatry, 178,* 556–560.

Van Kaam, A. (1966). *Existential foundations of psychology.* Pittsburgh, PA: Duquesne University Press.

Van Pampus, M. G., Wolf, H., Weijmar Schultz, W. C., Neeleman, J., & Aarnoudse, J. G. (2004). Posttraumatic stress disorder following preeclampsia and HELLP syndrome. *Journal of Psychosomatic Obstetrics and Gynecology, 25,* 183–187.

Index